INTRODUCTION TO COMMUNITY-BASED NURSING

4TH EDITION

INTRODUCTION TO COMMUNITY-BASED NURSING

ROBERTA HUNT RN, MSPH, PhD

Assistant Professor
College of St. Catherine
St. Paul, Minnesota

Wolters Kluwer Health | Lippincott Williams & Wilkins

Philadelphia • Baltimore • New York • London
Buenos Aires • Hong Kong • Sydney • Tokyo

Senior Acquisitions Editor: Margaret Zuccarini
Managing Editor: Michelle Clarke
Editorial Assistant: Brandi Spade
Production Project Manager: Cynthia Rudy
Director of Nursing Production: Helen Ewan
Senior Managing Editor / Production: Erika Kors

Design Coordinator: Holly Reid McLaughlin
Interior Designer: Lisa Delgado
Cover Designer: Bess Kiethas
Manufacturing Coordinator: Karin Duffield
Production Services / Compositor: Aptara, Inc.

4th edition

9 8 7 6 5 4

Printed in the United States of America

Library of Congress Cataloging-in-Publication Data
Hunt, Roberta.
    Introduction to community-based nursing / Roberta Hunt. — 4th ed.
        p. ; cm.
    Includes bibliographical references and index.
    ISBN-13: 978-0-7817-7247-1
    ISBN-10: 0-7817-7247-8
    1. Community health nursing. I Title.
    [DNLM: 1. Community Health Nursing.   2. Health Promotion. WY 106 H946i 2008]
    RT98.H86 2008
    610.73′43—dc22

                                        2007046590

LWW.com

Dedication

To my beautiful grandchildren, Josie, Gus, and Levi, with love.

RJH

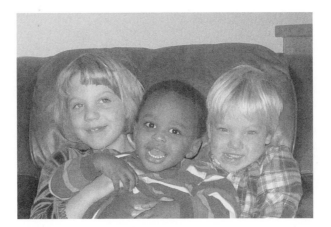

Marcia Derby, MSN, RN
Assistant Professor of Nursing
Nova Southeastern University
Fort Lauderdale, Florida

Paula Swiggum, MS, RN
Assistant Professor of Nursing
Gustavus Adolphus College
Saint Peter, Minnesota

Marva Thurston, MS, RN
Clinical Nurse Specialist
Hennepin County Mental Health Center
Minneapolis, Minnesota

Louise A. Aurilio, RNC, CAN, PhD
Associate Professor
Youngstown State University
Youngstown, Ohio

Karen Clark, RN, EdD
Dean of Nursing and Assistant Professor
Indiana University School of Nursing
    at Indiana University East
Richmond, Indiana

Sarah Covington, RN, MSN
Director of Nursing
Renton Technical College
Renton, Washington

Katherine Dewan, RN, MN, PNP
Associate Professor
Ohlone College
Fremont, California

Elizabeth A. Downes, MPH, MSN, APRN-BC, FNP
Clinical Assistant Professor
Nell Hodgson Woodruff School of Nursing,
    Emory University
Atlanta, Georgia

Marie O. Etienne, MSN, ARNP, PNP, FNP, GNP
Associate Professor, Senior
Miami Dade College, Medical Center
    Campus, School of Nursing
Miami, Florida

Pamela Gwin, RNC, BSN
Director, Vocational Nursing Program
Brazosport College
Lake Jackson, Texas

Rosemary F. Hall, RN, BSN, MSN, PhD
Associate Professor of Clinical Nursing
University of Miami School of Nursing
    and Health Studies
Coral Gables, Florida

Vicki L. Imerman, RN, MSN
Nursing Faculty
Des Moines Area Community College
Boone, Iowa

Karen Kelley, RN, MSN
Assistant Professor of Nursing
Harding University
Searcy, Arkansas

Nancy W. Mosca, RN, PhD
Professor and Coordinator, School Nurse
    Program
Coordinator, MPH Program
Youngstown State University
Youngstown, Ohio

Carel Mountain, RN, MSN
Faculty
Shasta College
Redding, California

Dr. Pammla Petrucka, BScN, MN, PhD
Assistant Professor
University of Saskatchewan
Regina, Saskatchewan

Debra Solomon
Instructor
Bethel University
St. Paul, Minnesota

Linda Spencer, RN, MPH, PhD
Director of Public Health Nursing
    Leadership Graduate Program
Nell Hodgson Woodruff School of Nursing,
    Emory University
Atlanta, Georgia

Mary Ann Thompson, RN, DrPH
Associate Professor of Nursing
McKendree College, Louisville Campus
Louisville, Kentucky

Sandra Kay Thompson, MEd, MSN, APRN, BC
Assistant Professor of Nursing
Bluefield State College
Bluefield, West Virginia

Jeanne Ann VanFossan
Professor of Nursing
West Virginia Northern Community
    College
Weirton, West Virginia

The changing health care delivery system presents new challenges for contemporary nurses. Schools of nursing are struggling to find the best way to restructure curriculum to meet current needs and to give students experiences in a variety of clinical situations and settings that will prepare them for their careers in the increasingly diversified field of nursing. This textbook, *Introduction to Community-Based Nursing*, fourth edition, is designed to fill that need. The fundamental concepts in this text spring from my experience of more than 25 years of teaching community health nursing and working in community settings. These concepts are articulated with careful attention to the National League for Nursing competencies.

PURPOSE OF THE TEXT

As the fourth edition of *Introduction to Community-Based Nursing* was developed, four major goals were considered:

1. *To give an informative and experiential introduction to nursing care in the community.*
   In the past, most schools of nursing focused on preparing students to provide care in the hospital. Increasingly, nursing care has moved out of acute care settings into a variety of settings and specialties throughout the community. Fundamental aspects of community-based care are presented to allow the nurse to develop a knowledge base applicable in any community setting.
2. *To illustrate the variety of settings and situations in which the community-based nurse gives care.*
   Because of the variety of settings in which a nurse may practice and the limitation of time in the curriculum of schools of nursing, it is often difficult to schedule sufficient diversified clinical experiences. A wide range of settings are discussed in this textbook: from home care nursing and specialized home care roles to school nursing; from emergency preparedness to chronic care; from parish nursing to advocacy in global health. One of the purposes of this text is to provide a variety of clinical applications in a range of settings with a diversity of populations. This is accomplished in several ways. First, examples of different settings and situations are scattered throughout the body of the text. Second, one of the special features of the text, *Client Situations in Practice*, integrates and synthesizes chapter concepts, showing the student step-by-step how the theory discussed in the chapter relates to the reality of clinical practice. Third, *Case Studies* appear in many of the *Learning Activities* at the end of each chapter and as part of the extensive instructors' resources available online at thePoint* (http://thePoint.lww.com), Lippincott Williams & Wilkins' popular web-based course and content management system. These case studies give students an opportunity to practice skills while applying chapter concepts. Last, questions for reflection for use with a clinical journal or individual assignments are found in the *Learning Activities* at the end of each chapter and at thePoint.
3. *To clarify the cultural diversification of the community in which nurses provide quality care.*

*thePoint is a trademark of Wolters Kluwer Health.

Another important emphasis of this edition of *Introduction to Community-Based Nursing* is cross-cultural care. Our society is diverse, with many racial, ethnic, and minority groups. The community-based nurse will care for clients from many different cultures, and must be prepared to give quality and culturally competent care to all clients and families. Chapter 3, "Cultural Care," is written by Paula Swiggum, who has extensive experience in cross-cultural nursing, in both recruiting and providing academic support for students from diverse cultural backgrounds, as well as in curriculum development. She is a member of the Transcultural Nursing Society and is a Certified Transcultural Nurse. Consideration of cross-cultural issues is woven throughout the text.

4. *To integrate throughout the text the importance of the individual to the family and the family to the individual.*

Most clients are part of a family. In this text, family is defined as those whom the client has identified as family or a significant other. The client's health and the client's care during illness are influenced by the family. In some cases, the client's health is influenced by lack of family and social support. The client's health status and outlook will influence the continuous growth and development of the family. Understanding this symbiotic relationship and incorporating this knowledge into care is an important focus of the text. Special attention is also given to nursing support of the lay caregiver.

ORGANIZATION OF THE TEXT

Introduction to Community-Based Nursing is divided into five units: basic concepts, nursing skills, application, settings, and implications for future practice.

◆ *Unit I, Basic Concepts in Community-Based Nursing,* includes the essential elements of community-based nursing. An introductory chapter discusses definitions of a community and a healthy community, components of community-based nursing, and nursing skills and competencies needed to give quality care in the community. The unit also provides information on health promotion and disease prevention, cultural considerations, and family implications.

◆ *Unit II, Skills for Community-Based Nursing Practice,* reviews the basics of assessment, health teaching, case management, and continuity of care, and addresses those skills specific to community-based settings.

◆ *Unit III, Community-Based Nursing Across the Life Span,* provides assessment guides, teaching materials, and strategies for addressing health promotion and disease prevention across the life span.

◆ *Unit IV, Settings for Practice,* discusses a wide sampling of practice settings and practice specialties. One chapter discusses home health care in depth and another focuses on specific roles in specialized home care nursing. Mental health nursing in community-based settings is also included in this unit. A new chapter addressing global health and community-based care discusses health issues that extend to the larger community, including environmental health, emergency preparedness, immigrants and refugees, and nursing advocacy in global health.

◆ *Unit V, Implications for Future Practice,* discusses trends in health care and implications for community-based nursing.

The text was designed using a consistent approach throughout the chapters. Many chapters include a short section giving a historical perspective on the subject. Most chapters address nursing skills and competencies, with information on the nursing process or on such topics as communication, health teaching, and case management. Any repetition of information among chapters is intended to reinforce knowledge or skills in light of each chapter's subject. Documentation is covered in many chapters because of its importance to community-based nursing. All chapters conclude with *Learning Activities*.

KEY FEATURES OF THE TEXT

The following features of the book were developed as pedagogical aids for the student. They help clarify text information, give the student guidelines for actions, or require the student to use critical thinking.

- ◆ Learning Activities: several activities at the end of every chapter that form a compact study and application guide. These comprise the following exercises:
  - ◆ Journaling: to be used for a clinical journal or as individual assignments to assist the student in applying theoretical content to clinical situations and becoming a reflective practitioner.
  - ◆ Client Situations in Practice: at least one in most chapters. A client situation is described, followed by critical thinking exercises.
  - ◆ Practical Applications: appear in many chapters. Not related to a specific client, these activities prepare the student for clinical application.
  - ◆ Critical Thinking Exercises: at least one in every chapter. A problem is presented in a sentence or two, with directions for critical thinking.
- ◆ Community-Based Nursing Care Guidelines: boxed information that includes specific interventions for the community-based nurse.
- ◆ Community-Based Teaching: boxed lists of information to give clients and their families.
- ◆ Research in Community-Based Nursing Care: boxed information that includes short paragraphs of descriptive research.
- ◆ Assessment Tools: many chapters provide sample assessment forms to be used in community-based nursing care.
- ◆ Healthy People 2010: health promotion and disease prevention materials in Chapters 8, 9, and 10, with addresses of Web sites from which numerous additional materials can be downloaded.
- ◆ What's on the Web: found in most chapters, this feature contains addresses and descriptions of Web sites related to the chapter material that provide additional resources. Chapter 16 includes a list of general Web sites helpful in community-based nursing.
- ◆ Other pedagogical aids: Objectives, Key Terms, Chapter Topics, References, and Bibliography.
- ◆ Glossary: helps the student review terminology or understand unfamiliar terminology used in the book.

We have tried to avoid sexist terms for the nurse and clients. Throughout the text, we have used the term "family" for consistency. However, the term refers to anyone who is concerned about and supportive of the client and can signify a relative or a significant other.

INSTRUCTOR'S RESOURCES

This book is accompanied by a set of Instructor's Resources that can be accessed on thePoint. These Instructor's Resources were prepared with an ongoing emphasis on practical application of the student's knowledge base. More than 200 assignments and discussion topics, more than 700 test questions, and additional client care studies are provided, all designed to help the associate-degree nurse develop the skills and knowledge essential for the unique role of community-based nursing. Many of the assignments have been used and improved over the years that I have taught community health nursing. In addition, quizzes are provided to test students' reading comprehension and review questions to test their learning. Answers are given for all of the tests, quizzes, assignments, discussion topics, and case studies. Point-by-point lecture outlines accompanied by PowerPoint presentations, all designed to support the instructor, are provided for each chapter.

Roberta Hunt, RN, MSPH, PhD
hunthean@comcast.net

ACKNOWLEDGMENTS

I am grateful to many individuals, especially family, friends, and colleagues, for their encouragement and assistance in the development of this textbook. It is impossible to acknowledge everyone, given the limitations of memory and space.

To all my colleagues who have given encouragement and validation and who have made the teaching of nursing an exciting and stimulating profession—you have contributed to this project. To the more than 2,000 students whom I have had the pleasure of working with in the classroom and in clinical settings in the community, who have provided feedback and suggestions about my teaching and assignments—you have each made an invaluable contribution to this book.

There are several people in the Nursing Education department of Lippincott Williams & Wilkins who have provided invaluable expertise and assistance. Jean Rodenberger, Executive Editor, has given professional guidance to craft and redefined the focus of this text. Michelle Clarke, Managing Editor of this edition, has been terrific with her quick, competent assistance. Thanks to Annette Ferran, Ancillary Editor, for being a patient mentor through the development of the ancillary products.

To my dear friend of many years, Paula Swiggum, I owe enormous thanks for writing Chapter 3, "Cultural Care." This expertly crafted and beautifully written chapter adds a great deal to the overall message of the importance of respectful care, which is the central premise of *Introduction to Community-Based Nursing*. To my former colleague and dear friend, Marva Thurston, a heart-filled thanks for writing Chapter 14. In this chapter, Marva shares her knowledge and her sensitive approach to care, gained through more than 20 years of working with individuals who have mental health issues. This chapter makes an important contribution in emphasizing that both mental and physical health are essential to comprehensive community-based care.

Finally, I am grateful to my family and friends, who provide day-to-day support and encouragement. To my colleagues at the College of St. Catherine—the most professional and supportive faculty group an educator could ever hope to work with—thanks for the opportunity to work with all of you. I especially want to thank Meg Carolan, Joann O'Leary, Sue Larson, and Susan O'Conner-Von for their ongoing friendships and listening ears. Thanks to my family, especially Becky Hunt Carmody and Steve Hunt, for your continuing encouragement. To Andrew and Mark, you guys are the most terrific young men—you make your Dad and me so proud of you. To my terrific son-in-law, David, and darling grandchildren, Josie, August, and Levi—you all really brighten up my life. To my wonderful daughters—Jackie, for your cheerful attitude plus valuable editorial assistance prodding me forward, and Megan, for your thoughtful advice and balanced view of the world—a heartfelt thank you. Most of all, I am grateful to my loving husband, Tim Heaney—your committed attitude towards me and all that I do has helped me become more than I ever imagined.

Roberta Hunt

CONTENTS

BASIC CONCEPTS IN COMMUNITY-BASED NURSING

B efore you practice nursing in a community-based setting, you must understand the basic concepts behind community-based health care. These concepts are introduced in Unit I as a knowledge base for further exploration as you begin to apply what you have learned. An overview of community-based nursing, beginning with a brief historical perspective of nursing is provided in Chapter 1. Also discussed are health care reform and health care funding, which have taken health care out of the hospital and into the community. Finally, components of community-based care and nursing skills and competencies round out the chapter.

Health promotion and disease prevention, as outlined by the federal government's Healthy People 2010 (U.S. Department of Health and Human Services, 2000), are the focus of Chapter 2.

Chapter 3 discusses the ever-changing makeup of our society and asks you to look at your own cultural background and attitudes about diversity. The chapter promotes culturally competent care.

Chapter 4 discusses family involvement, an important consideration in community-based care.

The remainder of the book will use these concepts to build your knowledge base and relate it to practical experiences.

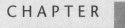
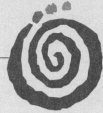

CHAPTER 1

Overview of Community-Based Nursing

ROBERTA HUNT

LEARNING OBJECTIVES

1. Identify major issues leading to the development of community-based nursing.
2. Discuss the current reimbursement system for health care services and its impact on nursing.
3. Describe the factors that define community.
4. Indicate the relationship between health and community.
5. Compare acute care nursing, community-based nursing, and community health nursing.
6. Discuss components of community-based care.
7. Examine the skills with which you perform necessary competencies.

KEY TERMS

acute care
advance directives
community
community-based nursing
continuity of care
demographics
diagnosis-related groups (DRGs)
extended family

health maintenance organizations (HMOs)
living will
nuclear family
preferred provider organizations (PPOs)
prospective payment
self-care
vital statistics

CHAPTER TOPICS

◆ Historical Perspectives
◆ Health Care Reform
◆ Health Care Funding
◆ The Community
◆ Community Nursing Versus Community-Based Nursing
◆ Focus of Nursing
◆ Components of Community-Based Care
◆ Nursing Skills and Competencies
◆ Nursing Interventions
◆ Conclusions

THE NURSING STUDENT SPEAKS

In general, having clinical in the community has broadened my horizons of what I am able to do as a nurse. Before this community experience, my mind-set was that you had to work in a hospital or a nursing home when you graduated. Acute care was the only setting that I could think about working in, and now I realize that these people in the community need me too. Public health, I have noticed, is short staffed too, just like hospitals. They only have one nurse at the shelter to see all of the families. It seems to be overwhelming. This experience has broadened my horizons to see the different roles that I can play as a nurse, most of which I have never seen myself in.

Before this experience, I could not believe that we had to do a community rotation. Once I was out there, I was shocked at how my views of community health were distorted. After the rotation was over, I was glad that we were able to experience the community setting. Working in the homeless shelter helped me to look at people in a more holistic way, which I now believe is the only way to look at people. Before this experience, it [my focus] was always the physical aspects of a person, such as blood pressure and pain. Now I can see the whole person—the physical, the mental, and the spiritual aspects. These are all of the parts that need to be healed. I appreciate what I have learned from the community experience. It is all coming together.

—KRISTIN OCKER, RN, Student Completing a BSN, College of St. Catherine

Over the last three decades nursing practice in the community has been transformed. These changes stem from public concern regarding our health care system. These concerns center on quality of, access to, and cost of health care, as well as fragmentation of health care. The resulting changes give nurses an opportunity to help shape health care at the dawn of the 21st century. National League for Nursing (NLN) has predicted 10 trends in health care that will affect nursing education and practice (Box 1-1).

These trends and the implications for nursing educational preparation and quality nursing practice are the focus of this book. This chapter provides an overview of nursing care and its historical background, introduces the reader to the community and community-based nursing, and describes components of community-based nursing practice, skills, and competencies.

HISTORICAL PERSPECTIVES

During most of the 20th century, nursing care was associated primarily with hospital settings (Bellack & O'Neil, 2000). However, historically, the setting for nursing care was the home. The first written reference to care of the ill in the home is found in the New Testament, in which mention is made of visiting the sick at home to aid in their care.

Florence Nightingale, credited as the mother of modern nursing, developed a classic model for educating nurses in hospital-based programs. Nightingale's curriculum

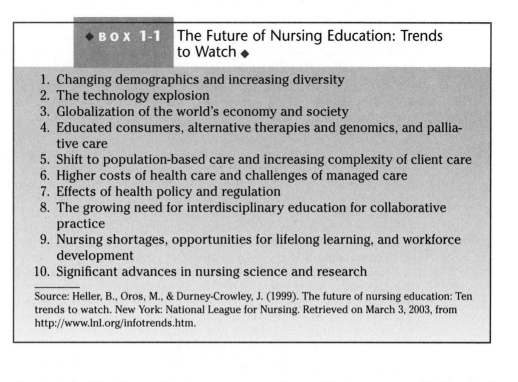

◆ **B O X   1-1**   The Future of Nursing Education: Trends to Watch ◆

1. Changing demographics and increasing diversity
2. The technology explosion
3. Globalization of the world's economy and society
4. Educated consumers, alternative therapies and genomics, and pallia- tive care
5. Shift to population-based care and increasing complexity of client care
6. Higher costs of health care and challenges of managed care
7. Effects of health policy and regulation
8. The growing need for interdisciplinary education for collaborative practice
9. Nursing shortages, opportunities for lifelong learning, and workforce development
10. Significant advances in nursing science and research

Source: Heller, B., Oros, M., & Durney-Crowley, J. (1999). The future of nursing education: Ten trends to watch. New York: National League for Nursing. Retrieved on March 3, 2003, from http://www.lnl.org/infotrends.htm.

also included the first training programs to educate district nurses, with 1 year of training devoted to promoting self-care and the health of communities (Monteiro, 1991).

William Rathbone, a resident of Liverpool, England, in the 1850s, established the modern concept of the visiting nurse (Kalish & Kalish, 1995). Lillian Wald and Mary Brewster began a program for visiting nurses in the United States in the early 1900s (Frachel, 1988). Wald, the founder of public health nursing, drew on con- temporary ideas that linked nursing, motherhood, social welfare, and the public. Her work was designed to respond to the needs of those populations at greatest risk by nursing the sick in their homes and providing preventive instructions to reduce illness. Wald argued that the nurse, through her "peculiar introduction to the patient and her organic relationship with the neighborhood," could be the "starting point" for wider service in the community. Wald believed that nurses could reach and educate their clients in the broadest sense, drawing on diversity of cultural beliefs and societal demands of the populace (Reverby, 1993).

Shift From Community to Hospital

In 1910, approximately 90% of all nursing care was provided in the home. After World War I, care of the sick started to shift to the hospital. In the early 1950s, the growing complexity in health care technology resulted in an increased need for hospital care. During the 1960s and 1970s, a person typically stayed in the hospi- tal for 7 to 10 days for uncomplicated conditions or for surgery (Craven & Hirnle, 2007).

This trend continued until the early 1980s, when escalating health care costs prompted changes in the health care delivery system and its financing. In brief, nursing care provided in the home in the 1800s migrated to the acute care hospital in the middle of the 20th century and then back to the home in the 1980s. From 1980, this trend intensified as the number of nurses working in public and community health, ambulatory care, and other institutional settings increased rapidly (Health Resources and Services Administration [HRSA], 2005).

An Era of Cost Containment

President Reagan signed the Tax Equity and Fiscal Responsibility Act (TEFRA) in 1982 and the Social Security Amendments in 1983. This legislation changed the way Medicare and Medicaid services were reimbursed, initiating a service called the **prospective payment** system. The prospective payment system calculates reimbursement to hospitals based on the client's diagnosis according to federally mandated **diagnosis-related groups (DRGs)**. The client's diagnosis is categorized according to the federal DRG coding system, and payment is bundled into one fee, which is then paid to the hospital. Payment by client diagnosis, therefore, was an attempt to contain Medicare and Medicaid costs.

Gradually, many insurance companies, **health maintenance organizations (HMOs),** and other third-party payers adopted the DRG method of payment. As the reimbursement system for health care changed, the average length of stay for a hospitalized client decreased substantially. In fact, it became financially advantageous for the hospital if clients had shorter stays. As a result, a scenario was created in which clients were discharged "quicker and sicker." With this transition, it became evident that it was more cost-effective to provide services outside the hospital. This trend continues to this day.

Shift From Hospital to Community

Acute Care Setting

Acute care is the term used for people who receive intensive hospital care. But hospital care is not always synonymous with acute care. In some cases community-based care is provided in the hospital where an ambulatory clinic or day surgery unit may be found. In general, individuals in acute care settings are very sick. Many are postsurgical clients or need highly technical care. Many of these clients have life-threatening conditions and require close monitoring and constant care. The care given these clients is specialized and requires considerable expertise in physical care giving. Acute nursing care is very different from **community-based nursing** care, as evidenced by differences between hospital and home environments shown in Table 1-1.

Community Setting

Clients affected by the transition into community-based health care are not in need of fewer services. Rather, the focus of services shifts from the hospital to the community. Care that once was considered safe only within the hospital has become routine in outpatient settings, such as ambulatory care centers, surgical centers, dialysis centers, rehabilitation centers, walk-in clinics, physicians' offices, and the home.

The change in health care services has resulted in changes in nursing care as well. In the past decade, the number of nurses working in every employment setting has increased. However, the rate of increase in hospitals is less than in previous years. The greatest increase occurred in community-based settings (Fig. 1-1). This trend of more nurses working in community-based settings continues (HRSA, 2005).

TABLE 1-1 Differences Between Hospital and Home		
Factors	**Hospital**	**Home**
Resources	Predetermined	Variable
Environment	Predictable	Highly variable
Locating client	Certain with captive audience	Requires planning
Access to client	Guaranteed	Not guaranteed, but determined by client and family
Focus	Individual client	Client in family system
Family support	Helpful in accomplishing client outcomes	Critical in accomplishing client outcomes
Client role	Relatively dependent	Highly autonomous
Safety	Under the auspices of agency oversight	Multiple unpredictable threats

Impact of the Nursing Shortage on Care in the Community

The Bureau of Labor Statistics estimates that job opportunities for RNs in all specialties are expected to be excellent with employment of registered nurses expected to grow much faster than average for all occupations through 2014. Employment is expected to grow more slowly in hospitals (Bureau of Labor Statistics [BLS], 2006). The U.S. Bureau of Labor Statistics predicts that the need for nurses will increase by 29% by 2014 while at the same time the number of U.S educated nursing school graduates decreased by 10% from 1995 to 2004. One of the main factors contributing to the decrease in the number of nursing school graduates is the shortage of nursing faculty. Unlike nursing shortages in the past, this shortage will be driven by a permanent shift in the labor market that is unlikely to

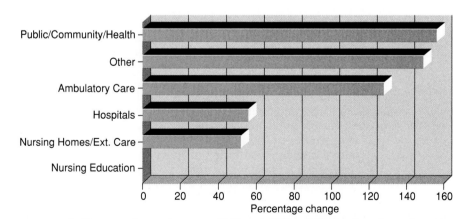

FIGURE 1-1. ▶ Percent change between 1980 and 2000 in RNs employed in selected settings. Source: Health Resources and Services Administration. Bureau of Health Professions. (2000). The registered nurse population: Findings from the national sample survey of registered nurses.

reverse in the next few years (Buerhaus, Staiger, & Auerbach, 2000). The federal government is projecting a shortfall of 800,000 registered nurses by 2020 (American Association of Colleges of Nurses, 2005).

These changes make it imperative for nursing educators to prepare graduates for positions outside the walls of the acute care setting and for roles in the community. The NLN recommends that all nursing education undergo a shift in emphasis to continue to ensure that all nurses from all education levels are prepared to function in a community-based, community-focused health care system. This means that nurses must be competent to practice in varied settings across the continuum of care.

HEALTH CARE REFORM

Health care in general is in transition. The United States is in the midst of reviewing and revising its health care system, and few people deny that some changes must occur. Legislation on state and national levels may result in the most dramatic changes of all. Healthy People 2010 (**www.healthypeople.gov** U.S. Department of Health and Human Services, 2000), which lists government goals (discussed further in Chapter 2), has stirred our imagination about meeting the needs of all Americans. Particular populations are targeted for care. The question has been raised: Is health care a right or a privilege? Who gets health care and who pays for this health care will be at the center of the debate for some time. These issues present challenges and opportunities for the nurse in the first decade of the new century.

Nurses have an important function to play in health care reform beginning by being prepared for practice in community settings. Further, nurses must understand the business aspects of health care. Last of all, nurses in community settings need highly developed skills in assessment, communication, interdisciplinary collaboration, and working with culturally diverse populations.

HEALTH CARE FUNDING

Health care is extremely expensive, and costs continue to rise. Increasing health care costs impact many health care agencies and organizations. They must now find funds, in addition to fee-for-service charges, in the form of voluntary donations and state and federal programs.

Few individuals can afford to pay their health care costs out of their own pockets. Many individuals belong to HMOs or rely on government-funded health care such as Medicare and Medicaid. Insurance plans, HMOs, and government programs provide a variety of coverage plans. Many, however, do not cover preventive care, psychiatric treatment, outpatient support services, and medications. Many limit the amount of service paid for a particular type of care, such as home health care visits. Some have a maximum cap for how much they will pay for an individual's care or for a specific condition.

Federally Funded Health Care

Primary government funding comes through Medicare and Medicaid. Under Medicare, home health care is an important service for the elderly, and concern about it will continue to grow as the elderly population increases in the United

States. Medicare covers nursing; physical, speech, and occupational therapies; home care aides; medical social services; and some medical supplies. With the Balanced Budget Act in 1997, changes were made to Medicare's payment system to contain cost. These changes affect the role of the nurse in the delivery of home care services.

Group Plans

Group plans include HMOs, **preferred provider organizations (PPOs),** and private insurance. **HMOs** are prepaid, structured, managed systems in which providers deliver a comprehensive range of health care services to enrollees. **PPOs** allow a network of providers to provide services at a lower fee in return for prompt payment at prenegotiated rates. Private insurance may be obtained through large, nonprofit, tax-exempt organizations or through small, private, for-profit insurance companies. This type of insurance is called third-party payment. Long-term care insurance may also be obtained through private insurance companies.

THE COMMUNITY

Nurses who practice community-based nursing benefit from understanding the community within which they practice. Knowledge of the community helps nurses maintain quality of care.

Defining Community

Community can be defined in numerous ways, depending on the application. This text uses the definition of community as "a people, location, and social system" (Josten, 1989).

People: Families, Culture, and Community
The variety of individuals, families, and cultural groups represented in a community contributes to the overall character of that community. The simplest way to understand a community is through **vital statistics** and **demographics.** These data may be thought of as the community's vital statistics, similar to an individual's vital signs. A community consisting primarily of senior citizens has totally different vital statistics from a community of young, unmarried adults.

The characteristics of the families living in a community contribute to the overall complexion of that community and, in turn, define the community health care needs. In communities where families are strong and nurturing, there is an opportunity for a strong and caring community. In communities where families fail to provide an adequate basis for individual growth, problems with physical abuse, neglect, substance abuse, and violence may arise. A strong family unit is the basic building block for strong communities.

Culture contributes to the overall character of a community and, in turn, influences its health needs. In most of the world, a scarcity of resources necessitates **extended family** residence together in one home. Included in the extended family are grandparents, aunts, uncles, and other relatives. When living together in one household, many members may be involved with child care and care of the sick or injured. In these communities, there are different needs related to child and health care than in communities such as those in the United States and Western Europe, where the **nuclear family** is the norm. In the 6% of the world where nuclear family structures prevail, isolation and self-reliance affect the needs and function of the family which, in turn, influence the design and delivery of services. A client, then, who has a nuclear family and no extended family often, has different needs from the client with numerous extended family members living in the same household or nearby.

The role within the family of individuals according to their ages is often dictated by culture. In some cultures, the older people retire from leadership and governing responsibilities, whereas in other cultures, these members are considered essential to the governing structure of the community. In this situation, the more prestigious positions of authority and responsibility are assigned to the older members of the community.

Health is affected by culture. Madeleine Leininger (1970) observed that "health and illness states are strongly influenced and often primarily determined by the cultural background of an individual." The culture of the individual and his or her family has an impact on the community's definition of health and on the service needs of that community.

Location: Community Boundaries

A community is usually defined by boundaries. Boundaries may be geographic, such as those defined as a city, county, state, or nation or may be political; precincts and wards may determine them. A community may have diffuse boundaries such as those that emerge as the result of a group of people identifying or solving a problem. Consequently, a community may establish a boundary within which a problem can be defined and solved. Figure 1-2 depicts this variety of community boundaries.

Community boundaries are important because they often determine what services are available to individuals living within a particular geographic area. Eligibility for services may be limited, or denied, depending on whether one resides within a certain geographic area. It is important for the nurse to realize that community boundaries limit availability of, and eligibility for, services. For example, suppose you are a nurse working at Ramsey County Hospital. Your patient is from Hennepin County. You will refer the client to services in Hennepin County. The client, however, may also be eligible for services with a home health care agency that serves multiple counties but is not located in Hennepin County. It is helpful for you to be familiar with the way that community boundaries may have bearing on eligibility requirements of organizations in your community.

It is important to have a working knowledge of service restrictions for agencies in a geographic area. In some counties, the first assessment visit by the county nurse is free; in other areas this may not be the case. Not only should the nurse be familiar with boundaries and basic eligibility criteria and restrictions, but also must know about the available resources within the specific area.

A community defined by its problems and solutions has a fluid boundary. The problems and those who are affected by those problems determine this boundary. This allows all those who may be affected by the problems to participate in the solutions and the resulting outcome. Thus, a more fluid boundary may allow for greater eligibility or opportunity for service.

The problem of air pollution in one community provides us with an example of a community of solution where the boundary is fluid. In the suburbs of Rosie Mountain and Awful Valley (Fig. 1-2), two school nurses in different elementary

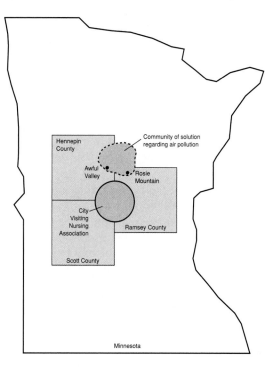

FIGURE 1-2. ▶ A community's boundaries may be many things: geographic, political, problematic. These boundaries are used in the example in this chapter.

schools notice that the percentage of children within their respective schools with symptoms of asthma is increasing. The school nurses talk to each other and note that most of the children with asthma in both school districts live west of a large oil refinery. The school nurses contact the Department of Health. The parents of the children from both schools are invited to a public meeting to discuss the increase in incidences of asthma in the two schools and the potential relationship air pollution in the community may have on this increase. After several meetings, a group of parents from both schools forms a constituency devoted to the identification of the problem and potential solutions. The theoretical boundaries of this community are shown in Figure 1-2. Established school boundaries become fluid in this scenario when a problem arises.

Social Systems
Social systems have an impact on a community and, consequently, the health of that community. Social systems include a community's economy, education, religion, welfare, politics, recreation, as well as its legal, health care, safety and transportation, and communication systems. Depending on the infrastructure, these systems may have a beneficial or detrimental impact on the health of individuals living in a given community. Where recreational facilities provide opportunities for health promotion activities, for instance, the health of the citizens will be enhanced.

It is a documented fact that the infant mortality rate is lower in communities where prenatal care is available and readily accessible to all pregnant women. Here is a social system at work within a community; it has a profound impact on the quality of health of its individual members.

Likewise, there is a relationship between the availability of grocery stores that sell fresh produce and recreational opportunities and childhood obesity within a given community. In communities where children have diets rich in nutritional, low-calorie snacks and safe places to participate in recreational activities, they are more likely to be of normal weight.

A Healthy Community

Just as there are characteristics of healthy individuals, so are there characteristics of healthy communities. These include the following:

◆ Access to health care services that focus on both treatment and prevention for all members of the community
◆ A safe environment
◆ Roads, schools, playgrounds, and other services to meet the needs of the people in that community
◆ Participation of subgroups in community affairs
◆ Emergency preparedness
◆ Ability to solve problems
◆ Communication through open channels
◆ Settling of disputes through legitimate mechanisms
◆ Participation by citizens in decision making
◆ A high degree of wellness among its citizens

A dynamic relationship exists between health and community. In this relationship, health is considered in the context of the community's people, its location, and its social system (Fig. 1-3). Healthy citizens can contribute to the overall health, vitality, and economy of the community. Similarly, if a large portion of individuals in a community is not healthy, not productive, or poorly nourished, the community can suffer from a lack of vitality and productivity (Fig. 1-4).

Location also influences the health of a community. If a toxic landfill or refinery contaminates the earth, water, or air, the health of the people in the area will obviously be detrimentally affected. Figure 1-5 illustrates the relationship between the location and the level of health in a given community.

Social systems and public policy also affect health. Figure 1-6 shows how a community's social systems affect its health. For example, there will be fewer smokers in communities where smoking is not allowed in public buildings or the sale of cigarettes to minors is restricted and strictly enforced. In a community where all pregnant women receive prenatal care, the infant mortality rate will be lower. In a community where immunizations are available and accessible to all children, the immunization rate will be higher and the communicable disease rates low.

Rather than being disease-free, the public sees lowering crime rates, strengthening families and their lifestyles, improving environmental quality, and providing behavioral or mental health care as critical elements to creating healthy communities. To build a healthy community individual health status and quality of life should be considered in every local government decision related to policy and resource allocation. A healthy community requires conventional values, such as quality education, jobs, a healthy environment, housing, and transportation as well as the more obvious need for health services. Some believe that ethical behavior, faith, governance, and early childhood development are also essential for a healthy community (Dennis & Liberman, 2004).

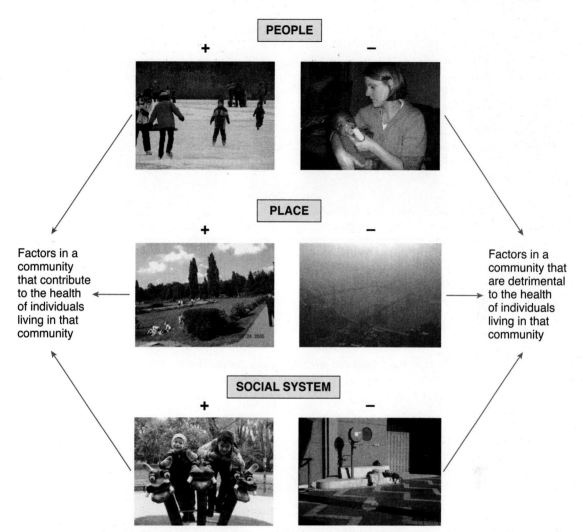

FIGURE 1-3. ▶ A community's health is considered in the context of its people, its location, and its social system.

COMMUNITY NURSING VERSUS COMMUNITY-BASED NURSING

More opportunities are created for nurses in the community as the setting for nursing care continues to move outside the acute care setting. Many of these settings, positions, and opportunities are discussed in Chapter 11. The prominent nursing role in the community in the past was that of public health or community health nurse. For over 35 years there has been a debate regarding the difference between community health and public health nursing. In this text the term community health nursing will be used synonymously with public health nursing. Although a monumental need for provision of nursing care in the community

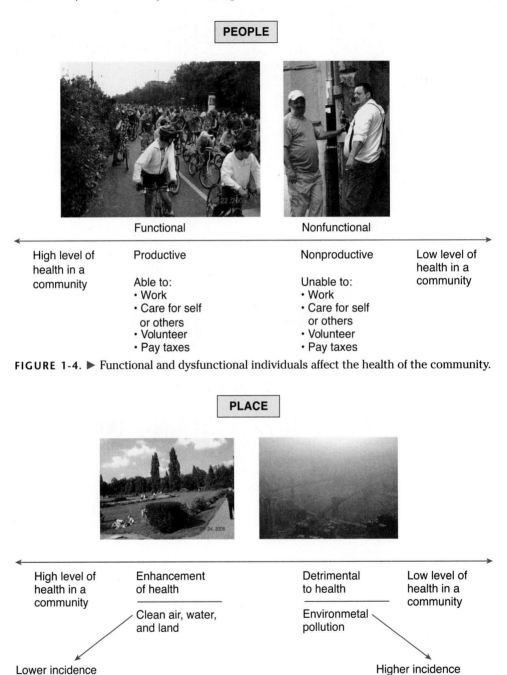

FIGURE 1-4. ▶ Functional and dysfunctional individuals affect the health of the community.

FIGURE 1-5. ▶ Location affects the health of the community.

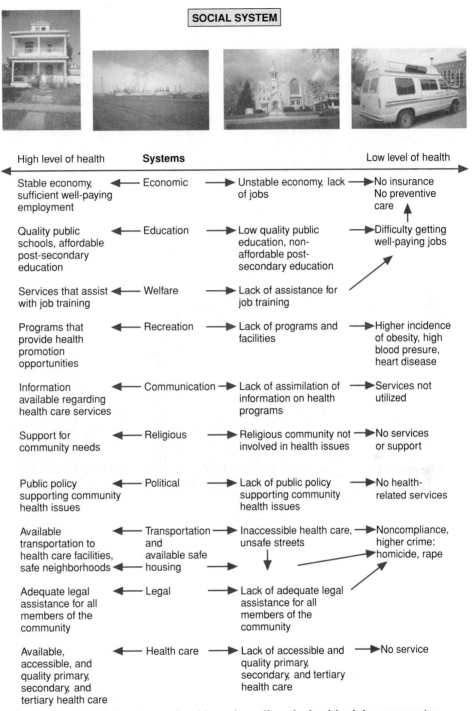

High level of health	Systems		Low level of health
Stable economy, sufficient well-paying employment	◄— Economic —►	Unstable economy, lack of jobs	—► No insurance No preventive care
Quality public schools, affordable post-secondary education	◄— Education —►	Low quality public education, non-affordable post-secondary education	—► Difficulty getting well-paying jobs
Services that assist with job training	◄— Welfare —►	Lack of assistance for job training	
Programs that provide health promotion opportunities	◄— Recreation —►	Lack of programs and facilities	—► Higher incidence of obesity, high blood presure, heart disease
Information available regarding health care services	◄— Communication —►	Lack of assimilation of information on health programs	—► Services not utilized
Support for community needs	◄— Religious —►	Religious community not involved in health issues	—► No services or support
Public policy supporting community health issues	◄— Political —►	Lack of public policy supporting community health issues	—► No health-related services
Available transportation to health care facilities, safe neighborhoods	◄— Transportation and available safe housing —►	Inaccessible health care, unsafe streets	—► Noncompliance, higher crime: homicide, rape
Adequate legal assistance for all members of the community	◄— Legal —►	Lack of adequate legal assistance for all members of the community	
Available, accessible, and quality primary, secondary, and tertiary health care	◄— Health care —►	Lack of accessible and quality primary, secondary, and tertiary health care	—► No service

FIGURE 1-6. ▶ Social system and public policy affect the health of the community.

resulted from the changes in the health care delivery system, this need has not been for more community health nurses but rather for additional nurses prepared to give community- based care.

While community health nursing practice includes nursing directed to individuals, families, and groups, the predominant responsibility is to the population as a whole (American Nurses Association [ANA], 1999). Thus, community, or public, health nursing is defined by its role in promoting the public's health. Community health nursing is a subset of community-based nursing. Community health nursing has a definitive philosophy of practice and requires specific knowledge and skill.

Community-based nursing is not defined by the setting or by the level of academic preparation but by a philosophy of practice (Hunt, 1998). It is about how the nurse practices, not where the nurse practices. Community-based nursing provides care along a continuum focusing on health promotion and rehabilitative primary health care through interdisciplinary collaboration for diverse populations (American Association of Colleges of Nursing [AACN], 2002; NLN, 1993). Community-based nursing is based on the assumptions that: the individual and the family have primary responsibility for health care decisions; health and social issues are interactive; and treatment effectiveness, rather than the technologic imperative, drives decisions related to health (NLN, 2000b).

Community-based nursing care can be defined as nursing care directed toward specific individuals and families within a community. It is designed to meet needs of people as they move between and among health care settings. The emphasis is on a "flowing" kind of care that does not necessarily occur in one setting.

High-technology care that previously was available only in acute care settings is now provided in the home. The community-based nurse must teach clients and families how to manage highly technical equipment and to be responsible for complex self-care.

FOCUS OF NURSING

Nursing, in any setting and with any nursing theory, involves a focus of four components: the client, the environment, health, and nursing (Fawcett, 1984). Each area is approached differently depending on whether the care is provided in the acute care setting or in the community-based setting (Table 1-1).

In the acute care setting, the client is typically identified by the medical diagnosis and is separated from the family. The environment is controlled by the facility with restriction of the family's access to the client and a limitation on the client's freedom. Health and illness are seen as separate and apart from one another. When the client is discharged, the goals of acute care are considered accomplished. Nursing functions are largely delegated medical functions that center on treatment of illness.

In community-based nursing, the client is in his or her natural environment, in the context of the family and community. Illness is seen as merely an aspect of life, and the goals of care are focused around maximizing the client's quality of life. Nursing in the community is an autonomous practice, for the most part, with nursing interventions determined by the client, family, and health care team and based on the values of the client or family and the community. The community model of care reflects the principles of community-based nursing where the goal of care is to encourage self-care in the context of the family and community with a focus on illness prevention and continuity of care.

COMPONENTS OF COMMUNITY-BASED CARE

Transitions in health care settings and consumer participation have brought about some changes in the directions of health care. Components of community-based care are: self-care, preventive health care, care within the context of the community, continuity of care, and collaborative care. These are described here and expanded on throughout the text.

Self-Care: Client and Family Responsibility

The consumer movement within the past several decades has enhanced awareness of the importance of self-care. The value of taking care of oneself to remain healthy, rather than neglecting health, with the consequence of illness or injury, has become a more accepted notion. Programs on stress management, nutrition, exercise and fitness, as well as smoking cessation and substance abuse prevention and treatment, are examples of how health-seeking behaviors have taken a more prominent role in health care. Self-care is also seen in disease management. Disease management programs are beginning to encompass providers across the continuum of care. This movement is also seen in political and government factions promoting seatbelt use, motorcycle and bicycle safety, pollution control, and handgun control.

Self-care charges the individual client and the family with primary responsibility for health care decisions and actions. Because health care is increasingly provided outside the acute care setting, by design the client, family, or other caregiver, such as a friend or neighbor, gives care rather than a health care professional. The burden of responsibility has shifted as the insurance companies and other third-party payers claim it is too expensive to do otherwise.

Empowering individuals to make informed health care decisions is an essential component of self-care. One example is **advance directives** that allow clients to participate in decisions about their care, including the right to refuse treatment. One type of advance directive is the **living will**, which is the client's statement regarding the medical treatment he or she chooses to omit or refuses in the event the client is unable to make those decisions for him or herself. Although the legislation for advance directives is over a decade old, there continues to be limited use of this important strategy. The nurse plays an essential role in ensuring that the client and family are informed about this important issue.

Although community-based nursing affords the opportunity for direct intervention, it also requires self-care teaching for the client and caregiver. The nurse's role in facilitating self-care requires use of the nursing process. In other words, assessment, planning, implementation, and evaluation revolve around this question: How much care can the client and other caregivers safely provide themselves?

Preventive Health Care

Treatment efficacy rather than technologic imperative promotes nursing care that emphasizes prevention. Community-based nursing considers all three levels of prevention (discussed in Chapter 2). Unlike community health nursing, community-based nursing focuses primarily on tertiary prevention. This emphasis is evident in all settings of community-based nursing.

For example, a nurse in the emergency room considers not only the impact of the child's poisoning, but also which preventive nursing interventions will maximize recovery and prevent a repeat of the incident. Careful teaching about wound care to avoid infection is an important preventive intervention for the client who is having a laceration sutured. Likewise, referral of a client for substance abuse assessment is an appropriate preventive nursing intervention for an intoxicated person who presents at the urgent care center after a fall.

Care Within the Context of the Community

Health and social issues are interactive. Nursing care is provided while considering the culture, values, and resources of the client, the family, and the community. If the client requests a particular religious or social ceremony before tube feeding, then the nurse attempts, within the constraints of safety, to comply with the client's request. In situations where family members want to participate in the client's care but their psychomotor skills restrict their ability to do so, the nurse will accommodate the desire within the constraints of time and safe care. If the client enjoys the social functions of religious services every week, the visiting nurse honors that community value by scheduling of visits around the religious functions.

Care in the context of the client, family, and community is affected by the location and social systems of each community. Location often defines eligibility for health care services. Consequently, access and availability of services affect the health of the community. For instance, access to care is impeded by location when an adolescent who does not drive lives in the suburbs where there is no public transportation and seeks information about family planning services offered only in the nearby metropolitan area. In such a case, the social systems of the community affect access to care.

Continuity of Care

Fragmentation of care has long been a concern of health care professionals. For instance, a client with a variety of problems may be seen by several physicians: the family physician, cardiologist, endocrinologist, consultants, and surgeon. A variety of other health care providers may also be involved in the client's care. This fragmentation of care can result in conflicting directions for care, overmedication or under medication, and a confused client. **Continuity of care** is a bridge to quality care.

Community-based care is essential when clients are seen by several health care practitioners and move from one health care setting to another. Continuity allows quality of care to be preserved in a changing health care delivery system. If all providers follow the basic principles of continuity of care, then the possibility of a detrimental impact from a decreased length of stay in the acute care setting, where care is coordinated, to a community setting, where care is provided through a variety of individuals, can be minimized. Continuity is the glue that holds community-based nursing care together and is one of the fundamental concepts of this book. Continuity of care is discussed in Chapter 7.

Collaborative Care

Closely related to continuity of care is collaborative care. Collaborative care among health care professionals is an essential part of community-based care in that the primary goal of each practitioner is to promote wellness and restore health. Regardless of the setting, the community-based nurse works with a variety of professionals as care for the client is assessed, planned, implemented, and evaluated.

The physician is responsible primarily for diagnosing an illness and initiating required medical or surgical treatment. Physicians have the authority to admit clients into a specific health care setting and to discharge them from that setting into another setting. Further, physicians determine the plan of care for the medical needs of the client with input from other professional caregivers. Various therapists (physical, occupational, respiratory, speech) may be involved in the client's care, providing therapy in the acute care setting, a rehabilitation setting, a residential care setting, or the home. The client may visit the facility, or the therapist may visit the home.

A dietitian may adapt a specialized diet to a specific individual and family or to counsel and educate clients and their families. The social worker helps clients and families make decisions related to use of community resources, life-sustaining treatments, and long-term care. A chaplain or the client's spiritual advisor will also counsel the client and family and give spiritual support. The pharmacist dispenses medications as directed by the physician.

Although each professional is responsible for a specialized concern, each is also responsible for sharing information with others or for evaluating how care is proceeding. If one person in the chain fails to communicate, the bridge of continuity is weakened. Usually one person is designated as coordinator of these communications. In many cases this coordinator is the nurse. This role is discussed in Chapter 7.

NURSING SKILLS AND COMPETENCIES

Health care has dramatically evolved in the past two decades as models of community-based care continue to develop. The Pew Health Professions Commission identified 21 competencies that health care professionals need in the 21st century. These competencies, listed in Box 1-2, emphasize community-based nursing care principles. Although these competencies apply to all health care professionals, the term "nurse" can be substituted in place of the term "practitioners" in the statements.

As mentioned nursing care in the acute care setting and the community differ greatly. Consequently, the nursing roles in each setting require different practice skills whether acute care, community-based health care or home care. A decades-old study by Hughes & Marcantonio (1992) studied the practice patterns among home health, community health, and hospital nurses. In the acute care setting, nurses spend the majority of their time in direct patient care and have little time for administrative, supervisory, or consultant roles.

The home care and community-based nurse spends almost three times as many hours as the acute care nurse in consultant roles (teacher, communicator). The community-based and home care nurses also spend five times as many hours in the administrator/manager role as the acute care nurse. In acute care, nurses spend 84% of their time doing direct client care; in community-based and home care nursing, only about 60% of time is spent on direct care.

The home care nurse spends more time in the supervision/management role than in the teaching or physical caregiver role. Home care incorporates critical aspects of both the hospital and community health nurse role. Nurses in home care express

---

◆ BOX 1-2 Pew Commission: Twenty-one Competencies for the 21st Century ◆

1. Embrace a personal ethic of social responsibility and service.
2. Exhibit ethical behavior in all professional activities.
3. Provide evidence-based, clinically competent care.
4. Incorporate the multiple determinants of health in clinical care.
5. Apply knowledge of the new sciences.
6. Demonstrate critical thinking, reflection, and problem-solving skills.
7. Understand the role of primary care.
8. Rigorously practice preventive health care.
9. Integrate population-based care and services into practice.
10. Improve access to health care for those with unmet health needs.
11. Practice relationship-centered care with individuals and families.
12. Provide culturally sensitive care to a diverse society.
13. Partner with communities in health care decisions.
14. Use communication and information technology effectively and appropriately.
15. Work in interdisciplinary teams.
16. Ensure care that balances individual, professional, system, and societal needs.
17. Practice leadership.
18. Take responsibility for quality of care and health outcomes at all levels.
19. Contribute to continuous improvement of the health care system.
20. Advocate for public policy that promotes and protects the health of the public.
21. Continue to learn and help others learn.

Source: Bellack, J. P., & O'Neil, E. H. (2000). Recreating nursing practice for a new century: Recommendations and implications of the Pew Health Profession's Commission's final report. *Nursing and Healthcare Perspectives, 21*(1), 14–18.

---

more job satisfaction than those working in acute care or community health (Simmons, Nelson, & Neal, 2001). Further, they are less likely to work weekends or nights.

Professional roles for the nurses in community-based care require both knowledge and skills in communication, teaching, management, and direct physical caregiving (Box 1-3).

Provider of Care Through Communication and Teaching

First and foremost, in community-based settings the nurse must establish practice as relationship-based. Developing the trusting, therapeutic relationship requires a knowledge about who we are, what we do, and how we do what we do (Dingman, 2005). Relationship-based care consists of three critical relationships: the nurse's relationship with self, the nurse's relationship with the client and family, and the nurse's relationship with colleagues (Beaty, 2006). The heart of relationship-based

---

◆ **BOX 1-3** Community-Based Nursing Competencies ◆

Communication

The nurse applies principles of interpersonal communication to inter-actions with clients, families, and other caregivers in all settings in the community.

Teaching

The nurse applies principles of teaching and learning to all learners, including the client, family member or caregiver, coworkers, and other care providers or community members.

Management

The nurse applies knowledge of leadership by performing the manage-ment functions of planning, organizing, coordinating, delegating, and evaluating care for a group of clients.

Physical Caregiving

The nurse applies knowledge of principles and procedures for providing safe and effective physical care.

---

care transpires when one human connects to another as compassion and care are communicated through touch, a kind act, competent clinical interventions, or through listening and seeking to understand another human being's experience. Healing is attributable to relationship-based care.

A competent nurse embraces the principles and techniques of interpersonal communication in relationship-based care and applies these in interactions with clients, family members, family caregivers, and other health care providers. In practice, the nurse identifies and interprets verbal and nonverbal communications. It is essential to recognize all recurring variables that influence the communication process. The nurse consistently and effectively uses interpersonal communication to establish, maintain, and terminate a therapeutic relationship. The interaction must effectively support the goals that are mutually established by the client and the multidisciplinary team.

The nurse in the community-based setting must have a working knowledge of the principles of teaching and learning as they relate to the scope of practice. The nurse collects and interprets information to assess the learner's need to learn or readiness to learn. Individualized learning outcomes are developed and implemented in the teaching plan. Learning outcomes are evaluated, and modifications are made as indicated. Teaching is discussed further in Chapter 6.

Manager or Coordinator of Care

As a manager of care in the community, the nurse uses his or her leadership abil-ity and carries out the management functions of planning, organizing, coordinating, delegating, and evaluating care for one client or a group of clients. This involves collecting and interpreting relevant data that leads to meeting priority needs of the client. The nurse assesses resources, capabilities of other providers, and the client or family's ability to provide ongoing care. This assessment and the established care plan goals provide the foundation used to develop a management plan geared toward the client's recovery.

The manager of care oversees the care of a group of clients, delegates nursing activities to coworkers, and assumes responsibility for care given under his or her direction. The manager may also work to maintain and improve the work environment by identifying opportunities for improvement and implementing change. The nurse as manager is responsible for evaluation of every aspect of care. Evaluation of the client's ability to assess his or her own situation and condition and to plan and implement care is an essential component of the recovery process. The manager role extends not only to clients but also to other nursing personnel who are providing care under the direction and leadership of the registered nurse. Care management is discussed in more depth in Chapter 7.

Provider of Care Through Assessment and Physical Caregiving

The nurse must know the principles and procedures required for safe and effective physical care. Some of these procedures are ordered by the physician. The nurse either performs these procedures or observes the client or caregiver in performing the tasks. The community-based nurse performs less physical care than does the nurse in the acute care setting.

Assessment is key to quality nursing care in all settings. Because the nurse in the community often functions in a more autonomous role than the nurse in the acute care setting, sound assessment skills are essential. The nurse, client, and family all work in tandem to assemble information about the health status of the client. After systematically collecting and interpreting data related to the client's condition, the nurse collaborates with the client and family to determine what care to initiate, continue, alter, or terminate. Likewise, the environmental variables in the home that may affect physical nursing care are acknowledged. In addition assessment includes identification of the factors in the community that may influence physical nursing care.

The client, caregiver, and nurse determine expected outcomes and outcome criteria and then develop a plan of care that will meet these goals. After the plan is implemented, effectiveness of the physical care, expected outcomes, and outcome criteria is evaluated, and modifications are made accordingly. The ability of other caregivers to provide adequate physical care for the client is also evaluated.

Critical Thinking

Although not a role, critical thinking is a skill that requires development as it is central to the role of the nurse in community-based settings. Critical thinking assists the nurse to identify options for solving client care problems. For example, a home care nurse encounters numerous problems to solve. He or she may identify symptoms that indicate an emergency situation where it is necessary to call 911 or merely a need to call the physician. The nurse may have to determine adaptations that can be made with resources within the client's home for one situation or how to address cultural or religious problems in another. The nurse may also

◆ **B O X 1-4**   Developing Self-Growth in Thinking Skills ◆

1. Make a list of your current thinking skills.
2. Keep a log (diary) of how you use thinking skills on a regular basis.
3. Share your log with a classmate. Learn from and applaud each other.
4. Read an article or book on thinking in nursing and discuss it with a classmate.
5. Draw a picture or write a paragraph that describes how you would like to enhance your thinking and the factors that hinder your thinking. Share it with a classmate.
6. Promise yourself always to consider at least three possible answers (hunches or conclusions) for every question.
7. Remind yourself that the path to responsible nursing care is along the path of critical thinking.
8. Give yourself a reward for your development of thinking skills.
9. Set goals for further development of your thinking skills.

Source: Craven, R. F., & Hirnle, C. J. (Eds.). (2007). *Fundamentals of nursing: Human health and function* (5th ed., p. 230). Philadelphia: Lippincott Williams & Wilkins.

help the client, caregiver, or family hone their own critical thinking skills to improve their problem solving skills.

The critical thinking process is similar to the nursing process. There are many definitions of critical thinking, but an ideal critical thinker has the following abilities: open mindedness, being inquisitive, truth seeking, analytical, organized in problem solving, and self-confident and self-aware of ability to use and critique scientific evidence to inform decisions (Simpson & Courtneay, 2002; Banning, 2006). Box 1-4 will help the student or nurse to strengthen and build natural skills.

Application of Nursing Process

Critical thinking as well as collaboration skills are necessary to effectively use nursing process. The nurse uses critical thinking to identify which assessments to make for each client as well as determining the meaning of assessment data. Assessments help the nurse determine the strengths and needs of the client, family, and caregiver as together they develop a problem statement or nursing diagnosis. They plan expected outcomes and outcome criteria. Interventions are identified that are reasonable and acceptable to all parties. The person who will carry out those interventions is designated. The nurse may teach a procedure. The client may be able to do the procedure, but a caregiver may need to buy the supplies or help set up the equipment for the procedure each time it is used. Analytical thinking is needed to evaluate a plan of care. Many community-based nurses follow a managed care plan or are given physician's orders to follow. These standard plans always must be individualized for the particular needs of each client and family as well as expanded by adding nursing care that may not be delineated on the standard plan. In community-based nursing the practice nursing process is used to develop therapeutic relationships with clients and caregivers. In the chapters that follow there are numerous opportunities to use nursing process in client situations in community-based settings.

Documentation

Complete, accurate documentation is an essential element of nursing care in any setting but it is of particular importance in community-based settings. Creating a clear account of what the nurse saw and did not only provides a record of care but also creates a log of client progress. Unlike the acute care setting where several caregivers may be documenting care simultaneously, in some community settings such as the home, only the nurse may be documenting care.

Charting is used to determine eligibility for reimbursement for care provided. If services rendered by the nurse fall within the requirements of Medicaid, Medicare, or other third-party payers, then the agency will be paid for the care rendered.

Charting is a legal document. In cases in which an agency and nurse are sued, charting of the incident in question will be used as the record of care provided and client response to that care. Litigation is often avoided or readily resolved if care is accurately and completely documented.

Ethical–Legal Concerns

In community-based nursing, ethical dilemmas present challenges that differ from those in the acute care setting. There may be lack of formal institutional support, such as an ethics committee or ethics rounds in community-based care. In the acute setting, the nurse has 24-hour contact with the client and family, whereas care is intermittent and brief in the community setting. Problem identification and problem solving are troublesome when communication is fragmented over several weeks or months. In theory collaborating with the client and family may sound like common sense but in reality can be exceedingly exasperating.

When care is provided in the home or other community settings, respecting the client and family's desire for self-determination is foremost. This may limit the nurse's influence in the decision-making process. In contrast, the acute care setting is often thought of as "the turf" of the nursing and medical staff. When the values of the family and nurse values collide, frustrating dilemmas may result. Some clients have limited resources and support systems. This may profoundly affect whether caregivers are accessible, available, and affordable. Interdisciplinary communication is difficult in community-based care; this fact may intensify difficulties with ethical issues.

The nurse may facilitate the discussion of ethical concerns as they arise, using an ethical framework and encouraging open dialogue between the client and appropriate family and friends. It is important to know one's own values. If conflicts arise when the nurse and family do not agree, the nurse may have to recommend that the family identify another party to facilitate discussions.

NURSING INTERVENTIONS

Nursing interventions in the community-based setting are both similar and different from those typical in the acute care setting. Nursing interventions in the community have been defined through the work of the Public Health Nursing Section of the Minnesota Department of Health. These interventions are organized to focus on three levels of practice: community-focused practice, system-focused practice, and individual-focused practice (Keller, Schaffer, Lia-Hoagberg, & Strohschein, 2002). This book will primarily highlight individual-focused practice and will be discussed in more detail in the next chapter.

CONCLUSIONS

Community-based nursing is not defined by a setting but by a philosophy of practice. Increasingly, health care is provided in community settings and not in acute care facilities. As a result, the client, family, friends, or neighbors provide care, rather than professional providers. The community-based nurse helps clients and families adapt to providing self-care.

Focusing on prevention, community-based nursing averts the initial occurrence of disease or injury and provides early identification and treatment or a comprehensive rehabilitation of a disease or injury. Continuity and collaborative care allow for quality care to be preserved in a changing health care delivery system. Community-based nurses use special skills and competencies to provide care within the context of the client's culture, family, and community.

References and Bibliography

American Association of Colleges of Nursing. (1998). *Essentials of baccalaureate education and professional nursing practice.* Washington, DC: Author.

American Association of Colleges of Nursing. (2002). *Moving forward with community-based nursing education.* Washington, DC: Author.

American Association of Colleges of Nursing. (2005). *With enrollment rising for the 5th consecutive year, U.S. nursing schools turn away more than 30,000 qualified applications in 2005.* Retrieved on September 7, 2007, from http://www.aacn.nche.edu/media/newsreleases/2005/enrl05.htm

American Nurses Association, Community Health Nursing Division. (1999). American Nurses Association standards of public health nursing practice.

Banning, M. (2006). Measures that can be used to instill critical thinking in nurse prescribers. *Nurse Education in Practice, 6,* 98–105.

Beaty, B. (2006). Relationship-based care: A true evolution of primary nursing. *Creative Nursing, 12*(1). Retrieved on July 5, 2006 from EBSCOHOST.

Bellack, J., & O'Neil, E. (2000). Recreating nursing practice for a new century: Recommendations and implications of the Pew Health Commission's final report. *Nursing and Health Care Perspective, 21*(1), 14–18.

Buerhaus, P., Staiger, D., & Auerbach, D. (2000). Implications of an aging registered nurse workforce. *JAMA, 283*(22), 2948–2952.

Bureau of Labor Statistics, U.S. Department of Labor, *Occupational Outlook Handbook, 2006-2007 Edition,* Registered Nurses. Retrieved on June 2, 2006, from http://www.bls.gov/oco/ocos083.htm

Craven, R. C., & Hirnle, C. J. (Eds.) (2007). *Fundamentals of nursing: Human health and function (5th ed.).* Philadelphia: Lippincott Williams & Wilkins.

Dennis, L. M., & Liberman, A. (2004). Indicators of a healthy and sustainable community. *The Health Care Manager, 23*(2), 145–155.

Dingman, S. (2005). A dialogue on relationship-based care: reflection on practice. *International Journal for Human Caring, 9*(2), 136.

Fawcett, J. (1984). *Analysis and evaluation of conceptual models of nursing.* Philadelphia: F. A. Davis.

Frachel, R. (1988). A new profession: The evolution of public health nursing. *Public Health Nursing, 51*(12), 84–91.

Health Resources and Services Administration. (2000). The registered nurse population: Findings from the national sample survey of registered nurses. Retrieved January 10, 2003, from http://bhpr.hrsa.gov/healthworkforce/reports/nursing/samplesurvey00/default.html

Health Resources and Services Administration. (2002). Projected supply, demand, and shortages of registered nurses: 2000–2020. Retrieved January 10, 2003, from http://bhpr.hrsa.gov/healthworkforce/rnsurvey04/

Health Resources and Services Administration. (2005). Preliminary findings; 2004 National Sample Survey of Registered Nurses. Retrieved May 30, 2006, from http://www.bhpr.hrsa.gov/healthworkforce

Heller, B., Oros, M., & Durney-Crowley, J. (1999). The future of nursing education: Ten trends to watch. New York: National League for Nursing. Retrieved March 3, 2003, from http://www.nln.org/nlnjournal/infotrends.htm

Hughes, K., & Marcantonio, R. (1992). Practice patterns among home health, public health, and hospital nurses. *Nursing and Health Care, 13*(10), 532–536.

Hunt, R. (1998). Community based nursing: Philosophy or setting. *American Journal of Nursing, 98*(10), 44–47.

Josten, L. (1989). Wanted: Leaders for public health. *Nursing Outlook, 37,* 230–232.

Kalish, P., & Kalish, B. (1995). *The advance of American nursing (3rd ed.).* Philadelphia: Lippincott.

Keller, L., Schaffer, M., Lia-Hoagberg, B., & Strohschein, S. (2002). Assessment, program planning, and evaluation in population-based public health practice. *Journal of Public Health Management Practice, 8*(5), 30–43.

Leininger, M. (1970). *Nursing and anthropology: Two worlds to blend.* New York: Wiley.

Monteiro, L. (1991). Florence Nightingale on public health nursing. In B. Spradley (Ed.), *Readings in community health nursing.* Philadelphia: Lippincott.

National League for Nursing. (1993). *A vision for nursing education.* New York: Author.

National League for Nursing. (1997). Final report: Commission on a workforce for a restructured health care system. New York: Author.

National League for Nursing. (2000a). A vision for nursing education. New York: Author.

National League for Nursing, Council of Associate Degree Nursing Competencies Task Force. (2000b). *Educational competencies for graduates of associate degree nursing programs.* Boston: Jones & Bartlett Publisher.

Reverby, S. M. (1993). From Lillian Wald to Hillary Rodham Clinton: What will happen to public health nursing? [Editorial]. *American Journal of Public Health, 83,* 1662–1663.

Simmons, B. L., Nelson, D. L., & Neal, L. J., (2001). A comparison of the positive and negative work attitudes of home health care and hospital nurses. *Health Care Management Review, 26*(3), 63–74.

Simpson, E., & Courtneay, M. (2002). Critical thinking in nursing education: Literature review. *International Journal of Nursing Practice, 8,* 89–98.

U.S. Department of Health and Human Services. (2000). Healthy people 2010: National health promotion and disease prevention objectives, full report, with commentary. Washington, DC: U.S. Government Printing Office. Available at http://www.healthypeople.gov

LEARNING ▼ ACTIVITIES

◆ JOURNALING ACTIVITY 1-1

In your clinical journal, discuss a community with which you are familiar and describe what defines that community.

1. Identify some of the health needs of that community.
2. Where do members of this community receive health care?
3. Are there people in the community who do not have access to health care? Who are they? What services are they not able to access?

◆ CLIENT CARE ACTIVITY 1-2

How can the nurse encourage self-care in the following client situations?

1. Jane is the 31-year-old mother of Jackie, a 4-month-old baby who has frequent apnea spells. Jane states, "I am afraid she will stop breathing at home. I can't figure out the monitor."
2. Stephan is a 60-year-old widower whose wife died 3 years ago. There is an increasing possibility that he will have to have his leg amputated below the knee as a result of a very large leg ulcer. Stephan has been hospitalized three times in the past 6 months because of uncontrolled diabetes. The last time, there were maggots in his leg ulcer.

◆ CLIENT CARE ACTIVITY 1-3

How can the nurse encourage disease prevention and health promotion in the following client situations?

1. Barb and Steve have a 10-month-old baby, Andy, who requires intermittent nursing care because of oxygen therapy and tracheotomy care. They have three other children, ages 2, 4, and 6. Andy has had three bouts of respiratory flu and two colds in the last 4 months. He has been hospitalized twice during that time. You are the home care nurse caring for Andy. You noticed on your last visit that Andy's brothers and sister kiss him, touch his trach tube, and cough on him. One of the children went in to use the bathroom and left the door open, and you noticed that he did not wash his hands afterwards.

   What is your priority nursing intervention with Barb, Steve and their family? What does the nursing literature say about the intervention that you identified? How will you proceed with your teaching using a prevention focus?
2. Meg and Bob have a 3-year-old child, Mark, who has cerebral palsy. Meg provides 24-hour care for Mark with no assistance from anyone. You notice on your last home visit that Meg has lost weight, is not sleeping, and complains that she has no energy. You suspect that she may be suffering from depression. You recommend several counselors and respite care for Mark so Meg can get out occasionally. Meg states, "I come from a very large family. We never use a baby-sitter in our family." What do you do and say?

◆ PRACTICAL APPLICATION ACTIVITY 1-4

Describe an incident from your clinical experience in which you believe continuity was interrupted.

- Indicate some things that could have been done to ensure continuity in these situations.
- Describe a time or circumstance that you observed or participated in where continuity of care was provided. What happened, and who and what made it happen?

◆ **PRACTICAL APPLICATION ACTIVITY 1-5**

1. Contact your local or state department of health. You can either call them or visit their web site. What are the current issues facing your department of health? How are these issues related to nursing?
2. Find an article in the paper that is related to one of the topics covered in this chapter. What new things did you learn about the issue or topic? How is the topic related to what is discussed in this chapter.

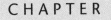

CHAPTER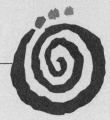

2

Health Promotion and Disease Prevention

ROBERTA HUNT

LEARNING OBJECTIVES

1. Describe the health–illness continuum.
2. Relate the two goals of Healthy People 2010 to community-based nursing.
3. After choosing one priority from each of the two major sections of Healthy People 2010, analyze it for a classmate.
4. Recognize the difference between health promotion and disease prevention.
5. Identify nursing roles for each level of prevention.
6. Describe nursing interventions in community-based settings.

KEY TERMS

disease and injury prevention services
function
health
health disparity
health promotion
health protection

health–illness continuum
nursing interventions in community-based settings
primary prevention
secondary prevention
tertiary prevention

CHAPTER TOPICS

◆ Health and Illness
◆ Healthy People 2010
◆ Health Promotion Versus Disease Prevention
◆ The Prevention Focus
◆ Nursing Competencies and Skills and Levels of Prevention
◆ Nursing Interventions in Community-Based Settings
◆ Conclusions

THE NURSE SPEAKS

When I went into nursing, I wanted to be a critical care nurse. I loved the idea of working with technology and having a lot of responsibility. Anatomy and physiology fascinated me, so critical care was a perfect fit for me. I worked for 5 years as a critical care nurse and really enjoyed it. The part about the job I liked the most turned out to be working with the families. When the families had questions, I was right there answering their questions. If a family member was feeling emotional and needed someone to listen, I actually enjoyed hearing their stories and trying to figure out how to be helpful. At the same time I was working in CCU, I was volunteering at the local senior citizens center, teaching classes on health topics that were identified by the clientele as being important to them. I began to make some home visits to some of the homebound seniors who had questions about their medications. I began to see the value of health promotion and disease prevention. Some of the people we saw in the CCU had conditions that could have been better managed at home, preventing an admission to the CCU. Some had diseases that could have been prevented. I also really enjoyed going to people's homes and taking care of them there. I looked into the home care agency in our hospital and learned that I could work one weekend a month as a home care nurse. I cut back on the CCU and began to gradually do more and more home care. That was 10 years ago, and I have never looked back. I love home care nursing.

—BECKY CARMONDY, RN, Home Care Nurse

The U.S. health care system is the most expensive in the world, using 15.2% of the U.S. gross national product (GNP), at a cost of nearly $5,711 per person. The next most expensive health care system is in Canada, where 9% of the GNP is used for health care, at a per capita cost of $2,980. A recent study found Canadians healthier than citizens in the United States despite spending almost half of what is spent on health care per person in the United States (Lasser, Himmelstein, & Woolhandler, 2006). Most industrialized nations spend 8% to 10% of their GNP on health care (World Health Organization [WHO], 2006).

Despite having the most expensive health care in the world, the United States lags behind other nations in key health indicators. The United States ranks 36th among nations in its infant mortality rate, at 7/1,000 births. This average does not show the higher rates for certain minority groups, such as 13.9/1,000 for Blacks, 8.6/1,000 for American Indians, and 5.8/1,000 for Caucasian Americans. Life expectancy in the United States ranks behind Sweden, Germany, Italy, France, and Canada. Twenty-one percent of the nation's 1 1/2- to 3-year-old children are inadequately immunized against diphtheria, tetanus, pertussis, polio, measles, mumps, and rubella. Disadvantaged populations rank significantly worse than average in these and other health indicators (Federal Interagency Forum on Child and Family Statistics, 2006; WHO, 2006).

Health care costs are a barrier to care for both the insured and the uninsured. According to a study by the Harvard School of Public Health, nearly one-quarter of Americans had problems paying medical bills in 2005, and more than 61% of those reporting problems paying medical bills were covered by health insurance (Kaiser Family Foundation & Harvard School of Public Health, 2005). Moderate- and low-income, working adults report significantly more problems paying for medical care compared with their higher-income peers. Uninsured adults (18% of the public) report more problems accessing health care because of costs and they say it is costs that keep them out of the health insurance market. Two-thirds (66%) of the insured adults say their health insurance premiums have gone up over the past 5 years, including 38% who say that their premiums have gone up "a lot." Every industrialized nation except the United States has a national health plan in place that covers all citizens.

Nursing is a reflection of society's needs. Although a great deal of money is spent on health care in the United States, the level of health of U.S. citizens is disappointing. The consumer movement toward increased participation in wellness, weight loss, smoking cessation, and exercising has resulted in the preventive care movement. Settings for practice have evolved naturally as nurses focus on health rather than illness. Nursing has taken on a new look as it assumes the role of health promotion and illness prevention. Community-based nursing calls for interventions distinct and different from many of those common in the acute care setting. Community-based nursing is a philosophy of care.

This chapter begins with a discussion of health and its place on the health–illness continuum. The goals and priorities in the federal government's program—Healthy People 2010—are presented. A large part of the chapter is devoted to illustrating the difference between health promotion and disease prevention and the major strategies nurses will use to meet the goals of Healthy People 2010, with emphasis on the preventive focus. Levels of prevention and nursing roles are outlined. The chapter ends with a description of nursing interventions appropriate for community-based nursing.

HEALTH AND ILLNESS

Rather than focusing on curing illness and injury, community-based care focuses on promoting health and preventing illness. **Health** is defined by the World Health Organization (1986) as a "state of physical, mental and social well-being and not merely absence of disease or infirmity." This holistic philosophy differs greatly from that of the acute care setting.

Considering health—rather than illness—as the essence of care requires a shift in thinking. The **health–illness continuum** illustrates this model of care (Fig. 2-1). Health is conceptualized as a resource for everyday living. It is a positive idea that emphasizes social and personal resources and physical capabilities. Wellness is a lifestyle aimed at achieving physical, emotional, intellectual, spiritual, and environmental well-being. The use of wellness measures can increase stamina, energy, and self-esteem. These then enhance quality of life.

Improvement of health is not seen as an outcome of the amount and type of medical services or the size of the hospital. Treatment efficacy, rather than technology, drives care in this model. Here health is viewed as a function of collaborative efforts at the community level.

Care provided in acute care settings is usually directed at resolving immediate health problems. In the community, care focuses on maximizing individual potential for self-care. The client assumes responsibility for health care decisions and

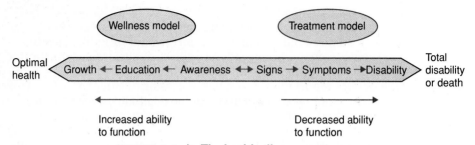

FIGURE 2-1. ▶ The health–illness continuum.

care provision. Where health is the essence of care, the client's ability to function becomes the primary concern. The intent of care is not to "fix" with treatment but to enhance the quality of life and support actions that make the client's life as comfortable and productive as possible.

Function is defined by subjective and objective measurements. Both the client's abilities to perform activities of daily living (ADL) and the client's perception of how well he or she is functioning are considered. Clients may state that they are satisfied with their ability to care for themselves; however, objective data from laboratory reports, diagnostic tests, and caregivers' observations may show that this is not the case. On the other hand, clients may report that they are concerned about their ability to perform ADLs, yet other information may indicate that they are functioning quite well. The following Client Situation in Practice reflects this dichotomy.

CLIENT SITUATIONS IN PRACTICE

◆ Perceptions of Health and Illness

Mary had a myocardial infarction 3 days ago. After two episodes of chest pain and dizziness, she reluctantly went to the emergency room. Laboratory values showed moderate heart damage. As a 46-year-old single parent, Mary is the sole provider for three adolescents. She is a physical therapist and works at an ambulatory clinic during the week and a nursing home on weekends. She tells the nurse caring for her that she feels fine and asks to go home so she can go back to work tomorrow.

Mary's mother, Shirley, is extremely distraught about her daughter's condition and believes Mary is dying. Figure 2-2 illustrates the objective data versus Mary's subjective point of view. The dissonance between subjective perceptions and objective data can interrupt and delay recovery.

A person's lifestyle is a dynamic process that involves needs, beliefs, assumptions, and values. Choices in life therefore can be seen as opportunities for moving toward optimal health or wellness.

Wellness involves more than simply good physical self-care. It also requires using one's mind constructively, expressing one's emotions effectively, interacting

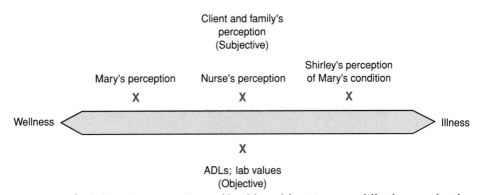

FIGURE 2-2. ▶ Subjective perceptions of health and function may differ from each other and from objective data.

constructively with others, and being concerned about one's physical and psychological environment. Regardless of the setting for health care, wherever nurses practice, their concern is for the whole person, and the care they provide is holistic (Fig. 2-3).

HEALTHY PEOPLE 2010

Healthy People 2010 offers a simple but powerful idea: Provide the information and knowledge about how to improve health in a format that enables diverse groups to combine their efforts and work as a team. It is a road map to better health for all, which can be used by many different people, communities, professional

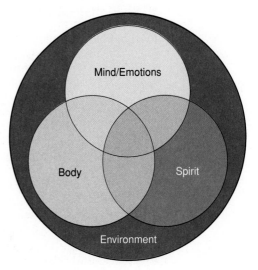

FIGURE 2-3. ▶ Schematic representation of holism. The system is greater than and different from the sum of the parts. Wherever the setting, the nurse's concern is for the whole person.

organizations, and groups whose concern is a particular population group or particular threat to health (U.S. Department of Health and Human Services [DHHS], 2000). Publication of this vision was the result of a national consortium of health care professionals, citizens, and private and public agencies from across the United States.

Healthy People 2010 states that its purpose is to commit the nation to the attainment of two broad goals:

1. To eliminate health disparities
2. To increase quality and years of healthy life

Measurable targets or objectives to be achieved are organized into 28 priority areas (see Healthy People 2010 2-1).

HEALTHY PEOPLE 2010 ▶ 2-1

Focus Areas

1. Access to quality health services
2. Arthritis, osteoporosis, and chronic back conditions
3. Cancer
4. Chronic kidney disease
5. Diabetes
6. Disability and secondary conditions
7. Education and community-based programs
8. Environmental health
9. Family planning
10. Food safety
11. Health communication
12. Heart disease and stroke
13. Human immunodeficiency virus (HIV)
14. Immunization and infectious diseases
15. Injury and violence prevention
16. Maternal, infant, and child health
17. Medical product safety
18. Mental health
19. Nutrition and obesity
20. Occupational safety and health
21. Oral health
22. Physical activity and fitness
23. Public health infrastructure
24. Respiratory diseases
25. Sexually transmitted diseases
26. Substance abuse
27. Tobacco use
28. Vision and hearing

Eliminate Health Disparity

The first goal of Healthy People 2010 is to eliminate health disparities. These include differences in health and access to health care services by gender, age, race or ethnicity, education or income, disability, geographic location, or sexual orientation. For example, men have a life expectancy that is 6 years less than women. Another example is that information about the biologic and genetic characteristics of African Americans, Hispanics, Native Americans, Alaska Natives, Asians, Native Hawaiians, and Pacific Islanders does not explain the health disparities experienced by these groups compared with the White, non-Hispanic population in the United States. See Box 2-1 for a summary of **health disparity** in the United States.

◆ **BOX 2-1** | Racial and Ethnic Disparities in Health Care ◆

The overall health of Americans has improved in the last few decades, but all Americans have not shared equally in these improvements. Among nonelderly adults, for example, 17% of Hispanic and 16% of Black Americans report they are in only fair or poor health, as compared with 10% of White Americans. One may ask: In people who receive health care, how much do differences in race and ethnicity contribute to disparities in that health care?

Primary care is central to the health care system in the United States. Research shows that having a source of care raises the chance that people receive adequate preventive care and other health services. Data from the Agency for Healthcare Research and Quality (AHRQ) Medical Expenditure Panel Survey shows that about 30% of Hispanic and 20% of Black Americans lack a usual source of health care, compared with less than 16% of White Americans. Further, Hispanic children are nearly two times as likely as non-Hispanic children to have no usual source of health care.

Race and ethnicity influence a patient's chance of receiving many specific procedures and treatments. Of nine hospital procedures investigated in one AHRQ study, five were significantly less common among African-American clients than among White patients; three of those five were also less common among Hispanics, and two were less common among Asian Americans. Other AHRQ research revealed additional disparities in client care for various conditions and care settings. Researchers found that African Americans are 13% less likely to undergo coronary angioplasty and one-third less likely to undergo bypass surgery than are Whites. Among preschool children hospitalized for asthma, only 7% of Black and 2% of Hispanic children, compared with 21% of White children, are prescribed routine medications to prevent future asthma-related hospitalizations.

Source: Agency for Health Care and Quality Research (2006). Addressing racial and ethnic disparities in health care fact sheet. Rockville, MD. Retrieved June 23, 2006, from http://www.ahrq.gov/research/disparit.htm

It is believed that these disparities are a result of the complex interaction among genetic variations, environmental factors, and specific health behaviors. Inequalities in income and education underlie many health disparities, with income and education often serving as a proxy measure for each other. In general, population groups that suffer the worst health status are also those that have the highest poverty rates and the least education. Disparities in health care can be eliminated through continued commitment to understanding why disparities exist. Effective strategies to eliminate and overcome disparities need to be identified. Nurses have a role in working more closely with communities to ensure that relevant research findings are implemented quickly. There is a need to evaluate transcultural competence (discussed in Chapter 3) as it relates to health care disparities. Last of all, capacity for health services research among minority institutions and minority investigators is lacking. Nurses have a role in seeing that these deficiencies are addressed (Agency for Healthcare Research and Quality, 2002).

Nurses can help reduce health disparities by doing the following:

◆ educating themselves regarding issues of disparity
◆ using evidence-based decision making
◆ identifying vulnerable populations in their communities
◆ helping clients pursue high-quality care
◆ advocating for vulnerable populations.

Increase the Quality and Years of Healthy Life

The fact that individual health is closely linked to community health was discussed in Chapter 1. Likewise, community health is affected by the collective behaviors, attitudes, and beliefs of everyone who lives in the community. The underlying premise of Healthy People 2010 is that the health of the individual is almost inseparable from the health of the larger community. One way to increase the quality and years of healthy life for communities is to follow the recommendations of Healthy People 2010. This road map for improving health is based on the concepts of health promotion, disease prevention, and health protection.

Health Indicators

The achievement of the Healthy People 2010 goals of reducing health disparity and increasing the quality and years of healthy life is determined through measuring and comparing health indicators. Each of the leading health indicators has one or more objectives from Healthy People 2010 associated with it. The health indicators reflect the major health concerns in the United States at the beginning of the 21st century. The health indicators were selected on the basis of their ability to motivate action, the availability of data to measure progress, and their importance as public health issues. Refer to Healthy People 2010 2-2 for a list of health indicators.

HEALTH PROMOTION VERSUS DISEASE AND INJURY PREVENTION

Sometimes people confuse health promotion and disease prevention. It is easy to do, because some approaches and interventions are the same or they overlap. **Health promotion** strategies relate to individual lifestyle, which has a powerful

▶ **HEALTHY PEOPLE 2010 ▶ 2-2**

Health Indicators

1. Physical activity
2. Overweight and obesity
3. Tobacco use
4. Substance abuse
5. Responsible sexual behavior
6. Mental health
7. Injury and violence
8. Environmental quality
9. Immunization
10. Access to health care

influence over one's long-term health. Educational and community-based programs, such as smoking cessation programs, are designed to address lifestyle. **Disease and injury prevention services** include counseling, screening, immunization, and chemoprophylactic interventions for individuals in clinical settings. Health promotion activities are used to promote and maximize health, and disease prevention activities are intended to prevent future illness. For example, Jill jogs every morning before work. She enjoys jogging, finding that it stimulates her for the day's activities, and makes her feel good. Jill jogs to promote wellness, so Jill is participating in a health promotion activity. By exercising, she may be preventing future illness, but she is primarily promoting trying to improve her health. On the other hand, Nancy jogs because her physician has told her to do so. She is overweight and has a family history of heart problems. Her physician tells her she needs exercise to help prevent future cardiovascular problems. Nancy jogs to prevent illness, so Nancy is participating in a disease prevention activity.

Health protection strategies relate to environmental or regulatory measures that confer protection on large population groups. Rather than the individual focus of health promotion, health protection involves a communitywide focus.

THE PREVENTION FOCUS

The prevention of disease and injury is a key concept of community-based nursing. Preventive services are a good investment for health (Coffield, 2006). Prevention is conceptualized on three levels: primary prevention, secondary prevention, and tertiary prevention. An overview of these levels of prevention appears in Table 2-1. Different preventive strategies are found at each level of prevention. These fall into a continuum of activities that prevent disease or injury, prolong life, and promote health. The following services are categorized as preventive strategies: counseling, screening, immunization, and chemoprophylactic interventions for clients in clinical settings.

TABLE 2-1	Levels of Disease Prevention and Examples of Activities	
Level	**Description**	**Activities[a]**
Primary	Prevention of the initial occurrence of disease or injury	Immunization, family planning, retirement planning, well-child care, smoking cessation, hygiene teaching, fluoride supplements, fitness classes, alcohol and drug prevention, seat belts and child seat car restraints, environmental protection
Secondary	Early identification of disease or disability with prompt intervention to prevent or limit disability	Physical assessments, hypertension screening, developmental screening, breast and testicular self-examinations, hearing and vision screening, mammography, pregnancy testing
Tertiary	Assistance (after disease or disability has occurred) to halt further disease progress and to meet one's potential and maximize quality of life despite illness or injury	Teaching and counseling regarding lifestyle changes such as diet and exercise, stress management and home management after diagnosis of chronic illness, support groups, support for caretaker, Meals On Wheels for homebound, physical therapy after stroke or accident, mental health counseling for rape victims

[a]Some prevention activities listed above overlap into health promotion or health protection.

Health protection and health promotion activities conducted by nurses in community-based settings usually occur at the primary level, although they may occur at secondary and tertiary levels also.

Some of the preventive activities listed in Table 2-1 are further developed in Table 2-2, which shows the goals of these selected activities.

There are numerous reasons for adopting a preventive focus to health care; cost benefit is one (Teutsch, 2006). Primary prevention strategies are particularly cost-effective. For every $1 spent on water fluoridation, $38 is saved in dental restorative treatment. The direct medical cost associated with physical inactivity was $29 billion in 1988 and $76.6 billion in 2000. Engaging in regular physical activity is associated with taking less medication and having fewer hospitalization and physicians visits (Centers for Disease Control and Prevention [CDC], 2006). Chronic disease is a significant contributor to the escalating health care costs; more than 90 million Americans are living with chronic illnesses. The medical costs of individuals with chronic illness account for more than 75% of the nation's $1.4 trillion medical care costs, with chronic disease causing 70% of all deaths (CDC, 2006). Nearly half of all cancer deaths are preventable (Jemal, 2006).

In 2004, hospital costs for preventable conditions totaled nearly 29 billion dollars. This means that one out of every 10 dollars of the total hospital costs were preventable. In that year, 4.4 million hospital stays could have been prevented with better ambulatory care, improved access to effective treatment, or improved self care practices. From 1997 to 2004, there was a 31% increase (adjusted for inflation) in hospital costs for potentially preventable admissions, while the number of admissions rose by only 3 percent. The conditions in which the greatest increases

TABLE 2-2	Activities at Each Level of Prevention	
Level	**Activities**	**Goal of the Activity**
Primary	Immunization clinics	Prevention of communicable diseases such as polio, pertussis, rubella
	Smoking cessation	Prevention of lung and heart disease, cancer
	Tobacco chewing prevention	Prevention of cancer of the mouth, tongue, and throat
	Sex education with emphasis on condom use	Prevention of acquired immunodeficiency syndrome (AIDS) and other sexually transmitted diseases (STDs)
Secondary	Programs to teach and motivate men to do self-exam for testicular masses	Early identification and treatment of testicular cancer
	Blood pressure screening	Early identification and treatment of hypertension to prevent strokes and heart disease
	Programs to teach and motivate women to do breast self-exams	Early identification and treatment of breast cancer
Tertiary	Counseling, low-sodium diet, exercise for management of hypertension	Minimize the effects of hypertension
	Exercises and speech therapy after a cerebrovascular accident	Restore function and limit disability

in preventable admissions were seen included diabetes, circulatory diseases, and chronic respiratory disease (Russo, Jiang, & Barrett, 2007).

As more technology and treatment choices are developed, the cost of health care as well as potential cost savings increases. The lifetime costs of health care associated with human immunodeficiency virus (HIV), in light of recent advances in diagnostics and therapeutics, has grown from $385,200 to $618,900 or more per person (Schackman, et al., 2006). These costs mean that HIV prevention efforts may be even more cost-effective, providing cost savings to society. The most cost-effective preventive health services are shown in Box 2-2.

In addition to being cost-effective, appropriate prevention interventions result in enhanced client satisfaction and faster recovery. Historically, the major portions of primary, secondary, and tertiary prevention services are provided by nurses in community-based settings. This is still true today. **Nursing interventions** in primary, secondary, and tertiary prevention play an important role in preventing and minimizing the impact of chronic conditions on individuals, families, communities, and nations.

Primary Prevention

Primary prevention is commonly defined as prevention of the initial occurrence of disease or injury. Primary prevention activities include immunizations, family

---

◆ BOX 2-2   Cost-Effective Preventive Health Services ◆

1. Aspirin therapy
2. Childhood immunizations
3. Tobacco use screening, intervention
4. Colorectal cancer screening
5. Measurement of blood pressure in adults
6. Influenza immunizations
7. Pneumococcal immunization
8. Alcohol screening and counseling
9. Vision screening for adults
10. Cervical cancer screening
11. Cholesterol screening
12. Breast cancer screening
13. *Chlamydia* screening
14. Calcium supplement counseling
15. Vision screening in children
16. Folic acid
17. Obesity screening
18. Depression screening
19. Hearing screening
20. Injury prevention counseling
21. Osteoporosis screening
22. Cholesterol screening for high-risk patients
23. Diabetes screening
24. Diet counseling
25. Tetanus–diphtheria boosters

Coffield, A. (2006). Preventive services a good investment for health. *The Nation's Health, 36*(6), 2.

---

planning services, classes to prepare people for retirement, and counseling and education on injury prevention. These are categorized as primary prevention because they prevent the initial occurrence of a disease or injury. Tables 2-1 and 2-2 list examples of specific primary prevention activities.

Also included in primary prevention are health promotion and health protection activities. Health promotion focuses on activities related to lifestyle choices in a social context for individuals who are already essentially healthy. Examples of health promotion include exercise and nutrition classes and prevention programs for alcohol and other drug abuse. Smoking cessation programs are often targeted at healthy individuals, offering them a lifestyle choice.

Prevention is also accomplished through health protection. Health protection focuses on activities related to environmental or regulatory measures that provide protection for large population groups. This category would include activities directed at preventing unintentional injuries through motor vehicle accidents, occupational safety and health, environmental health, and food and drug safety.

Other examples of health protection include seat-belt and child car seat restraint laws and laws prohibiting smoking in public places. Implementation of child car seat restraint laws has prevented a significant number of deaths and disabilities among children in the United States over the past 20 years. It has been effective as a health protection activity. Environmental protection and pollution control are other primary prevention strategies.

Secondary Prevention

The intent of **secondary prevention** is the early identification and treatment of disease or injury to limit disability. Identification of health needs, health problems, and clients at risk is the inherent component of secondary prevention. Activities of secondary prevention include screening programs for blood pressure, breast cancer, scoliosis, hearing, and vision. Intervention does not prevent scoliosis, but it does provide early identification and subsequent treatment of a condition that already exists in school-age children. Likewise, mammography does not prevent breast cancer, but it provides an opportunity for early identification and treatment. Typically, screening efforts should address conditions that cause significant morbidity and mortality in the target age group. Tables 2-1 and 2-2 list other examples of specific secondary prevention activities.

Tertiary Prevention

Tertiary prevention maximizes recovery after an injury or illness. Most care provided in acute care facilities, clinics, and skilled nursing facilities focuses on tertiary care. Rehabilitation is the major focus in this level of prevention. Rehabilitation activities assist clients to reach their maximum potential despite the presence of chronic conditions. Teaching a client who has had a hip replacement how to create a safe home environment that prevents falls is an example of tertiary prevention.

Shelters for battered women and counseling and therapy for abused children are further examples of tertiary prevention. Other examples are listed in Tables 2-1 and 2-2.

NURSING COMPETENCIES AND SKILLS AND LEVELS OF PREVENTION

Despite an increasing emphasis on disease prevention and health promotion, and despite ample evidence demonstrating the effectiveness of preventive services, such services are underutilized, with many researchers speculating on the contributing factors (Benjamins, Kirby, & Bond Huie, 2004; Benjamins, (2005). This emphasis has generated numerous opportunities for nurses to participate in health promotion and disease prevention activities at all levels of prevention. Now that you understand the levels of prevention, this section discusses the role of the nurse at each level of prevention in two types of community-based care: the ambulatory and home care settings. Typically, the prominent nursing competencies in these settings are those of communicator and teacher. Competencies as manager and physical care provider also are essential in the home setting. This can be true of ambulatory care as well, depending on the setting.

Primary Prevention

Ambulatory Health Care

Nurses provide information about primary prevention in the ambulatory setting. For example, a nurse may provide information on the importance of infant seats, child restraints, and helmets to all the mothers at a well-child clinic. School nurses may communicate with families through written flyers sent home with the children. Subjects may include the communicability and the methods of transmission of diseases such as chickenpox, influenza, and head lice. Parents of preschool children can obtain vital information and clarification from school nurses about when, where, and why their children can receive periodic checkups and immunizations.

Teaching in clinics, schools, and occupational settings may be directed to individuals or groups. Topics can cover a wide range and include such things as immunizations, family planning, and prenatal care. At adult clinics, nurses provide current information about diet, exercise, stress management, and weight reduction. Women of childbearing age may attend classes on family planning and prenatal topics. Occupational health nurses provide information about injury prevention, repetitive motion injuries, and sensory losses secondary to job tasks. They disseminate information about shift work, offer strategies to avoid sleep disturbances, and provide information about the importance of health promotion activities such as exercise. Many companies provide recreational programs and physical activities at work or in the community through their occupational health programs.

The physical caregiver role in the clinic, school, occupational health setting, and home is usually provided at the tertiary level of prevention. Evaluation of the physical care provided to a client may be a function of either or both the physical caregiver and the manager of care. A manager of care in these settings applies knowledge about the principles of management for a group of clients or staff. This includes managing all aspects of care and involves communication, teaching, and physical care specific to clients and staff in community-based settings. However, there will be some common elements in the responsibilities of this role in the community with that of the manager in the hospital. For instance, the manager evaluates the teaching, physical care, and communication skills of the home health aide, for instance, or the care manager teaches a licensed practical nurse in the clinic and school.

Home Health Care

Clients in the home frequently require episodic care for acute health care conditions. Opportunities for primary prevention are limited. Home care nurses communicate information to the client and family regarding primary prevention strategies because in community-based care, the nurse considers the client in the context of the family. The nurse influences the family's health behaviors in many areas that are not directly related to the client's condition. For example, if the client's spouse asks about immunizations for their children, the nurse has the opportunity to teach about the immunization schedule and where to get affordable care. Or if the client's adult child mentions that he or she would like to stop smoking, the nurse may provide information about resources for smoking cessation.

Secondary Prevention

Ambulatory Health Care

Secondary prevention can involve alerting clients about the time frames for health screening (e.g., mammography, Pap smears, glaucoma screening, breast examinations, lipid levels). The clinic nurse may see clients who are at risk for certain conditions, alert them to their risk, and provide information about community services that may be able to assist them.

Preschool screening, vision and hearing testing, and scoliosis screening are secondary prevention strategies provided in the school. In addition, school nurses teach secondary prevention by educating parents about the screening programs available for their children.

The workplace may be the site where screening is done for hypertension, hearing loss, exposure to hazardous substances, and breast cancer. The nurse disperses information about the services and provides educational programs.

Client need determines in which setting information may be presented. For example, as a manager of care in the clinic, the nurse may not have the opportunity to assess the family caregiver's abilities in assisting a client with insulin injections. However, the nurse in the home can better assess how well the family can assist and support the client. The nurse, as the manager of care in the home, may decide that the family caregiver needs additional teaching to administer the insulin because he or she could not accurately draw up the insulin during an early morning nursing visit.

Home Health Care

Care in the home usually involves short visits. Thus, opportunities for communicating secondary prevention information are limited. However, home health care nurses do inform the client and family about services in the community that may help them with the client's care, early identification and treatment of conditions related to the client's diagnosis, and general health promotion and disease prevention.

Tertiary Prevention

Ambulatory Health Care

Clinic nurses often give their clients information about community resources. Parents of children with a chronic disease, for instance, may receive a list of organizations that provide emotional support, respite care, and information and referral. Clients with chronic conditions benefit from teaching that is directed at successful rehabilitation and prevention of related complications. Physical care in the clinic may include changing a dressing, wrapping a sprained ankle, and giving an intravenous infusion.

Through the schools, parents can learn about community services available for children with chronic conditions. In some states, children with disabilities are mainstreamed into the public schools. These children and their families need tertiary prevention education. In all states, children with less severe chronic conditions attend school and benefit from health care instructions.

Some schools provide a significant amount of physical caregiving through school-based clinics. Services may include physical examinations, routine screenings, venipuncture for laboratory studies, family planning, and even prenatal care. Nurses may also provide direct nursing care to some children on an ongoing basis (e.g., children who use a mechanical ventilator or children with conditions that result in frequent urinary catheterization). The school nurse also dispenses prescription medications and provides first aid in emergencies.

In the occupational setting, physical care is primarily first aid. The nurse may tell personnel with chronic conditions or recent acute conditions about the opportunities and advantages of returning to work. Return-to-work programs assist personnel with chronic injuries or illnesses and illustrate the tertiary prevention approach of maximizing individual potential for health through teaching.

Home Health Care

A primary role of home health care nurses is to provide health instruction to clients and family members. Because home health care clients usually have a chronic condition, only episodic care is generally needed, and most teaching is directed toward tertiary prevention. Teaching may focus on rehabilitation or restoration for those with a recent stroke, head injury, fractured hip, diagnosis of a chronic condition, or surgery.

Physical care provided in the home is usually at the tertiary level of prevention. To qualify for payment for services, most home health care nursing includes a physical care component, such as completing dressing changes, while teaching and implementing good infection control techniques with the client and the family.

Although in home care the client is the main focus of care, a holistic nursing style means that nurses also provide care for family and other support persons. Chapter 13 covers this topic in more detail.

TABLE 2-3	Three Levels of Public Health Practice	
Levels	**Definition**	
Population-based	Public health interventions are population-based if they consider all levels of practice. This concept is represented by the three inner rings of the Intervention Wheel. The inner rings of the model are labeled community-focused, systems-focused, and individual/family-focused. A population-based approach considers intervening at all possible levels of practice. Interventions may be directed at the entire population within a community, the systems that affect the health of those populations, and/or the individuals and families within those populations known to be at risk.	
Community-focused practice	Changes community norms, community attitudes, community awareness, community practices, and community behaviors. They are directed toward entire populations within the community or occasionally toward target groups within those populations. Community-focused practice is measured in terms of what proportion of the population actually changes.	
Systems-focused practice	Changes organizations, policies, laws, and power structures. The focus is not directly on individuals and communities but on the systems that impact health. Changing systems is often a more effective and long-lasting way to impact population health than requiring change from every single individual in a community.	
Individual-focused practice	Changes knowledge, attitudes, beliefs, practices, and behaviors of individuals. This practice level is directed at individuals, alone or as part of a family, class, or group. Individuals receive services because they are identified as belonging to a population at risk.	

Minnesota Department of Health. Division of Community Health Services: Public Health Nursing Section. (2001). Public health nursing interventions: Application to public health nursing practice. Minneapolis, Minnesota: Author. Used with permission.

NURSING INTERVENTIONS IN COMMUNITY-BASED SETTINGS

The differences between the philosophy of acute care nursing and community-based nursing have been discussed. These necessitate nursing interventions that are consistent with the philosophy of community-based care. Community-based care incorporates three levels of practice. Public health interventions are population-based at all levels of practice. Table 2-3 describes the three levels of population-based practice. The interface between the levels of practice and the levels of prevention are shown in Table 2-4. The Intervention Wheel is a practice model that encompasses three levels of practice and 17 community nursing interventions for use in community settings (Fig. 2-4). Interventions are defined as what the nurse can do at the individual, family, and community level. All 17 interventions and definitions are found in Table 2-5. These will be discussed in greater depth in Units II and III.

TABLE 2-4	Community-Based Nursing at Three Levels of Prevention for Individuals, Families, Groups, and Communities		
	Levels of Prevention		
Client Served	**Primary**	**Secondary**	**Tertiary**
Individual client	Sexuality; teaching about using condoms	Counseling and HIV testing	Nutrition teaching to the client with AIDS to maximize health
	Family planning	Early prenatal care	Support groups for parents of low-birth-weight infants
	Dietary teaching and exercise programs to assist clients with obesity	Screening for early identification of diabetes	Teaching to a newly diagnosed diabetic about diet and how to administer insulin
Family	Education about infection control in the home of a family member on a ventilator there	Tuberculosis screening for a family at risk	Teaching to a family caregiver about how to follow sterile procedure for a dressing change
Systems	Prenatal classes for pregnant adolescents	Vision screening for first graders	Support groups for children with asthma
	Sexuality teaching about AIDS and other STDs	Hearing screening at a senior center	Swim therapy for physically disabled
Communities	Fluoride water supplementation	Organized screening programs such as health fairs	Shelter or relocation provision for victims of natural disasters
	Environmental cleanup of paint and other substances containing lead	Lead screening of children in a community	Development of programs to assist children with developmental delays caused by lead exposure

TABLE 2-5	Public Health Interventions With Definitions
Public Health Intervention	**Definition**
Surveillance	Describes and monitors health events through ongoing and systematic collection, analysis, and interpretation of health data for the purpose of planning, implementing, and evaluating public health interventions. [Adapted from MMWR, 1988]
Disease and other health event investigation	Systematically gathers and analyzes data regarding threats to the health of populations, ascertains the source of the threat, identifies cases and others at risk, and determines control measures.
Outreach	Locates populations-of-interest or populations-at-risk and provides information about the nature of the concern, what can be done about it, and how services can be obtained.
Screening	Identifies individuals with unrecognized health risk factors or asymptomatic disease conditions in populations.
Case-finding	Locates individuals and families with identified risk factors and connects them with resources.
Referral and follow-up	Assists individuals, families, groups, organizations, and/or communities to identify and access necessary resources in to prevent or resolve problems or concerns.
Case management	Optimizes self-care capabilities of individuals and families and the capacity of systems and communities to coordinate and provide services.
Delegated functions	Direct care tasks a registered professional nurse carries out under the authority of a health care practitioner as allowed by law. Delegated functions also include any direct care tasks a registered professional nurse entrusts to other appropriate personnel to perform.
Health teaching	Communicates facts, ideas and skills that change knowledge, attitudes, values, beliefs, behaviors, and practices of individuals, families, systems, and/or communities.
Counseling	Establishes an interpersonal relationship with a community, a system, family or individual intended to increase or enhance their capacity for self-care and coping. Counseling engages the community, a system, family or individual at an emotional level.
Consultation	Seeks information and generates optional solutions to perceived problems or issues through interactive problem solving with a community, system, family or individual. The community, system, family or individual selects and acts on the option best meeting the circumstances.
Collaboration	Commits two or more persons or organizations to achieve a common goal through enhancing the capacity of one or more of the members to promote and protect health. [Adapted from Henneman, L., and Cohen (1995). Collaboration: A concept analysis. *Journal of Advanced Nursing* (*21*)103–109.]
Coalition building	Promotes and develops alliances among organizations or constituencies for a common purpose. It builds linkages, solves problems, and/or enhances local leadership to address health concerns.
Community organizing	Helps community groups to identify common problems or goals, mobilize resources, and develop and implement strategies for reaching the goals they collectively have set. [Adapted from Minkler, M. (Ed.) (1997). *Community organizing and community building for health.* New Brunswick, NJ: Rutgers University Press.]

TABLE 2-5 Public Health Interventions with Definitions (*Continued*)	
Public Health Intervention	**Definition**
Advocacy	Pleads someone's cause or act on someone's behalf, with a focus on developing the community, system, individual or family's capacity to plead their own cause or act on their own behalf.
Social marketing	Utilizes commercial marketing principles and technologies for programs designed to influence the knowledge, attitudes, values, beliefs, behaviors, and practices of the population-of-interest.
Policy development	Places health issues on decision-makers' agendas, acquires a plan of resolution, and determines needed resources. Policy development results in laws, rules and regulation, ordinances, and policies.
Policy enforcement	Compels others to comply with the laws, rules, regulations, ordinances and policies created in conjunction with policy development.

Minnesota Department of Health, Public Health Nursing Section (2001). *Public health nursing interventions: Application for public health nursing practice.* Minneapolis, Minnesota: Author. Used with permission.

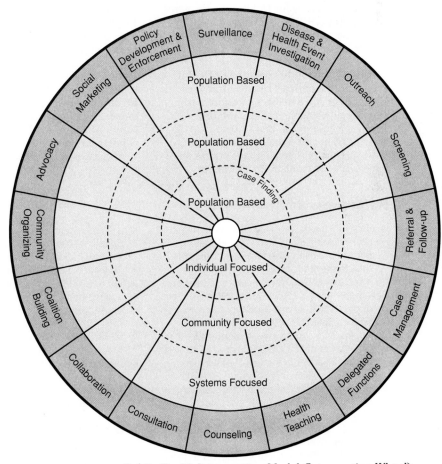

FIGURE 2-4. ▶ Public Health Intervention Model (Intervention Wheel).

CONCLUSIONS

Settings for nursing practice have evolved as a reflection of society's need to focus on health rather than illness. State and local health departments are using Healthy People 2010 as a framework to put disease prevention into action. The prevention focus is a key concept of community-based nursing. Different preventive strategies are found at three levels of prevention. The public health nursing Intervention Wheel and its 17 corresponding nursing interventions are introduced.

What's on the Web

National Guideline Clearinghouse (NGC)
Internet address:
http://www.guideline.gov
The NGC is a comprehensive database of evidence-based clinical practice guidelines and related documents. NGC is an initiative of the Agency for Healthcare Research and Quality (AHRQ), U.S. Department of Health and Human Services. NGC was originally created by AHRQ in partnership with the American Medical Association and the American Association of Health Plans (now America's Health Insurance Plans [AHIP]). The NGC's mission is to provide physicians, nurses, and other health professionals, health care providers, health plans, integrated delivery systems, purchasers, and others an accessible mechanism for obtaining

objective, detailed information on clinical practice guidelines and to further their dissemination, implementation and use.

Consumer Assessment of Health Plans (CAHPS)
Internet address:
https://www.cahps.ahrq.gov/default.asp
This program is a public-private initiative to develop standardized surveys of patients' experiences with ambulatory and facility-level care. Consumers and researchers use CAHPS data to select a health plan through the research on the site that: (1) assesses the patient-centeredness of care; (2) compares and reports on performance; and (3) improves quality of care.

References and Bibliography

Agency for Health Care and Quality Research (2006). Addressing racial and ethnic disparities in health care fact sheet. Rockville, MD. Retrieved June 23, 2006, from http://www.ahrq.gov/research/disparit.htm

Benjamins, M. R. (2005). Social determinants of preventive service utilization. *Research on Aging, 27*(4), 475–497.

Benjamins, M. R., Kirby, J. B., & Bond Huie, S. A. (2004). County characteristics and racial and ethnic disparities in the use of preventive services. *Preventive Medicine, 39,* 704–712.

Centers for Disease Control and Prevention. (2006). Chronic disease prevention: Chronic disease overview. Retrieved on June 24, 2006, from http://www.cdc.gov/nccdphp/overview.htm

Coffield, A. (2006). Preventive services a good investment for health. *The Nation's Health, 36*(6), 2.

Federal Interagency Forum on Child and Family Statistics. (2006). America's children: Key national indicators of well being, 2006. Washington, DC: U.S. Government Printing Office.

Jemal, A. (2006). Simple precautions protect against many cancers. HealthDay. Retrieved on August 15, 2006, from http://www.medicineonline.com/news/10/9258/Simple-Precautions-Protect-Against-Many-Cancers.html

Kaiser Family Foundation & Harvard School of Public Health. (2005). Washington, DC: Author. (Doc # 7371). Retrieved on June 26, 2006, from www.kff.org

Lasser, K., Himmelstein, K., & Woolhandler, S. (2006). Access to care, health status, and health disparities in the United States and Canada: Results of a cross-national population-based survey. *American Journal of Public Health, 96*(5), 1300–1307.

Minnesota Department of Health. Division of Community Health Services. Public Health Nursing Section. (2001). Public health nursing interventions: Application for public health nursing practice. Minneapolis, Minnesota: Author.

Russo, A., Jiang, J., & Barrett, M. (2007). Trends in Potentially preventable hospitalizations among adults and children, 1997–2004. Statistic Brief #36. Healthcare Cost & Utilization Project. Agency for Healthcare Research and Quality. Retrieved on Octrober 25, 2007, from http://www.hcup-us.ahrq.gov/reports/statbriefs/sb36.pdf

Schackman, B., et al. (2006). The lifetime cost of current human immunodeficiency virus care in the United States. *Medical Care, 44*(11), 990–997. Retrieved on October 26, 2007, from http://www.lww-medicalcare.com/pt/re/medcare/abstract.00005650-200611000-00005.htm; jsessionid=HvzHCGYHGHwyhzY YJSHQ2LMj9b5gG8vt2ZCG15Dk9Q2dCW3 dQLMT!1899110359!181195628!8091!-1

Teutsch, S. (2006). Cost-effectiveness of prevention. *Public Health & Prevention, 4*(2). Retrieved on August 15, 2006, from http:// www.medscape.com/wiewarticle/540199

U.S. Department of Health and Human Services. (2006). Document 13 HIV. Retrieved on September 10, 2007, from http://www.healthypeople.gov/document/html/volume1/13hiv.htm

U.S. Department of Health and Human Services. (2006). Document 14 Immunization and infectious diseases. Retrieved on September 10, 2007, from http://www.healthypeople.gov/document/html/volume1/14immunization.htm

U.S. Department of Health and Human Services. (2006). Fact sheet on health care disparities in rural areas. Retrieved June 24, 2006, from www.ahrq.gov

World Health Organization. (1986). Twelve yardsticks for health. New York: WHO.

World Health Organization. (2006). Country information. Retrieved on June 23, 2006, from www.who.int/countries.

LEARNING ▼ ACTIVITIES

◆ JOURNALING 2-1

1. In your clinical journal, identify issues you have observed in your clinical experiences that relate to health rather than to illness.
2. Discuss how this differs from what you previously thought of as health.
3. How does this observation affect your impression of the role of the nurse in the community?
4. In your clinical journal, identify issues you have observed in your clinical experiences that relate to Healthy People 2010 goals.
5. What can you do as a nurse to affect these health issues?

◆ CLIENT CARE 2-2

1. Levels of prevention determine the primary nursing role(s) and interventions for each of the following clients.
   - **Jack**. Jack is a 43-year-old man with a colostomy. He has evidence of early skin breakdown around the stoma site despite the fact that he has followed the established protocol. The clinic nurse notes the problem at Jack's first visit to the clinic after his surgery. She teaches him about a new product that may interrupt the skin breakdown.
     a. Determine the primary nursing role and intervention.
     b. Identify the level of prevention the nurse is using.
   - **Stephen**. Stephen is a 12-year-old boy with a neurologic condition that requires self-catheterization every 2 hours. He has had three bladder infections in the past 2 months. The school nurse has taught Stephen about the

infectious cycle and the importance of hand washing and has watched Stephen self-catheterize in an attempt to identify the reason for the frequent infections.
 a. Determine the primary nursing role and intervention.
 b. Identify the level of prevention the nurse is using.

◆ PRACTICAL APPLICATION 2-3

You have been asked to start a support and education group for people in your community who have had strokes.

1. Describe how you will decide who in the community should participate in the group.
2. What would be the objectives for the sessions?
3. Discuss how the components of community-based nursing apply to these problems:
 a. Self-care
 b. Preventive care
 c. Care within the context of the community
 d. Continuity of care
 e. Collaborative care
4. Identify levels of prevention on which you will focus. Determine if there are levels you will not include.
5. State two likely basic or physical needs at each level of prevention.
6. List two behavioral outcomes and nursing interventions for the basic or physical needs you have chosen.
7. State two likely psychosocial needs at each level of prevention.
8. List two client outcomes and nursing interventions for the psychosocial needs at each level of prevention.

◆ PRACTICAL APPLICATION 2-4

1. You work in an emergency department. An older woman and her husband enter. The woman is loud and combative, and her blood alcohol level is elevated.
 a. Identify the level of prevention on which you will focus.
 b. Determine if any level of prevention will not be included at all.
 c. List the reasons for focusing on tertiary prevention in home health care.

◆ PRACTICAL APPLICATION 2-5

Read the following examples and identify the nursing intervention from the definitions of the public health nursing interventions on pages 46-47.

1. Parents of premature infants participate in a program that identifies children from birth to 5 years of age who are at risk for developing health or developmental issues. At discharge the child is assessed and the parents are asked if they are interested in participating in the program. Every 4 months for the first 2 years and every 6 months after 2 years of age, the parents are asked to complete a mailed questionnaire about the child's development and are contacted if any delays are noted.
2. Every 6 months, nursing students and their instructor administer the DDSTII to children at a preschool for homeless families. Students discuss the results of the screening with parents. Children found to have delays are referred to programs for early intervention.

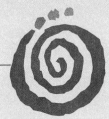

CHAPTER 3

Cultural Care

PAULA SWIGGUM
AND ROBERTA HUNT

LEARNING OBJECTIVES

1. Define culture, cultural care, transcultural nursing, ethnocentrism, cultural blindness, acculturation, assimilation, lifeways, and emic and etic care.
2. Describe the history of transcultural care in nursing.
3. Describe how culture influences worldview, communication, time orientation, family, society, and health.
4. Describe the components of a cultural assessment.
5. Discuss transcultural nursing skills and competencies in community settings.
6. Describe the nursing role as advocate for those clients from diverse cultures.
7. Identify transcultural nursing resources.

KEY TERMS

acculturation
assimilation
cultural awareness
cultural blindness
cultural encounter
cultural knowledge
cultural skill

culturologic assessment
emic care
ethnocentrism
etic care
lifeways
transcultural nursing

CHAPTER TOPICS

◆ Historical Perspectives
◆ Cultural Awareness
◆ Cultural Knowledge
◆ Cultural Skill
◆ Cultural Encounter
◆ Conclusions

THE NURSING STUDENT SPEAKS

Although I had been having experiences with those from other cultures all of my life, my first true immersion into the lives of another culture occurred when I volunteered to help children who had recently come to America from Somalia. I became involved with helping them to both read and speak better English, as well as how to count money and tell time. Most importantly, we were just friends trying to help them assimilate into a culture so very different from their own.

Before my first day "on the job" I went through my text and reviewed the Somali culture, trying to increase my knowledge so that I would know just how to act. The more I thought about it, the more nervous I became. How was I going to remember everything? How was I going to communicate with a child who looks and speaks so differently from myself?

In nursing class you learn so many things, but it was through this experience that I learned perhaps my most important lesson. Although not as profound as Einstein's theory of relativity, it is a lesson that I hold close to my heart. In watching these children play, it occurred to me how similar we all are. Many times we get so focused on the differences that lie between us, that we forget that we are all human, with many of the same basic needs. Sometimes we just have different means to our ends. We all need to be loved, nurtured, and cared for; we all desire and strive to achieve that sense of wellness, wholeness, and belonging. It is in keeping these principles close to heart that I have been able to provide the best cross-cultural care to all of my clients. Respecting our differences and embracing our similarities are what's important.

—STEPHANIE LARSON, **Nursing Student, Gustavus Adolphus College**

The increasing diversity of people in the United States is becoming more evident each day. One needs only to walk the streets of urban areas and farming communities to notice the changing face of America. Recent immigrants have come from the far reaches of the world, primarily Southeast Asia, East Africa, and Latin American countries. It is predicted that by 2050 the number of Hispanics and Asians will triple and non-Hispanic Whites will comprise 50.1% of the population, down from 69.4% in the 2000 census (U.S. Census Bureau, 2004). New groups bring with them a variety of languages, customs, modes of dress, and other cultural practices. Nurses in the 21st century are challenged to provide care to persons whose customs are unfamiliar. Because culture influences health and well-being in a myriad of ways, the professional nurse must understand what that means for each client encountered.

Nurses have always been concerned with the whole person, their physical, emotional, psychological, spiritual, social, and developmental dimensions. With the increasing numbers of immigrants coming to the United States, especially in the last 30 years, the new challenge is to understand the cultural dimension. Culture incorporates not only customs, but also beliefs, values, and attitudes shared by a group of people and passed down through generations.

Healthy People 2010 (U.S. Department of Health and Human Services [DHHS], 2000) calls for the elimination of disparity among groups in access to quality health care services and an increase in community-based programs that are culturally and linguistically appropriate. It states, "The U.S. population is composed of many diverse groups. Evidence indicates a persistent disparity in the health status of racially and culturally diverse populations as compared with the health status of the overall U.S. population." Information about the disparity of health outcomes for minority groups is essential for nurses who plan and carry out nursing interventions in community settings. For example, the infant mortality rate among Alaskan Natives, Native Americans, and African Americans is double that of Whites. The death rate for heart disease is 40% higher for African Americans than for Whites. The knowledge of these and other disparities noted in Healthy People 2010 can lead community-based nurses to learn about diverse cultural factors that must be taken into account to improve health status within cultural groups (Leininger & McFarland, 2006). Transcultural nursing knowledge is essential to attain the goals of understanding and improving health, as outlined in the document.

This chapter will discuss transcultural nursing and its historical beginnings. In addition, key concepts will be explored related to cultural care, cultural awareness, and culturally appropriate nursing competencies involving assessment and intervention. Because there is such a multitude of cultural groups and practices, nurses cannot have knowledge of each and every one. Therefore, a culturally sensitive approach will be discussed, one that incorporates how to discover important cultural beliefs affecting health and wellness and the available resources.

HISTORICAL PERSPECTIVES

Discussions of cultural competence in nursing are not new. In fact, the field of transcultural nursing had its roots in the early 1900s, when public health nurses cared for immigrants from Europe who came from a wide range of cultural backgrounds and had diverse health care practices. Since the late 1940s Madeleine Leininger has been a nurse pioneer in establishing the theory and research in transcultural nursing. Leininger believes that care is the essence of nursing or what makes nursing what it is or could be in healing, wellbeing, and to help people face disabilities and dying (Leininger & McFarland, 2006, p. 3). Over the last five decades she has seen the importance of nursing care that is based on the client's culture, that is, their unique values, beliefs, practices, and **lifeways** passed down from one generation to the next. The idea that culture and care are inextricably linked led her to study other cultures, and she became the first nurse to obtain a PhD in anthropology. **Transcultural nursing** (a term coined by Leininger) is a body of knowledge and practice for caring for persons from other cultures.

Since those early days, the theory of cultural care diversity and universality, developed by Dr. Leininger, has generated substantive knowledge for the discipline of nursing. The world has been on a fast track to multiculturalism, and nurses have not had the knowledge to provide care that was culturally appropriate. Having this knowledge is a moral and ethical obligation for nurses as they strive to provide the best care possible to all their clients. Community nurses have been particularly interested in this field because they work directly with individuals and families in their own settings and see the need firsthand.

Although the large groups of immigrants came to America primarily from Europe in the early 1900s, the recent wave of immigrants to the United States has come from all over the world, including Latin America, Asia, Africa, and other areas. Figure 3-1 depicts the country of origin for immigrants from 1850 to 2000.

Percent distribution. For 1960-90, resident population. For 2000, civilian noninstitutional population plus Armed Forces living off post or with their families on post.

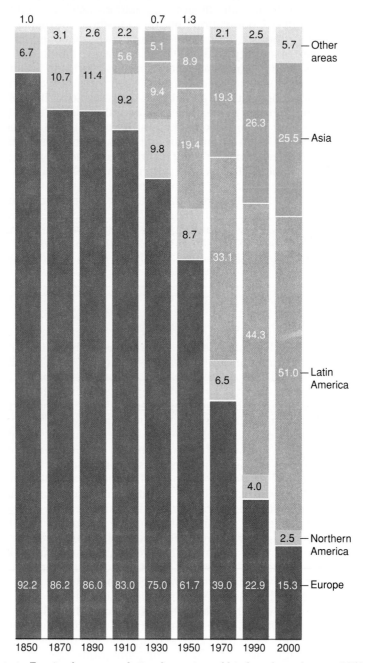

FIGURE 3-1. ▶ Foreign-born population by region of birth: selected years 1850 to 2000. Source: U.S. Census Bureau Web Site.

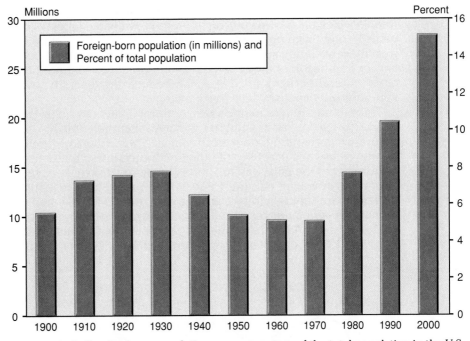

FIGURE 3-2. ▶ Foreign-born population as a percentage of the total population in the U.S. Source: U.S. Census Bureau, Decennial Censuses, 1900 to 1990 and Current Population Survey, March 2000. Retrieved on November 2, 2007, from www.census.gov/population/pop-profile/2000/chap17.pdf

Today, both urban and rural communities have significant numbers of members whose country of origin is not the United States. In addition the percentage of the U.S. population that is foreign-born has increased in the last 30 years (Fig. 3-2). The Native American population has significant numbers who live off the reservation and contribute to the multicultural makeup in cities and towns.

Many nurse leaders and educators have embraced the need for culture-specific care, and various approaches to gaining this knowledge have been developed. Dr. Josepha Campinha-Bacote, a Cape Verde native who now lives and works in the United States, developed one such model. Her model involves the components of cultural awareness, cultural knowledge, cultural skill, and cultural encounter (Campinha-Bacote, 2003). It will be used here as a framework to help nurses learn the concepts necessary to gain cultural competence working within the community setting.

CULTURAL AWARENESS

Before nurses can intervene appropriately with clients from another culture, they must first understand their own, that is, have a self-awareness of their own cultural background, influences, and biases. Only with this **cultural awareness** can they appreciate and be sensitive to the values, beliefs, lifeways, practices, and problem-solving methods of a client's culture.

One exercise that can be illuminating for nurses is to respond to a "cultural tree" in which one's own cultural heritage is evaluated in terms of the various components that make up a culture. Figure 3-3 depicts the components of a cultural tree. By considering specific examples and anecdotes about family traditions and beliefs, one becomes aware of beliefs and practices that are highly influenced by one's cultural background. There can be amazing diversity, even within a group that outwardly appears very much alike.

This new awareness of one's own cultural influences helps the nurse avoid attitudes that can be detrimental to the nurse–client relationship. **Cultural blindness** occurs when the nurse does not recognize his or her own beliefs and practices, nor the beliefs and practices of others. **Ethnocentrism** refers to the idea that one's own ways are the only way or the best way to behave, believe, or do things. For example, a dominant cultural value in the United States is planning for the future. Calendars are kept religiously, goals are set, events are planned weeks and months in advance, and money is saved for retirement. In other cultures, value is placed on the present, and there is a belief that life is preordained, so there is no point in planning or trying to change the future. Future-oriented individuals may feel that

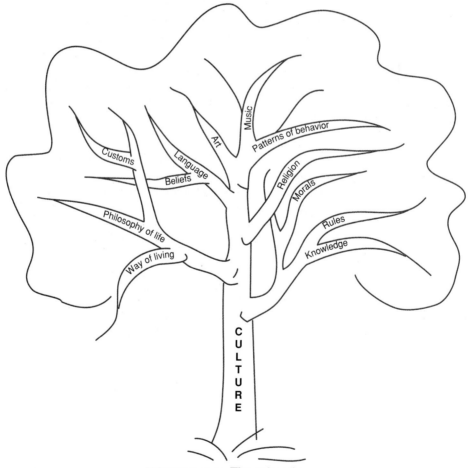

FIGURE 3-3. ▶ The cultural tree.

this is the only correct way to live and may be disdainful of those with another time orientation. This is ethnocentrism.

Another concept in mainstream American culture that is taken for granted as normal is the concept of time. Americans live by the clock, make time, waste time, kill time, want to know what time, and worry about having enough time. In many cultures, one's daily activities take place as the need arises without regard to a prescribed time of day. For members of these cultures, "being on time" for an appointment may have a range of several hours. The community nurse must be aware of these views and accommodate them accordingly.

The reliance on self is another dominant cultural value in the United States. There are more than 100 words in the English language that begin with the word "self." In many languages there is no translation for the word "self." Individual needs are secondary to the needs of the group. This has strong implications for the concept of self-care. Mainstream American culture places high value on taking care of one's self. People are reluctant to have someone do for them what they think they can do for themselves. This is not so for all cultures.

CLIENT SITUATIONS IN PRACTICE

◆ The Meaning of Self-Care

Maria, a Mexican woman, gave birth 2 days ago. For a period of time called "la cuarentena" or "la dieta," specific rules apply regarding the postpartum woman's activity and diet (Andrews & Boyle, 2007). During this time, she is not to do any heavy lifting, exercise, or housework. Family and community members take over the chores of the household, including child care and meal preparation (Fig. 3-4). Jane, a community nurse visiting during this postpartum period, is aware of this cultural practice and provides teaching according to her client's values, which are different than the more active approach to a mother's recovery from childbirth practiced in her own culture.

Because nurses working in the community are frequently visiting postpartum mothers and their newborns, it is essential that they understand how strongly culture influences postpartum self-care and how much that may vary from Western practices.

The way that health decisions are made is culturally based. These decisions are private and individual for some, while others wouldn't think of making a treatment decision without first consulting their extended families.

CLIENT SITUATIONS IN PRACTICE

◆ Client's Right to Know

In the Pakistani culture, the individual's autonomy is secondary to the family's responsibility for health care decisions. Abby is the nurse assigned to a Pakistani woman who has metastatic liver cancer in a home care setting. She would be obligated not to divulge the serious nature of the client's terminal illness. Pakistanis believe that this prevents distress and allows the client to die in peace (Andrews & Boyle, 2007).

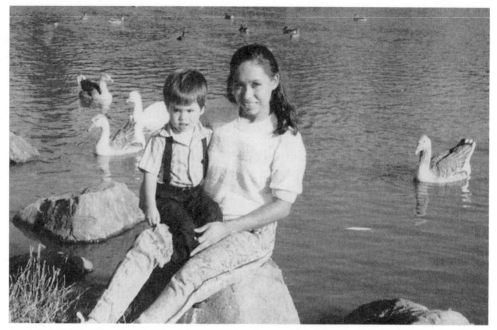

FIGURE 3-4. ▶ Family relationships and child care are strongly influenced by cultural traditions.

Just as cultural norms dictate much of our daily behavior, attitudes, and values, it is not surprising that culture influences the individual's response to pain. Pain is the second most common reason people seek health care and has significant socioeconomic, health, and quality-of-life implications. Racial and ethnic minorities tend to be undertreated for pain when compared to non-Hispanic Whites (Research in Community-Based Nursing Care 3-1).

It is important that nurses develop an understanding of the interaction between culture and the expression of pain (Giger & Davidhizar, 2004). Some people come from backgrounds where stoicism is the norm and pain is not expressed, while others have the view that openly verbalizing pain is expected. It is important for the nurse to be knowledgeable about possible cultural variations and the cultural influences on pain tolerance, expression of pain, and alternative practices used to manage pain. At the same time it is important to consider individual differences and use caution not to make assumptions or have stereotypes about pain expressions (Table 3-1). Strategies for developing culturally appropriate assessment and management of pain are seen in Table 3-2.

CLIENT SITUATIONS IN PRACTICE

◆ Pain Expression

Eva, a community-based nurse, is caring for a Vietnamese client. She knows this culture idealizes stoicism that may suppress the verbalization of pain in disease states where the nurse would expect pain to be expressed. This awareness leads Eva to make a physician referral before her client's disease is in an advanced stage (Lasch, 2000).

RESEARCH IN COMMUNITY-BASED NURSING CARE ▶ 3-1

Research Informs Practice

This study was initiated to provide health care providers, researchers, health care policy analysts, government officials, patients, and the general public with pertinent evidence regarding differences in pain perception, assessment, and treatment for racial and ethnic minorities. A selective literature review was completed by experts in pain management. Racial and ethnic disparities in pain perception, assessment, and treatment were found in all settings for pain in situations with postoperative care, cancer care, and chronic nonmalignant pain. The sources of pain disparities among racial and ethnic minorities were found to be complex, involving patient (e.g., patient/health care provider communication, attitudes), health care provider (e.g., decision making), and health care system (e.g., access to pain medication) factors. The researchers recommended that there is need for improved training for health care providers and educational interventions for patients to address disparities among racial and ethnic minorities.

Source: Green, C. R., Anderson, K. O., Baker, T. A., Campbell, L. C., Decker, S., & Fillingim, R. B., et al. (2003). The unequal burden of pain: Confronting racial and ethnic disparities in pain. *Pain Medicine, 4*(3), 277–294.

In each example, cultural self-awareness is essential to help the nurse recognize and value the right of others to follow their cultural beliefs and practices. Awareness of one's own cultural values opens the nurse's mind to the possibility that the client's values, beliefs, and practices may vary in ways that are very different from his or her own, which can significantly impact the provision of care. The effective nurse will recognize other cultural beliefs and practices as valid and accommodate the client's ways in providing care. The nurse should ask, "How will knowing these things about my client influence my care?"

CULTURAL KNOWLEDGE

Once nurses are more sensitive and aware of their own cultures and biases, they are ready to discover the culture and lifeways of the community within which they work. **Cultural knowledge** encompasses the familiarity of the worldview, beliefs, practices, and problem-solving strategies of groups that are ethnically or culturally diverse (Campinha-Bacote, 2003).

Community-based nursing practice requires that the nurse have cultural knowledge of the community. This knowledge allows the nurse to use a preventive approach and facilitate self-care according to the client's particular culture. Collaboration and continuity are also enhanced when the nurse knows the cultural community in which he or she is working with the client. Having cultural knowledge about the community will influence what is seen, leading to a more thorough and appropriate assessment and intervention.

TABLE 3-1 Pain Expression in Selected Ethnocultural Groups	
Ethnic Group	**Some Common Responses to Pain**
African Americans	Often viewed as a sign of illness or disease Some believe that pain and suffering are inevitable Spiritual and religious beliefs may contribute to high tolerance for pain Some believe that praying and laying on of hands may aid in deliverance from pain and suffering
Arab Americans	Often view pain as unpleasant and something that should be controlled Tend to express pain openly with family members but may act in a more restrained manner in the presence of health professionals May expect positive response from Western medical intervention to control pain
Chinese Americans	Expression of pain typical similar to those of Native Americans Often believe pain is related to the influence of imbalances in yin and yang Usually cope with pain using externally applied oils and massage as well as warmth; sleeping on the area of pain; relaxation; and aspirin
Greek Americans	Pain (*panos*) is viewed by many as an evil that needs to be eradicated Physical and emotional pain are usually shared with the family Family is considered a resource for pain relief because they act as advocates and provide emotional support
Mexican Americans	May delay seeking medical help for pain and hope, instead, that it will go away; consider it a necessary part of life Seem to experience more pain than other ethnic groups but report it less frequently Often see a direct relationship between pain and suffering and immoral behavior
Navajo Indians	May not openly express their pain or request pain medication Adequate pain control is often difficult because they may mask the actual intensity of their pain May prefer herbal medicines and use them without the knowledge of the healthcare provider

Source: Taylor, C., Lillis, C., & LeMone, P. (2006). *Fundamentals of nursing: The art and science of nursing care.* Philadelphia, PA: Lippincott Williams & Wilkins (p. 1204).

Lack of cultural knowledge stands in the way of cultural competence. Nurses can have wonderful intentions and be sensitive and caring, but if there is a lack of specific knowledge about the client's culture, then mistakes are bound to be made.

CLIENT SITUATIONS IN PRACTICE

◆ The Use of Touch

John, a community health nurse, is visiting a family in the Hmong community of St. Paul. As John walks in the door, a young boy is standing there, and John reaches out to touch his head in greeting and as an expression of caring. Lacking cultural knowledge of the Hmong, the nurse is unaware of a strong taboo against touching the head, which is considered the most sacred part of the body, where the brain is, and thinking processes take place. This unintentional affront compromises the nurse's ability to provide care to the family.

TABLE 3-2	Strategies for Developing Culturally Appropriate Assessment and Management of Pain	
Utilize assessment tools to assist in measuring pain	The Brief Pain Inventory has been found to have a high degree of reliability and validity in countries outside the United States for level of pain and impact on functions even when behavioral expressions of pain vary. Some pain-rating scales have been translated into several languages.	
Appreciate variation in affective response to pain	Cultural responses to pain are typically divided into the categories of stoic or emotive.	
Be sensitive to variations in communication styles	Pain assessment and intervention presents a challenging problem not resolved by simple yes or no questions.	
Recognize that communication of pain may not be acceptable within a culture	Some cultural groups view asking for assistance as lack of respect while other cultures see expression of pain as an act of weakness.	
Appreciate that the meaning of pain varies between cultures	Pain is personal, and expression of pain is altered by circumstances and cultural values.	
Utilize knowledge of biological variation	There are significant differences in drug metabolism, dosing requirements, therapeutic responses, and side-effects in racial and ethnic groups.	
Develop personal awareness of values and beliefs that may affect responses to pain	Beliefs, assumptions, and values about pain and about various cultural groups may influence how pain is treated.	

Davidhizar, R., & Giger, J. N. (2004). A review of the literature on care of clients in pain who are culturally diverse. *International Nursing Review, 51*, 47–55.

CLIENT SITUATIONS IN PRACTICE

◆ Postpartum Care

Concesca is a new immigrant to the United States from Guatemala. She takes her 2-week-old infant in for a checkup. As the umbilical cord has dried and is ready to fall off, the physician plucks it away and tosses it into the trash as Concesca looks on in horror. In her culture, the umbilical cord is precious and is saved in a special place by the mother.

The physician wasn't being cruel, but he was ignorant of cultural knowledge related to postpartum practices in Guatemalan culture. A simple question asked by the doctor or nurse such as, "What cultural practices are important to you in the care of your newborn?" would have alleviated the trauma to this young woman.

Generic and Professional Knowledge

Dr. Madeleine Leininger uses the terms "emic" and "etic" to describe types of care (Leininger & McFarland, 2006). **Emic** refers to the local or insider's views and values about a phenomenon. **Etic** refers to the professional or outsider's views and values about a phenomenon. The community-based nurse uses both these types of care knowledge and verifies with the client and family those areas that are meaningful and acceptable to them. Discovering how generic (emic) and professional (etic) systems are alike or different assists the nurse in providing culturally congruent care to individuals or groups.

In Mexican–American culture, there are several levels of healers within the *curanderismo* folklore system. At one level is a *curandero*, or folk healer, who is believed to have God-given gifts of healing. This folk healer may treat those with a wide range of physical and psychological problems, ranging from back pain and gastrointestinal distress to irritability or fatigue. After a diagnosis is made, the *curandero* may use treatments such as massage, diet, rest, indigenous herbs, prayers, magic, or supernatural rituals (Andrews & Boyle, 2007). The nurse working in a Mexican–American community should know about the levels of folk healers used by her clients and inquire as to the consultation and treatment already rendered.

Using this emic understanding of the client's beliefs about health issues, the community nurse can coordinate that care with professional (etic) care that would be acceptable to the client. If massage or a specific diet treatment has been successful, then those interventions can be incorporated into a plan of care. When cultural practices are acknowledged and respected by the professional nurse, clients are more willing to incorporate Western medicine that may augment and enhance the response to treatment.

Components of Cultural Assessment

Six phenomena related to a cultural assessment are discussed in this section (Assessment Tools 3-1).

Communication

Because the community-based nurse spends much of his or her time teaching and communicating roles, knowledge of communication styles and meanings is essential. Verbal and nonverbal behavior, space between persons talking, family member roles, eye contact, salutations, and intergender communication patterns vary significantly among cultures. For example, lack of eye contact to Western cultures is seen as impolite and may indicate indifference or no interest. In Native American and Southeast Asian cultures, on the other hand, lack of eye contact is a gesture of respect. In conversations, European Americans tend to answer quickly, often before the person speaking has finished; however, Native Americans use silence before answering to carefully absorb what the other has said and to formulate their own response. A nurse working within this community must be aware of this and allow time for these interactions.

In many Eastern cultures, agreeing by nodding or saying "yes" is considered polite, whether or not the individual really agrees or understands what has been asked. To a Hmong person, saying, "yes" to a medical explanation may simply mean that the person is politely listening, not that they have agreed to or even understood what was said. The Hmong appear passively obedient to protect their own dignity by not appearing ignorant and also to protect the doctor's dignity by acting deferential (Fadiman, 1997).

ASSESSMENT TOOLS 3-1

Six Phenomena of Cultural Assessment

- *Communication*. A continuous process by which one person may affect another through written or oral language, gestures, facial expressions, body language, space, or other symbols.
- *Space*. The area around a person's body that includes the individual, body, surrounding environment, and objects within that environment.
- *Social organization*. The family and other groups within a society that dictate culturally accepted role behaviors of different members of the society and rules for behavior. Behaviors are prescribed for significant life events, such as birth, death, childbearing, child rearing, and illness.
- *Time*. The meaning and influence of time from a cultural perspective. Time orientation refers to an individual's focus on the past, the present, or the future. Most cultures combine all three time orientations, but one orientation is more likely to dominate.
- *Environmental control*. The ability or perceived ability of an individual or persons from a particular cultural group to plan activities that control nature, such as illness causation and treatment.
- *Biologic variations*. The biologic differences among racial and ethnic groups. It can include physical characteristics, such as skin color, physiologic variations, such as lactose intolerance, or susceptibility to specific disease processes.

Giger, J. N., & Davidhizar, R. E. (1991). *Transcultural nursing: Assessment and intervention.* St. Louis. Mosby–Year Book.

CLIENT SITUATIONS IN PRACTICE

◆ Client Teaching

Nicole is a nurse teaching about medication regimens and wound care in a community setting. Being familiar with the cultural beliefs of her clients, she uses other means of ensuring understanding rather than simply asking, "Do you understand?" She expects return demonstrations or verbal explanations back to her, helping to ensure that her teaching is effective. For example, Nicole may say, "To be sure that your mother will get her medication in the best way to help her, tell me the times you will give her this pill." Or she may say, "Give me some examples of the kinds of foods that you can prepare for your father so that he will minimize the amount of grease in his diet." A respectful and caring approach is a universal dimension of care.

Space and Physical Contact

The concept of space is another important dimension of cultural knowledge. How close people stand by each other in conversation, overt expressions of affection or caring with touch, and rules relating to personal space and privacy vary greatly among cultures. For example, in Italian and Mexican cultures, physical presence and touching is valued and expected. Family members of both genders embrace, kiss, and link arms when walking. In Middle Eastern cultures, close face-to-face conversations where one can almost feel the breath of the other person is the norm, whereas in the United States, the normal space for conversation between persons is an arm's length. In Muslim cultures, it is inappropriate for males and females to even shake hands before marriage. It would be highly improper and distressing for a female Somalian client to be assessed by a male nurse.

CLIENT SITUATIONS IN PRACTICE

◆ Physical Contact

An Iranian child of the Muslim faith is brought in to the local clinic by his parents. The office nurse refrains from shaking hands with the child's father when greeting him. This ensures a feeling of being respected for the father, and a trusting relationship is fostered.

The professional nurse learns about these cultural traditions and beliefs by reading, observing, and asking questions. When in doubt, it is always appropriate to ask, "In your culture, what is considered proper relating to touching and physical space?"

Time

The Western orientation to time and its value was discussed previously. Because the concept of time has such different meanings in various cultures, it is important for the nurse to know of this dimension within the cultural group receiving care. Implications for making appointments, follow-up care, and proper medication administration need to be considered. For example, a physician may prescribe a medication to be taken three times a day with meals. Three meals a day is the norm for most Americans, but this is not so in all other cultures. The nurse should find out when the family has a meal and how much time there is between meals to determine how to explain the regimen within this client's normal patterns of eating.

When scheduling a home visit, 2:00 PM is an exact time to a nurse accustomed to Western orientation to time, but it may mean "sometime in the afternoon" to a person who doesn't share that value of exactness to clock time. Clarifying with the client and family what is meant by a designation of an appointment time saves frustration for both parties.

Another aspect of time is that of past, present, or future orientation. As described already, traditional American culture is future-oriented. Calendars and plans for the future are a part of everyday American life. In contrast, Native-American cultures tend to be past oriented, with a focus on ancestors and traditions. African-American culture tends to focus on the present, with an emphasis on "now" and day-to-day activities. Persons without a future orientation need a different approach when discussing preventive care. The nurse may involve the client by saying, "Because of the strong tendency toward developing diabetes that exists in your family, in what ways can we work together to help you avoid this disease in the future?"

Social Organization

The community-based nurse must understand the family patterns of the groups within the community being served. The family is the basic unit of society. Cultural values can determine communication within the family group, the norm for family size, and the roles of specific family members (Taylor, Lillis, & LeMone, 2006). Nurses should consider, learn about, and assess for these things:

◆ What is the definition of family in this cultural group; does it include primarily the nuclear family, or is the extended family considered the basic unit?
◆ Are there gender or age roles that affect the choice of whom the nurse should address when entering the home or in consultation about a client's health?
◆ What are the traditional roles within the family that affect caregiving?
◆ What value is placed on children and the elderly, and how does that affect health care decision making within the family?
◆ What is the status of females within the culture, and how does that affect the acceptability of a health care provider?
◆ What is the expected family involvement in health care decisions, and who is the primary decision maker within the family?
◆ How is information regarding the health of a family member shared with others in the community?
◆ What role does religion play in health care practices and decision making within the culture and the family unit?

Biologic Variations

To perform a thorough assessment and provide culturally congruent care, the community-based nurse who knows biologic variations specific to his or her clients will be most effective. Although some biologic variations are obvious (e.g., skin color, hair texture, facial features, stature, and body markings), others require knowledge based on medical information and research. For example, Africans and African-American persons have a much higher incidence of sickle cell disease than other groups. Much of the world's population (many Asians, Africans, Hispanics, and Native Americans) is lactose intolerant, or unable to digest milk sugars. To provide health teaching related to a diet that includes milk and milk products to people in these groups is ethnocentric. Native Americans have a high incidence of diabetes mellitus. Health assessment by community-based nurses working with this population should include screening for high blood-sugar levels and culturally appropriate preventative teaching.

The action, absorption, excretion, and dose parameters of many pharmacologic agents also vary among ethnic groups. Genetic differences, structural variation in binding receptor sites, and environmental conditions may affect the drug action in different groups of people. Blood pressure medications, analgesics, and psychotropic drug doses may be significantly different depending on the ethnic group requiring the medication (Andrews & Boyle, 2007). Adult doses for many medications are not determined by weight as for pediatric doses; instead, body mass should be considered for groups of small stature, such as people of Japanese and Korean descent. The nurse should also ask about herbal remedies that the client might be taking that could affect the action or metabolism of certain medications. Table 3-3 lists some common diseases and their effect on different populations.

TABLE 3-3	Biocultural Aspects of Disease
Disease	**Remarks**
Alcoholism	Native Americans have double the rate of Whites; lower tolerance to alcohol among Chinese and Japanese Americans
Anemia	High incidence among Vietnamese due to presence of infestations among immigrants and low-iron diets; low hemoglobin and malnutrition found among 18.2% of Native Americans, 32.7% of Blacks, 14.6% of Hispanics, and 10.4% of White children under 5 years of age
Arthritis	Increased incidence among Native Americans Blackfoot 1.4% Pima 1.8% Chippewa 6.8%
Asthma	Six times greater for Native American infants < 1 year; same as general population for Native Americans ages 1–44 years
Bronchitis	Six times greater for Native American infants < 1 year; same as general population for Native Americans ages 1–44 years
Cancer	Nasopharyngeal: High among Chinese Americans and Native Americans Breast: Black women 1 1/2 times more likely than White Esophageal: No. 2 cause of death for Black males ages 35–54 years *Incidence:* White males 3.5/100,000 Black males 13.3/100,000 Liver: Highest among all ethnic groups are Filipino Hawaiians Stomach: Black males twice as likely as White males; low among Filipinos Cervical: 120% higher in Black females than in White females Uterine: 53% lower in Black females than White females Prostate: Black males have highest incidence of all groups Most prevalent cancer among Native Americans: biliary, nasopharyngeal, testicular, cervical, renal, and thyroid (females) cancer Lung cancer among Navajo uranium miners 85 times higher than among White miners Most prevalent cancer among Japanese Americans: esophageal, stomach, liver, and biliary cancer Among Chinese Americans, there is a higher incidence of nasopharyngeal and liver cancer than among the general population
Cholecystitis	*Incidence:* Whites 0.3% Puerto Ricans 2.1% Native Americans 2.2% Chinese 2.6%
Colitis	High incidence among Japanese Americans
Diabetes mellitus	Three times as prevalent among Filipino Americans as Whites; higher among Hispanics than Blacks or Whites Death rate is 3–4 times as high among Native Americans ages 25–34 years, especially those in the West such as Utes, Pimas, and Papagos *Complications:* Amputations: Twice as high among Native Americans versus general U.S. population Renal failure: 20 times as high as general U.S. population, with tribal variation (e.g., Utes have a 43-times higher incidence)
G6PD	Present among 30% of Black males

TABLE 3-3 Biocultural Aspects of Disease *(Continued)*	
Disease	**Remarks**
Influenza	Increased death rate among Native Americans ages 45+
Ischemic heart disease	Responsible for 32% of heart-related causes of death among Native Americans; Blacks have higher mortality rates than all other groups
Lactose intolerance	Present among 66% of Hispanic women; increased incidence among Blacks and Chinese
Myocardial infarction	Leading cause of heart disease in Native Americans, accounting for 43% of death from heart disease; low incidence among Japanese Americans
Otitis media	7.9% incidence among school-age Navajo children versus 0.5% in Whites; up to ⅓ of Eskimo children <2 years; increased incidence among bottle-fed Native Americans and Eskimo infants
Pneumonia	Increased death rate among Native Americans ages 45 +
Psoriasis	Affects 2–5% of Whites, but <1% of Blacks; high among Japanese Americans
Renal disease	Lower incidence among Japanese Americans
Sickle cell anemia	Increased incidence among Blacks
Trachoma	Increased incidence among Native Americans and Eskimo children (3–8 times greater than general population)
Tuberculosis	Increased incidence among Native Americans Apache 2.0% Sioux 3.2% Navajo 4.6%
Ulcers	Decreased incidence among Japanese Americans

Based on data reported in Overfield, T. (1995). *Biologic variation in health and illness: Race, age, and sex differences.* New York: CRC Press; Office of Minority Health. (1995). *Cancer in minority communities. Closing the gap.* Washington, DC: U.S. Government Printing Office; and Andrews, M., & Boyle J. (1999). *Transcultural concepts in nursing care* (pp. 46–47). Philadelphia: Lippincott Williams & Wilkins.

Environmental Control

There are three predominant views on the relationship between the environment and health: magicoreligious, biomedical, and humoral. The magicoreligious view sees illness as having a supernatural force; that is, malevolent or evil spirits cause disease, or illness is a punishment from God. People from Hispanic and Caribbean cultures may have this health belief system. Because the belief is that a supernatural influence (rather than organic) caused the health problem, people with this perspective will look for a supernatural counterforce to rid them of the problem. People with this belief will seek a voodoo priestess or spiritualist who has the powers to remove "spells" from a variety of sources. Although Western medicine has classified voodoo illness as a psychiatric disorder, nurses who practice cultural care will understand this view of illness and intervene accordingly.

In the biomedical view, disease and illness are believed to be caused by microorganisms or a malfunction of the body. People with this health view look to medicines, medical treatment, or surgery to cure their illness.

The humoral health belief looks for a balance or harmony with nature. Many Eastern cultures ascribe to the theory of yin and yang being opposite forces that must be kept in balance. Imbalance results in illness or disease. The hot and cold theory of many Latino and Asian cultures is similar. The treatment of disease becomes the process of restoring the body's humoral balance through the addition or subtraction of substances that affect each of these humors. The healthy body is characterized by evenly distributed warmth and that illness results when the body is attacked by an increase of either hot or cold (Andrews & Boyle, 2007).

CLIENT SITUATIONS IN PRACTICE

◆ Humoral Health Theory

To the Chinese, childbirth is seen as an experience in which the body loses heat balance that must be restored. Mrs. Yiu, a postpartum Chinese woman, will refuse ice water and will accept only foods that are seen as "warm," such as chicken and rice. Bathing would contribute to the loss of body warmth and would be refused for a period of time after childbirth. The nurse visiting this client in a community setting would be sensitive to these practices and provide care accordingly.

Many variations exist among cultural groups as to how health care is managed and decisions are made. It is important to also keep in mind that individual families may have their own roles, beliefs, and practices that differ from the larger cultural group. This may reflect the degree to which the family has been acculturated to Western cultural patterns and beliefs, or it may be a regional or familial variation. Professional nurses who desire to provide effective care that is culturally congruent to the beliefs of the client are aware of the potential for variations and know what questions to ask. While it is helpful to have a holding knowledge (i.e., knowledge of a group learned from transcultural nursing texts, literature, and previous encounters) of cultural groups, the nurse must always verify with each client which beliefs and practices are personally relevant to him or her. In this way, cultural sensitivity and respect are conveyed even when the nurse is not well versed in the lifeways of a particular group.

Acculturation and Assimilation
Two other concepts are important for nurses to keep in mind as they learn about the culture of particular groups. Individuals within a group may adhere to the traditional culture to varying degrees; this variation may result from acculturation or assimilation.

As new groups enter a different society, **acculturation** may occur as they learn the ways to exist in a new culture. This may include learning to drive, going to school, negotiating public transportation, getting a job, and interacting in an environment unlike that of the home country. As these activities become more comfortable, individuals become more acculturated to the dominant society, yet they may retain much of their own cultural traditions within their communities. For example, a young Somalian girl may continue to wear her traditional Muslim attire (*hijab*) and retain the tradition of gender roles while going to an American high school and getting a job at a fast-food restaurant on weekends.

Assimilation takes place when individuals or groups identify more strongly with the dominant culture in values, activities, and daily living. This usually occurs over longer periods of time, sometimes generations. These assimilations are important for the nurse to keep in mind as there may be a wide variation in how cultural traditions are carried out, even within the same family. The parents may have emigrated from another country, but the children have been raised surrounded by the dominant culture and have, therefore, assimilated more aspects of the dominant culture.

CULTURAL SKILL

Campinha-Bacote describes **cultural skill** as the ability to collect relevant cultural data regarding the client's health history. Up to this point we have discussed the need for nurses to examine their own cultural traditions, beliefs, values, and practices to increase awareness of how influential their culture is on their view of the world and to open their mind to the valid variations in worldviews of varying cultures. This helps to avoid cultural blindness, cultural imposition, and ethnocentrism. It is then the nurse's responsibility to learn as much as possible about the ethnic or cultural groups encountered in the community where the nursing care is being delivered. A holding knowledge of the emic or folk care practices along with the etic or professional care practices gives the community nurse a basis from which to individualize care that is culturally sensitive to the client as an individual or as a family. Practices within cultural groups or families may vary significantly from general descriptions; therefore, knowing the questions to ask for culturally specific care is essential to avoid stereotyping. Having cultural skill is essential to that process.

Leininger defines a **culturologic assessment** as a "systematic identification and documentation of culture care, beliefs, meanings, values, symbols and practices of individuals or groups with a holistic perspective" (Leininger & McFarland, 2002, p. 117). Community-based nurses focus on preventive care. These nurses assess the health risks of a particular group and consider cultural practices and beliefs to plan teaching and activities to prevent disease or health risks (primary prevention). Using culturally based knowledge of generic or folk health care practices in the group, community-based nurses then incorporate their **etic** and **emic care** knowledge to diagnose and treat threats to health and wellness (secondary prevention). Tertiary prevention in the community seeks to rehabilitate or prevent recurrence of health problems. Through a skillful culturologic assessment, the community nurse has listened to the clients' perception of the health problem and compared it to his or her own perception, explaining and acknowledging the similarities and differences. Involving members of the community, the nurse then negotiates a treatment plan that will be seen as beneficial to the community.

Numerous models for culturologic assessment have been developed by various authors in the field of transcultural nursing (Andrews & Boyle, 2007; Giger & Davidhizar, 2004; Leininger & McFarland, 2006). Each organizes assessment data in a different manner, and individual nurses will determine which model works best within their scope of practice and the community served. A cross-cultural assessment tool (Assessment Tools 3-2) can be useful with any client (Kemp, 2005). The questions are open ended and provide the opportunity for the client to describe his or her perception of the health problem. For example, in response to the second question, "How would you describe this problem you have?" The parents of a Hmong child with epilepsy might respond, "The spirit catches you and you fall down" (Fadiman, 1997).

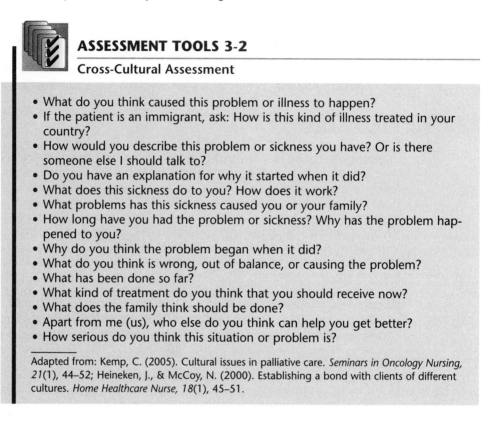

ASSESSMENT TOOLS 3-2

Cross-Cultural Assessment

- What do you think caused this problem or illness to happen?
- If the patient is an immigrant, ask: How is this kind of illness treated in your country?
- How would you describe this problem or sickness you have? Or is there someone else I should talk to?
- Do you have an explanation for why it started when it did?
- What does this sickness do to you? How does it work?
- What problems has this sickness caused you or your family?
- How long have you had the problem or sickness? Why has the problem happened to you?
- Why do you think the problem began when it did?
- What do you think is wrong, out of balance, or causing the problem?
- What has been done so far?
- What kind of treatment do you think that you should receive now?
- What does the family think should be done?
- Apart from me (us), who else do you think can help you get better?
- How serious do you think this situation or problem is?

Adapted from: Kemp, C. (2005). Cultural issues in palliative care. *Seminars in Oncology Nursing, 21*(1), 44–52; Heineken, J., & McCoy, N. (2000). Establishing a bond with clients of different cultures. *Home Healthcare Nurse, 18*(1), 45–51.

The culturologic assessment gives the nurse good information with cultural implications to use as a basis for planning teaching and treatment plans. All clients have a right to have their values, beliefs, and practices considered, respected, and incorporated into the plan of care.

CULTURAL ENCOUNTER

The **cultural encounter** is the opportunity for the nurse to engage in direct contact with the members of cultural communities. Through frequent contact with numerous members of a cultural group, the nurse keeps in mind that variations will exist within the community and stereotypical expectations are to be avoided. Trust builds over time between the caregiving nurse and members of the community, and it is essential to the well-being of both.

Using knowledge of etic and emic care practices and having completed a culturologic assessment, the nurse now uses the skills and competencies necessary to effect healthful outcomes for the clients in the community. Leininger has identified three modalities that "guide nursing judgments, decisions or actions so as to provide cultural congruent care that is beneficial, satisfying and meaningful to people nurses serve" (Leininger & McFarland, 2006, p. 8). These three modalities are defined in Table 3-4.

TABLE 3-4	Leininger's Guidelines for Providing Culturally Congruent Care
Modality	**Definition**
Cultural care preservation and/or maintenance	Refers to those assistive, supporting, facilitative, or enabling professional actions and decisions that help people of a particular culture to retain and/or preserve relevant care values so that they can maintain their well-being, recover from illness, or face handicaps and/or death
Cultural care accommodation or negotiation	Refers to those assistive, supporting, facilitative, or enabling creative professional actions and decisions that help people of a designated culture (or subculture) adapt to or negotiate with others for a beneficial or satisfying health outcome with professional care providers
Cultural care repatterning or restructuring	Refers to those assistive, supporting, facilitative, or enabling professional actions and decisions that help a client reorder, change, or greatly modify lifeways for new, different, and beneficial health care patterns while respecting the client's cultural values and beliefs and still providing beneficial or healthier lifeways than before the changes were coestablished with the client(s)

Leininger, M. N., & McFarland, M. (2002). *Transcultural concepts, theories, research, practice* (p. 84). New York: McGraw-Hill.

Cultural Care Preservation

The first of the modalities is cultural care preservation and/or maintenance. After careful assessment and observation, the nurse identifies those cultural care practices that are helpful to the client. The nurse then assists, supports, facilitates, or enables the client and family to preserve those actions or behaviors. For example, in the Amish community, the extended family, neighborhood, and church expect to assist and care for members within the community. The nurse working in this community encourages and supports ways to enlist the help of the extended community and facilitates ways to let the care needs be known.

Cultural Care Accommodation

The second mode of cultural care accommodation or negotiation refers to those nursing actions and decisions that assist or enable the client and family to continue with practices that are meaningful to them but may be altered due to circumstances. For example, the nurse in the community may be setting up a referral for a client to be seen in a clinic for follow-up care. The client is Muslim and must adhere to the practice of praying five times a day. The nurse will negotiate with the client as to times of day that would provide enough time between prayers for an appointment or assist in helping the client find a place within or near the clinic where these prayers may be said.

In another example, the community-based nurse is doing a follow-up visit to a Jewish child recently diagnosed with type 1 diabetes. Knowing the Jewish restriction of pork products, the nurse might intervene to ask the physician to prescribe a nonporcine insulin product.

In addition to assisting the client in carrying out his or her religious practices, the respect and care shown by the nurse toward these clients enhances trust and feelings of caring support.

Cultural Care Repatterning

The third way in which nurses make decisions or intervene is cultural care repatterning or restructuring. When the nurse assesses the client, family, and community and finds practices that may be detrimental to health and well-being, he or she will work with the client to change behaviors that are harmful.

CLIENT SITUATIONS IN PRACTICE

◆ Dietary Repatterning

Joan is working within the Navajo community, where members observe the practice of eating bread fried in fat as a staple in the diet. Knowing that this much fat soaked into the bread is detrimental to a community at risk for heart disease, Joan works with the Navajo women to explore ways to decrease the amount of fat in servings of fry bread. Together they may decide that placing the fry bread vertically or on paper towels before serving may decrease the amount of fat as it drips off before eating. Because the nurse works with the client(s) to diminish risks to health, the changes are more likely to take effect.

Box 3-1 presents research that led nurses to provide culturally responsive care using three modes of action in an ambulatory care setting. Note how knowing the culture and learning the emic care can lead to simple but important nursing actions and decisions that will be perceived by the clients as cultural care.

Whether the nurse is validating and supporting helpful existing practices, helping clients to negotiate ways to maintain their health care practices, or working to identify and change harmful behaviors, it is essential that he or she work with the community as a partner. Because optimum health care for all clients is the goal of nursing, these three modes of nursing actions and decisions, in close cooperation with the clients, can be enormously beneficial and satisfying to both the community and the nurse.

◆ BOX 3-1 Research Related to Community-Based Nursing Care ◆

Cultural Care Modalities for the Puerto Rican Client in an Ambulatory Care Setting

The purpose of this study was to examine the cultural beliefs and practices of Puerto Rican families that influence feeding practices and affect the nutritional status of infants and young children. The goal of the study was to outline strategies that would enable nurses to provide culturally congruent care for this population. Resulting cultural care modalities are listed on p. 73.

(continued)

◆ B O X 3-1	Research Related to Community-Based Nursing Care (*Continued*) ◆

Cultural Care Preservation Modalities

Reinforce family caring values of nurturance and succorance.

Respect and understand use of religious symbols and protective care symbols.

Touch the infant or child and say "God bless you" if complimenting the child.

Treat the family with respect, use professional demeanor, maintain eye contact.

Promote continuity of care.

Cultural Care Accommodation Modalities

Use the Spanish language to include the grandmother; reinforce intergenerational caregiving.

Promote *respeto* (respect) and *confianza* (confidence, trust) by accommodation (or deference) to family and community values.

Encourage introduction of traditional, healthy foods—rice, beans, and eggs—at the appropriate time, linking their use with green vegetables and meat.

Encourage the generic folk practice of *Ponche* as needed, with additional health considerations.

Develop a comprehensive bilingual feeding assessment guide to improve anticipatory guidance.

Cultural Care Repatterning Modalities

Include grandmother and kin in a collaborative participatory approach to feeding.

Emphasize the cultural ideology and beliefs. Explain how a new approach will contribute to a big, healthy baby.

Anticipatory guidance about overfeeding formula should begin at 2–4 weeks.

Anticipatory guidance about not adding solids to the bottle should be given at 4–8 weeks before the practice is initiated. Stress the ease of feeding solids by mouth at 4–6 months of age.

Develop Spanish-language pamphlets linking emic and etic feeding practices.

Provide nutrition and cooking demonstration classes with a cultural theme, linking emic and etic foods for mothers, fathers, and grandmothers.

Advertise classes on Spanish-speaking radio and TV stations.

Develop a nutritional outreach program including bilingual Puerto Rican mothers who are interested in nutrition and health.

Higgins, B. (2000). Puerto Rican cultural beliefs: Influence on infant feeding practices in western New York. *Journal of Transcultural Nursing, 11*(1), 19–30.

CLIENT SITUATIONS IN PRACTICE

◆ Planning for a Cultural Encounter

Sarah is a home health care nurse assigned to visit Ahmed and her 2-week-old new-born son. This Somalian family consists of Ahmed, her husband, 3-year-old daughter, and the new baby. The family has been in the United States for 4 months, after spending a year in a refugee camp in Kenya. Both Mohammed and Ahmed were residents of Mogadishu before the civil war and were from middle-class traditional Somalian families. Both speak English, although not fluently. Prenatal history indicates the baby was born by C-section after a reported uneventful pregnancy, notable only for the fact that Ahmed's first prenatal visit with a physician was 1 week prior to the child's birth. She experienced false labor and was brought to the physician's office by her neighbor.

Sarah is preparing to visit Ahmed and her new baby for the first time. What are some considerations she should think about prior to her visit?

Sarah should consider the traditional Somali practice of female circumcision and her own cultural beliefs related to that practice. She cannot assume Ahmed is circumcised or to what degree, but the decision to have a C-section may have been a result of this possibility (although circumcised women can give birth vaginally as well).

Sarah knows that most Somalians are Muslims. Where can she find out some basic beliefs and practices of those who practice Islam?

Sarah can review current literature and transcultural nursing books as well as access information on-line related to Muslim religious practices. She notes that 99% of Somalians are Sunni Muslims. She knows this will be an important question to ask as culture and religion are highly intertwined in Somalia.

What basic cultural practices are important for Sarah to know prior to visiting this Somalian family?

Gender roles are quite specifically defined in traditional Somali culture. Sarah will know that she must not offer to shake hands with Mohammed, as physical contact with a woman other than a close family member is forbidden. She will also know that female modesty is a high priority when assessing Ahmed's incision.

Sarah plans to discuss family planning. What is important for her to know in providing culturally sensitive care?

In the Muslim religion, children are seen as gifts from Allah, and many children are considered a blessing. Preventing conception is not acceptable, but the concept of family "spacing" to preserve the mother's health and provide adequate time for weaning the youngest child is an appropriate approach to take (Turkoski, 2005; Callister, 2002).

As in any cultural encounter, Sarah must proceed slowly, know some basic cultural practices and beliefs she is likely to encounter, verify the degree to which the client is acculturated, and establish a climate of trust using cultural sensitivity and respect.

CONCLUSIONS

All nurses, regardless of their own cultural background, are obligated to learn what is important to their clients. "Health and illness states are strongly influenced and often primarily determined by the cultural background of the individual" (Leininger, 1970, p. 22). Cultural awareness of one's own background, beliefs, values, and practices opens the nurse's mind to value and support the diversity of others. Cultural knowledge learned from books, formal coursework, and discussions with community members gives the nurse a background or framework in which to understand the cultural health care beliefs of a group. This information can then be validated or altered based on individual interactions. Cultural skill is the ability to conduct a culturologic assessment that will guide nursing actions and decisions. In the cultural encounter, the nurse reinforces, negotiates, or assists clients to repattern care practices for optimum health care.

An attitude of sensitivity, acceptance, and sincere desire to work with culturally diverse clients results in continuity and collaborative care and promotes a trusting relationship with the client. Nurses in the community setting must establish a bond based on trust with the home health care client to provide excellent care and do so cost effectively (Heineken & McCoy, 2000). Using knowledge of the generic or emic care practices of the cultural community and integrating these with professional or etic knowledge, the nurse assists in self-care by encouraging existing healthy behaviors and establishing preventive measures that are culturally congruent and acceptable in creating a healthy future for each community served.

What's on the Web

Center for Cross-Cultural Health
Internet address:
http://www.crosshealth.com
The mission of the Center for Cross Cultural Health is *"to integrate the role of culture in improving health."* The vision of this organization is increased health and well-being for all through cross-cultural understanding. To achieve this goal, the Center promotes the education and training of health and human service providers and organizations as well as a research and information resource. Through information sharing, training, organizational assessments, and research the Center works to develop culturally responsive individuals, organizations, systems, and societies.

Center for Healthy Families and Cultural Diversity
Internet address:
http://www2.umdnj.edu/fmedweb/chfcd/index.htm

The Center is dedicated to leadership, advocacy, and excellence in promoting culturally responsive, quality health care for diverse populations. It began as a program focused primarily on multicultural education and training for health professionals, but has grown to an expanded resource for technical assistance, consultation, and research/evaluation services.

Ethnomed
Internet address:
http://www.ethnomed.org
This Web site, through the University of Washington, offers excellent information on a wide range of cultures.

The Provider's Guide to Quality and Culture
Internet address: http://erc.msh.org/mainpage.cfm?file=1.0.htm&module=provider&language=English
This site has content on culture care as well as numerous links to a variety of sites and resources.

National Center for Cultural Competence (NCCC)
Internet address: http://gucchd georgetown.edu/nccc/
The mission of the National Center for Cultural Competence (NCCC) is to increase the capacity of health and mental health programs to design, implement, and evaluate culturally and linguistically responsive service delivery systems.

Transcultural Nursing Society
Internet address: http://www.tcns.org
This is an excellent Web site, with links to other resources, information about membership in the Transcultural Nursing Society, and transcultural nursing workshops, courses, and certifications. The site also provides an on-line index for all articles published in the *Journal of Transcultural Nursing* since 1989.

References and Bibliography

Andrews, M., & Boyle, J. (1999). *Transcultural concepts in nursing care.* Philadelphia: Lippincott Williams & Wilkins.

Andrews, M., & Boyle, J. (2007). *Transcultural concepts in nursing care.* (5th ed.). Philadelphia: Lippincott Williams & Wilkins.

Callister, L. C. (2001). Culturally competent care of women and newborns: Knowledge, attitude and skills. *Journal of Obstetric, Gynecologic and Neonatal Nursing, 30*(2), 9–15.

Callister, L. C. (2002). Toward evidence based practice. Culture care conflicts among Asian-Islamic immigrant women in United States hospitals. *American Journal of Maternal Child Nursing, 27*(3), 194.

Campinha-Bacote, J. (2003). Many faces: Addressing diversity in health care. *Online Journal of Issues in Nursing, 8*(1), 3. Retrieved on July 3, 2006, from http://nursingworld.org/MainMenuCategories/ANAMarketplace/ANAPerodicals/OJIN/TableofContents/Volume82003/Num1Jan31_2003/AddressingDiversityinHealthCare.aspx

Davidhizar, R., & Giger, J. N., (2004). A review of the literature on care of clients in pain who are culturally diverse. *International Nursing Review, 51,*47–55.

Fadiman, A. (1997). *The spirit catches you and you fall down.* New York: Noonday Press.

Giger, J. N., & Davidhizar, R. E. (1991). *Transcultural nursing: Assessment and intervention.* St. Louis: Mosby-Year Book.

Giger, J. N., & Davidhizar, R.E. (2004). *Transcultural nursing: Assessment and intervention* (4th ed.). St. Louis: C.V. Mosby.

Green, C. R., Anderson, K. O., Baker, T., Campbell, L. C., Decker, S., & Fillingim, R. B., et al. (2003). The unequal burden of pain: Confronting racial and ethnic disparities in *pain. Pain Medicine, 4*(3), 277–294.

Heineken, J., & McCoy, N. (2000). Establishing a bond with clients of different cultures. *Home Healthcare Nurse, 18*(1),45–51.

Higgins, B. (2000). Puerto Rican cultural beliefs: Influence on infant feeding practices in western New York. *Journal of Transcultural Nursing, 11*(1), 19–30.

Kemp, C. (2005). Cultural issues in palliative care. *Seminars in Oncology Nursing, 21*(1), 44–52.

Lasch, K. E. (2000). Culture, pain and culturally sensitive pain care. *Pain Management in Nursing, 1*(3)(Suppl. 1), 16–22.

Leininger, M. M. (1970). *Nursing and anthropology: Two worlds to blend.* Columbus, OH: Greyden Press.

Leininger, M. M. (2002). Culture care theory: a major contribution to advance transcultural nursing and practice. *Journal of Transcultural Nursing, 13*(3), 189–192.

Leininger, M. M., & McFarland, M. (2002). *Transcultural nursing concepts, theories, research, practice.* New York: McGraw Hill.

Leininger, M. M., & McFarland, M. (2006). *Culture care diversity and universality: A worldwide nursing theory.* Boston: Jones & Bartlett.

Office of Minority Health. (August 1995). *Cancer in minority communities. Closing the gap.* Washington, D.C.: U.S. Government Printing Office.

Overfield, T. (1995). *Biologic variation in health and illness. Race, age, and sex differences.* New York: CRC Press.

Stewart, E. C. & Bennett, M. J. (1991). *American cultural patterns: In a cross-cultural perspective (revised edition).* Yarmouth, Maine: Intercultural Press.

Taylor, C., Lillis C., & LeMone, P. (2006). *Fundamentals of nursing: The art and science of nursing care.* Philadelphia, PA: Lippincott Williams & Wilkins.

Turkoski, B. B. (2005). Ethical support for culturally sensitive healthcare. *Home Healthcare Nurse, 23*(6), 355–358.

U.S. Census Bureau. (2004). Chronical Graphic. Retrieved on June 29, 2006, from http://sfgate.com/cgi-bin/article.cgi?file=/ chronicle/archive/2004/03/18/ MNGTB5MUOG1.DTL

U.S. Department of Health and Human Services. (2000). Healthy people 2010: National health promotion and disease prevention objectives, full report, with commentary. Washington, DC: U.S. Government Printing Office.

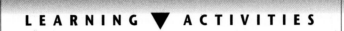

L E A R N I N G ▼ A C T I V I T I E S

◆ JOURNALING ACTIVITY 3-1

1. In your clinical journal, write about either a personal or professional encounter you have had working with someone who you are different from ethnically, racially, or from life experience.
   a. Describe what happened.
   b. What did you learn about yourself and the other person?
   c. Was the other person as similar or as different from you as you expected?
   d. How did this encounter change the way you think about transcultural nursing?
   e. What would you do differently next time?
2. Keep a journal of your nursing encounters with persons from cultures different than your own.
   a. Discuss how prepared you felt in each interaction and what cultural beliefs, values, or lifeways you discovered in each encounter.
   b. How did that knowledge affect the care you provided?

◆ LEARNING ACTIVITY 3-2

Using the cultural tree in Figure 3-3, write the ways in which your family of origin or your cultural background influence each area depicted on a branch. Discuss your findings with another student.

1. In what areas was culture a strong influence?
2. In what areas has acculturation or assimilation influenced your beliefs and preferences compared to what your grandparent may have answered?
3. What similarities and differences did you note in comparing your tree to another student's responses?
4. By participating in this activity, what awareness did you gain that may be helpful to you in caring for clients from other cultures?

◆ LEARNING ACTIVITY 3-3

Make a list of various ethnic and minority or cultural groups (e.g., Native Americans, Asians, the elderly, Latinos, WASPs [White Anglo–Saxon Protestants], Jews) and write a stereotype you have or have heard about each group.

1. How does knowing these stereotypes exist make you more sensitive to clients about potential barriers in daily living and access to health care?
2. In what way can nurses break through stereotypes to deliver the best possible care?

◆ **LEARNING ACTIVITY 3-4**

Read the following list of American cultural values and reflect on how these values may vary significantly from those of other cultural groups.

◆ **American Cultural Values**
Doing: value of activity, i.e., keeping busy
Problem solvers: conceive of more than one course of action
Achievement: personal, visible, measurable, materialistic
Choices: effects are preferably measurable, visible, materialistic
Practical: adjust to immediate situations without much thought for long-term effects
Exploration of values: "oughtness," "should"
Self-centered
Equality and fairness
Majority rule
Decision makers are responsible for subsequent action, rational order to the world; cause and effect, world and nature are controllable
Separation of work from play
Hard work ethic
Time is money
Temporal orientation: toward the future, can improve on the present with effort and optimism; action and hard work = goal achievement (positive)
Training and education very important
Source of motivation lies in individual, not society
Need feedback: sensitive to praise/blame; need to be liked
Competitive: individual and ascriptive (team, country, etc.)
Failure is the result of lack of will and effort of the individual
Individualism vs. individuality
Limits role of authority: to providing services, protecting rights of individuals, inducing cooperation and adjudicating differences
Equality of opportunity
Social equality
Don't like obligations socially
Competition within cooperation
Cooperation to get things done more important than social relationship of doers
Physical comfort and health
Private property and free enterprise
(Excerpted from Stewart & Bennett, 1991)

◆ **Follow these instructions in your clinical journal:**
1. Describe several of the values that are part of your everyday way of living.
2. How do those values influence how you see other cultural ways that differ?
3. Knowing that significant value orientation differences may exist between you and your clients in the community, describe accommodations you might make to provide culturally sensitive care within that setting.

◆ **LEARNING ACTIVITY 3-5**

Using a cultural assessment guide referenced in the chapter, conduct a cultural assessment on a client from a cultural group that differs from your own. What specific information did you learn that would guide your nursing actions related to (1) cultural preservation, (2) cultural accommodation, and (3) cultural repatterning?

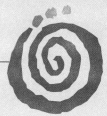

4

Family Care

ROBERTA HUNT

LEARNING OBJECTIVES

1. Recognize the relationships among family structure, family roles, family functions, and culture.
2. Differentiate between the concept of the family as the client and the care of the client in the context of the family.
3. Identify family developmental tasks throughout the life span.
4. Describe characteristics of healthy family functioning.
5. Discuss the health–illness continuum and family needs during illness.
6. Describe the role of the nurse in family assessment.
7. Identify the steps of planning, implementing, and evaluating in family-focused community-based nursing.
8. Identify community agencies for family interventions at each level of prevention.

KEY TERMS

affective interventions	family role
behavioral interventions	family structure
cognitive interventions	family systems theory
culturagram	functional assessment
developmental assessment	genogram
family developmental tasks	healthy family functioning
family functions	role conflict
family health	structural family assessment

CHAPTER TOPICS

◆ Significance of Family Care
◆ Nursing Competencies and Skills in Family Care
◆ Conclusions

THE NURSE SPEAKS

For many years, the nursing students at our college had the opportunity to see patients in a pediatric primary care clinic. To meet the needs of working parents, this clinic was open during the week from 5:00 to 9:00 PM. One evening, one of my students completed the initial assessment with Ty, a 3-year-old boy. Ty was accompanied by his mother and father and two younger siblings.

Ty had a history of frequent otitis media and was being seen that evening for ear drainage, ear pain, and a low-grade fever. Ty was accustomed to the routine and allowed the student to do the initial assessment as he sat on his mother's lap.

The pediatrician did her evaluation and diagnosed otitis media of the right ear. Because the pediatrician was familiar with the family, she asked if they had kept the referral appointment she had made for Ty to see an ear, nose, and throat (ENT) specialist the month before. The mother, who spoke very little English, shook her head no.

After leaving the room, the pediatrician voiced her concern with us because she noted hearing impairment as a result of the otitis media. Next, she wrote a prescription for an oral antibiotic, which was filled at the clinic, and found a sample bottle of oral analgesic. The nursing student and I went back to see the family and to review the home care instructions. I encouraged the student to have the mother and father administer the first dose of antibiotic and analgesic before the family left the clinic. The student questioned why she would need to observe this as Ty had a long history of otitis media. I again encouraged her to observe the mother and father administer the medications. The student asked the parents to administer the first dose of medications while at the clinic. The parents agreed, so Ty's mother washed her hands, read each medication bottle, and precisely measured the exact amount to be administered. Next, Ty's mother placed him across her lap and attempted to administer the oral antibiotic into his right ear. In utter surprise, the nursing student stopped the mother before she was able to place the medication into Ty's ear. The student politely explained how the medications worked and the need to administer both medications orally. At this point, a staff person who could serve as an interpreter was able to visit with the family, and it was discovered that the parents had routinely given the oral medications into whichever ear was affected.

Through the assistance of the interpreter, the student reviewed the home care instructions with the parents. The parents verbalized their understanding of the route of administration, and each medication was correctly administered by the mother before leaving the clinic. The parents agreed to a follow-up by a community health nurse and the ENT specialist.

We all learned an important lesson that evening in the midst of a very busy pediatric clinic—that is, the value of making time for discharge teaching along with a return demonstration, especially when administering medications to children.

— SUSAN O'CONNER-VON, DNSc, RNC, Assistant Professor, School of Nursing
University of Minnesota, Minneapolis, Minnesota

Not only is the family the basic social unit in American society, but also it is the most influential and dynamic unit. It has been the primary focus of nursing care in the community since the establishment of public health nursing in the late 19th century. The family performs a variety of key functions and has a central role in promoting and maintaining the health of its members.

Understanding family structure, roles, and functions is paramount in providing comprehensive nursing care. Knowledge of **healthy family functioning** allows the nurse to identify unhealthy functioning and take appropriate actions. In the current health care climate, the nurse must be cognizant of the needs, feelings, problems, and views of the family when providing care to the individual client.

Numerous models depict the relationship between nursing care and the family. These models reflect three ways to consider the family as it relates to nursing care:

Care of the individual in the context of the family. This point of view considers the family as it relates to the recovery of the individual client. Consequently, the client is the focus, and the context is the family.

The family's impact on the recovery of the client. In this model, the influences that family structure, function, development stage, and interpersonal interactions have on the recovery of the client are considered.

Improvement of the family's collective health. This method focuses on the family as the unit of service. In this model, the nurse assesses the family, determines the family's health problems or diagnoses, and develops goals with the family that are intended to improve its collective health.

This chapter discusses all three models by which nursing care is provided to families. However, **family health** will be considered primarily in the context of the impact of the family on the health of the individual. Nursing process skills will focus on the health of the family as it relates to the health recovery of the individual client.

SIGNIFICANCE OF FAMILY CARE

Regardless of which method is used, it is evident the family and individual are closely interrelated. The individual's health affects the family, and the family's health affects the client.

Concepts

Definitions of family have evolved over the past several decades. Definitions usually include family structure, roles, and function. The definition currently accepted by most health care professions is that of a social group whose members share common values and interact with each other over time. Usually, but not always, they live together. In this text, we will use this definition but also consider those whom the client has identified as family or significant others.

Family Structure

Traditionally, the family has been defined as the nuclear family, or a family with a mother, father, and two or more children. The characteristics of the "typical" family in the United States have changed markedly over the past 20 years. During that time,

TABLE 4-1 Family Structures	
Structure	**Participants**
Nuclear family	Married couple with children
	Unmarried couple, heterosexual or same sex with children
Nuclear dyad	Couple, married or unmarried; heterosexual or same sex
Single-parent family	One adult with children (separated, divorced, widowed, or never married)
Single adult	One adult
Multigenerational family	Any combination of the first four family structures
Kin network	Two or more reciprocal households (related by birth or marriage)

the typical family has evolved to the point where the traditional nuclear family—mother, father, and 2.2 children—no longer represents the majority of the population. Many different family structures exist. Table 4-1 lists the various **family structures** and their components; Figure 4-1 depicts different family structures.

In 1970, 85% of all children under age 18 were living with two parents; in 1993, only 71% were, and in 2004, 68% of all children were living with two parents. The proportion of children living with only one parent almost doubled between 1970 and 2004, rising from 12% to 23%. For White children, 77% were living with two parents in 2004; however, only 35% of African American children and 65% of Hispanic children lived with both parents (Federal Interagency Forum on Child and Family Statistics, 2006).

Marked differences in income are apparent among the different family structures. Children in married-couple families are much less likely to be living in poverty than children living only with their mother. In 2004, 9% of children in married-couple families were living in poverty, compared with 42% in female-householder families. The contrast by family structure is especially pronounced among certain racial and ethnic groups. For example, in 2004, 11% of African American children in married-couple families lived in poverty, compared with 50% of African American children in female-householder families. Twenty-one percent of Hispanic children in married-couple families lived in poverty, compared with 51% in female-householder families. Most children living in poverty are White and not Hispanic. However, the proportion of African American or Hispanic children in poverty is much higher than the proportion of White, non-Hispanic children.

To complicate matters, 13% of all children had no health insurance (Federal Interagency Forum on Children and Family Statistics, 2006). These statistics are important because the level of health and the quality of health care are affected by poverty. Those living in poverty, and consequently receiving poor health care, represent a large number of families in the United States.

Family Roles

A **family role** is an expected set of behaviors associated with a particular family position. Roles can be formal or informal. Formal roles are recognized by expectations associated with the roles, such as wife, husband, mother, father, or child. Examples of formal roles include breadwinner, housekeeper, child caretaker, financial manager, or cook. Informal roles are those that are casually acquired

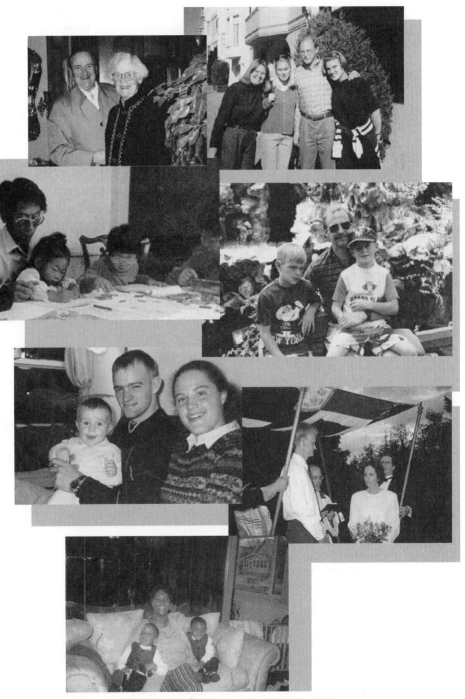

FIGURE 4-1. ▶ Various family structures.

within a family. An example of an informal role would be the family member who plans the social schedule or who takes out the garbage.

Role conflict may occur when the demands of one role conflict with or contradict another. This may also occur when one family member's expectations conflict with another's expectations. Role overload occurs when an individual is confronted with too many role responsibilities at one time. For instance, when a woman with children returns to school, she may have difficulty managing the roles of cook, driver, housekeeper, wife, and child care provider while keeping up with her schoolwork. The new role of student competes with the prior roles, and role overload occurs.

Illness or hospitalization of a family member causes role conflict or overload for all family members. Flexibility with family roles becomes particularly important during crises. Hospitalization and illness often require shifts in family roles and responsibilities. If one family member is ill, other family members may have to assume certain roles temporarily or permanently. In some situations, this may mean that a child assumes a parental role if one of the parents becomes ill or is hospitalized. During illness, various family members' ability to take on different roles facilitates the family's adaptation or return to homeostasis. Role flexibility also allows the family to provide support to the family member who is recovering from an illness or injury. Similarly, role flexibility in a family may allow the ill family member to be more comfortable with giving up roles, thus facilitating recovery.

Family Functions

Family functions are defined as outcomes, or consequences, of family structure. They are the reason families exist. Functions are divided into several categories: affective, socialization, reproductive, economic, and health care, as shown in Figure 4-2.

The affective function of the family is defined as the family's ability to meet the psychologic needs of family members. These needs include affection and understanding. This is considered by some as the most vital function of families.

Socialization or social placement is the second function. Socialization is the process of learning to adapt to life in a family and a community. This involves helping children adapt to the norms of the community and become productive members of society. This socialization process is built into all cultures. Specific functions include a variety of day-to-day family and social experiences that prepare children to assume adult roles. These may include learning the norms of dress and hygiene and preparing and eating food.

The third function, reproductive, is procreation. It may be thought of as the family's provision of recruits for society to ensure the continuity of the intergenerational family and society.

Economic functions encompass the allocation of adequate resources for family members. This entails the provision of sufficient income to provide for basic necessities. It also includes the allocation of these resources to all family members, especially those unable to provide for themselves.

Providing for health care and the physical necessities is the final family function. Physical care is the provision of material necessities, such as food, clothing, and shelter. Family health care includes health and lifestyle practices, such as nutrition, chemical use and abuse, recreation, and exercise and sleep practices.

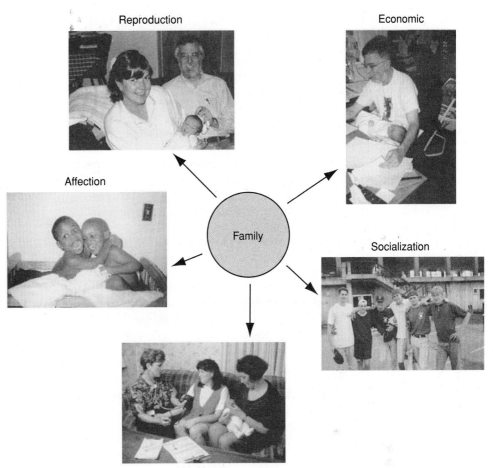

FIGURE 4-2. ▶ Basic family functions.

Family functions can also be viewed in relation to Maslow's hierarchy of needs. Maslow's theory is directionally based and presents the concept that the needs at the bottom of the model must be met before the next level can be addressed (Fig. 4-3). According to Maslow, the family must first meet physiologic needs (e.g., food, fluids, shelter, sleep) before members can consider any other opportunities in life.

Safety needs include both physiologic and psychologic safety of family members. The infant experiences safety when held securely in the arms of the parent. The young child experiences safety in the family when the environment is sufficiently structured to protect the child from harm. Adolescents feel safe in an environment that allows freedom and provides responsibility and structure.

Physiologic and psychologic safety remains important to adults. Physical safety includes living in a safe community. Increasingly, urban neighborhoods are more and more violent, resulting in residents feeling unsafe. Psychologic safety evolves

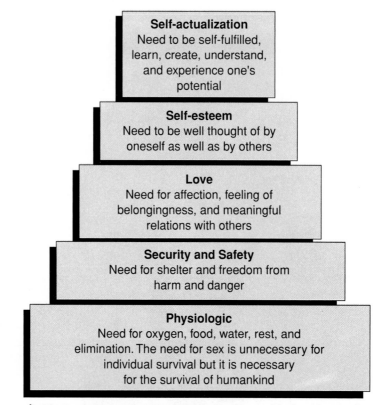

FIGURE 4-3. ▶ Maslow's hierarchy of needs. According to Maslow, basic physiologic needs must be met before the person can move on to higher-level needs. Adapted from Maslow, A. H. (1954). *Motivation and personality*. New York: Harper & Row.

from living a relatively structured life with some definite social expectations of one's self and those around us.

Another family function is meeting love-and-belonging needs. We all need meaningful relationships with other people. In classic research by Spitz (1945), two groups of infants and children were studied. Both groups received excellent physical care, but the second group received little demonstrative affection. Members of the first group were talked to, held, and caressed. There was a higher mortality rate as well as impaired development among the infants and children of the second group who received no physical affection. This demonstrates the vital importance of meeting the love-and-belonging need.

Fulfillment of esteem needs is also a family function. Self-esteem comes from feeling that we are valued by those around us. The family introduces the child to self-esteem. Family members may assist one another to feel good about themselves through acceptance and approval. Self-actualization is being "true to oneself," to fulfill one's potential. Self-actualization is not what one chooses to do in life, but how one feels about that choice. To joyfully do in life what one wants and is suited to do is self-actualization.

Family Systems Theory

The identification of the family as the unit of care is an emerging trend in family systems theory. **Family systems theory** defines family as a collection of people who are integrated, interacting, and interdependent. The actions of one member influence the actions of other members. The family system has a boundary; people recognize the family members. This boundary is selectively permeable according to the family's wishes, so items such as material goods, people, and information are allowed in or out according to the perceived needs of the system. Families with closed boundaries in one area may, for instance, be reluctant to use community resources.

After a crisis or during a transition from one developmental stage to another, the family system may experience disequilibrium. This imbalance causes a large amount of energy to be expended by individual family members in an attempt to cope with the discomfort. The family will attempt to return to the previous state of equilibrium. A nurse who is knowledgeable about family systems theory can facilitate healthy functioning.

The nurse considers the actions of family members as they apply to the health of the individual client. Family boundaries can be assessed to determine the likelihood that the family will use needed services. Similarly, disequilibrium of the family system as it pertains to the client can also be assessed.

Family Health

The Health–Illness Continuum

The family's structure, roles, ability to fulfill family functions, culture, and developmental tasks all affect the way the family functions. When a family member is ill, adaptation depends on each of these areas. An individual's place on the wellness–illness continuum affects all members of the family and all interactions within the family.

Family structure also affects the health recovery of an individual. In a family with two adult members, recovery may be different from that in a family headed by one adult. Certainly, when an individual lives alone, there is a greater need to tap extended family and friends for support and assistance than when the family has other adult members.

Family roles have an impact on the health recovery of the individual, and the health of the individual affects family roles. It is difficult to fulfill the usual functions of the family during times of stress or illness. When a family member is hospitalized, it may be difficult to fulfill the family's basic physical necessities and care. Examples include the inability to provide meals, maintain a regular bedtime, or wash laundry.

Family Needs Before and During Illness

Health care professionals are placing increased emphasis on the needs and roles of the family during a loved one's critical illness. Studies show that although nurses are often in the best position to meet families' needs, their needs are not always met (Holden, Harrison, & Johnson, 2002). The standards for comprehensive and effective family care by the Association for the Care of Children's Health focus on the immediate emotional and practical needs of the family in crisis. These recommendations may be adapted to all family care:

◆ Recognizing that the family is the primary constant in the client's life, which requires nurse and family collaboration
◆ Sharing information

◆ Providing support
◆ Recognizing family strengths
◆ Respecting different methods of family coping

There are some practical steps that every family can take to be prepared in the event that a family member becomes seriously injured or ill (Wagner-Cox, 2005). Families can be coached to consider these suggestions. First, families should pay attention to the health insurance plan and choose one that offers: 1) a catastrophic limit they can afford to spend, 2) a home care provision, 3) a medication plan, and 4) the doctors and hospitals they can trust. Second, when family members are well they should talk to their primary physician to establish rapport and sign an advance directive. Next, every family should get legal affairs in order such as a will, power of attorney, 401Ks, individual retirement accounts (IRAs), life insurance, care titles, and house titles. Cross training is important for families as well as in the work place. Having a basic understanding of all aspects of running a household ensures that if one member is incapacitated the basics will continue to be addressed. Last of all, prepare for death and dying emotionally and psychologically by talking about what should be done in the event of a severe illness and death.

Once a health crisis occurs, there are steps that a family can take to navigate the stormy waters. The family can act as an advocate for the ill family member by creating a duplicate chart with medical history, test reports, and medication record. Often a family member must keep tract of newly ordered tests and procedures so it is helpful to know: 1) the test that is ordered; 2) the location, date, and time; 3) what preparation is needed; 4) what reports/laboratory tests are required to be completed prior to the new test; 5) when the results will be ready; and 6) how to get a copy of the test (Wagner-Cox, 2005).

It is essential that when a family member is ill that the rest of the family mobilizes their support system. These resources may be friends and extended family that can be counted on to listen, assist them to face their fears, and encourage them to be kind to themselves and the rest of the family. Each individual family member will have his or her own manner of coping and benefits from employing healthy coping mechanisms. It is helpful if family members enjoy the good times that are still there (Wagner-Cox, 2005).

Families require similar assistance from nursing staff during the course of a lifelong chronic condition. There are several ways to increase resilience in families with an ill family member (O'Connell, 2006). These common needs include support, informational and skill training, advocacy, and referral to resources. This research showed a relationship between the quality of information given to families and their feelings of insecurity and helplessness.

In addition to these needs, families experience stages or landmarks when a family member is ill (Freeman, O'Dell, & Meola, 2000; Marino & Kooser, 1986). As with any stage theory, these landmarks are not rigid pathways but, rather, fluid progressions. These stages could apply to chronic, acute, or terminal illnesses. Family needs during illness vary according to these stages and the family roles and relations to the person experiencing illness. Table 4-2 outlines these needs.

In the first stage, the prediagnostic period, signs, and symptoms of the disease appear. The client and family often perceive this stage as a threat. There may be concern about the future, along with misconceptions and misinformation that compound existing fears. The nurse's role is that of counselor and educator.

TABLE 4-2	Family Needs During Stages of Illness			
Stage Priority	**Family Needs**	**Education Needs**	**Role of the Nurse**	**Psychosocial Issues**

Prediagnosis	Information
	Relief from anxiety
	To be with and
	    helpful to the client
	Support and personal
	    needs
			Counselor
			Educator
				Presurgery fear
				Empathy

Diagnosis	Relief from anxiety
	Information
	To be with and
	    helpful to the client
	Support and personal
	    needs
		Complications
		Postdischarge
		    care
			Support system
			Educator
			Assessor of family
			    systems	

Treatment	Relief from anxiety	Treatment op-
		    tions and
		    outcomes
			Support for com-
			    fort measures
			Resource person
			Support for personal
			    needs
			Support for emotions
				Diminished support of
				    friends
				Decreased work hours
				Limited time with family
				Socialization at hospital
				Peer support
				Community support
				Changes, jealousy
				Cause of disease
				Isolation
				Special treatment
				Health fears
				Overprotection
				Empathy

End of life	Relief from anxiety
	To be with and
	    helpful to the client
	Support
		Terminal care
		    planning
			Support for
			    emotions
				Confrontation of
				    possible death
				Maturational lag
				Spirituality
				Social support
				Need to help similar
				    families
				Long-term outcome
				Preparation
				Continued counseling

Adapted from Marino, L., & Kooser, J. (1986). *The psychosocial care of clients and their families: Periods of high risk.* In L. Marino (Ed.), *Current Nursing* (pp. 53–56). St. Louis: Mosby.
Adapted from Freeman, K., O'Dell, C., & Meola, C. (2000). Issues in families of children with brain tumors. *Oncology Nursing Forum, 27*(5), 843–848.

In the second stage, a diagnosis is made. The client and family may experience a variety of responses—from denial and anger to guilt—as they attempt to cope with the diagnosis. During this stage, the role of the nurse requires that the nurse educate, assess the family system, and assist the family in identifying and garnering their support system. They may have education needs in the areas of complications and postdischarge care if they are hospitalized.

The third stage, the treatment period, may be characterized by optimism, despair, anger, dependency, feelings of powerlessness, and fear of recurrence or long-term impairment. This is the stage of the "long, hard pull," which may last for months, but more often for years. Frequently, the nurse's role during the treatment period involves providing physical comfort measures, assisting with contacting and referring to resources, and giving positive feedback and encouragement.

The last stage is the end of life. Both terminal and chronic illnesses apply in this final stage. The client may have feelings of hopelessness and fear of abandonment; the family feels guilt, relief, or a profound sense of loss. The nurse provides support during this grieving process.

NURSING COMPETENCIES AND SKILLS IN FAMILY CARE

Nurses are in a unique position among health care professionals in their close proximity to clients. As nursing has moved away from a task orientation, it has adopted a more holistic view of clients as individuals with a life beyond their illness. A holistic perspective allows the nurse to address the cadre of needs families experience when lives have been irrevocably changed by the illness of one member. Providing nursing care to families is a logical development of the holistic approach to care of the client and is an important cornerstone of nursing practice.

The essential considerations when caring for individuals in the context of their families are as follows:

- ◆ One part of the family cannot be understood in isolation from the rest of the system.
- ◆ A family's structure and organization cannot be understood in isolation from the rest of the system.
- ◆ Communication patterns between family members are essential in the functioning of the family.

Competence in using the nursing process with families requires different skills and knowledge as compared to care of the individual client.

Family Assessment

The intent of the assessment process as it applies to the client within the context of the family in community-based nursing is to determine the nursing needs and intervene for the client. Initially a nurse collects information about the family to treat the client. The entry level nurse working with individuals and families in the community uses family interviewing as a technique for intervention.

The Family Interview

The same principles used in an effective interview with a client apply to a family interview. Effective communication is essential in the first step of establishing a trusting relationship. The interview might start with an informal conversation so all participants are put at ease. It is helpful to have all the family members present during this interview. It is also beneficial to encourage them all to participate.

Numerous family assessment tools are available. A short family assessment form is shown in Assessment Tools 4-1. Many agencies have a standard form that they use for all family interviews.

(text continues on page 94)

ASSESSMENT TOOLS 4-1

Family Assessment Guide

Family Members

Member	Birth Date	Sex	Marital Status	Education

Genogram

Stage of Illness

In what stage of illness is this family? (See Table 4-2.)

_____

_____

What are this family's priority needs?

_____

_____

What is the role of the nurse in this stage?

_____

_____

_____

(continued)

ASSESSMENT TOOLS 4-1

Family Assessment Guide (*Continued*)

Development Assessment

What is this family's developmental stage?

_____

Is the family meeting the tasks of its stage?

_____

_____

_____

Does, or will, the client's health problem interrupt the family's ability to meet the developmental tasks? If yes, how does it interrupt it?

_____

_____

_____

State nursing interventions to assist family members in meeting their developmental tasks.

_____

_____

_____

Functional Assessment

Does the family meet the individual's need for affection, love, and understanding?

_____

_____

_____

Does the family meet the individual's need for physical necessities and care?

_____

_____

_____

_____

(continued)

ASSESSMENT TOOLS 4-1

Family Assessment Guide (*Continued*)

Does the family have the economic resources necessary to provide for the basic needs of the family?

_____

_____

_____

Is the family meeting the function of reproduction as defined by the family?

_____

Is the family meeting the family function of socialization? Is the family fulfilling the function to socialize children to become productive members of society?

_____

_____

_____

Does the family attempt to actively cope with problems?

_____

_____

_____

_____

Assessment of Presence of Characteristics of a Healthy Family

Is communication between members open, direct, and honest, and are feelings and needs shared?

_____

_____

_____

Do family members express self-worth with integrity, responsibility, compassion, and love to and for one another?

_____

_____

_____

(continued)

ASSESSMENT TOOLS 4-1

Family Assessment Guide (*Continued*)

Are family rules known to all members?

_____

_____

Are rules clear and flexible, and do they allow individual members freedom?

_____

_____

_____

Does the family have regular links to society that demonstrate trust and friendship?

_____

_____

_____

Do family members belong to various groups and clubs?

_____

_____

_____

The assessment may determine if a family's response to the current situation is adaptive or maladaptive. This permits the nurse to identify problem areas and the need for additional assessment and referral. For example, after a family interview, the nurse may encourage family members to share their individual concerns with the entire family. For example, one family member may share his or her concerns with the nurse about difficulties with family communication. With the entire family present the nurse may bring up and suggest that everyone share his or her observations about how the family is communicating. Based on this discussion, the nurse may then suggest that the family explore this topic with a social worker, public health nurse, physician, clergy member, or counselor. Family assessment may lead the nurse to recommend additional assistance by a professional, such as a family therapist or social worker with special expertise in family therapy. The intervention in this example is a referral.

The type of family assessment used depends on the focus of the treatment and the knowledge level of the care provider, as illustrated in Figure 4-4. Family members

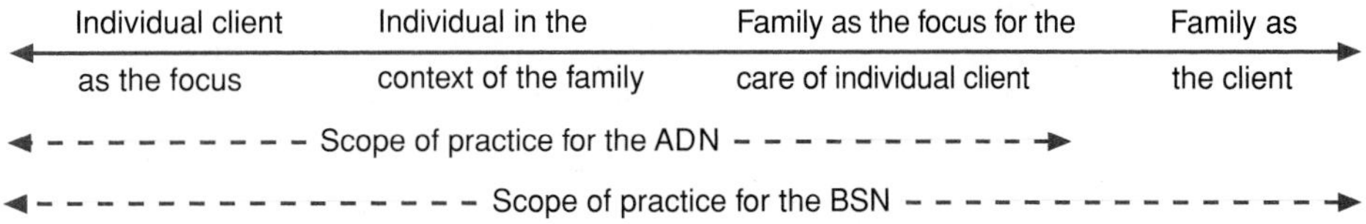

Individual client	Individual in the	Family as the focus for the	Family as
as the focus	context of the family	care of individual client	the client

◄ – – – – – – – – – Scope of practice for the ADN – – – – – – – – – – ►

◄ – – – – – – – – – – – – – – Scope of practice for the BSN – – – – – – – – – – – – – – – ►

FIGURE 4-4. ▶ Focus of nursing care for individuals and families.

are asked questions regarding the client and the client's condition. The client is assessed within the context of the family with questions such as the following:

◆ Question to the client: What is your understanding of a diabetic diet?
◆ Question to the mother: What is your understanding of your son Jon's diabetes?
◆ Question to the father: What is your understanding of your son Jon's diabetes?

When the family is the client, other realms need to be assessed. These include family functions such as financial role responsibilities, the family's emotional system, and the meaning to the family of the health event and its outcome. Consequently, when the family is viewed as the client, individual members of the family are asked questions:

◆ Question to the client: What impact do you think your illness has had on your family?
◆ Question to the parents: How do you feel your family has adjusted to your son's illness?
◆ Question to the parents: How has your son's illness affected your family's finances?

The first step in assessing the family as the client is to determine the family's impact on the recovery of the client. This is appropriate especially when the family's functioning is clearly impeding the recovery. Figure 4-5 illustrates the levels that are necessary in a comprehensive family assessment.

Family as client
Assess family structure, function, stage of development as affected by health of the family

Family as it impacts health of individual
Assess family structure, function, developmental stage as it affects health of the individual client

Individual in the context of the family
Assess biopsychosocial needs of each family member as it impacts on health of the individual

Individual as client
Assess biopsychosocial needs of the individual

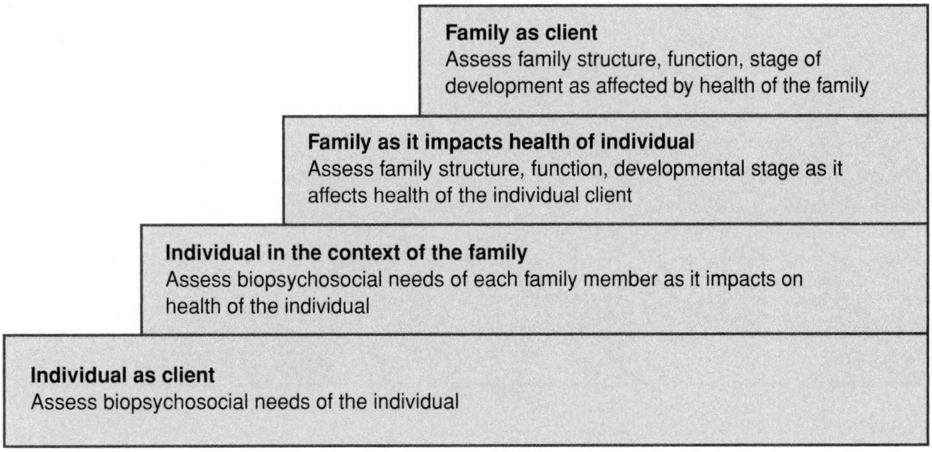

FIGURE 4-5. ▶ Levels necessary to assess in a comprehensive family assessment.

Overall, the intent of evaluating the family is to analyze the client's potential for recovery and self-care, given the familial conditions. To facilitate the client's return to the highest level of wellness, the circumstances in which the client lives must be considered.

Models of Family Assessment

DEVELOPMENTAL ASSESSMENT

The health of a family's functioning may be evaluated by a family **developmental assessment** considering normal **family developmental tasks**. As individuals have development stages that they must go through to move to the next stage of development, so do families. Duvall (1977) developed a commonly used theory of development stages of family life as it relates to nursing care. According to Duvall, there are predictable stages within the life cycle of every family; each stage includes distinct family developmental tasks (Table 4-3). Stages of the family life cycle follow no rigid pattern. The family enters each stage with the birth of the first child or according to the age of the oldest child in the family. This model can be used as a guide to assessment by following these steps:

1. Determine the family's developmental stage. This can be done by determining the age of the oldest child in the family and correlating it with the level in Table 4-3.
2. Consider the family members' health problems in the context of the tasks in their developmental stage. Is it likely that the health condition will interrupt the family's developmental tasks?

TABLE 4-3	Stages of the Family Life Cycle	
Stage	**Scope of the Stage**	**Family Developmental Tasks**
Married couple	Couple makes commitment to one another	Establishing a mutually satisfying marriage Fitting into the kin network
Childbearing	Oldest child is infant through 30 mo	Adjusting to infants and encouraging their development Establishing a satisfying family life for both child and parent
Preschool	Oldest child is 2½–6 y	Adapting to the needs of preschool children in growth-producing ways Coping with lack of privacy and energy
School age	Oldest child is 7–12 y	Fitting into age-appropriate community activities Encouraging the children's achievement
Teenage	Oldest child is 13–20 y	Balancing freedom with responsibility as teens mature and emancipate Establishing outside interests and career
Launching	First child leaves home to last child leaving home	Assisting young adults to work, attend school or military, with marriage, with appropriate rituals
Middle-aged parents	Empty nest to retirement	Rebuilding marital bond Cultivating kin ties with younger and older family
Aging family	Retirement to moving out of family home	Coping with loss and living alone Adapting to retirement and aging

Adapted from Allender, J. A., & Spradley, B. W. (2001). *Community health nursing: Concepts and practice* (5th ed., p. 440). Philadelphia: Lippincott Williams & Wilkins.

3. Determine if family members are meeting the tasks at their levels of development.
4. Identify the nursing interventions that would assist the family in meeting these developmental tasks.

Because of the wide variety of family structures, not all families fit neatly into this family stage theory. For individuals who do not marry, remain childless, divorce, remarry to form a blended family, or are in same-sex unions, the stages are viewed differently. In families in which the stages of the family life cycle are disrupted, the emotional processes and issues relating to transition and development also differ from those set out in Duvall's stages.

Disruption of the family cycle because of a divorce causes additional steps to be taken to re-stabilize the family for further development. Family life cycle stages for divorced or disrupted families are compared with healthy families in Figure 4-6. In the postdivorce phase, the single custodial parent experiences a different emotional process and transition than does the noncustodial parent. The developmental issues differ as well (Table 4-4). Further there is now evidence that post divorce many woman experience financial stress which in turn has a negative effect on physical health and morbidity (Wickrama, Lorenz, Conger, Elder, Todd Abraham, & Fang, 2006). Further, the stress of divorce directly influences a woman's morbidity independent of family financial difficulties. Family assessment must regard the impact that divorce may have on families over time. These families may have needs for disease prevention and health promotion interventions that differ from other families.

Families with remarriage may experience emotional transitions or developmental issues as well (Table 4-5). Emotional transitions include attaining an adequate emotional separation from the previous marriage and accepting and dealing with fears about forming a new family. In addition, when beginning a blended family, members must find the time and patience necessary to permit another emotional adjustment. Resolving the feelings of attachment to a previous spouse and accepting the new family model require transitions by individuals. Developmental issues are also seen in each phase of the new marriage.

Family developmental tasks involve meeting the basic family functions discussed earlier in this chapter. The needs of the individual family members, family developmental tasks, and family functions must mesh.

Meeting these needs is not necessarily easy in families. The conflict that often occurs in families with adolescents illustrates this point. Typically, adolescents are attempting to break away from parents and spend more time with friends than family. Yet, parents may wish for the adolescent to participate as more of an adult in family activities. This conflict may be compounded, for instance, when family members need adequate rest to provide health care to a family member, but the adolescent's need is to stay out late and get support and approval from peers.

STRUCTURAL FAMILY ASSESSMENT
Structural family assessment considers the family's composition. A structural assessment defines the immediate family members, their names, ages, and the relationship among those who live together. A **genogram** is constructed to clarify the relationship and information about each member of the family. Symbols often used for the genogram are shown in Figure 4-7.

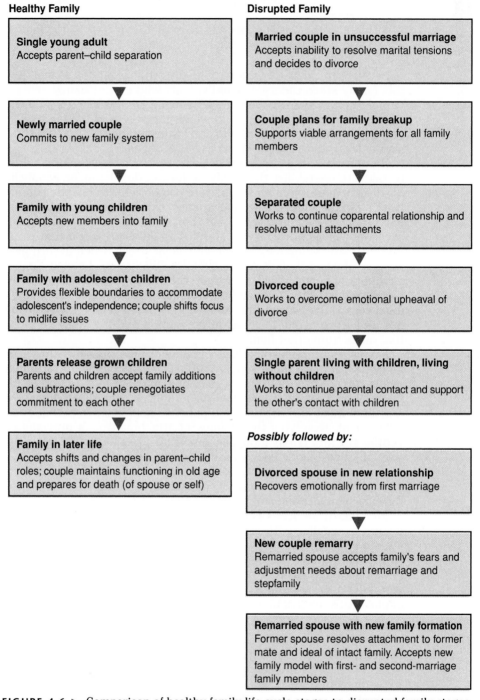

Healthy Family

Single young adult
Accepts parent–child separation

▼

Newly married couple
Commits to new family system

▼

Family with young children
Accepts new members into family

▼

Family with adolescent children
Provides flexible boundaries to accommodate adolescent's independence; couple shifts focus to midlife issues

▼

Parents release grown children
Parents and children accept family additions and subtractions; couple renegotiates commitment to each other

▼

Family in later life
Accepts shifts and changes in parent–child roles; couple maintains functioning in old age and prepares for death (of spouse or self)

Disrupted Family

Married couple in unsuccessful marriage
Accepts inability to resolve marital tensions and decides to divorce

▼

Couple plans for family breakup
Supports viable arrangements for all family members

▼

Separated couple
Works to continue coparental relationship and resolve mutual attachments

▼

Divorced couple
Works to overcome emotional upheaval of divorce

▼

Single parent living with children, living without children
Works to continue parental contact and support the other's contact with children

Possibly followed by:

Divorced spouse in new relationship
Recovers emotionally from first marriage

▼

New couple remarry
Remarried spouse accepts family's fears and adjustment needs about remarriage and stepfamily

▼

Remarried spouse with new family formation
Former spouse resolves attachment to former mate and ideal of intact family. Accepts new family model with first- and second-marriage family members

FIGURE 4-6. ▶ Comparison of healthy family life cycle stages to disrupted family stages. Liebermann, A. (1990). *Community and home health nursing.* Springhouse, PA: Springhouse Corporation.

TABLE 4-4	When Families Divorce	
Phase	**Emotional Responses**	**Transitional Issues**
1. Stressors leading to marital differences	Reveal the fact that the marriage has major problems	Accept the fact that the marriage has major problems
2. Decision to divorce	Accept the inability to resolve marital differences	Accept one's own contribution to the failed marriage
3. Planning the dissolution of the family system	Negotiate viable arrangements for all members within the system	Cooperate on custody, visitation, and financial issues Inform and deal with extended family members and friends
4. Separation	Mourn loss of intact family Work on resolving attachment to spouse	Develop coparental arrangements/ relationships Restructure living arrangements Adapt to living apart Realign relationship with extended family and friends Begin to rebuild own social network
5. Divorce	Continue working on emotional recovery by overcoming hurt, anger, or guilt	Give up fantasies of reunion Stay connected with extended families Rebuild and strengthen own social network
6. Postdivorce	Separate feelings about ex-spouse from parenting role Prepare self for possibility of changes in custody as children get older; be open to their needs Risk developing a new intimate relationship	Make flexible and generous visitation arrangements for children and noncustodial parent and extended family members Deal with possibilities of changing custody arrangements as children get older Deal with children's reaction to parents' establishing relationships with new partners

Adapted from Allender, J. A., & Spradley, B. W. (2005). *Community health nursing: Concepts and practice* (6th ed., p. 511). Philadelphia: Lippincott Williams & Wilkins.

Genograms can be helpful to nurses in many settings. An inpatient nurse can quickly sketch a genogram and identify family members; this helps to define which family members should be involved in the collaboration of planning care, including being present at care conferences with professional staff. Genograms may also be used in discharge planning by identifying the need for support and assistance when the client returns home. Genograms may help the home care nurse clarify the dynamics of the family in relation to the recovery of the client.

FUNCTIONAL ASSESSMENT
Six family functions must be considered during **functional assessment:** affective, health care and physical necessities, economics, reproduction, socialization and placement, and family coping.

Through interviews, the nurse collects information about the family members' perceptions of how well the family is fulfilling basic functions. To assess

TABLE 4-5	Remarriage and Blending Families	
Phases	**Emotional Responses**	**Developmental Issues**
1. Meeting new people	Allowing for the possibility of developing a new intimate relationship	Dealing with children's and ex-family members' reactions to a parent dating
2. Entering a new relationship	Completing an "emotional recovery" from past divorce and loss of marriage Accepting one's fears about developing a new relationship Working on feeling good about what the future may bring Discovering what you want from a new relationship Working on openness in a new relationship	
3. Planning a new marriage	Accepting one's fears about the ambiguity and complexity of entering a new relationship such as the following: New roles and responsibilities Boundaries: space, time, and authority Affective issues: guilt, loyalty, conflicts, unresolvable past hurts	Recommitting to marriage and forming a new family unit Dealing with stepchildren as custodial or noncustodial parent Planning for maintenance of coparental relationships with ex-spouses Planning to help children deal with fears, loyalty conflicts, and membership in two systems Realigning relationships with ex-family to include new spouse and children Restructuring family boundaries to allow for new spouse or stepparent
4. Remarriage and blending of families	Forming a final resolution of attachment to previous spouse Accepting of new family unit with different boundaries	Realigning relationships to allow intermingling of systems Expanding relationships to include all new family members Sharing family memories and histories to enrich members' lives

Adapted from Allender, J. A., & Spradley, B. W. (2005). *Community health nursing: Concepts and practice* (6th ed., p. 511). Philadelphia: Lippincott Williams & Wilkins.

family functions, the nurse may ask questions from each of the following categories.

◆ Is the family meeting the individual's need for affection, love, and understanding?
◆ Is the family meeting the individual's need for physical care?
◆ Does the family have the economic resources required to provide for basic needs of the family?
◆ Is the family meeting the function of reproduction, as defined by the family?
◆ Is the family meeting the family function of socialization? Is the family fulfilling the function of socialization of its children for them to become productive members of society?
◆ Does the family attempt to actively cope with problems?

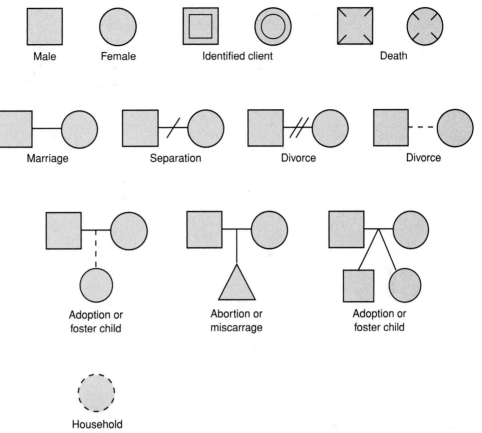

FIGURE 4-7. ▶ Symbols used in genograms.

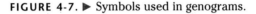

Using Characteristics of a Healthy Family for Assessment

The characteristics of a healthy family can be used as the baseline for family assessment. Family health depends on the ability of family members to share and to understand the feelings, needs, and behavior patterns of each individual (Satir, 1972). Healthy families demonstrate the following characteristics:

◆ There is a facilitative process of interaction among family members.
◆ The family enhances the development of its individual members.
◆ Role relationships are structured effectively.
◆ The family actively attempts to cope with problems.
◆ The family has a healthy home environment and lifestyle.
◆ The family establishes regular links with the broader community.

In addition, interactions in a healthy family display the following qualities:

◆ Communication among members is open, direct, and honest, with shared feelings.

◆ Family members express self-worth with integrity, responsibility, compassion, and love to, and for, one another.
◆ All members know the family rules. Rules are clear and flexible and allow individual members their freedom.
◆ The family has regular links with society, which demonstrate trust and friendship.
◆ Family members belong to various groups and clubs.

Culturagram as a Family Assessment Tool

The **culturagram** is a family assessment tool that attempts to individualize care for culturally diverse families (Congress & Kung, 2005). By completing a culturagram on a family the nurse will develop a better understanding of the sociocultural context of the family as well as identify appropriate interventions for the family. Administered in a manner similar to an ecomap or genogram, the culturagram examines the following areas (Congress & Kung, 2005):

◆ Reasons for relocation
◆ Legal status
◆ Time in the community
◆ Language spoken at home and in the community
◆ Health beliefs
◆ Crisis events
◆ Holidays and special events
◆ Contact with cultural and religious institutions
◆ Values about education and work
◆ Values about family structure (power, hierarchy, rules, subsystems, and boundaries)

An example of a culturagram is seen in Figure 4-8.

Nursing Diagnosis: Identifying Family Needs

After the family interview and assessment are completed and analyzed, the nurse can identify family strengths and needs. Again, the primary focus presented in this text is the care of the client. Assessment and identification of the needs of the family are focused on the family's effect on the care and recovery of the client.

The process of identifying the needs of the family follows the same steps as those used for the client. By comparing the collected data about the family with defining characteristics of the North American Nursing Diagnosis Association (NANDA) diagnosis, the nurse can arrive at the appropriate diagnosis for the client in the context of the family.

Maslow's model is valuable in individualizing and prioritizing care for individuals in the context of the family. Again, food and shelter, the most basic family needs, must be met first. When these needs are met, the priority of care can shift to safety and then up the hierarchy of needs. The priorities of the family can change as the circumstances of the family change.

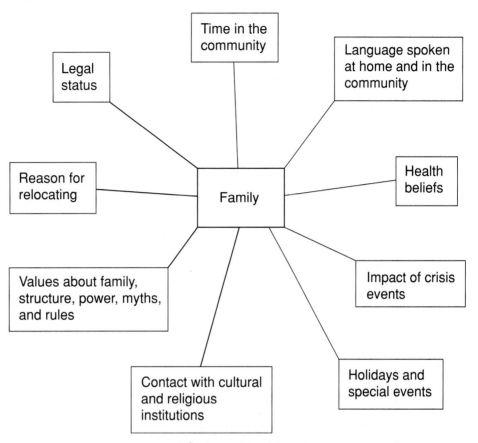

FIGURE 4-8. ▶ An example of a culturagram.

Planning: Goals

The process of planning care for families is similar to planning for an individual's care. The primary intent is to define goals in relation to the recovery of the client. The family may benefit from these established goals; however, the primary intent is to enhance the recovery of the client.

Mutual goal setting in which the client and the family are included is the cornerstone of effective planning in relation to families. Examples of goals for family interventions are listed in Box 4-1. It is essential that both the client and family members be a part of the planning process because, ultimately, it is the client and family members who are the primary caregivers and implement the plan of care. The process of goal setting has a positive effect on the health care provider's interactions with families. Mutual goal setting also has a positive effect on family interactions and compliance and accountability with the plan of care. Like individual clients, family members tend to resist being told what

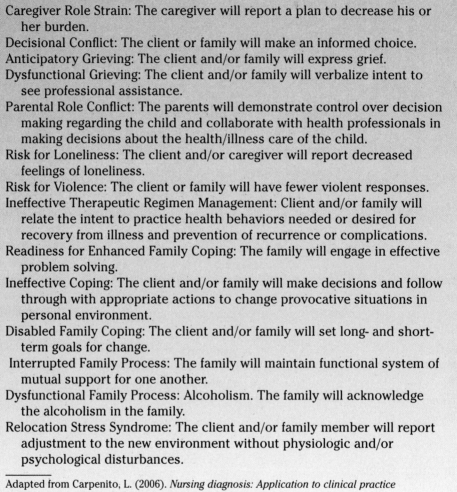

◆ **BOX 4-1** Examples of Goals for Commonly Used Nursing Diagnoses ◆

Caregiver Role Strain: The caregiver will report a plan to decrease his or her burden.

Decisional Conflict: The client or family will make an informed choice.

Anticipatory Grieving: The client and/or family will express grief.

Dysfunctional Grieving: The client and/or family will verbalize intent to see professional assistance.

Parental Role Conflict: The parents will demonstrate control over decision making regarding the child and collaborate with health professionals in making decisions about the health/illness care of the child.

Risk for Loneliness: The client and/or caregiver will report decreased feelings of loneliness.

Risk for Violence: The client or family will have fewer violent responses.

Ineffective Therapeutic Regimen Management: Client and/or family will relate the intent to practice health behaviors needed or desired for recovery from illness and prevention of recurrence or complications.

Readiness for Enhanced Family Coping: The family will engage in effective problem solving.

Ineffective Coping: The client and/or family will make decisions and follow through with appropriate actions to change provocative situations in personal environment.

Disabled Family Coping: The client and/or family will set long- and short-term goals for change.

Interrupted Family Process: The family will maintain functional system of mutual support for one another.

Dysfunctional Family Process: Alcoholism. The family will acknowledge the alcoholism in the family.

Relocation Stress Syndrome: The client and/or family member will report adjustment to the new environment without physiologic and/or psychological disturbances.

Adapted from Carpenito, L. (2006). *Nursing diagnosis: Application to clinical practice* (11th ed.). Philadelphia: Lippincott Williams & Wilkins.

to do; they are much more likely to work toward goals they have chosen and support.

Nursing Interventions

Nursing interventions for families in community-based settings primarily are the same as those discussed for individuals (Table 4-5). These fall into three levels: cognitive, affective, and behavioral. **Cognitive interventions** involve the act of knowing, perceiving, or understanding. An example is teaching a client or family member about the exchange system for a diabetic diet. This intervention is health teaching. **Affective interventions** have to do with feelings, attitudes, and values. Helping family members to understand their fears about a loved one's diagnosis of diabetes is an illustration of an affective intervention. Another would be to discuss concerns about drawing up and injecting insulin. These two are counseling interventions. **Behavioral interventions** are those that have to do with skills and behaviors. Teaching clients and family members about giving insulin injections is one example of a behavioral intervention. Another is a group exercise program for newly diagnosed diabetic clients. Both of these interventions are health teaching. Similar to other steps of the nursing process, interventions must be directed primarily toward the health recovery of the client.

Nursing interventions provide specific directions and a consistent, individualized approach to the client's care. They are written as instructions for others to follow. Obviously, interventions in community-based care require the active involvement of the client and the family to determine the appropriate interventions. The client or family will often be responsible for implementing the interventions at home. As with goal setting, the client and family are more likely to comply with the plan of care if they are active participants in the planning of interventions. Examples of goals and nursing interventions appear in Table 4-6.

The Internet is an excellent resource for researching appropriate nursing interventions for families. For example, the Bright Futures for Families Web site (http://www.brightfutures.org), supported by the Maternal and Child Health Bureau of the U.S. Department of Health and Human Services, offers tools to prepare families for health supervision to make them full participants in the process, to

TABLE 4-6 Examples of Goals and Nursing Interventions for Commonly Used Nursing Diagnoses for Family Intervention		
Nursing Diagnosis	**Goals**	**Nursing Intervention**
Decisional conflict	The client or family will make an informed choice.	Establish a trusting and meaningful relationship that promotes mutual understanding and caring. Facilitate a logical decision-making process.
Parental role conflict	The parents will demonstrate control over decision making regarding the child and collaborate with health professionals in making decisions about the health/illness care of the child.	Allow parents to share frustrations. If indicated, refer for counseling for management of stressors and role changes.
Disabled family coping	The client and/or family will set long- and short-term goals for change.	Be direct and nonjudgmental. Encourage a realistic appraisal of the situation; dispel guilt and myths.
Interrupted family process	The family members will maintain a functional system of mutual support for each other.	Assist the family with appraisal of the situation. Acknowledge strengths of the family when appropriate.

Adapted from Carpenito, L. (2006). *Nursing diagnosis: Application to clinical practice* (11th ed.). Philadelphia: Lippincott Williams & Wilkins.

demonstrate the value of health supervision, and to teach families what to expect from health professionals.

Nursing interventions for families may include strategies in primary, secondary, and tertiary prevention. Primary prevention encompasses nursing interventions that obviate the initial occurrence of a disease. When attempting to implement interventions for individual clients, it is often necessary to involve family members because they are affected as well. An example is family planning. In some cultures, partners make decisions together about birth control and the spacing of children. In other cultures, the female or male partner decides independently of the other about family planning.

CLIENT SITUATIONS IN PRACTICE

◆ Intervention at the Primary Prevention Level

Pam is a nurse working in a clinic whose clients are primarily from Southeast Asia. When she first began teaching female clients about family planning, Pam did not include the husband or significant other. Over time, she discovered that the use of birth control, for many of her clients, was decided by the male partner. By involving the male partner in planning (choosing a method of birth control and teaching the couple about its use), the couples were more likely to comply.

Secondary prevention is early detection and treatment of a condition. In some families, lack of information may be a barrier to seeking services related to secondary prevention.

CLIENT SITUATIONS IN PRACTICE

◆ Intervention at the Secondary Prevention Level

Tom is a nurse working in a day care center for older adults. One of the clients who comes to day care, Irene, is having problems with her eyesight and comes from a family with a history of glaucoma. Tom has been encouraging her to have her eyes tested. Although Irene has severe arthritis, she is alert and cognitively intact. Irene tells Tom that she does not want to ask her son to take her to any more clinic visits. The son is unaware of his mother's vision problems. Tom learns that only by involving another family member (Irene's son) will the secondary prevention strategy (vision screening) occur.

Tertiary prevention is seeking treatment and rehabilitation for maximizing recovery. In some situations, the family is compliant with nursing care but is not aware of resources in the community that may support the client's care.

CLIENT SITUATIONS IN PRACTICE

◆ Intervention at the Tertiary Prevention Level

Kristi is a staff nurse working on a medical–surgical unit in a hospital. Her situation illustrates tertiary prevention. Kristi is in charge of Barb's discharge planning. Barb has had a fusion of three cervical vertebrae and will be discharged from the hospital in 4 days. She lives alone; however, her daughter (the mother of 5 children) lives an hour's drive from Barb's home. After discharge, Barb will need assistance with activities of daily living for at least 2 weeks at home, will not be permitted to drive for 6 weeks, and will receive physical therapy 4 times a week starting 2 weeks after discharge. Kristi, Barb, and Barb's daughter sit down together to plan for the care and assistance Barb will need at home. They also discuss the community services that may be able to transport Barb to physical therapy until she is permitted to drive.

Evaluation

Evaluation has a profound effect on the quality of care in community-based nursing. It is a joint effort among the nurse, family, and other caregivers. As is true in an acute care setting, evaluation leads to more assessment or refinement of the goals set out in the care plan and results in the identification of additional diagnoses, goals, or interventions.

The following questions for reflection may be useful during evaluation of the family care plan:

- ◆ What additional data are required to evaluate progress?
- ◆ Did the nursing diagnosis focus on the most important problem for this family as it relates to the potential for the client to do self-care?
- ◆ What other nursing problems apply to this family and client?
- ◆ What other strengths are apparent in this family?
- ◆ Were the diagnosis, goals, and interventions realistic and appropriate for this client and family?
- ◆ Were the family strengths considered when the goals and interventions were defined? If not, how could these strengths be used to enhance the outcome?
- ◆ Are the nurse, client, and family satisfied with the outcome? If not, what would provide satisfaction?
- ◆ The nursing process continues in an ongoing, circular, and dynamic manner. Information gained from asking the above questions is used to define a new problem and identify new or additional goals and interventions as the ongoing process of providing care and evaluating its effect continues.

Documentation

Complete and accurate information is an essential element of nursing care of the client or family. Creating a clear account of what the nurse saw and did related to the family's care provides a record of that care. This includes documentation of the client and family's strengths and needs. Charting is used to determine eligibility for care needed and for reimbursement for care provided.

CLIENT SITUATIONS IN PRACTICE

◆ The Family and Nursing Process

Tamesa, a home health care nurse, is assigned to care for Becky, a 30-year-old home-maker who is the mother of three preschool children (Joe, age 4, Kevin, age 2, and Michael, age 2 months). Becky has been diagnosed with liver cancer. Jack, Becky's husband, is a 32-year-old accountant with his own accounting firm. Jack's parents are in good health and live in another city. Ila, Becky's mother, lives in the same neighborhood as Jack and Becky. Becky's father died 10 years ago, and Ila remarried Stephen last year. Ila has severe arthritis. Becky also has a sister and brother who both live out of state.

As Becky's home care nurse, Tamesha completes a family assessment during the first visit. She begins the family interview by getting acquainted with all of the family members. Joe shows her the new toy his grandmother sent for his birthday; Kevin is very shy and sits in Becky's lap during the home visit. Jack holds the baby. Tamesha hopes to be able to identify how much support the family will be able to provide to Becky from this family assessment. She is also interested in identifying any problem areas where intervention is needed. The completed family assessment is shown in Assessment Tools 4-2.

Identification of the Nursing Diagnosis

Tamesha reviews her family assessment as well as Becky and Jack's responses. She identifies these family strengths:

- *The family and a large number of supportive friends are willing to assist with care of the children and the home.*
- *A strong marital bond between Becky and her husband is apparent; they show mutual support and love.*
- *The family has a stable financial status.*

She identifies these family needs:

- *There is difficulty managing the home and child care of three preschool children. This was evident when Becky stated she needed help managing the family's daily needs. Tamesha also observed that the house was very disorganized.*
- *There is the potential for ineffective family coping. This was evident when Becky and Jack were unable to be honest and open when discussing Becky's illness and prognosis.*
- *Becky has difficulty in performing her role of child caretaker because of her disabling illness.*

Setting Priorities

To identify the priority of family needs, Tamesha uses Maslow's hierarchy of needs. Recognizing that the family and client must have their basic needs addressed first, she concentrates on the family's difficulty in managing the home and the child care.

As a result, Tamesha believes that this is Becky and Jack's priority problem:

- *Impaired Home Maintenance Management related to Becky's complex care regimen as evidenced by a disorderly home environment and Becky's statement, "I can only care for the kids a few minutes at a time. We need help."*

Planning

At the second home visit, Tamesha, Becky, and Jack discuss the family assessment. Tamesha shares her conclusion about their primary need. She asks Becky and Jack for their impressions, and they agree that the major concern is the care of the home and the children. Becky adds, "I am concerned about being able to continue to provide care for the kids. I'm also worried about Jack and me having time together and being able to talk."

Through the intervention of counseling, Tamesha assists the family to enhance their capacity for self-care. The three decide to address the problems about home management and save the discussion about communication for the third visit. Tamesha suggests that if some of the issues regarding care of the home and family are addressed, Becky may have more energy for the children.

Goals

Tamesha, Becky, and her husband define the following goals that address impaired home maintenance. The goal is to accomplish them by the third visit:

1. Becky and Jack will identify home maintenance tasks that need to be done daily and weekly.
2. Becky and Jack will compile a list of family members and friends who are able and willing to assist with these tasks.
3. Becky and Jack will match the list of tasks with the list of people and contact them within the next 3 days.
4. Becky will call Tamesha with the list of tasks that their family and friends can do.
5. Jack will contact the list of community agencies that Tamesha gave him to see what assistance they can provide.

Nursing Implementation

Tamesha lists the specific nursing interventions she has identified for the plan of care:

1. Through counseling Tamesha will assist the family in determining a realistic plan for both health care and home maintenance.
2. Through the intervention of referral Tamesha will identify resources in the community that can assist with the tasks that the family and friends cannot do. She will contact Jack and give him the list of resources and telephone numbers.
3. Tamesha will use case management and schedule periodic home visits to evaluate the effectiveness of the plan and identify any changes that occur in Becky's condition that may need intervention.

Evaluation

At the third home visit, Tamesha uses the nursing intervention of case management as she assists Becky and Jack to evaluate the plan to date. The first four goals were met; however, Jack did not contact the community agencies. He will contact them next week. Tamesha and the family agree on the plan and the method for evaluating the plan. Tamesha also reviews the list of community resources with Becky and Jack. They all agree on which one to contact. They agree to discuss Becky's concern about caring for her children at the next visit.

ASSESSMENT TOOLS 4-2

Family Assessment

Family Members

Member	Birth Date	Sex	Marital Status	Education
Becky	7/15/78	♀	Married	College grad
Jack	11/10/76	M	Married	College grad
Joe	9/18/04	M		
Kevin	2/15/06	M		
Michael	2/22/08	M		

Culturagram

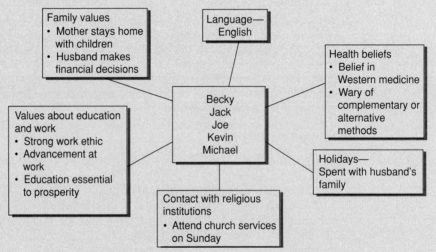

Stage of Illness

In what stage of illness is this family? (See Table 4-2.)

Diagnosis stage

What are this family's priority needs?

Relief from anxiety information, to be with and helpful to the client, and support for personal needs

What is the role of the nurse in this stage?

Emotional support, educator, assessor of family

(continued)

ASSESSMENT TOOLS 4-2

Family Assessment (*Continued*)

Developmental Assessment

What is this family's developmental stage?

Preschool age stage

Is the family meeting the tasks of its stage?

No, the added energy depletion of Becky's illness has caused profound exhaustion for all members of the family

Does, or will, the client's health problem interrupt the family's ability to meet the developmental tasks? If yes, how does it interrupt it?

Becky's illness has interrupted the family's ability to meet the developmental tasks. Becky and Jack state they are "unable to keep up with the demands of the kids, the baby, and rigors of daily living."

State nursing interventions to assist family members in meeting their developmental tasks.

1. Identify specific parental roles that Becky and Jack want to retain.
2. Identify parental responsibilities that they are willing to give up to someone else.
3. Identify possible support persons who could assist more with child care.
4. Determine other household tasks that can be assumed by family members or community services.

Functional Assessment

Does the family meet the individual's need for affection, love, and understanding?

Both Becky and Jack continue to be very affectionate and loving to each other and their children. This is evident in the way they interact with each other and with the children, hold the children, explain things to them, and comfort them. The children are in turn affectionate to Becky. Becky states, "My sister has provided me with a lot of emotional support."

(continued)

ASSESSMENT TOOLS 4-2

Family Assessment (*Continued*)

Does the family meet the individual's need for physical necessities and care?

Jack is able to continue working, and he still has the opportunity to take some time off if necessary. Becky is unable to fulfill her prior role responsibilities of homemaker, which included cooking, cleaning, marketing, and most of the child care. Becky states that she is "exhausted and able to participate only in a limited manner in the care of the children and the work of running the household." Becky states, "I want to be able to bathe the kids and read them their bedtime story. I also want to continue to give Michael his bottles." Note disorderly surroundings with the children's toys, dirty clothes, and dirty dishes scattered in all of the rooms. The children are cranky, and the baby cries most of the visit.

Does the family have the economic resources necessary to provide for the basic needs of the family?

Jack states, "My job is very secure. I have been lucky that I have a job which allows me to provide so well for my family. I have a lot of vacation time saved up because we were going to take a big family vacation next summer."

Is the family meeting the function of reproduction as defined by the family?

Yes

Is the family meeting the family function of socialization? Is the family fulfilling the function to socialize children to become productive members of society?

Becky states, "It is very hard to provide guidance and discipline for Joe because I am so tired. He wears me down. Maybe he should be in day care a few days a week. There is a day care at our church, which is only a few blocks away."

Does the family attempt to actively cope with problems?

Becky says, "Jack does not want to talk about the future and what the doctor has said about my prognosis. He believes that I will be better by summer. He has been so angry since the diagnosis." Jack says, "I believe that Becky will be better by summer. She has the best doctor in the Midwest, and people survive from cancer all the time."

(continued)

ASSESSMENT TOOLS 4-2

Family Assessment (*Continued*)

Assessment of Presence of Characteristics of a Healthy Family

Is communication between members open, direct, and honest, and are feelings and needs shared?

Becky says, "It is hard for Jack to share his feelings with me. I think he talks to his dad but not to me. Sometimes his dad tells me what he has said. It's hard for me to tell him what I really think because it seems like then I am giving up." Jack says, "I have a close relationship with my dad. It is so hard for me to talk to Becky about my fears because I want to be upbeat and hopeful; I don't want her to have to comfort me."

Do family members express self-worth with integrity, responsibility, compassion, and love to and for one another?

Both Becky and Jack express love and concern for each other. They are so concerned about each other that Becky states, "Our concern for each other gets in the way of open communication."

Are family rules known to all members?

Becky and Jack describe the family in precisely the same way—"Becky is responsible for the care of the children and the home and Jack is the bread winner."

Are rules clear and flexible, and do they allow individual members freedom?

Both state that before Joe was born, Becky worked full time and the home maintenance was shared. Becky says that since she became ill, Jack has assumed many of the responsibilities at home. Becky states, "He is working too hard and is exhausted. We need help!"

Does the family have regular links to society that demonstrate trust and friendship?

During the home visit, three neighbors came over with food, and two people called. There were many plants, cards, and flower arrangements in the house. Becky stated, "Our friends have been wonderful. They have offered to take the kids, brought food, and visited."

Do family members belong to various groups and clubs?

The family is active in a church, and Jack is involved in an environmental group. Becky has many friends in the neighborhood.

CONCLUSIONS

The family is the basic social unit of American society and has long been the primary focus of nursing care in the community. Understanding family structure, roles, and functions is essential in providing comprehensive nursing care both in the acute care and community-based setting. Knowledge of healthy family functioning permits the nurse to identify unhealthy functioning and take appropriate action, including referrals to community resources. Often, families with an ill family member are in crisis and require nursing intervention or referrals.

Today, more than ever, the nurse must be cognizant of the needs, feelings, problems, and views of the family when providing care for the individual client. Community-based nursing requires the nurse to provide care in the context of the client's family to enhance self-care. This is accomplished by assessing the client in the context of the family.

To provide continuous care with a preventive focus, the nurse must consider the family's ability and needs. The care of the client in the context of the family is enhanced by following the principles of community-based care.

What's on the Web

Bright Futures for Families
Internet address:
http://www.brightfutures.org
This Web site is supported by the Maternal and Child Health Bureau of the U.S. Department of Health and Human Services.

Using Family History to Promote Health
Internet address: http://www.cdc.gov/genomics/public/famhistMain.htm
This Web site provides fact sheets, case studies, tools, presentations, and other resources that may be used with family histories to promote health. Very informative resource.

Centers for Disease Control and Prevention: National Office of Public Health Genomics
Internet Address: http://www.cdc.gov/genomics/default.htm
This site provides updated information on how human genomic discoveries can be used to improve health and prevent disease. It also provides links to CDC-wide activities in public health genomics.

References and Bibliography

Allender, J. A., & Spradley, B. W. (2005). *Community health nursing: Concepts and practice* (6th ed.). Philadelphia: Lippincott Williams & Wilkins.

Carpenito, L. (2006). *Nursing diagnosis: Application to clinical practice* (11th ed.). Philadelphia: Lippincott Williams & Wilkins.

Congress, E. P., & Kung, W. W. (2005). Using the culturagram to assess and empower culturally diverse families. In E. P. Congress & M. J. Gonzales (Eds.) *Multicultural perspectives in working with families* (pp. 4–21). New York: Springer.

Duvall, E. M., & Miller, B. (1985). *Marriage and family development* (6th ed.). New York: Harper & Row.

Federal Interagency Forum on Children and Family Statistics. (2006). *American's children: Key national indicators of well-being, 2006.* Washington, DC: U.S. Government Printing Office.

Freeman, K., O'Dell, C., & Meola, C. (2000). Issues in families of children with brain tumors. *Oncology Nursing Forum, 27*(5), 843–848.

Holden, J., Harrison, L., & Johnson, M. (2002). Families, nurses and intensive care patients: A review of the literature. *Journal of Clinical Nursing, 11*(2), 140–148.

Marino, L., & Kooser, J. (1986). The psychosocial care of cancer clients and their families: Periods of high risk. In L. Marino (Ed.), *Cancer Nursing* (pp. 53–66). St. Louis: Mosby.

Maslow, A. H. (1954). *Motivation and personality.* New York: Harper & Row.

O'Connell, K. L. (2006). Needs of families affected by mental illness. *Journal of Psychosocial Nursing and Mental Health Services, 44*(3), 40–48.

Satir, V. (1972). *People making.* Palo Alto, CA: Science and Behavioral Books.

Spitz, R. (1945). Hospitalization: Inquiry into genesis of psychiatric conditions in early childhood. Psychoanalytic Study of the Child, 1.

Wagner-Cox, P. 2005. Lessons learned: From the other side of the nurse-patient family relationship. *Homecare Nurses, 23*(4), 218–223.

Wickrama, K. A., Lorenz, F. O., Conger, R. D., Elder, G. H. Jr., Todd Abraham, W., & Fang, S. A. (2006). Changes in family financial circumstances and the physical health of married and recently divorced mothers. *Social Science & Medicine (1982), 63,* 123–136.

LEARNING ▼ ACTIVITIES

◆ LEARNING ACTIVITY 4-1

You are working in a chemical dependency day treatment unit for adolescents. Your primary client is Chris, a 16-year-old boy, admitted yesterday. His father, Michael, and his stepmother, Joanna, brought in Chris after a family fight. Michael says that Chris' grades in school have been on a downhill slide since his sophomore year began 6 months ago. Both parents have noticed that Chris' behavior has changed. He is spending more time in his room; his appearance has become disheveled; and he is increasingly more listless, fatigued, hostile, and erratic. Michael describes his son as a cheerful, focused boy—until this year.

Chris has a 13-year-old brother, and both boys live for a week with their mother, Lori, and a week with their father, Michael, and his second wife, Joanna. Lori and Michael have been divorced for 4 years. Michael and his new wife have a 1-year-old daughter. Lori visited Chris this morning. While at the treatment center, she mentions that she is suing Michael for money he owes her. After lunch, you are visiting with Michael, and he relates to you that two of Lori's brothers are lawyers, and the family is always suing someone for something. Last year, he says, Lori claimed that she had lupus and collected disability payments until the insurance company discovered it was a phony claim.

During the initial family conference, Lori blames Michael for Chris's problems, maintaining that Michael has suffered from depression over the past years. Michael talks about his feelings: that the ongoing battle between him and Lori is stressful for their children. He wants the conflict to end.

1. Construct a genogram for this family.
2. Identify which stage of illness this family is experiencing. List data that led you to this conclusion.
3. Describe additional information you will need to plan care.
4. Identify the developmental stage of each member of the family. Explain how you will use this information.

5. Identify the developmental stage of each family. Explain how you will use this information when planning care for Chris.
6. Detect which family functions are not being met.
7. Develop goals you hope to see with this family.
8. Propose referrals you could initiate.

◆ LEARNING ACTIVITY 4-2

Complete a family assessment on the family of a client you are caring for in clinical who has a nontraditional family structure. Use the family assessment tool in the text of this chapter (Assessment Tools 4-1) to collect basic information on the family. After you have completed the family assessment, respond to the following questions.

1. Identify the family problem or need that may interfere with the client's recovery.
2. Identify the family problem or need that may interfere with the client's ability to maximize his or her functioning within the limitations of his or her health condition.
3. Identify the family strengths that will enhance the client's recovery.
4. What client or family goals do you hope to see based on the family's needs stated in the first question?
5. List nursing interventions that will help you, the client, and the family achieve the goals you have identified.
6. Describe ways you will evaluate your nursing plan for the family.

◆ LEARNING ACTIVITY 4-3

Identify three agencies in your community that provide health services for families. Using the form in the Instructor's Manual for Chapter 2, group project No. 2, analyze the agency you have selected.

◆ LEARNING ACTIVITY 4-4

Locate a local, state, or federal program that assists families. Call the state or county department of health in your community for suggestions or the public health or public health nursing division. Common federal programs are Headstart; the Women, Infants, and Children (WIC) Program; and immunization programs. These all have Web sites and are administered through county or state agencies. What are the goals of the program you contacted? Do you think the program creates benefits for families? What are the benefits? (This can be a program in your own community, such as an after-school program for children or a federal program like Headstart.)

◆ LEARNING ACTIVITY 4-5

1. In your clinical journal, create a genogram of your family showing three generations.
   • What patterns do you see regarding health issues as you analyze your own genogram?
   • Determine which developmental stage your family is in by using Table 4-3 or Table 4-5. Examine whether your family members are meeting the developmental tasks of the stage. If not, analyze which is preventing this from occurring.
   • What was the most important thing you learned from doing this activity?

2. In your clinical journal, discuss a situation you have observed or served as the caregiver in which the family enhanced or interrupted the client's self-care or return to maximum functioning. What was the family doing to influence the client's health? What else could they have done? Use theory from this chapter to support your ideas.
   • What did you do (or would you have done) as a nurse to facilitate family involvement in this situation? What did you learn from this experience? What would you do differently next time? Use a theory from this chapter to support your ideas.

SKILLS FOR COMMUNITY-BASED NURSING PRACTICE

N ow that you understand the concepts of community-based nursing, including the importance of a healthy community, understanding cultural surroundings, and care of the family, you are ready to explore how you can develop skills in applying your knowledge. Skills in assessment, teaching, case management, and continuity of care are all important in community-based nursing. Although you probably have studied these concepts previously, they are discussed in this unit in the context of their specific relationship to community-based health care. Nursing interventions directed to the care of individuals, families, and communities or populations in community-based care will be emphasized. This chapter is only intended to be an introduction to using nursing process in community-based settings. Chapters 8, 9, and 10 discuss in more depth the topics of health promotion, disease prevention, and the corresponding nursing interventions for community-based care.

Chapter 5 opens with a discussion of the use of nursing process including assessment, planning, intervention, and evaluation of the individual client, family, and community in community-based care. An evolving case study illustrates the principles and concepts of nursing process related to the care of the client and family in community settings. Population-based care of communities highlight community assessment including concepts, methods, and applications.

The importance of client teaching along with teaching theory and developmental considerations in Chapter 6 leads to a discussion of the relationship of the nursing process to the teaching process.

Chapter 7 discusses continuity of care and the role of the case manager in community-based settings. It is all too common for clients and families to experience gaps in care as they move from one setting to another. It is the responsibility of the nurse to work in collaboration with the client, family, and other professionals to build bridges between settings, caregivers, and other resources. Entering and exiting the various agencies and providers along with the skills and competencies involved in continuity of care are covered.

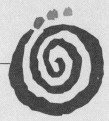

CHAPTER 5

Assessment: Individual, Family, and Community

ROBERTA HUNT

LEARNING OBJECTIVES

1. Identify components essential to assessment of the client, family, and communities in community-based settings.
2. Discuss health needs common to community-based settings.
3. Identify the components of the 15-minute family interview.
4. Discuss the value of population-based care.
5. Utilize nursing interventions designed for community-focused population-based care.
6. Describe assessment, planning, intervention, and evaluation of community-focused population-based care.
7. Discuss methods for collecting community data.
8. Apply nursing process to situations including the care of the client, the family, and the community.

KEY TERMS

activities of daily living (ADL)
assessment
community assessment
community health need
constructed surveys
demographics
environmental assessment
epidemic
functional assessment
holistic assessment

informant interviews
instrumental activities of daily living (IADL)
mortality
morbidity
participant observations
power systems
secondary data
social system
spiritual assessment
windshield survey

CHAPTER TOPICS

- ◆ Nursing Process in Community-Based Settings
- ◆ History of Nursing Process in Community Settings
- ◆ Nursing Process for the Care of the Individual Client in Community Settings
- ◆ Assessment of the Family
- ◆ Population-Based Care: Assessment of the Community
- ◆ Public Policy Making
- ◆ Conclusions

THE NURSE SPEAKS

While working as a staff nurse in a children's hospital, I had the opportunity to care for a 13-year-old young man on his day of discharge. Josh was an "old pro" when it came to the hospital environment, as he had endured 12 reconstructive surgeries on his right ear since birth. When I entered his room, Josh was lying in bed with the head of the bed slightly elevated. He was alone in the room and had turned off the radio and TV. He had a large dressing over his right ear, and a bandage wrapped around his head to hold the dressing in place. On assessing his vital signs, I noted that he was afebrile; however, his blood pressure and pulse were slightly elevated. After assessing his vital signs, I asked Josh to rate his pain on a numeric scale of 0 to 10. Without hesitation, Josh replied a 9. I was quite concerned about his pain intensity level as the surgeons had already examined his ear and decided that he was ready to go home. In addition, they recommended over-the-counter analgesics for postoperative ear pain.

Before consulting with his physicians, I continued with my pain assessment. I asked Josh about the quality and duration of his pain, along with analgesic effectiveness. Then I asked Josh what the color of pain was, and he replied red. Lastly, I asked Josh to use my red pen to mark on a body outline pain tool the exact location of the pain. Much to my surprise, when Josh handed the pain tool back to me, there was a large red mark on his left leg, the donor site for his ear grafting!

When I inquired about the pain in his right ear, he replied, "What pain? My ear feels fine." Josh taught me an important lesson about the subjectivity of pain.

Although the obvious site of pain was his right ear, as a nurse, I cannot assume the obvious. I needed to be holistic in my pain assessment and remember to assess the location(s) of pain. Based on the valuable information from Josh, I was able to consult with his physicians and arrange for an effective analgesic to cover the pain at his donor site that would allow him to have pain control once he was home.

—SUSAN O'CONNER-VON, DNSc, RNC, Assistant Professor, School of Nursing
University of Minnesota, Minneapolis, Minnesota

NURSING PROCESS IN COMMUNITY-BASED SETTINGS

There are similarities and differences in the way that nursing process is used in community-based settings as compared with the acute care setting. It is important that nurses in community settings emphasize that it is a deliberate, adaptable, cyclic, client-focused, and interactive process. Further, in community settings nursing process is used with wider application to guide care of individuals, families, and populations or communities. Whatever the setting the basic construct is the same: Assessment, diagnosis, outcomes, planning/intervention, and evaluation.

HISTORY OF NURSING PROCESS IN COMMUNITY SETTINGS

Nursing has long understood the significance of the community in the health of the individual and family. Florence Nightingale set the scene early for involvement of health care professionals in assessing and intervening in establishing healthy communities. Her analysis of 1861 census data became the foundation of England's sanitary reform acts which is an excellent example of use of nursing process to identify a community diagnosis (Woodham-Smith, 1950). Nightingale accomplished this end by focusing on assessment of the physical and social environment and its role in causing or contributing to illness. She identified how sanitation, nutrition, and rest contribute to successful recovery from injury and illness as well as determined the relationship among adequate housing, recreation, employment, and health. From this data she identified community-wide problems (diagnosis); determined what changes needed to be made (outcomes); formulated plans to address the problem, the sanitary reform act, (intervention); and evaluated the results.

NURSING PROCESS FOR THE CARE OF THE INDIVIDUAL CLIENT IN COMMUNITY SETTINGS

Assessment, the first step in nursing process, is a dynamic, ongoing process that uses observations and interactions to collect information, recognize changes, analyze needs, and plan care. Physicians primarily use assessment to determine pathology. Hospital-based nurses use assessment as the first step in the nursing process, for ongoing monitoring of acute conditions, and as an essential component in ensuring continuity with discharge planning. In community-based settings, assessment provides baseline information to help evaluate physiologic and psychologic normality and functional capacity, and to identify environmental factors that may enhance or impair the individual's health status. Because the community-based nurse sees clients only periodically and the status of conditions varies over time, thorough assessment is the cornerstone of quality community care.

To perform an accurate assessment, the nurse must communicate effectively, observe systematically, and interpret the collected data accurately (Carpenito, 2006). Typically, the health assessment consists of the interview and health history. The focus and parameters of the assessment depend on the scope of the service provided by the agency and the role of the nurse in that service. However, the first contact is always extremely important because it acts as the foundation for the nurse–client relationship. Establishing trust beginning with the first contact is imperative.

Community care differs from nursing care provided in tertiary care settings. Because the client and family are in charge of most aspects of care most of the time, the nurse is primarily a facilitator of self-care rather than solely a care provider. Thus, the assessment process is intended to assess the client, whether it be the individual client, family, or community, and to identify needs and strengths and proceed accordingly. It is a continuous process that occurs in the context in which the response occurs. Thus, the response must be considered within the environment, whether it be family, culture, immediate physical environment, or community environment. A holistic assessment often requires collaboration of many professionals. This approach expands the usual definition of **holistic assessment**—body, mind, and spirit—to an even broader view.

This comprehensive view is used across the life span. The nurse in community-based settings is always diligent to complete a comprehensive assessment but is particularly attentive when caring for vulnerable populations. Thus, when assessing a newborn during a home visit, the nurse will bear in mind that a holistic assessment of the physical and psychological condition of the newborn, the immediate environment, and the skill of the primary caregivers is essential to the infant's normal growth and development and protection from harm. The newborn is unable to speak on his or her behalf, so a thorough assessment is the primary way the nurse initiates advocacy for the infant. Thus, comprehensive assessment is essential to injury and disease prevention as well as health promotion and maintenance.

Infants and Children

When assessing the infant and toddler, the nurse should begin by interviewing the primary caregiver. Typically the areas covered include nutrition, growth and development, and vision and hearing. When working with families with infants, it is essential to assess and promote attachment. Community-Based Nursing Care Guidelines 5-1 presents some helpful suggestions.

Monitoring growth and development is easily done by weighing the infant, measuring length and head circumference, and plotting the results on a growth grid (National Center for Health Statistics, 2006 @www.cdc.gov/growthcharts/). Psychologic status should also be assessed. Development of the infant, toddler, and preschooler is assessed by using the Denver Developmental Screening Tool (Figure 5-1).

COMMUNITY-BASED NURSING CARE GUIDELINES ▶ 5-1

Nursing Interventions to Promote Attachment

The following are interventions that are directed to parents to assist them to develop an attachment with their newborn.

- Explore the mother and partner's feelings of moving from pregnancy to postpartum.
- Ask the parents what they see in the newborn that were behaviors from the baby in utero.
- Remind the parents that the newborn knows their voices from hearing them when the baby was in utero.
- Tell the parents that newborns like being flexed and close to them as they were positioned before they were born.
- Emphasize the partner's role in nurturing the mother to nurture the newborn.
- Encourage the partner to get support as needed.
- Compliment the mother on her ability to read her newborn's cues, for example, the need for comfort, nourishment, and diaper change. Bring to the mother's attention the infant's response to her care.
- Comment positively regarding the newborn's progress.
- Ask about the mother's well-being.

O'Leary, J. (2006). *After loss: Parenting in the next pregnancy.* Minneapolis: Allina Publishing.

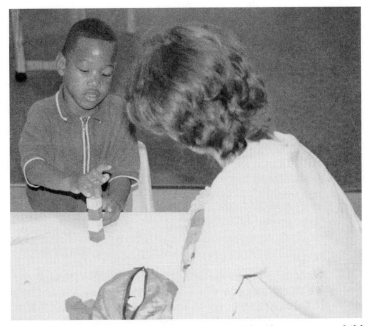

FIGURE 5-1. ▶ Developmental screening uses a series of tasks to screen children for developmental delays.

Once variations from normal development are identified, whether assets or needs, the nurse identifies the outcomes, interventions, and criteria for evaluation. For example, if an infant's weight does not tract within the norms of the growth chart the nurse may ask the mother about the child's feeding patterns. Determining what, how, how much, and when the infant is eating, the nurse may be able to suggest some alternatives. The nurse and the mother of the infant may devise a feeding plan and determine how much weight they would like the infant to gain before the next visit. At the next visit if the outcomes are reached, the nurse and the mother may continue with the same plan. Alternatively, if the infant does not gain weight, the nurse may assess for other problems or refer for additional assessment by a nurse practitioner or physician.

Infants and toddlers are not routinely screened for vision and hearing until 3 years of age. However, a parent's observations may indicate the possible presence of vision and hearing problems. One out of every 20 infants may be at risk for abnormal vision, according to the American Optometric Association (Huggins, 2006). This is troubling because impaired vision can affect a child's cognitive, emotional, neurological, and physical development by potentially limiting the type and amount of information to which the child is exposed (Bauer, 2005). For assessment of vision with an infant older than 6 weeks of age, ask the parent the following questions:

◆ Does the infant return your smile?
◆ Do the infant's eyes follow you as you walk past or move around the room?
◆ Do you have any concerns that the infant is unable to see?

To assess for evidence of the need to screen the vision of toddlers, ask the parents the following questions:

◆ Does the child cover one eye when looking at objects?
◆ Does the child tilt his or her head to look at things?

◆ Does the child hold toys, books, or other objects very close or very far away to look at them?
◆ Does the child rub his or her eyes, squint, frown, or blink frequently?

If the parent responds affirmatively to one or more of these questions, the nurse may use the intervention of referral to an eye doctor so that the child has additional assessment.

Infants at high risk for hearing impairment should be screened at birth. These include infants with the following:

◆ Family history of childhood hearing impairment
◆ Perinatal infection (e.g., cytomegalovirus, rubella, herpes, toxoplasmosis)
◆ Anatomic malformations of the head or neck
◆ Low birth weight (<1,500 g)
◆ Hyperbilirubinemia exceeding indications for exchange transfusion
◆ Bacterial meningitis
◆ Birth asphyxia, infants with an Apgar score of 0 to 3, failure to breathe spontaneously in 10 minutes, or hypotonia of 2 hours past birth

Even if an infant's hearing has already been tested, the parents should be aware of signs that hearing is intact. During the first year, most babies react to loud noises, imitate sounds, and begin to respond to their name. By the age of 2 most children play with their voice, imitate simple words, and enjoy games like peek-a-boo and pat-a-cake. They may also use two-word sentences to talk about and ask for things. To determine if a toddler should be screened for hearing impairment, ask if the child has had frequent ear infections or has the same risk factors listed previously for infant screening. Also assess the child's speech. Hearing impairments often become apparent when the child begins to talk and are evidenced by the child's difficulty with pronunciation, resulting in speech that is hard to comprehend. If there are deficits in any of these areas, the parent should be referred for additional assessment.

Periodic assessment of preschool- and school-age children includes a health history and physical and developmental evaluation. As with the infant and toddler, height, weight, and head circumference are important indicators of growth. Not only do these measurements determine if the child is following a normal growth curve, but they also reflect whether the child's weight is proportional to his or her height. If the child does not follow within the parameters of the growth chart, referral to a pediatric nurse practitioner, pediatrician, or other physician is necessary.

It is important to assess and intervene in the area of nutrition when caring for infants, children, and adolescents. Screening tools for infants, children, and adolescents are found in Appendix A. Obesity is on the increase, with more than 16% of children between the ages of 6 and 19 years overweight (Centers for Disease Control and Prevention (a) [CDC], 2006). Because obesity substantially increases the risk of illness from high blood pressure, high cholesterol, type 2 diabetes, heart disease and stroke, arthritis, sleep disturbances, and cancer (breast, prostate, and colon), it is important to identify overweight children early to allow for early intervention.

Adults and Elderly Adults

Increasingly, the caseload of nurses working in community-based settings will reflect the graying of the population. By 2030, 20% of the population will be older than 65 years, and by 2050 the number of persons 65 and over will more than double to 80 million. The fastest growing segment of the elderly population into the next century is individuals over 85 years of age (United States Census Bureau, 2006). Because contact with the nurse is intermittent in community-based settings, it is essential that nursing care be comprehensive. Holistic care addresses environmental, cultural, spiritual, and nutritional factors, as well as functional and physical aspects of the client.

Assessing and Intervening With Functional Status

The **functional assessment** requires the nurse to determine whether there are environmental, cognitive, neurologic, or behavioral barriers to independent function and self-care. Societal and cultural factors may also create barriers. The primary consideration of the functional assessment is whether the client needs the assistance of another person for daily function. The client's ability to conceptualize an activity is just as important as the client's physical ability to perform the activity. Once functional status is assessed the needs and strengths or assets of the client are identified and the outcomes determined.

Using nursing process through a functional assessment begins with an **environmental assessment** or evaluation of the client's home and neighborhood environment. The client may be physically, cognitively, or emotionally disabled yet able to function independently except for the limitations created by barriers in the home. The next areas assessed are neurological status, cognitive and emotional status, integumentary status, and respiratory status. Last, the individual's abilities to complete **activities of daily living (ADL)** and **instrumental activities of daily living (IADL)** should be assessed. Analyzing a client's ADL is a standard method for evaluating ability to perform the activities that are essential for independent living. They include grooming, dressing, bathing, toileting, transferring, walking, and feeding or eating. IADL involve planning and preparing light meals, traveling, doing laundry, housekeeping, shopping, and using the telephone. Assessment Tools 5-1 presents a complete functional assessment.

CLIENT SITUATIONS IN PRACTICE

Richard, a 63-year-old widower who has just had a hip replacement is going home from the hospital tomorrow. Richard is 5′ 9″ tall and weighs 216 pounds. He also has extensive rheumatoid arthritis which makes it difficult for him to manage self-care at home and he is diabetic. When the nurse assesses ADL/IADLs and asks him about how he will manage when he is home he says, "With the walker and the trouble I have with my hands, I am not sure how I will be able to dress myself, take a bath, or prepare food let alone go to the grocery store." When the nurse asks Richard about his typical diet in a normal day he states "I live a block from a bakery and I like to walk down there at 5:00 PM every day to buy the day old doughnuts, cookies, and pies. I have a sweet tooth." Functional assessment indicates Richard may have potential for ineffective therapeutic regimen management. When the nurse assesses the neighborhood she learns that Richard can seek services through the Block Nurse program in his neighborhood. The goal will be that Richard will relate intent to practice healthy behaviors (in this case adequate nutrition) needed to recover from his surgery. Through the nursing interventions of counseling, case management, and referral and follow-up, Richard is referred to the Block Nurse program in his neighborhood (see page 339 in Chapter 11). A nurse from the Block Nurse program will visit him the day after he is discharged from the hospital.

ASSESSMENT TOOLS 5-1

Functional Assessment

Environmental Assessment

Structural Barriers

Do stairs in the home limit the client's independent mobility
to reach the bathroom, kitchen, and bedroom?
Check for presence of the following:

Handrails on stairs and in the bathroom and tub	Inadequate lighting
	Safe gas and electrical appliances
Narrow doorways	Improperly stored hazardous
Unsafe flooring or floor covering	materials

Neurologic Status

Perceptual Function

Is the client able to perceive his or her immediate environment?

Sensory Function

Does the client have impaired vision?
Does the client have impaired hearing and ability to understand spoken
language?
Is the client able to participate in an appropriate conversation 10 to 15 minutes
long?
Is the client experiencing chronic pain?

Cognitive and Emotional Status

Does the client make eye contact with the visitor, greet the visitor, and appear
to be well groomed or have made an attempt to be?
Assess if the client is oriented to person, place, and time. Work these questions
into the conversation.
Ask the client to perform a simple task such as getting the nurse a glass of
water (but without putting the client on the spot or acting as if this is a test).

Integumentary Status

If the client is unable to perform ADL or IADL because of a wound, dressing,
or pain, then the wound impairs the client's functional ability.

Respiratory Status

Respiratory status is impaired if the client's respiratory status, typically shortness of breath or dyspnea, prevents functioning. Here are some indications:

If the client stops or slows down the activity before it is completed
If the client sits down midway through or after the activity
If the client complains of chest tightness or pain or breathes in quick
shallow breaths

Adapted from Neal, L. J. (1998). Functional assessment of the home health client. *Home
Healthcare Nurse, 16*(10), 670–677, and Hunt, R. (Ed.). (2000). *Readings in community-based
nursing* (pp. 168–177). Philadelphia: Lippincott Williams & Wilkins.

Nutrition

Nutrition screening is an important part of providing care for clients across the life span in community-based settings. An example of a nutrition screening tool for adults is found in Assessment Tools 5-2. After assessing the client's nutritional risk, the nurse, client, and family will devise a plan together to address the identified needs. If the client requires additional assessment, a nurse specially trained in nutrition or a Dietitian assesses the client.

Assessing Medication Knowledge

Assessing medication knowledge and practice is an important aspect of comprehensive assessment. Polypharmacy, the use of multiple medications, is common among anyone with a chronic condition but particularly in older people because of the multiple chronic illnesses they experience. Fifty percent of individuals over the age of 65 have multiple chronic conditions. Studies show that these elderly take an average of two to six prescribed medications routinely and concurrently use one to three. Predictors for polypharmacy include complex drug therapy, multiple prescribers, elderly client, psychosocial contributors, and adverse drug reactions (Austin, 2006). However, correct use of medication is a concern across the life span. The tool in Assessment Tools 5-3 can be used in a community-based setting to assess a client's medication use. After assessing the client's knowledge base, the nurse and client then devise a plan to address identified learning needs. Interventions to address medication safety range from teaching the individual client to developing a teaching program for all clients cared for on a specific unit

CLIENT SITUATIONS IN PRACTICE

Marge, the nurse from the Block Nurse program, visits Richard the day after his morning discharge from the hospital. He is sitting in a chair in the living room. He is unshaven and looks like he has slept in his clothes. He stands up and says he is weak, in pain, and has not eaten since yesterday. He did not take his medication today. Pain and medication assessment indicates Richard has need for nursing intervention due to ineffective therapeutic regimen management. First, Marge does a quick medication assessment. He states he wants to take his medication but is neither able to open the new bottle of medication that he received the day before nor does he have a family member or friend to help him take his medications. Marge's goal is that Richard will regularly take his medication to promote postoperative healing. Using health teaching, Marge puts his medication in an egg carton and labels the time and day they are to be taken. On her next visit she will bring a plastic medication case. Marge knows the services in the neighborhood. Through the nursing interventions of case-finding, care management, and referral, Marge calls Meals on Wheels to deliver a meal that day and for a neighbor to get some simple groceries for him for the next few days. The goal is that Richard will have access to adequate nutrition needed to recover from his surgery and facilitate incision healing. Richard states that his other main concern now is to be able to have a bath twice a week. Using the nursing intervention of case management, and referral, Marge calls and arranges for a home health aid to come in to give him a bath twice a week. She and Richard then discuss how often he would like her to visit him in the next few weeks and other help that he believes he needs.

ASSESSMENT TOOLS 5-2

Level I Nutrition Screen

LEVEL I NUTRITION SCREEN	CLIENT		
	PAYER	TEAM	MR#
	DATE		TIME

BODY WEIGHT AND HEIGHT (Measure height to the nearest inch and weight to the nearest pound):
PRIMARY DIAGNOSIS: _____ Weight (lb): _____ Height (in): _____
OTHER DIAGNOSIS: _____ Special diet. Type: _____ Calorie limitations: _____

Check any boxes that are TRUE for the individual:
- ■ ☐ Has lost or gained 10 pounds (or more) in the past six (6) months without wanting to.

EATING HABITS

■ ☐ Has appetite changed?	● ☐ Has difficulty chewing or swallowing.
■ ☐ Consumes dairy or dairy products once or not at all daily (and does not take calcium supplement).	◆ ☐ Has pain in mouth, teeth, or gums.
	☐ Anorexia.
■ ☐ Consumes fruits or drinks fruit juice once or not at all daily.	☐ Has more than one alcoholic drink per day (woman); more than two drinks per day (man).
■ ☐ Does not have adequate fluid intake (less than 4 glasses [8 oz] per day).	☐ Usually eats alone.
◆ ☐ Eats vegetables two or fewer times daily.	● ☐ Does not have enough food to eat each day.
◆ ☐ Eats breads, cereals, pasta, rice, or other grains five or fewer times daily.	◆ ☐ Does not eat anything on one or more days each month.

LIVING ENVIRONMENT

◆ ☐ Lives alone.	☐ Does not have a stove and/or refrigerator.
■ ☐ Are there more than six people living in household?	☐ Lives in a home with inadequate heating or cooling.
■ ☐ Is housebound.	■ ☐ Is unable or prefers not to spend money on food (< $25–$30 per person spent on food each week).
■ ☐ Does not have significant caregiver.	

FUNCTIONAL STATUS

Usually or always needs assistance with these activities: (check each that apply)	Other Problems:
◆ ☐ Walking or moving about.	● ☐ Nausea. ☐ Vomiting.
■ ☐ Eating.	● ☐ Diarrhea (> 3–5 per/day for > 2 days).
■ ☐ Preparing food.	◆ ☐ Constipation (> 2 weeks).
● ☐ Shopping for food or other necessities.	◆ ☐ Over 80 years of age.

INSTRUCTIONS: To be completed within 5 days from start of care date.   TOTALS:
Repeat Level I screen at least every 120 days (every other recertification).
HIGH RISK:
- ● Proceed to Level II Nutritional Screen.   ● _____
- ◆ 5 or more "◆," proceed to Level II Nutritional Screen.   ◆ _____
- ■ 8 or more "■," go to Level II Nutritional Screen.   ■ _____

Categories left blank should be addressed by the signature nutrition screener or go to Level II.

Signature of Screener: Date:

ASSESSMENT TOOLS 5-3

Medication Assessment

Note to administrator: The sequence of the interview, along with the instructional statements, are merely suggestions, and should be considered guidelines when using the interview. It is acceptable to reword statements or change the format to better meet the needs of the individual, yet all topics must be included in the assessment.

Start Time: _____

Who is the respondent? ☐ Client ☐ Spouse ☐ Other (list) _____

Please Check the Appropriate Response

Administrator: *"I need to see all of your medications. Please show me those you take every day and those you take occasionally. Don't forget to show me eyedrops, insulin, laxatives, vitamins, antacids, ointments, or any over-the-counter drugs you sometimes use. Are there any other medications that you regularly take that are not here today?"* (Attach copies of medication profiles to document drugs.)

I. Medication Administration and Storage

☐ Yes ☐ No Can client open a pill bottle? (Have client demonstrate.)
☐ Yes ☐ No Can client break a pill in half? (Have client demonstrate. Omit if not applicable.)
☐ Yes ☐ No Does someone help you take your medicine?
☐ Yes ☐ No Do you use any type of system to help you take your pills, such as a pillbox or a calendar?
List: _____
☐ Yes ☐ No Do you have problems swallowing your pills?
Where do you store your medicines? _____

II. Medication Purchasing Habits

What drugstore do you use? _____
☐ Yes ☐ No Does the drugstore you use deliver the medications to your home?
If no, then how do you get your medications? _____
☐ Yes ☐ No Do you always use the same drugstore? If no, explain: _____
☐ Yes ☐ No Do financial difficulties ever prevent you from buying your medications?

III. Attitudes

☐ Excellent How would you describe your health? _____
☐ Good What do you see as your health needs? _____
☐ Fair
☐ Poor
☐ Yes ☐ No Does taking your medications upset your daily routine? If yes, explain: _____
☐ Yes ☐ No Do side effects from your medications upset your daily routine?
☐ Yes ☐ No Do your medications help you?
☐ Don't know
☐ Yes ☐ No Do you ever share your medications with anyone else?

(continued)

ASSESSMENT TOOLS 5-3

Medication Assessment (*Continued*)

IV. Lifestyle Habits

TIMES PER WEEK

_____ How often do you drink coffee, tea, or colas, or eat chocolate?

_____ How often do you use cigarettes, snuff, or tobacco products?

_____ How often do you consume beer, wine, or liquor?

_____ How often do you use recreational drugs, such as marijuana?

V. Home/Environment

Who else stays at your residence? (List relationship and age) _____

_____

If someone else lives in your home, does that person participate in your health care? _____

VI. Medication Profile

Record each medication separately on the following form: (Attach additional sheets as necessary.) _____

_____

_____

(Medicine Name, Dosage, Route, Expiration Date Exactly as Printed on Label)

☐ Yes ☐ No Can you read the name, dosage, and expiration date of this medicine? Why do you take the medication? _____

_____

How long have you taken this dosage? _____

When do you take the medicine and how many do you take?

_____

Do you know what the side effects are? List: _____

_____

☐ Yes ☐ No Does the medicine cause you any problems or side effects?

_____

What do you do if you experience side effects? (Stop the pills, call the doctor, etc.) _____

_____

Adapted with permission from DeBrew, J. K., Barba, B. E., & Tesh, A. S. (1998). Assessing medication knowledge and practice in older adults. *Home Healthcare Nurse, 16*(10), 686–692.

to developing hospital policy to require medication teaching (see Research in Community-Based Nursing Care 5-1).

Psychosocial Factors and Culture

Culture and the impact culture has on health and health beliefs are discussed in Chapters 3 and 4. A cultural assessment is always a part of the health history as it is imperative to incorporate the client's understanding of health-related issues,

RESEARCH IN COMMUNITY-BASED NURSING CARE ▶ 5-1

Evaluation of a Medication Education Program for Elderly Hospital In-Patients

The purpose of this study was to improve elderly patients' understanding and safe use of their medications. Patients 65 years old or older who spoke English were recruited to participate in the study. They were taking at least one medication on a daily basis and had a Mini-Mental State Examination score of at least 20 of 30, indicating that each participant was not significantly cognitively impaired. Each patient was taught about his or her medication on 3 consecutive days. A pretest of the patient knowledge about the medication was done prior to the education sessions and at a home visit following discharge from the hospital. Before the teaching sessions, patient medication knowledge showed that they knew 50% of the brand names, dosage, and times; 55% of medication purpose; and 15% of major side effects. At the follow-up home visit, the participants knew 90% of the names, dosage, and times ordered; 85% the purpose of the medicine; and 25% of the side effects. The researchers concluded that a simple, practical, nursing constructed program worked in improving medication knowledge even with patients with mild cognitive impairment.

Source: Shen, Q., Karr, M., Ko, A., Chan, D. K., Kahn, R., & Duvall, D. (2006) Evaluation of medication education program for elderly hospital in-patients. *Geriatric Nursing, 27*(3), 184–192.

the family's cultural perspective, and the various cultural viewpoints within neighborhoods, communities, and regions into all health care. A simple cultural assessment guide is seen in Assessment Tools 5-4. After the assessment is complete, the nurse, client, and family devise a plan of care, which is built around the identified cultural considerations.

Further, a psychosocial assessment in tandem with the cultural assessment will help the nurse understand the client in the context of family, as defined by the client's culture. This may involve exploring the topics of family decision maker, sick role behavior, language barriers, and community resources as they relate to the client's culture. This assessment may simply address the following issues:

◆ Who is the decision maker in the family?
◆ What are the characteristics of the sick role in the client's culture?
◆ Do any language barriers exist?
◆ What resources are available in the community that are sensitive to the client's culture?

Assessing Environment

An environmental assessment is an essential aspect of any assessment across the life span and across settings. Figure 5-2 and Assessment Tools 5-5 are useful when completing an environmental assessment.

The primary consideration of any environmental assessment is to identify safety concerns. Again, vulnerable populations, the very young and very old, and

(*text continues on page 139*)

ASSESSMENT TOOLS 5-4

Cultural Assessment Guide

Client _____

Cultural/ethnic identity_____

Religion _____ Spiritual rituals _____

Primary language _____ Speaks English?   Yes   No

Language resources _____

Health beliefs _____

Client's explanation of health problem _____

Traditional healer_____

   Contact information _____

Traditional treatments _____

   Where obtained and prepared _____

Do cultural health practices conflict with current medical practice?

   If so, how? _____

Expectations of nurse/care providers _____

Pain Assessment

Cultural patterns/client's perception of pain response _____

Nutrition Assessment

Ethnic preferences _____

Religious prohibitions and preferences _____

Sick foods _____
_____

Food intolerances/taboos _____

Medication Assessment

Client's perceptions of medications _____
_____

Possible pharmacogenetic variations _____
_____

Psychosocial Assessment

Family structure and decision-making patterns _____
_____

Sick role behavior _____
_____

Cultural/ethnic/religious resources/supportive systems _____
_____

Environmental Assessment Checklist

Patient _____ Patient Number _____ Team/Person Completing Form _____

Date and initial as each assessment area is addressed. Describe unsafe/unmet needs. Suggest modifications.

Assessment Areas	Safe/Meets Client's Needs	Unsafe/Needs Adaptation	Recommended Modifications and Possible Referral
Physiologic and Survival Needs Food/Fluids/Eating			
Elimination/Toileting			
Hygiene/Bathing/Grooming			
Clothing/Dressing			
Rest/Sleeping			
Medication			
Shelter			
Safety and Security Mobility and Fall Prevention			
Fire/Burn Prevention			
Crime/Injury Prevention			
Love and Belonging Caregiver			
Communication			
Family/Friends/Pets			
Self-Esteem, Self-Actualization Enjoyable/Meaningful Activities			

FIGURE 5-2. ▶ Environmental assessment checklist (see Assessment Tools 5-5 for questions for each category). Adapted from Narayan, M. C., & Tennant, J. (1997). Environmental assessment. *Home Healthcare Nurse, 15*(11), 799–805.

ASSESSMENT TOOLS 5-5

Questions to Complete: Environmental Assessment Checklist

Physiologic and Survival Needs

Food and Fluids/Eating

What does the client plan to eat? Drink? Who will prepare the food?
Is there food in the home? Who will do the grocery shopping?
Is the food properly stored? Does the refrigerator work?
Is there drinkable water?
Does the kitchen have barriers to the client actually preparing the food?
Are the pathways clear? Can the items be reached? Are there clean dishes?

Elimination/Toileting

Can the client get to the bathroom? Is the pathway clear? Is a bedside
  commode indicated?
Do assistive devices (wheelchairs, walkers) fit through the doorways and can
  the client turn?
Will the client have a hard time getting up and down from the commode?
  Would a raised toilet seat help? Grab bars? (Towel racks, if used for steadying,
  can pull away from the wall.)
Will the client be able to wash hands? Able to turn water off and on?

Hygiene/Bathing/Grooming

What is the plan for bathing? Bathtub? Shower? Shower chair? At the sink?
  Requires help?
Is there hot and cold running water? Is the water temperature 120° or less?
Are there grab bars next to the tub and shower?
Are there nonskid tiles/strips/appliques/rubber mats on tub bottom and
  shower floor?
Are the bathroom and fixtures clean?
What provisions are there for mouth care? Hair care?

Clothing/Dressing

Does the client have shoes or slippers that are easy to put on, fit properly with
  nonskid soles?
Will the client be able to change clothes?
Are the clothes so baggy that they could trip the client?
Are there clean clothes? How will the laundry be washed?

Rest/Sleeping

Where will the client sleep? Would the client benefit from a hospital bed?
  A trapeze?
How far is the bed from the floor? Can the client get in and out of
  the bed?
How much time will the client spend in bed? Does the client need a special
  mattress?
How far is the bed from the bathroom? From other family members?

(continued)

ASSESSMENT TOOLS 5-5

Questions to Complete: Environmental Assessment Checklist *(Continued)*

Medications

Does the client have a plan for taking the right medications at the right time?
Is there a secure place to store the medications? Are they safe from children and the cognitively impaired?
Can the client reach the medications needed? Open the container? Read the label?
Is there adequate lighting where the client will be preparing medications?
Is there a safe way to dispose of syringes? Medical supplies?

Shelter

Is the house clean and comfortable for the client? Who will do the housework?
Are the plumbing and sewage systems working?
Is there a safe heat source? Are space heaters safe? Are the electrical cords in good condition?
Is there adequate ventilation?
Is the house infested with roaches, other insects, or rodents?

Safety and Security

Mobility/Fall Prevention

Is the client able to get around the home? Does the client have good balance? Steady gait?
Is the caregiver thinking of using restraints? What sort of restraints? Are they necessary?
Does the client use assistive devices (walkers, canes) correctly? Are they the right height?
Do the devices fit through the pathways without catching on furnishings?
Are the pathways, hallways, and stairways clear? Are there throw rugs?
Are there sturdy handrails on the stairs? Are the first and last steps clearly marked?
Is there adequate lighting in hallways and stairways? Is the path to the bathroom well lighted at night?
Are the floors slippery? (Floors should not have a high gloss or be highly waxed.)
Are there uneven floor surfaces?
Are the carpets in good repair without buckles or tears that could cause tripping?
Can the client walk steadily on the carpets? (Thick pile carpets can cause tripping if the client has a shuffling gait.)
Are the chairs the client uses sturdy? Are they stable if the client uses them to prevent a fall?
Does the client use furniture or counters for balance when walking? Are these sturdy enough to withstand the pressure?
Are there cords or wires that could cause the client to trip?

(continued)

ASSESSMENT TOOLS 5-5

Questions to Complete: Environmental Assessment Checklist *(Continued)*

Fire/Burn Prevention

Is there a smoke detector on each level of the home? Is there a fire extinguisher?
Is there an escape plan for the client to get out of the house in case of fire?
Is the client using heating pads and space heaters safely?
Are wires and plugs in good repair?
If the client smokes, are there plans to make sure the client smokes safely?
Are there signs of cigarette burns? Burns in the kitchen?
Are oxygen tanks stored away from flames and heat sources?

Crime/Injury Prevention

Are there locks on the doors and the windows?
Can the client make an emergency call? Is the telephone handy? Are
    emergency numbers clearly marked?
Are firearms securely stored in a locked box? Is the ammunition stored and
    locked away separately?
Is there evidence of criminal activity?

Love and Belonging

Caregiver

Is there a caregiver? Is the caregiver competent? Willing? Supportive?
Does the caregiver need support?
Can the caregiver hear the client? Should there be an intercom? "Baby
    monitor?" Handbell?

Communication

Is the telephone within easy reach of the client?
Should the telephone have an illuminated dial? Oversized numbers? Memory
    feature? Audio enhancer?
Are needed numbers clearly marked? Police? Fire? Ambulance? Nurse? Doctor?
    Relatives? Neighbors?
Is there a daily safety check system? Should there be an alert system like Lifeline?
How will the client obtain mail?

Family/Friends/Pets

Are the neighbors supportive?
Does the client have family, friends, church/synagogue/mosque members to help
and visit?
Is the client able to take proper care of any pets? Are pets well behaved?

Self-Esteem and Self-Actualization

Are there meaningful activities the client can do? Listening to music/book
    tapes? Interactive activities?
What kind of activities does the client enjoy? Are there creative ways that these
    activities can be brought to the client?

Adapted with permission from Narayan, M. C., & Tennant, J. (1997). Environmental assessment. *Home Healthcare Nurse, 15*(11), 799–805.

those with serious chronic conditions are most at risk for safety issues. Many communities have home safety check kits available through the Red Cross or local fire department to assess for unsafe conditions in the home.

Assessing Spirituality

Numerous studies show that religious practice is correlated with greater health and longer life. Assessing spiritual health and intervening according to the client's values may be one of the most important areas to address in community-based care. A **spiritual assessment** allows the nurse to determine the presence of spiritual distress or identify other spiritual needs. A spiritual needs protocol is shown in Assessment Tools 5-6. The nurse, client, and family can mutually use the results of this assessment to identify spiritual issues and incorporate them in the plan of care. Another reason for completing a spiritual assessment on all clients stems from the requirement by the Joint Commission on Accreditation of Healthcare Organizations (JCAHO) that all clients cared for by accredited health care organizations must have a spiritual assessment (JCAHO, 2006).

CLIENT SITUATION IN PRACTICE

Marge has been seeing Richard for 3 weeks. At the last visit his incision was healing well and with Marge setting up his medications he was taking them every day. He was able to do his ADLs and his IADLs except grocery shopping. Today when Marge knocks and walks in the house, Richard is sitting on the sofa with his head in his hands. When he looks up his eyes are red and teary. Marge says, "Richard, what is wrong?" He says, "I am so lonely. Maryanne and I use to go to Mass every day together. I have missed that so much." Marge immediately recognizes that Richard is experiencing spiritual distress. Marge problem solves with Richard and helps him to identify a local parish that provides rides to Mass to homebound people. Her goal is that Richard will be able to attend Mass and her nursing intervention is counseling and case management. She completes her assessment and learns that his incision is healed, and he continues to take his medication. His nutritional status is stable but his blood sugars continue to be labile. They schedule the next visit for the following week when his daughter is visiting from another state.

ASSESSMENTS OF THE FAMILY

Assessment of the ability of the family of the client to provide caregiving that may keep the client at home and out of the hospital or nursing home is often imperative.

Changes in health care delivery, budget constraints, and staff cutbacks have all contributed to enormous pressure on nurses to do more in less time. A simple family assessment, completed in 15 minutes or less, may actually save the nurse time, allowing the nurse to identify issues early and prevent problems later. The key ingredients to a simple family interview are speaking politely and respectfully, using therapeutic communication, constructing a family genogram,

ASSESSMENT TOOLS 5-6

Spiritual Needs Protocol

Illness often triggers spiritual wrestling in addition to emotional, mental, and physical pain. Spiritual care is an integral part of holistic care. The health care team must be comfortable with and receptive to these needs for them to emerge and be addressed. The concept of presence implies self-giving by the health care provider to the client. It means being available and listening in a meaningful way. It also means having an awareness that it is a privilege to be invited into a person's life in this way, as well as an ethical responsibility.

Assessment

Assess spiritual or religious preference and note any request to see the chaplain. Use admission database.

Listen for verbal cues regarding spiritual or religious orientation:

• Client refers to God or higher power
• Client talks about prayer, church, synagogue, mosque, spiritual or religious leader

Look for visual cues on the client and in his or her room regarding spiritual or religious orientation:

• Bible, Torah, Koran, or other spiritual books
• Symbols such as the cross, Star of David, or prayer rug.
• Articles such as prayer beads, medals, or pins

Listen for significant comments, such as, "It's all in God's hands now" or "Why is this happening to me?"

Assess for signs of spiritual concerns:

• Discouragement
• Mild anxiety
• Expressions of anticipatory grief
• Inability to participate in usual spiritual practice
• Expressions of concern about relationship with God or higher power
• Inability to obtain foods required by beliefs

Assess for signs of spiritual distress:

• Crying
• Expressions of guilt
• Disturbances in sleep patterns
• Disrupted spiritual trust
• Feeling remote from God or higher power
• Moderate to severe anxiety
• Anger toward staff, family, God, or higher power
• Challenged belief or value system
• Loss of meaning and purpose in life

(continued)

ASSESSMENT TOOLS 5-6

Spiritual Needs Protocol *(Continued)*

Assess for signs of spiritual despair:

* Loss of hope
* Refusal to communicate with loved ones
* Loss of spiritual belief
* Death wish
* Severe depression
* Flat affect
* Refusal to participate in treatment regimen

Assess for special religious concerns such as diet, refusal of blood.

Interventions

Convey a caring and accepting attitude.
Provide support, encouragement, and respect.
Provide presence.
Listen actively.
Use therapeutic communication techniques such as restatement, clarification, or silence.
Join in prayer or reading scripture if comfortable.
Use therapeutic touch with the client's permission.
Include family or significant other in spiritual care.
Consult physician for medications as needed for anxiety or depression.

Reportable Conditions

Notify physician of severe anxiety or depression that may require pharmacologic or psychiatric intervention.
Notify chaplain, priest, rabbi, pastor, or spiritual leader of spiritual concerns, distress, or despair with client's permission.

Documentation

Document assessment on database and flow sheet.
Document in nurse's notes significant comments, behaviors of client, family, or significant other; interventions; physician notification; and referrals to chaplain or other religious leader.
Document initiation of protocol on plan of care.

Adapted with permission from Sumner, C. (1998). Recognizing and responding to spiritual stress. *American Journal of Nursing, 98*(1), 26–30.

asking therapeutic questions, and commending the family and individual on their strengths (Wright & Leahey, 1999).

In many ways, modern culture has experienced a decline in civility and good manners. Nursing has not been immune to this phenomenon. The professional relationship requires that the nurse introduce himself or herself to the client and family and set a contract with the client and family. Setting a contract involves developing mutual goals and outcomes for every encounter. Following basic elements of establishing a therapeutic relationship, such as calling the client and family by name and involving the client and family in the care, are essential to establishing a trusting relationship with the client (Wright & Leahey, 1999).

Therapeutic communication is the second element of a simple family assessment. From the start of a brief family assessment, conversation is purposeful and time limited. Often, listening, showing compassion, and emphasizing assets are the most powerful therapeutic interventions that a nurse can use. Some of the most basic suggestions include the following (adapted from Wright & Leahey, 1999, p. 264):

◆ Invite families to accompany the client to the unit/clinic/hospital.
◆ Involve families in the admission procedure or interview.
◆ Encourage families to ask questions during the client orientation or first visit.
◆ Acknowledge the client and family's expertise in self-care or assisting in self-care.
◆ Ask about routines at home and incorporate them in the plan of care.
◆ Encourage the clients to practice interactions that may come up in the future related to health regimens (e.g., have a parent practice telling a diabetic child that she may not eat ice cream at a birthday party).
◆ Consult with clients and family about their ideas for treatment and discharge.

CLIENT SITUATIONS IN PRACTICE

When Marge arrived for the visit the next week, Richard answered the door and invited her into the living room. As Marge and Richard sat down Marge heard someone doing dishes in the kitchen. She asked Richard, "Did your daughter arrive?" "Yes, she is in the kitchen," Richard replied. Marge went into the kitchen and invited his daughter to join the conversation. After Richard's daughter Kathy sat down, Marge introduced herself, told her that she was a nurse working for the Block Nurse program and explained that she had been visiting Richard since the day after he was discharged from the hospital. She asked if Kathy had any questions. Marge went on to praise Richard for how he had managed his own care after his surgery and summarized his progress for Kathy. Marge then asked Richard if he had anything to add and he indicated he did not. She asked Kathy what she would like to know about Richard's health care needs. Kathy replied that because she had been transferred back and had purchased a house two blocks from her father she expected that she would be as involved as her father desired. Richard replied that he was having a lot of trouble regulating his diet, blood sugars, and insulin and needed help with this. Marge then suggested that they start by talking about his usual routine and how his diet and diabetes regulation could be based on it. She then asked what Kathy and Richard knew about diabetes and the treatment of diabetes and what they wanted to know. Marge's intervention of health teaching began based on what Kathy and Richard already knew and wanted to know about diabetes. Kathy, Richard, and Marge decided that they would meet the next week. Their goal next week would be to talk about the diabetic diet and recipes that were within the diabetic diet.

A genogram is an essential element of the quick family interview. See Chapter 4 for detailed information on completing genograms.

Asking therapeutic questions is the next element of the brief family interview. Numerous examples are found in Chapter 4. Additional questions are listed below (Wright & Leahey, 1999):

◆ Of your family or friends, who would you like us to share information with, and who should we not?
◆ How can we be most helpful to you and your family or friends as we provide care for you?
◆ What has been most or least helpful to you in past hospitalizations, home visits, or clinic visits?

The last aspect of the simple family interview is to focus on strengths rather than on needs and problems. Strength-based nursing validates the client and family's assets. In every encounter with a family, the acknowledgment of the resources, competencies, and efforts observed allows the family and client to realize their assets and develop new perspectives of themselves and their abilities.

In summary, this framework recommends the following steps:

1. Use good manners to engage or reengage the client's family; introduce yourself by offering your name and role and orienting family members to the purpose of a brief family interview.
2. Assess key areas of internal and external structure and function; obtain genogram information and key external support data.
3. Ask three key questions to family members.
4. Commend the family on two strengths.
5. Evaluate the usefulness of the interview and conclude (Wright & Leahey, 1999, p. 272).

POPULATION-BASED CARE: ASSESSMENT OF THE COMMUNITY

All nurses have a role in community assessment, ranging from identifying appropriate resources for referral to determining the need for a new hospital. Because community assessment varies in levels of complexity, the role of the nurse depends on the nurse's educational preparation and expertise. The person with an associate's degree in nursing (ADN) uses community assessment primarily as it relates to the care of the individual client in the context of the community. For example, a nurse working in the acute care setting may want to find placement for a client with mental illness, but the agencies generally used by the referring facility are not appropriate. Thus, the nurse may conduct a simple community assessment to determine available, accessible, and appropriate community resources for referral. In another example, interventions to address medication safety range from developing a teaching program for all clients cared for on a specific unit to developing hospital policy to require medication teaching (see Research in Community-Based Nursing Care 5-1.). In population-based care of communities addressing medication safety may involve state or federal recommendations or regulation regarding medication safety.

Another example of population-based care of communities is seen in the nurse who recognizes that many children are overweight within a certain neighborhood. She or he may lead a group of citizens to encourage the local school to reinstate

RESEARCH IN COMMUNITY-BASED NURSING CARE ▶ 5-2

A Community Intervention Reducing Inactivity

This effort involved local political and lay leaders, health and social workers in planning and implementing a set of strategies to increase physical activity in a low-income, multi-ethnic community. The urban community where the program was implemented had high rates of health disease, obesity, and physical inactivity. The strategies involved planning and promoting organized long walks; distributing leaflets and other reminders about the health benefits of physical activity such as using stairs; and offering free diet, nutrition, and smoking cessation counseling. After 3 years compared with the control community, the get-fit community lost weight, reducing their risk of type 2 diabetes, and had improvements in cholesterol, blood pressure, and blood sugar levels. The net increase in activity in the get-fit group was 9% and significant changes in lipid levels, smoking habits, and blood sugar levels. This community program "led to significant health effects on risk actors for type 2 diabetes and cardiovascular disease," according to the researchers. This population-based community intervention showed that low cost community-based strategies that get people moving have the potential to reverse the epidemic of obesity and type 2 diabetes.

Source: Jenum, A. K., Anderssen, S. A., Birkeland, K. I., et al. (2006). Promoting physical activity in a low-income multiethnic district: Effects of a community intervention study to reduce risk factors for type 2 diabetes and cardiovascular disease: A community intervention reducing inactivity. *Diabetes Care, 29,* 1605–1612.

recess and lunch play time on the playground. Or the group may ask the school board to add physical education to the school curricula. An example of a population-based community-wide program to increase physical activity in a neighborhood is seen in Research in Community-Based Nursing 5-2. Public health nurses typically use community assessment to determine needs for particular services or programs in a given geographic area or neighborhood. An example is the community health nurse who uses community assessment to determine the need for flu shot clinics in a neighborhood.

A more complex example is the use of community assessment in influencing public policy. The nurse with a graduate degree, or a nurse statistician or epidemiologist, may be contracted by a state or local government to do a community assessment to determine the number and percentage of citizens in a particular geographic area who are uninsured or underinsured.

Through population-based care and community assessment, the nurse determines how a community influences the health of its residents. Community assessment is a technique that may be used to determine the health status, resources, or needs of a group of individuals. Similar to basic nursing process, **community assessment** consists of information about the physiological, psychological, sociocultural, and spiritual health of the community. Community assessment allows the nurse to explore the relationship between a variety of community variables and the health of its citizens. Professionals from a number of disciplines participate in community assessment activities. These professionals include nurses, social workers, therapists, community health workers, public health nurses, physicians, epidemiologists, statisticians, and public policy makers.

Components of Community Assessment

Chapter 1 describes the community as an entity made up of people, a place, and social systems, and it discusses the characteristics of a healthy community. Just as the characteristics of healthy families can be used in assessment, the characteristics of a healthy community can be used as a simple tool to assess a community's level of health.

Community assessment reflects a problem-solving process similar to the nursing process and uses steps similar to those used to assess the individual client or family. All three dimensions of the community are assessed: the people, the place, and the social systems.

People

A community can be assessed by analyzing the characteristics of the people in that community. These characteristics are defined through the **demographics** of the community, which include the number, composition by age, rate of growth and decline, social class, and mobility of the people in the community. Other vital statistics include the birth rate, overall death rate (**mortality**), mortality by cause and by age, and infant mortality rate. Of these, the infant mortality rate is considered to be the most important statistical indicator regarding the level of maternal–infant health in a community. Vital statistics also include **morbidity** or rate of a particular disease within a community. These vital statistics are the "vital signs" of the community. They tell a very important story about the health of a community or population.

Place

Place or location is where the community is located and its boundaries. It may include the type of community, such as rural or urban; location of health services; and climate, flora, fauna, and topography. Assessment of location is important because it determines what services are accessible and available to the people living within that area. Place also impacts the mortality and morbidly from certain conditions. For example, the rates of Lyme disease are considered as an epidemic in some parts of the country; sections of Wisconsin and Connecticut. Similarly, deaths from hypothermia or severe frostbite are more common in regions of the United States where there may be temperatures below 0°F for long periods of time.

Social Systems

Social systems are assessed as economic, educational, religious, political, and legal systems. Further, human services, opportunities for recreation, and communication systems are components of a community's social systems. **Power systems** within a community must also be assessed as part of the overall social system—how power is distributed throughout a particular social system. Determining how decisions are made and how change occurs is essential in planning. Power systems impact health and health care. There is wide disparity in the rate of those without health insurance by state, which is mostly a result of the existence or quality of the social systems. For example, in Minnesota the percentage of poor children who do not have health insurance is 3.9% and in Texas 14.9% (U.S. Census Bureau, 2006).

Methods in Community Assessment

Many methods can be used to collect data in a community. Five methods are discussed here: windshield survey, informant interviews, participant observations, secondary analysis of existing data, and constructed surveys. These assessments are typically in the domain of the public health nurse; however, it is helpful for community-based nurses to understand these methods because they may be asked to participate in community assessment. As with care of the family or individual in community settings, assessment looks for both needs and assets.

Windshield Survey

A common method of community assessment is a windshield survey. The **windshield survey** is the motorized equivalent of a simple head-to-toe assessment. The observer drives through a chosen neighborhood and uses the five senses and powers of observation to conduct a general assessment of that neighborhood. Conclusions from a windshield survey show common characteristics about the way people live, where they live, and the type of housing that exists in a given neighborhood. An example of a windshield survey is seen in Assessment Tools 5-7.

Informant Interviews

Informant interviews involve community residents who are either key informants or members of the general public. Key informants are individuals in positions of power or influence in the community, such as leaders in local government, schools, and the religious or business community. General public interviews may include random telephone or person-on-the-street interviews. Interviews are typically unstructured and are conducted to collect general information.

Nurses working in acute care settings use the equivalent of informant interviews to elicit information from the client, family members, social workers, and spiritual counselors. Nurses may also use this technique as they talk to other nurses about potential community resources that may be appropriate for referral purposes. If the hospital or agency uses follow-up telephone calls after discharge, informant information about referral sources is elicited.

Participant Observations

The third method of data collection is **participant observations**. The nurse observes formal and informal community activities to determine significant events and occurrences. This leads to conclusions about what is happening in selected settings. Formal gatherings include government, city council, county board, and school board meetings. Informal gatherings occur at the local coffee shop or cafe, barbershop, or school. Participant observations can be effective in determining the values, norms, and concerns of a community. It may also offer an opportunity to identify the power systems within the community. Recognizing how power is distributed throughout the community social system and how decisions are made provides important insight into how change occurs in a community.

Nurses in in-patient settings use participant observation when they watch a client in physical therapy, occupational therapy, or any activity off the unit. These observations may tell the staff nurse something about the client's values and

ASSESSMENT TOOLS 5-7

Windshield Survey

This assessment has been designed to assist the nurse traveling around the neighborhood to identify objective data related to people, places, and social systems that help define the community. This information may help identify trends, stability, and changes that may affect the health of the individual living in the community.

People

Who is on the street (e.g., women, children, men)?
How are they dressed?
What are they doing?
Are the people African American, White, Asian?
How are the different racial groups residentially located?
How would you categorize the residents: upper, upper middle, middle, lower class? How did you come to this conclusion?
Is there any evidence of communicable diseases, alcoholism, drug abuse, mental illness? How did you come to this conclusion?
Are there animals on the street? What kind?

Place

Boundaries

Where is the community located?
What are its boundaries?
Natural boundaries?
Human-made boundaries?

Location of Health Services

Where are the major health institutions located?
What health institutions may be necessary for a community of this size but are not located in the community (e.g., a large community with few or no acute care or ambulatory care facilities)?
Are there geographic features that may pose a threat?
What plants or animals could pose a threat to health?

Human-Made Environment

Do you see major industrial areas with heavy industrial plants?
Do the roads allow easy access to health institutions? Are those roads marked by easily seen and understandable signs?

Housing

What is the quality of the housing?
How old are the houses?
Are there single or multifamily dwellings?
Are there signs of disrepair and decay? If so, explain.
Are there vacant dwellings? If so, explain.

(continued)

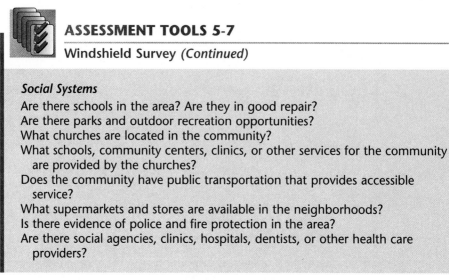

ASSESSMENT TOOLS 5-7

Windshield Survey *(Continued)*

Social Systems

Are there schools in the area? Are they in good repair?

Are there parks and outdoor recreation opportunities?

What churches are located in the community?

What schools, community centers, clinics, or other services for the community are provided by the churches?

Does the community have public transportation that provides accessible service?

What supermarkets and stores are available in the neighborhoods?

Is there evidence of police and fire protection in the area?

Are there social agencies, clinics, hospitals, dentists, or other health care providers?

behavior. Home visits, conducted with clients after discharge from the acute care setting to assess their ongoing needs or before admission to an acute care setting, are examples of participant observation. During the home visit, the nurse collects information about the client in the context of the family and the community.

Secondary Data

Sources of **secondary data** include records, documents, and other previously collected information. Depending on the community, an abundance of demographic data may be available to describe the health status of its members. These may include databases from schools, departments of health at the city and state levels, county data, private foundations, and state universities. Health data kept by the state may be thought of as the health record of the citizens of that state. Secondary data provides the statistics that are the vital signs of the community.

An example of secondary data may be seen in a clinic setting. Let's say that you are working in a clinic. Last week you noticed that many of the adults seen in the clinic were admitted with the diagnosis of bronchitis. You calculate that within the last week 30 of 100 clients who came to the clinic had bronchitis. You wonder if this is an **epidemic** (the occurrence of a disease that exceeds normal or expected frequency in a community or region). To determine if it is, you look at the clinic statistics for the year before and find that during the same week last year, 20 of 60 adults were admitted for bronchitis. Are you seeing an epidemic this year? Nurses in acute care and clinics use secondary data when they consult old charts and past notes, vital signs, orders, and other indicators of client progress documented in the client's chart.

Constructed Surveys

Constructed surveys may be used to collect information about communities. This model is typically time consuming and expensive. A random sample of a targeted population asks a list of specific questions. Data collected are analyzed for patterns and trends. This type of assessment is beyond the scope of this book, but is an important aspect of the role of the nurse with a graduate degree working in community-based settings.

Nursing Process and Population-Based Care

Population-based community care occurs through partnerships between all constituents just as nursing care of the individual and family is a mutually formulated process. A partnership exists when two or more persons are in the same enterprise, sharing the profits and risks (Webster's, 1996). This partnership requires ongoing dialogue in a reciprocal relationship between all stakeholders. Population-based community care is not something that the nurse does "for" a community, rather "with" a community.

Community assessment may be accomplished by using any one, or a combination, of the methods just discussed. These methods are applied to the three dimensions of community: people, place, and social systems. One simple method of assessment is to use the characteristics of a healthy community. Another way to assess a community is to use an assessment guide with specific assessment questions. Once information is collected, the nurse reviews it for repeating patterns that may appear in all three areas of assessment: people, place, and social systems. At this point, a community health need may be identified. A third way to assess people, place, and social systems is to use the components of community-based care, as outlined in Table 5-1.

TABLE 5-1 Examples of Community Assessment in Community-Based Care		
People	**Place**	**Social Systems**
Self-Care		
Assess the client related to people in immediate-environment and surrounding community to determine ability to enhance or detract from the client's ability to maintain self-care.	Determine where the client lives and how the home, neighborhood, and community may contribute to the client's ability to maintain self-care.	Assess available, appropriate, and accessible community resources to support self-care.
Context of Client, Family, and Community		
Assess the values, attitudes, and norms of people in the client's immediate environment and surrounding community.	Determine where the client lives, both the immediate environment and surrounding community.	Identify if social systems provide support or detract from the individual's potential for recovery.
Prevention		
Consider the people in the immediate environment and surrounding community to determine support or disregard for a preventive focus.	Assess the location and whether it supports or disregards a preventive focus.	Assess the social systems for evidence of a preventive focus.
Continuity		
Determine if the people in the immediate and surrounding community support continuity.	Identify if the location enhances or detracts from continuity.	Describe the available, accessible, and appropriate community resources that support continuity.

POPULATION-BASED COMMUNITY-FOCUSED SITUATIONS IN PRACTICE

For example, you are a nurse who just moved from South Dakota to Washington County, Ohio. You notice that there seemed to be many more children in the clinic where you work as a pediatric nurse who have asthma, compared to South Dakota. In your community you see young children on the street using inhalers. You ask a friend who is a school nurse and he tells you that in the last decade the number of children with asthma has increased dramatically in the school district. He says that some of the community members believe that the problem is a containment waste dump near the oil refinery. You do a web search and compare the state statistics with those from other states and notice a higher rate of asthma in Ohio. The state average is 13/100 children age 0 to 17 (Environmental Health Watch, 2006). The school nurse tells you that she thinks that in her school the rate is around 30/100 in children age 5 to 12. Further, you see that your region has three times the rate of high pollution days as compared to the national average. You wonder if the oil refinery located nearby could contribute to the high rate of asthma.

You find more information on the internet and also learn that in the United States asthma prevalence has increased overall by 75% in the last decade and that 7% of children live with the disease. In 1 year, asthma accounts for 12.7 million doctor visits, 1.9 million emergency department visits, almost 500,000 hospitalizations, more than 4,000 deaths, and millions of dollars in health care spending (Krisberg, 2006). Over 25% of American children live in areas that regularly exceed the U.S. Environmental Protection Agency's limits for ozone, more than one quarter of which comes from auto emission (CDC (b), 2006).

Nursing Diagnosis for Population-Based Community-Focused Care

Common nursing diagnosis for community include: ineffective community coping; readiness for enhanced community coping; or ineffective community therapeutic regiment management. One way to state the nursing diagnosis would be: at risk for ineffective community therapeutic regiment management as manifested by an unexpected increase in the rate of asthma among children. Community nursing diagnosis statements may be stated as *potential for enhanced* _____, in a one-part diagnosis; in two parts as *risk diagnosis related to risk factor,* stated as in the example above; and in three parts with *diagnostic label, contributing factors, and signs and symptoms* (Carpenito, 2006). In the real world the diagnosis is stated as a problem statement. Formatting statements of the community's health concerns or problems, as well as its assets, concludes the assessment phase. It is important to document the data that support the problem and the overall processes used for the identification of the problem.

Planning/Goals and Outcomes

Planning follows the formulation of the nursing diagnosis. Planning involves prioritizing the community needs, establishing goals and objectives, and determining an action plan.

POPULATION-BASED COMMUNITY-FOCUSED SITUATIONS IN PRACTICE

You decide that the nursing diagnosis for the need you have identified in your community is risk for ineffective management of therapeutic regime related to the high number of pollution alert days and as oil refinery located in the region, as manifested by the high rate of asthma among children age 5 to 12 years of age as compared to national rates. This may also be stated as a problem statement: In Washington County, Ohio, in 2008 compared to the national average there are twice as many pollution alert days with three times the rate of asthma among children ages 5 to 12 years.

Interventions

Common nursing interventions in community-based settings are community organizing and coalition building. Coalition building promotes and develops alliances among organizations or constituencies for a common purpose by building linkages, solving problems, and enhancing local leadership to address health concerns. Through community organizing the nurse assists community groups to identify common problems or goals, mobilize resources, and develop and implement strategies for reaching these goals. In this case you are organizing and building coalitions to build awareness of the issue and investigate the causes of the high rate in asthma among children in your community. Coalition building and community organizing may be accomplished by using an asset-based community development model seen in Box 5-1.

Evaluation

Community interventions are evaluated, just as nursing interventions for individual clients and families are evaluated. The expected outcome is compared with the outcome achieved at the end of the established time frame. Some questions that may be asked when evaluating a population-based community assessment include:

1. Were all the key stakeholders satisfied with the program?
2. What additional data do we need to collect to evaluate the program?
3. Did the problem statement focus on the most important problems for the individuals living in the community?
4. What other problems are important to this community?
5. Were the problem statement, expected outcome, and interventions realistic and appropriate for this community?
6. Are other members of the community satisfied with the outcome?

Similar to the nursing process, community assessment is cyclical and continuous. Evaluation is not an end point. It usually begins the assessment step of the next phase of community assessment.

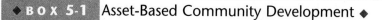

◆ **BOX 5-1** Asset-Based Community Development ◆

Asset-based community development is a process that focuses on the strengths of a community. The intention of asset-based community development is to mobilize assets for community improvement. Each community has unique assets upon which to work toward a better future. One model suggests five steps to facilitate community building.

1. Mapping the capacities and assets of individuals, citizens' associations, and local institutions that exist and that can be marshaled in the community.
2. Building and strengthening partnership among local assets for mutually beneficial problem solving within the community.
3. Mobilizing the community's assets for economic development and information sharing purposes.
4. Convening as broadly representative a group as possible for purposes of building a community vision and plan.
5. Leveraging activities, investments, and resources from outside the community to support asset-based, locally-defined development.

Source: McKnight, J., & Kretzmann, J. (2006). Tip sheet: Asset-based community development. Retrieved on September 14, 2007, from http://www.health.state.mn.us/communityeng/intro/models.html

POPULATION-BASED COMMUNITY-FOCUSED SITUATIONS IN PRACTICE

In Washington County, you have enlisted several other nurses and parents interested in this issue. The group meets in your living room and determines that the priority need is to form a task force of representatives from various constituencies (e.g., local department of public health, school districts, parents of children with asthma, nurses and physicians from the local hospital and clinic, individuals from the local industries and business communities). The goal or outcome is for the task force to study the issue and if deemed necessary, develop recommendations to be presented to the county department of health. Within the frame work of the task force your main interventions will be to promote and develop alliances among the constituents as well as build linkages and enhance local leadership to address the concern of the increased rate of asthma. Further, through community organizing you will mobilize resources, develop and implement strategies for reaching the goals the task force sets. Once the study and recommendations are complete they are presented to the County Department of Health and County Board. After the presentation the Department of Health and County Board suggests that the task force proceeds with a public health assessment (Box 5-2).

◆ **B O X 5-2** Public Health Assessment ◆

A public health assessment (PHA) examines hazardous substances, health outcomes, and community concerns at a hazardous waste site to determine whether people could be harmed from coming into contact with those substances. The PHA also lists actions that need to be taken to protect public health. The process is that a health assessor is called in from the federal government to review site-related environmental data and general information about toxic substances at the site. The assessor estimates the dose of the substance to which people in the community might be exposed and compares this with regulatory standards. A PHA functions like a clinical evaluation of a community by examining the relationship between actual exposures to contaminants and subsequent signs of disease and illness. Then cases of those diseases and injuries with regard to potential site-specific exposure situations in the community are evaluated. The conclusions address the likelihood that those living near a site were exposed, are being exposed, or might be exposed at some future time to harmful levels of hazardous substances from the site. Community input is valued in this process as community members may have useful information about the community history, the site history, and human activities and land use near the site. Information from members of the community can improve estimates of exposure, risks, and health threats.

Source: Searfoss, R., & Stupak, L. (2004). A citizen's guide to risk assessment and public health assessments. Agency for Toxic Substances and Disease Registry. Retrieved on July 12, 2006 from http://www.atsdr.cdc.gov/publications/CitizensGuidetoRiskAssessments.html

---

CLIENT SITUATIONS IN PRACTICE

◆ Addressing Community Needs in the School

Maria is the school nurse for Harmony High School, which has an enrollment of 2,300 students. To determine the health needs of the students attending Harmony, she is conducting an assessment of the school community. She has collected the following information about the school district and the students at Harmony High.

Windshield Survey

Maria began her assessment of the community by spending time traveling around the school district completing a windshield survey. This is what she discovered:

Most of the people on the street during the day are women and small children. Based on the way they are dressed and the cars they are driving, they appear to be middle class.

Most of the people are Mexican American or White. There is no evidence of drug abuse or blatant sale of drugs on the street observed and no problems with communicable diseases, as may be evidenced by people with hacking coughs or a wasted appearance.

Harmony is a community of 20,000 people located at the outer suburban ring of Metropolitan City, which has a population of 3,000,000; it is a predominantly suburban community with 10% of the citizens in rural areas. The racial mix is 20% Hispanic, 30% African American, and 50% White. There is little pollution of any type in the area. There are no hospitals or clinics in the community. The houses are primarily well-kept, single-family dwellings between 5 and 20 years old.

In evaluating the social systems, Maria found that there are primary, secondary, and tertiary health care services nearby. However, because there is no public transportation, it is difficult for students to gain access to these services. In addition, none of the health services offers services for adolescents. For instance, 100% of the participants in the prenatal classes offered at the closest hospital are suburban, middle-class couples. The closest facility in which adolescents can receive confidential pregnancy testing, prenatal care, or prenatal classes is 45 minutes away by car. There is no public transportation available to this clinic.

Informant Interviews

Maria then interviews some of the key informants in the community. She asks them what they think are the primary health issues among high school students in their community. The county public health nurses, counselor, principal of the high school, and parish nurse all agree that many pregnant adolescents do not receive prenatal care. The fire chief and mayor believe there is a need for more emergency medical services.

Participant Observations

Based on the students who come to her office for care, Maria has identified two categories of students who frequently need health care. One group consists of students with somatic complaints related to personal or family stress. The second group consists of students who have questions about sexuality or who are pregnant and need information about available services. The girls who are pregnant have a great deal of difficulty getting early prenatal care.

Maria attends the school board meetings where issues of health are occasionally discussed. All of the school board members are concerned about cost containment, and two members are particularly sensitive about including sexuality in the school's curriculum. The superintendent is committed to curricula sensitive to community values and reluctant to consider curricula that may include sexuality if the board members' concerns are representative of the community.

Secondary Data

Maria collects secondary data on the community from the state health department. She discovers demographic facts about Harmony and compares them with data on all the high school students in the state. Harmony has a lower rate of prenatal care among adolescents and a higher infant mortality and rate of low-birth-weight newborns for students of color.

Community Health Need or Problem Statement

Maria decides that the **community health need** in Harmony High School is early identification of pregnancy and provision of prenatal care for pregnant adolescent girls. The community problem is: Harmony High students have a lower rate of prenatal care and a higher infant mortality rate and rate of low-birth-weight newborns for students of color as compared to the state statistics due to lack of early identification of pregnancy and access to prenatal care.

Outcome and Interventions

Maria defines the outcomes she hopes to establish and the interventions to the school board and public health nurses, teachers, counselors, and other community stakeholders.

Outcome After 6 Months

Establish a task force made up of a teacher, a counselor, a public health nurse, and a member of the school board to determine how the school and community can address this need.

Interventions for the Next 6 Months

1. Establish and convene a task force every 2 weeks.
2. Present a summary of the results of the community assessment to the school board, public health nurses, teachers, and counselors.
3. Keep the key players apprised of the progress of the task force.

After 1 year the task force presents the results to the school board, public health nurses, teachers, and counselors. The task force recommends that the school offer a prenatal course to all pregnant students at the high school. They recommend the following outcomes after 1 year.

1. Develop a method for referring all pregnant adolescents seen by school and community personnel to the school's prenatal program.
2. Develop a prenatal course to be offered in the school.
3. Develop a list of community referral sources for prenatal adolescents.
4. Develop a mechanism for follow-up after birth.
5. Ask for input and involvement of all key players.

Once the method for referral process, prenatal course, list of community referrals sources, and follow-up process is complete they report back to the school board and other key stakeholders. The task force recommends and the school board agrees to the following interventions for the next year.

1. Begin the program
2. Evaluate the prenatal program, including the number and percentage of pregnant students attending the classes, satisfaction with the program, and total percent now receiving prenatal care, infant mortality rate, and rate of low-birthweight infants.
3. Increase community awareness about the prenatal program.

Evaluation

Are the outcomes met?

1. Yes: Continue with the interventions.
2. No: Revise the interventions: Reconvene the task force; reassess the community.

Reassessment

To reassess the community, Maria determines if the key constituents were satisfied with the program. She explores if there is additional information necessary in order to evaluate the program. Marie affirms that the problem statement focused on the most important problems for the individuals living in the community. She asks if there were other problems important to this community. She establishes that the problem statement, expected outcome, and interventions were realistic and appropriate for this community. Last, Marie explores if there were other members of the community who were satisfied with the outcome.

Population-based community-focused care is an important aspect of community-based nursing. It utilizes nursing process to direct interventions toward entire populations within a community to change community norms, attitudes, awareness, practices, and behaviors.

CLIENT SITUATIONS IN PRACTICE

Examples of nursing process applied to planning care of the individual, family, or community are seen below.

Statement of a Concern or Problem and Goals

From the problem statement, the nurse defines goals or expected outcomes. These outcome statements are specific and based on measurable criteria. Examples with possible outcomes follow.

Example 1: When the Individual Is the Client
Nursing diagnosis: Ineffective airway clearance related to asthma as manifested by a respiratory rate of 28 breaths/min and wheezes in all lung fields.

Goals: The client will demonstrate a respiratory rate of 16 breaths/min and cessation of wheezes in all lung fields.

Example 2: When the Community of the School District Is the Client
Problem statement: The number of children between the ages of 5 and 18 years with asthma in the school district of Rosie Mountain increased from 50/1,000 in March 1995 to 100/1,000 in March 2005.

Expected outcome: Reduce the number of children between the ages of 5 and 18 years in Rosie Mountain with the diagnosis of asthma from 100/1,000 in 2005 to 50/1,000 by the year 2010.

Example 3: When the Community of the County Is the Client
Community problem: The infant mortality rate for Normaldale County was 11/1,000 births in 2010, compared with the state infant mortality rate of 8/1,000 and the national rate of 7/1,000.

Expected outcome: Reduce the infant mortality rate for Normaldale County to 9/1,000 births by 2015.

Example 4: When the Community of the Hospital Is the Client
Community problem: In March 2010, at Normaldale County Hospital, 65% of the nursing staff washed their hands between clients. The recommended percentage is 90%.

Expected outcome: By March 2015, 90% of the nursing staff will wash their hands between clients.

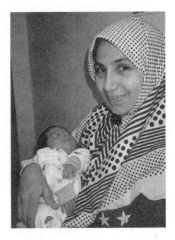

FIGURE 5-3. ▶ Public opinion and advocacy led to increased postpartum care.

PUBLIC POLICY MAKING

Public policy may appear, at first glance, to evolve primarily from the government. However, policy makers consider many sources when developing public policy. Nurses are valued professionals whose opinions and input are often sought by those who participate in the policy-making process. The nurse may participate in policy making in a variety of ways. These activities may range from calling or sending a letter to a city, state, or federal lawmaker; to testifying at a public hearing; to informing a client about proposed changes in the law related to health care. Often, through public education, the nurse may influence public opinion and, in turn, public policy. It is a professional responsibility of the graduate nurse to stay current on health care issues and to share that expertise with other members of the community.

Evidence of public opinion affecting public policy is seen in maternal care (Fig. 5-3). Until the late 1970s, third-party payers allowed a postpartum woman to stay in the hospital from 3 to 5 days. Gradually, reimbursement reduced the length of stay to 2 to 4 days and, eventually, to 24 hours to 3 days. As the negative consequences of early discharge on the mother and newborn became common knowledge through the medical and nursing community's disapproval and advocacy for longer stays, this policy was changed. By the late 1990s, many states extended the 24-hour stay to 48 hours.

Numerous issues offer nurses the opportunity to act as advocates for individuals, families, and communities. Through advocacy and education, the nurse may influence public opinion and health care public policy.

CONCLUSIONS

Assessment in community settings has long been a part of nursing practice. Assessment is directed toward individual clients across the life span, families, and communities. Holistic assessment considers not only physical and psychosocial factors, but also cultural, functional, nutritional, environmental, and spiritual aspects of the client. Family assessment may be abbreviated but is always essential to quality community care. Community assessment helps the nurse become aware of problems in the community that directly or indirectly affect the lives of clients and their families. Although the community-based nurse is infrequently asked to do a formal community assessment, the nurse may, along with other health care professionals, participate in some aspect of community assessment. Communities are assessed by using the nursing process to determine how people, place, and social systems influence health. As health care and nursing shift from the acute care setting to the community setting, the role of the nurse in community assessment will continue to expand.

What's on the Web

Mayo Clinic/Make Weight Loss a Family Affair
Internet address:
http://www.mayoClinic.com/health/childhood-obesity/FL00058

This page on the MayoClinic Web site has slide shows, tools including a child and adolescent body mass index (BMI) calculator and teaching materials for weight control. There are also numerous links to information on nutrition and activity.

The Community Tool Box
Internet address: http://ctb.ku.edu/
The Tool Box for population-based community-focused care includes practical guidance for the different tasks necessary to promote community health and development. Sections on leadership, strategic planning, community assessment, grant writing, and evaluation to give just a few examples of what is found on this website. Each section includes a description of the task, advantages of doing it, step-by-step guidelines, examples, checklists of points to review, and training materials.

Healthy People in Health Communities: A Community Planning Guide Using Healthy People 2010.
Internet address: http://www.healthypeople.gov/Publications/HealthyCommunities2001/default.htm or

http://www.healthypeople.gov/Publications/
This guide provides information for building community coalitions, creating a vision, measuring results, and creating partnerships dedicated to improving the health of a community. Includes "Strategies for Success" to help in starting community activities.

Centers for Disease Control and Prevention/Health Impact Assessment
Internet address:
http://www.cdc.gov/healthyplaces/hia.htm
This site describe an innovative process for addressing the potential impact that projects that affect land use or expansion of existing industries could have on the health of communities. *Health impact assessment* (HIA) can be used to evaluate objectively the potential health effects of a project or policy *before* it is built or implemented. It can provide recommendations to increase positive health outcomes and minimize adverse health outcomes. A major benefit of the HIA process is that it brings public health issues to the attention of persons who make decisions about areas that fall outside of traditional public health arenas, such as transportation or land use. This process has been used extensively in Europe, Canada, and Australia and is beginning to be used in the United States.

References and Bibliography

Austin, R. P. (2006). Polypharmacy as a risk factor in the treatment of type 2 diabetes. *Diabetes Spectrum, 19*(1), 13–24. Retrieved on July 12, 2006, from infotract.

Bauer, J. (2005). Simple test is not done often enough in kids. *RN, 68*(7), 20.

Carpenito, L. (2006). *Nursing diagnosis: Application to clinical practice* (11th ed.). Philadelphia: Lippincott Williams & Wilkins.

Centers for Disease Control and Prevention, National Center for Health Statistics (a). (2006). Prevalence of overweight among children and adolescents: United States, 1999–2002. Retrieved July 7, 2006, from http://www.cdc.gov/nchs/products/pubs/pubd/hestats/overwght99.htm

Centers for Disease Control and Prevention (b). Respiratory health and air pollution. Retrieved July 10, 2006, from http://www.cdc.gov/healthyplaces/healthtopics/airpollution.htm

DeBrew, J. K., Barba, B. E., & Tesh, A. S. (1998). Assessing medication knowledge and practices of older adults. *Home Healthcare Nurse, 16*(10), 686–692.

Dunn, C. (2002). Assessing and preventing medication interactions. *Home Healthcare Nurse, 20*(2), 104–111.

Environmental Health Watch: Asthma. (2006). Retrieved on July 12, 2006, from http://www.ehw.org/Asthma/ASTH_home1.htm

Huggins, C. (2006). Early screening spots vision problems in infants. Retrieved on October 28, 2007, from http://www.infantsee.org/ or http://www.iol.co.za/general/newsview.php?click_id=692&art_id=qw1151011086798B243&set_id=16

Hunt, R. (Ed.). (2000). *Readings in community-based nursing* (pp. 168–177). Philadelphia: Lippincott Williams & Wilkins.

Jenum, A. K., Anderssen, S. A., Birkeland, K. I., Holme, I., Graff-Iversen, S., Lorentzen, C., Ommundsen, Y., Raastad, T., Ødegaard, A. K., & Bahr, R. (2006). Promoting physical activity in a low-income multiethnic district: Effects of a community intervention study to reduce risk factors for type 2 diabetes and cardiovascular disease: A community intervention reducing inactivity. *Diabetes Care, 29*, 1605–1612.

Joint Commission on Accreditation of Healthcare Organizations. (2004). Spiritual assessment. Retrieved July 12, 2006, from http://www.jcaho.org/

Krisberg, K. (2006). Poor air quality, pollution endangers health of children: Designing healthier communities for kids. *The Nation's Health, 36*(2). Retrieved on July 10, 2006, from http://www.medscape.com/viewarticle/523845_print

McKnight J., & Kretzmann, J. (2006). Tip sheet: Asset-based community development. Retrieved on September 14, 2007, from http://www.health.state.mn.us/communityeng/intro/models.html

Narayan, M. C., & Tennant, J. (1997). Environmental assessment. *Home Healthcare Nurse, 15*(11), 799–805.

National Center for Health Statistics, 2006 @www.cdc.gov/growthcharts/

Neal, L. J. (1998). Functional assessment of the home health client. *Home Healthcare Nurse, 16*(10), 670–677.

O'Leary, J. (2006). After loss: Parenting in the next pregnancy. Minneapolis: Allina Publishing.

Searfoss, R., & Stupak, L. (2004). A citizen's guide to risk assessment and public health assessments. Agency for Toxic Substances and Disease Registry. Retrieved on July 12, 2006, from http://www.atsdr.cdc.gov/publications/CitizensGuidetoRiskAssessments.html

Shen, Q., Karr, M., Ko, A., Chan, D. K., Kahn, R., & Duvall, D. (2006) Evaluation of medication education program for elderly hospital in-patients. *Geriatric Nursing, 27*(3), 184–192.

Sumner, C. H. (1998). Recognizing and responding to spiritual stress. *American Journal of Nursing, 98*(1), 26–30.

U.S. Census Bureau. (2006). Health Insurance Data: Low Income Uninsured Children by State. Retrieved on July 9, 2006, from http://www.census.gov/hhes/www/hlthins/liuc04.html

Webster Online Dictionary. Retrieved on October 28, 2007, from http://merriam-webster.com/

Webster Online Dictionary. Retrieved on October 28, 2007, from http://census.gov/hhes/www/hlthins/lowinckid.html

Woodham-Smith, C. (1950). *Florence Nightingale, 1820–1910*. London: Constable.

Wright, L., & Leahey, M. (1999). Maximizing time, minimizing suffering; The 15-minute (or less) family interview. *Journal of Family Nursing, 5*(3), 259–274.

LEARNING ▼ ACTIVITIES

◆ LEARNING ACTIVITY 5-1

Nhu is a home care nurse who is making a home visit to Marion, an 85-year-old woman who has just been discharged from a transitional hospital after a hip replacement. After completing the agency admission intake interview, Nhu takes a few minutes to assess Marion's functional capacity.

What areas will Nhu assess?

Nhu learns that Marion is able to perform all ADL, her home environment is basically safe, her sensory and perceptual function is intact, and her cognitive, emotional, integumentary, and respiratory status are all within normal limits and sufficient to allow her to live independently. However, as Nhu is assessing function, Marion tells her, "I was doing fine until the physician changed my medication for high blood pressure. Now I am dizzy all the time."

What does Nhu assess next?

◆ LEARNING ACTIVITY 5-2

Conduct a windshield survey of your community. Consider people, place, and social system using Assessment Tools 5-5.

What community needs and assets did you identify?
What would you identify as the priority need or community problem?
What goals or outcomes would you suggest for this problem?

◆ LEARNING ACTIVITY 5-3

Complete a functional assessment (see Assessment Tools 5-1) for a vulnerable client in his or her home or apartment. Determine one or more appropriate nursing diagnoses, goals and outcomes, and nursing interventions. Identify interventions from the public health intervention wheel. Summarize the safety concerns you identified for this client as well as the client's strengths or assets. Identify resources in the community that provide safety devices, such as the safety council. Share all of the information with the client and his or her family and suggest that he or she share it with the appropriate community providers, such as the client's physician, nurse practitioner, or public health nurse.

◆ LEARNING ACTIVITY 5-4

Make a home visit to a family with a newborn baby. Use Community-Based Nursing Care Guidelines 5-1 to assess and intervene with issues related to attachment. Identify family strengths or assets and needs and formulate one or more short- and long-term nursing diagnoses. Use at least one of the nursing interventions listed in the guidelines and evaluate how well it worked, why it did or didn't work, and what other things you would do on the next visit. Document your care.

◆ LEARNING ACTIVITY 5-5

◆ Individual Client Assessment

In your clinical journal, describe a situation in which you used an assessment guide from this chapter to assess a client in a community-based setting:

What was your nursing diagnosis?
What were the outcomes and nursing interventions?
What benefit do you think you created for your client?
What did you do that didn't work?
What did you learn from this activity?
What will you do differently next time?

◆ Family Assessment

In your clinical journal, describe a situation in which you used an assessment guide from this chapter to assess a family in a community-based setting.

What family needs and assets did you identify?
What was your nursing diagnosis?
What were the outcomes and nursing interventions?
What did you learn from this activity?
What benefit do you think you created for the family?
What did you do that didn't work?
What will you do differently next time?

◆ Community Assessment

In your clinical journal, describe a situation in which you used an assessment guide from this chapter to assess a community.

What community needs and assets did you identify?
What was your nursing diagnosis?
What were the outcomes and nursing interventions?
What did you learn from this activity?
What benefit do you think you created for the community or could create for the community?
What did you do that didn't work?
What will you do differently next time?

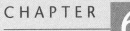
6

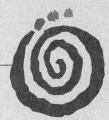

Health Teaching

ROBERTA HUNT

LEARNING OBJECTIVES

1. Discuss teaching and learning theory, learning domains, and successful teaching techniques as related to community-based nursing.
2. Define health teaching.
3. Discuss assessment, planning, and teaching methods required in determining learning needs.
4. Summarize Medicare reimbursement guidelines for teaching.
5. Identify barriers to successful teaching.
6. Explore the characteristics of successful teaching.
7. State methods used in teaching the client who is not adhering to the treatment plan.
8. Discuss specific teaching techniques for each level of prevention.

KEY TERMS

affective learning
cognitive learning
health teaching
health literacy
learning domains
learning needs

learning objective
need to learn
psychomotor learning
readiness to learn
reimbursement requirements

CHAPTER TOPICS

- Health Teaching in the 21st Century
- Teaching and Learning Theory
- Learning Domains
- Developmental Considerations
- Teaching and Levels of Prevention
- Nursing Competencies and Skills in the Teaching Process
- Conclusions

THE NURSING STUDENT SPEAKS

As a student, I find that often the value of interpersonal communication and cultural competence in our role of teaching patients and families is overlooked, diminished, and not regarded as important when compared to all of the other information that must be learned. However, as you start your clinical rotations and begin working with more diverse populations, you begin to realize that these aspects are just as important as the physiological issues. Every time you think someone else is "different," you need to remember they feel the same way about you. I've had two incredible experiences traveling to foreign countries and working with diverse patient populations: in Guatemala and in England. The important lesson I've learned is that I need to learn from the patients about their families, social structures, values, and beliefs before I can provide nursing care for them. It is just as important for me to learn from them as it is for them to learn from me.

—KASSIE STECKER, **Nursing Student, Gustavus Adolphus College**

At no other time in history has client teaching been so important. Owing to the decreased length of stay in all acute care settings and increased amount of care provided in community settings, teaching is a central role for nurses in all settings. At the same time there is a low rate of health literacy that acts as a barrier to self-care. Lack of health literacy affects both health and health care and has significant economic implications. **Health literacy** is the degree to which individuals have the capacity to obtain, process, and understand based on information and services needed to make appropriate health decisions (U. S. Department of Health and Human Services [DHHS] 2000). Increasingly, health literacy allows one to navigate complex health systems and better manage self-care (Pawlak, 2006). The consequences of inadequate health literacy include poorer health status, lack of knowledge about medical conditions and care for the conditions, lack of understanding and use of preventive services, poorer self-reported health, poorer compliance rates with treatment modalities, increased hospitalizations, and increased health care costs (Andrus & Roth, 2002).

One consequence of inadequate health literacy is seen in the knowledge that hospitalized clients have about their medication before they are discharged from acute care settings. Studies show that 20% of clients discharged from hospitals do not even fill their prescriptions after discharge. Of those who do, between 40% and 60% do not follow the prescribed regimen, either increasing or decreasing the dose, not taking the correct dose at the prescribed time, or not taking the entire dose. This issue is illustrated in that with people who are prescribed high blood pressure medication, only 50% continue to take it after 1 year, and of those, only 75% take enough to fully control their blood pressure (Consumer Health Information Corporation [CHIP], 2006). These errors may result in serious health complications as well as unnecessary hospitalization, treatment, and lost work time. Education services could save the United States nearly $100 billion a year in health care and lost productivity by improving prescription medication compliance and health outcomes (CHIP, 2006).

In the last decade, management of chronic conditions has become an important health need. Studies repeatedly show that client education prevents up to 50% of medication errors for clients in community settings where they self-administer their medications. As health care is more community-based, an illness is primarily managed by clients or family members. Nurses have an important role in promoting quality self-care through health teaching.

With this in mind, this chapter addresses health teaching. **Health teaching** is defined as "communicating facts, ideas, and skill that change knowledge, attitudes, values, beliefs, behaviors, and practices of individuals, families, systems, and/or communities" (Minnesota Department of Health, 2001). The benefits of teaching and strategies for successful health teaching are presented in light of the current health care system. Teaching and learning theory are discussed along with learning domains. A large section of the chapter is devoted to helping the nurse develop skills and competencies in teaching, discussing teaching as it follows the nursing process, and sharing useful teaching techniques. The chapter ends with activities to be used in further developing understanding and skills in teaching.

HEALTH TEACHING IN THE 21st CENTURY

In the 21st century, care will increasingly be provided outside the acute care setting. In addition to the economic arguments already presented there are other reasons to support prioritizing health teaching within the health care system. The most important goal of health teaching in community-based care is to assist the client and family in achieving independence through self care. When client learning needs are considered within the context of the client, family, and community care is improved, recovery facilitated, and postoperative complications reduced. Good teaching improves client and family satisfaction and confidence about discharge and follow-up care. A client's sense of control is enhanced through mutual participation in the teaching process.

Likewise, staff satisfaction improves when teaching results are positive. It is professionally satisfying to prepare a client for discharge and receive subsequent feedback that the discharge was satisfactory. Likewise, it is professionally satisfying for the home care nurse to prepare a client to successfully manage self-care at home. On the other hand, it is stressful when a nurse sees a client with inadequate preparation trying to manage home care unsuccessfully.

Quality health education provides continuity between settings of care. Providing information about diet, activity, medications, equipment, and follow-up appointments enhances self-care capacity. For over a decade there has been evidence that it is not only cost effective to provide health education for the client but also for lay caregivers. More than 2% of all hospital readmissions are a result of a need to reeducate caregivers (Leske & Pelczynski, 1999). In addition to the financial costs to the client, family, and third-party payers, it is frustrating when teaching has to be repeated several times because it was not done well the first time. Furthermore, concern for cost containment requires that all teaching incorporates prevention strategies, which further allow resources to be used efficiently. Teaching begins at whatever point the client enters the system.

TEACHING AND LEARNING THEORY

To be a successful teacher in any setting, one must understand and apply basic teaching and learning principles. Learning depends on both the **need to learn** and the **readiness to learn** and is influenced by the individual's life experiences (Knox, 1986).

Learning is facilitated when the client perceives information as needed or relevant for immediate application. For example, a postoperative client is scheduled to go home in 2 hours with a client-controlled analgesia pump. The client learns quickly how to use the pump and administer medication to control postoperative pain. This learning is facilitated by the need for pain relief and the immediate application of learning.

Learning depends on readiness. Readiness involves such factors as emotional state, abilities, and potential. Examples of these are listed in Community-Based Teaching 6-1. An example of lack of learning readiness follows. You are doing preadmission teaching with a 30-year-old woman, an attorney with a busy law practice who has outpatient surgery scheduled for the next day. She is thinking about the important trial she has beginning the afternoon following surgery. She may not hear you when you tell her she should not drive or make important decisions for a full day after surgery with general anesthesia. Because of her distracted mental state, she is not ready to learn.

Motivation is a strong determinant of learning readiness. Motivation starts with the client's need to know and then provides the drive or incentive to learn. Because so many things can affect motivation, it can change from day to day. For instance, a young woman who drinks alcohol becomes pregnant, and her health care provider tells her alcohol is harmful for the fetus. Because she is concerned for her baby's welfare, she discontinues drinking. The motivation is strong enough to make her stop. However, at a party her friends insist that she join them in a drink.

COMMUNITY-BASED TEACHING ▶ 6-1

Factors That Affect Readiness to Learn

- Physiologic factors: Age, gender, disease process currently being treated, intactness of senses (hearing, vision, touch, taste), preexisting condition
- Psychosocial factors: Sociocultural circumstances, occupation, economic stability, past experiences with learning, attitude toward learning, spirituality, emotional health, self-concept and body image, sense of responsibility for self
- Cognitive factors: Developmental level, level of education, communication skills, primary language, motivation, reading ability, learning style, problem-solving ability
- Environmental factors: Home environment, safety features, family relationships/problems, caregiver (availability, motivation, abilities), other support systems

"One drink won't hurt you," they say. Now the woman may be motivated to drink. Her decision depends on which motivation is stronger.

Both differences and similarities between past and present life experiences influence learning. For example, you are doing discharge planning from a maternity center for a multipara who delivered her second child yesterday evening. Her delivery was complicated by a 1,000-mL blood loss and a fourth-degree laceration. She has an 18-month-old toddler at home. Her husband is an accountant. It is tax season, and he presently works 12 or 13 hours a day. Neither set of grandparents nor any other family nor friends live nearby. Your client is going home this afternoon and insists that she does not need help at home because she did not need help after her first child. The client does not understand the difference between her first delivery and the circumstances complicating the second one.

LEARNING DOMAINS

Teaching and learning occur in three **learning domains**: cognitive, affective, and psychomotor. All three domains must be considered in all aspects of the teaching and learning process. Thus, the nurse must assess the client's need, readiness, and past experience in the cognitive, affective, and psychomotor domains.

Cognitive learning involves mental storage and recall of new knowledge and information for problem solving. Sometimes this domain is referred to as the critical thinking or knowledge domain. An example of cognitive learning is seen in the client who has recently been diagnosed with insulin-dependent diabetes. Not only will this client need information about diet, insulin, and exercise, but he or she will also need to use the information to formulate menus and an exercise plan. In addition, as blood sugar levels fluctuate, a client with diabetes must alter food intake and exercise. All this requires cognitive learning.

Affective learning involves feelings, attitudes, values, and emotions that influence learning. This is also referred to as the attitude domain. In the last decade the role emotion plays in learning has been speculated to be the most influential of all the domains in impacting motivation, thus the first domain that educators should assess. For example, the client who has just been identified as having diabetes may have to talk about his or her feelings about having diabetes before being ready to learn about insulin. Some of the client's feelings may stem from his or her prior knowledge and preconceived ideas about diabetes.

Psychomotor learning consists of acquired physical skills that can be demonstrated. This may be referred to as the skill domain. For example, the client with newly diagnosed insulin-dependent diabetes must learn to give self-injections, which will require learning the skill of using syringes.

DEVELOPMENTAL CONSIDERATIONS

It is helpful for the nurse to understand various theories of development. Implications for Teaching at Various Developmental Stages (Appendix B) outlines intellectual development as well as other developmental stages and nursing implications related to them. Just as the need to learn will be different at various age levels, the cognitive domain will differ and life experiences will differ. For example, teaching a

6-year-old girl about insulin administration will be different from teaching a 24-year-old woman, which would in turn be different from teaching a 69-year-old woman. The nurse must consider these factors when developing teaching plans.

Affective learning and psychomotor learning will also differ depending on developmental stage. The 6-year-old girl will approach insulin administration differently emotionally than will the 24-year-old woman. The 6-year-old girl may not have the fine motor skills needed to administer insulin. On the other hand, the older woman may have arthritis and not have the dexterity needed to fill the syringe or insert the needle in the site. Box 6-1 shows signs and symptoms associated with visual age-related changes and diseases that can interfere with the client's teaching–learning process. Chronologic age does not always indicate maturity. A young child may respond more maturely to health teaching than a 28-year-old client. Much depends on the client's responses to changes and stress in life experiences.

When nurses instruct parents about administering medication to their children, parents may not always understand instructions. One study reported that when parents gave their child the pain medications acetaminophen and ibuprofen, 51% of the children received inaccurate doses because most parents had difficulty deciding which dose to give. Another study was designed to determine if parental errors in administering liquid medication to their child with otitis media could be decreased through education. One group of parents received a dosage demonstration, in addition to receiving the prescription and verbal instructions, whereas the other group received only the prescription and verbal instructions. The group

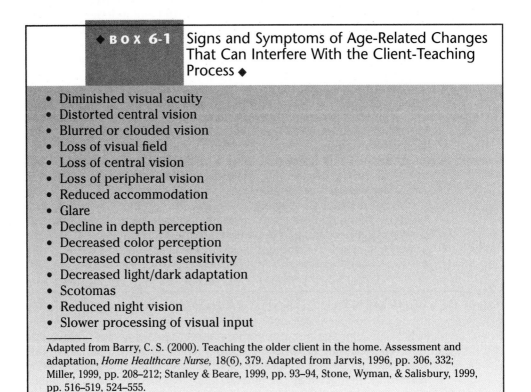

◆ **BOX 6-1**   Signs and Symptoms of Age-Related Changes That Can Interfere With the Client-Teaching Process ◆

- Diminished visual acuity
- Distorted central vision
- Blurred or clouded vision
- Loss of visual field
- Loss of central vision
- Loss of peripheral vision
- Reduced accommodation
- Glare
- Decline in depth perception
- Decreased color perception
- Decreased contrast sensitivity
- Decreased light/dark adaptation
- Scotomas
- Reduced night vision
- Slower processing of visual input

Adapted from Barry, C. S. (2000). Teaching the older client in the home. Assessment and adaptation, *Home Healthcare Nurse,* 18(6), 379. Adapted from Jarvis, 1996, pp. 306, 332; Miller, 1999, pp. 208–212; Stanley & Beare, 1999, pp. 93–94, Stone, Wyman, & Salisbury, 1999, pp. 516–519, 524–555.

that received the demonstration fared much better as 83% to 100% of their children received the correct dose (Magoon, 2002).

Nurses may need to show adults why they need to learn before the actual teaching can begin. Many adults have not been involved in an educational process for many years. They may show a hesitancy to learn something new, perhaps because they are afraid of failing. Added to this is the older client's concern about memory loss.

The nurse should never assume that all clients can understand verbal directions or read and write. Illiteracy is found in every walk of life, among all races and cultures, and at all socioeconomic levels. Nurses should also not assume that all the individuals they care for speak English. Minority clients are more likely to have difficulties communicating with health care providers, with over 20% of Spanish-speaking Latinos not seeking medical advice due to language barriers. Of older clients, two thirds have inadequate or marginal literacy skills. One study in a public hospital revealed that 81% of clients over 60 could not read or understand basic materials such as prescription labels (American Public Health Association, 2004). Educational level is not a true determinant of a person's ability to read or write. Literacy or illiteracy must be assessed as part of the client's readiness to learn.

TEACHING AND LEVELS OF PREVENTION

Teaching, whether it is in the acute care or community-based setting, occurs at all levels of prevention. An important goal of teaching is to prevent the initial occurrence of disease or injury through health promotion and prevention activities. A nurse teaching a nutrition class to parents and day care providers is an example of health promotion. A school nurse teaching parents about preventing childhood injuries is focusing on health protection. Teaching parents and day care providers about the importance of immunization is primary prevention, as is teaching about community resources that provide free or inexpensive immunization.

Secondary prevention is teaching targeted toward early identification and intervention of a condition. A home care nurse teaching the parents of a ventilator-dependent child about early signs of upper respiratory infection and when to contact the nurse on call is focusing on secondary prevention.

Most teaching in the home setting addresses tertiary prevention because most home care clients have chronic conditions or are postsurgical. Tertiary prevention arises from teaching that attempts to restore health and facilitate coping skills (Fig. 6-1). The home care nurse provides clients with a new diagnosis of diabetes instruction in changing the diet, handling syringes, giving themselves injections, and measuring their blood sugar. Teaching family or caregivers about community resources that are available for respite care facilitates coping skills and falls in the category of tertiary prevention.

NURSING COMPETENCIES AND SKILLS IN THE TEACHING PROCESS

The process of teaching and learning follows several prescribed steps, similar to the steps of the nursing process, as shown in Table 6-1. A comprehensive assessment

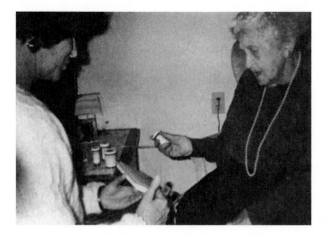

FIGURE 6-1. ▶ Tertiary prevention involves helping restore the client to health. On this visit, the nurse uses a weekly medication container to help an older woman with limited vision devise a plan for compliance in taking her medications.

determines the client and/or family members need to learn, readiness, and past life experiences. Learning outcomes, which direct the learning plan and provide outcome criteria, arise from the learning needs. Once the learning objectives or outcomes are defined, then the teacher will determine teaching strategies or tools and methods appropriate for the learner. After implementation of the plan, evaluations are made to determine the success of teaching. A diagram of this process is shown in Figure 6-2.

Assessment

The assessment begins by looking at the learning needs, readiness, and life experiences of the client, family, and caregiver in all three learning domains. It is also essential to consider the nursing implications for various developmental

TABLE 6-1	Relationship Between Nursing Process and Teaching and Learning	
Steps	**Nursing Process**	**Teaching and Learning**
Assessment	Assessment of client/family/ caregiver determines need for nursing care.	Assessment of client/family/ caregiver determines need for nursing care.
Diagnosis	Statement of nursing problem	Statement of learning need
Goals/expected outcome	Goals for client or family	Learning objectives/goals for the learner
Planning	Nurse and client work together to develop plan of nursing care.	Nurse and client work together to develop learning plan.
Interventions	A variety of actions can be used to implement the plan.	A variety of actions in cognitive, affective, and psychomotor learning are used to augment plan.
Evaluation	Nurse and client evaluate success of outcomes; nurse determines why plan was not successful (if so); nurse and client revise and set new objectives and plan.	Nurse and client evaluate success of outcomes; nurse and client determine weakness of plan; new objectives and plan are written.

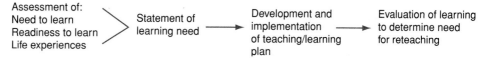
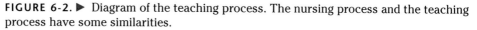

FIGURE 6-2. ▶ Diagram of the teaching process. The nursing process and the teaching process have some similarities.

stages listed in Appendix B. Successful teaching is positively associated with a nonjudgmental attitude. This is especially true when the nurse's culture is different from the client's. A nonjudgmental attitude is cultivated when the nurse:

◆ Recognizes and accepts differences between the nurse and client
◆ Tries to understand the cultural or value basis for the client's behavior
◆ Listens and learns before advising or teaching
◆ Empathizes with the client regardless of differences in attitudes and values

A cultural assessment tool will help the nurse determine how learning need is influenced by culture. Cultural assessment tools are discussed in Chapter 3 and 5.

An assessment guide can be used to assess the learning need of the client. Such a guide is printed in Assessment Tools 6-1. After assessments on the client, family, and caregiver needs; readiness to learn; and past life experiences have been assessed and documented, the learning need can be determined.

Identification of the Learning Need

The nurse draws inferences based on the information found in the assessment. Table 6-2 shows this process. A list of **learning needs** emerges, from which priority needs are identified. When lack of knowledge, motivation, or skill hinders a client's self-care, a nursing diagnosis can be used to name the need or strength. The list of the North American Nursing Diagnosis Association (NANDA) diagnoses can help identify the learning needs of the individual, family member, or caregiver. According to Carpenito (2006), knowledge deficit can not be used as a separate diagnosis category because it does not represent a human response, alteration, or pattern of dysfunction. Rather knowledge deficit should be used in a nursing diagnosis as a related factor. Most nursing diagnoses incorporate teaching as a part of the diagnosis. This is illustrated in the following:

◆ Risk for Ineffective Management of Therapeutic Regimens related to lack of knowledge of management, signs, and symptoms of complications of diabetes mellitus
◆ Decisional Conflict related to lack of knowledge about advantages and disadvantages of infant circumcision
◆ Risk for Impaired Home Maintenance Management related to lack of knowledge of home care and community resources
◆ Risk for Injury related to lack of knowledge of bicycle safety

Learning needs can be determined in one, two, or all of the learning domains. Consider the learning domains in the example on page 173.

ASSESSMENT TOOLS 6-1

Learning Assessment Guide

Client name_____

Health condition requiring health education_____

Primary caregiver _____

Learner _____ Relationship to client _____

Age _____ Gender _____ Occupation _____

Developmental stages and implications for learner _____

Psychosocial stage _____

_____

Cognitive stage _____

Language _____

_____

How does the caregiver or client feel about the responsibilities of self-care?

_____

_____

Describe any disabilities or limitations of the learner (including sensory

disabilities) _____

_____

Describe any preexisting health conditions of the learner _____

_____

List sociocultural factors that may impede learning _____

_____

State learner behaviors that indicate motivation to learn _____

_____

_____

Can the learner read and comprehend at the reading level required by the

task? _____

_____

Does the learner show an ability to problem solve at a level that provides

safe care in the home? _____

_____

Is the home environment conducive to the learning required by the care?

_____

_____

If not, what modifications are necessary? _____

_____

(continued)

ASSESSMENT TOOLS 6-1

Learning Assessment Guide (*Continued*)

If the learner is not able to carry out the care, are other caregivers available for backup support? _____

_____

If so, please name. _____
Phone number _____
Address _____
What other support is available for the client and caregiver? _____

_____

_____

CLIENT SITUATIONS IN PRACTICE

◆ Discharge Teaching With Newborn Circumcision

Pat, a primipara, delivered a boy yesterday afternoon. The newborn is to be circumcised this afternoon before Pat and her newborn are discharged. Despite the fact that you have gone over the teaching outline about circumcision twice with Pat, she states, "How will the penis look in 3 days?" She is also unable to demonstrate the application of the dressing to the site and states, "Maybe we shouldn't have the baby circumcised if it will hurt the baby."

For this scenario, the following is an example of a learning need in the affective domain:
Anxiety related to lack of knowledge as manifested by the mother's statement, "Maybe we shouldn't have the baby circumcised if it will hurt the baby."

Here is an example of a learning need in the psychomotor domain:
Risk for Impaired Home Maintenance Management related to lack of knowledge and ability to demonstrate dressing change.

The following is an example of a nursing diagnosis in the cognitive domain:
Altered Parenting related to lack of knowledge and inexperience as manifested by the mother's statement, "How will the penis look in 3 days?"

◆ Reimbursement for Teaching in the Home

After the learning need is identified, the nurse determines if the teaching needed by the client is reimbursable. In the example above teaching is an expected part of the role of the nurse in discharge planning and is a reimbursed activity. However, nursing care in the home that is only focused on teaching is reimbursed only if it meets certain requirements. Medicare, Medicaid, and most other third-party payers reimburse only skilled nursing care that falls within specific parameters. Consequently, referrals for health education needs depend on **reimbursement requirements** of the payer of the services. Most insurance companies, health maintenance organizations, and other third-party payers follow Medicare Guidelines. The specific requirements are defined in the Medicare Guidelines, Revision 222, Section 205.13 summarized in Box 6-2.

An example is seen in a client who is newly diagnosed with diabetes. The client's learning needs must meet the requirements seen in Assessment Tool 6-1; otherwise

Medicare or the insurance company, depending on the coverage, will not reimburse for the home visit for health teaching. It is imperative that the nurse knows the reimbursement requirements of the various third-party payers as agencies will not receive payment for teaching if the nurse does not follow the requirements specified by the particular payer.

TABLE 6-2 Examples of Inferences Made From Assessment Data		
Factors to Consider When Assessing Readiness to Learn	**Data**	**Inference**
Physiologic Factors		
Age	85	Elderly client may have special needs
Gender	Male	Men and women each have special needs
Disease process currently under treatment	Newly diagnosed diabetic	New diabetics have many teaching needs
Intactness of senses—hearing, vision, touch, taste	Hearing and vision are impaired	Teaching must be modified considering sensory deficit
Preexisting conditions	Cataract surgery 2 y ago	Vision may still be partially impaired or may be corrected
Psychosocial Factors		
Sociocultural	Hmong refugee	Teaching must consider diet common to this culture
Occupation	Retired	Does the client have health insurance?
Cognitive Factors		
Motivation	Learner states, "I am interested in learning about _____"	Learner is motivated
Reading ability	Observed reading the newspaper	Shows ability to read
Learning style	Observer, doer, or listener	Tailor teaching to style
Problem-solving ability	Learner can come up with concepts and alternatives	Learner can problem solve
Environmental Factors		
Home environment	Home cluttered with no place to sit or set up teaching	Environment must be modified before teaching
Caregiver		
Availability	Client is a widow or spouse works full time	No caregiver available
Motivation	Caregiver states, "I can't handle hearing about that device"	Caregiver not motivated
Abilities	Caregiver is unable to follow simple instructions or directions	Caregiver has limited ability to provide care
Other support	Client is active in his or her church	Church may be another source of care and support

---

◆ **B O X 6-2** Medicare Guidelines ◆

"... activities which require skilled nursing personnel to teach a beneficiary, the beneficiary's family or care givers how to manage his treatment regimen constitutes skilled nursing services. Where the teaching or training is reasonable and necessary to the treatment of the illness or injury, skilled nursing visits for teaching would be covered. The test of whether a nursing service is skilled relates to the skill required to teach and not to the nature of what is being taught. ... Skilled nursing visits for teaching and training activities are reasonable and necessary where the teaching or training is appropriate to the beneficiary's functional loss, or his illness or injury." From *Medicare Guidelines Coverage of Services* Revision 222, Section 205.13.

Summary of Medicare Reimbursement Requirements for Teaching

Teaching is reimbursed when it is considered in these ways:
    Teaching how to manage treatment
    Reasonable and necessary to the treatment of the illness or injury
"Reasonable and necessary" means teaching to the client's functional loss
    or his or her illness or injury.
To determine the number of necessary and reasonable visits, use the
    following criteria:
    Initial teaching = number of visits depends on the *complexity* of the
        tasks and the *ability* of the learner
    Reinforcement teaching = number of visits depends on *retained*
        knowledge and anticipated learning progress
Teaching is not generally reimbursed under these conditions:
    It becomes apparent after a reasonable period of time the client, family,
        or caregiver is *not* able to learn.
    The reason that learning did not occur is *not* documented.

Adapted from *Medicare Guidelines Coverage of Services* Revision 222, Section 205.13.

Planning

Planning for learning involves developing a teaching plan. Teaching plans are similar to nursing care plans—both follow the steps of the nursing process. Some agencies use standardized or computerized teaching plans. If standardized plans are used, the plan must always be individualized to the client and his or her needs. Teaching plans are also incorporated into critical pathway documentation.

The teaching plan identifies learning objectives that reflect the specifics of the ongoing care at home. Methods of documentation vary, but the trend is toward the use of clinical pathways that outline teaching needs by diagnosis or procedure and include learning outcomes, content, methods, and strategies for teaching.

Often, the goal of teaching is to ensure the client's safety and total reliance on self-care. Planning care is a mutual process among the nurse, client, and family caregivers using the three learning domains.

◆ Cognitive objectives: Relate to learning activities that strengthen comprehension regarding the illness and its treatment
◆ Affective objectives: Relate to learning activities that enhance the acceptance of the illness and subsequent treatment
◆ Psychomotor objectives: Relate to learning activities that demonstrate management of the treatment procedures

A **learning objective** is similar to a client goal or expected outcome used in the nursing process. Each objective includes a subject, action verb, performance criteria, target time, and special conditions (Box 6-3).

The following learning objective contains these components:

◆ Client will state three signs and symptoms of infection by (date)_____ and know which complications require contacting the nurse on call.
◆ Subject: client
◆ Action verb: state
◆ Performance criteria: signs and symptoms of infection
◆ Target time: (date)
◆ Special conditions: when to contact the nurse on call

Examples of learning objectives in the three learning domains are as follows:

◆ Cognitive objectives: Family or caregiver will state three signs and symptoms of infection by (date)_____.

◆ **BOX 6-3** Active Verbs for Learning Objectives ◆

Cognitive Domain	Affective Domain	Psychomotor Domain
categorize	answer	adapt
compare	choose	arrange
compose	defend	assemble
define	discuss	begin
describe	display	change
design	form	construct
differentiate	give	create
explain	help	manipulate
give example	initiate	move
identify	join	organize
label	justify	rearrange
list	relate	show
name	revise	start
prepare	select	work
plan	share	
solve	use	
state		
summarize		
write		

◆ Affective objectives: Family or caregiver will express feelings about having to be in charge of client's Port-a-Cath care by (date)_____.
◆ Psychomotor objectives: Family or caregiver will demonstrate aseptic technique when cleaning and flushing sites on Port-a-Cath by (date)_____.

In most situations, the nurse and the client plan a series of small, incremental learning objectives based on the specific needs of the client. The overall goal of planning is to assist the client or family caregiver to have enough understanding to be safe with self-care. For many clients, the ultimate goal of independence is achieved through reliance on family or other caregivers. The goal of teaching is to maximize individual potential and quality of life of individuals and families.

Intervention

The nurse carries out the teaching plan according to the client or family caregiver's learning needs accomplished in one or more teaching sessions. Interventions may vary according to learner readiness, perceived need, and past life experience, all of which fluctuate throughout an individual's life span. Specific approaches for teaching children are shown in Appendix C, and nursing implications for various developmental stages are given in Appendix B. With clients across the life span the nurse needs to develop rapport and be an honest and open communicator to encourage, or give the client self-confidence, to learn something new. General principles to guide teaching with older learners are seen in Box 6-4.

Evaluation

In the last phase both learning and teaching are evaluated to determine if the learning outcomes were met and if the teaching methods were effective. The plan is then modified as necessary.

◆ BOX 6-4 General Principles to Guide Community-Based Teaching With the Older Learner ◆

- Meet in a quiet, well-lit room where there is no background noise.
- Face the learner and speak in a low, slow voice so lip-reading is possible.
- With the client's permission, include family members.
- Limit sessions to no more than 20 to 30 minutes and watch for cues indicating inadequate hearing, lack of attention, or tiredness.
- Relate new information to past experiences if possible. Repeat information frequently; use frequent summaries.
- Encourage autonomous decision making to support ego integrity.
- Provide written materials as reinforcement, when possible, with visual aids with large letters and bright colors.
- Compliment the client for adaptability to learning session.

Learning is evaluated by deciding if the learning outcomes were met. The following questions may be asked to assess the level of learning:

◆ What additional data do I need to collect to evaluate the progress made toward the learning objectives?
◆ What other learning needs apply to this client and family?
◆ Were the objectives met? If not, why not?
◆ How do I know that my client learned what I planned to teach?
◆ Did the timing of the teaching impede or enhance learning?
◆ Is the nurse, client, and family satisfied with the outcome? If not, what would provide satisfaction?

Second, evaluation of teaching appraises the efficacy of the teaching plan and methods. Evaluation of teaching considers the barriers to, and characteristics of, successful teaching. The nurse may ask these questions:

◆ Did the teaching focus on the most important problem for this family in relation to the potential of the client for self-care?
◆ Was the plan collaborative?
◆ Was there reinforcement?
◆ Was the home environment appropriate? If not, how was it modified?
◆ Was the equipment adequate?
◆ Was the nurse prepared?
◆ Did the nurse use a variety of teaching methods?
◆ Did the learner have the opportunity for hands-on practice?
◆ Was the visit structured to reduce anxiety and enhance learning?
◆ Was the teaching plan realistic?
◆ Were the learning objectives, teaching plan, and methods realistic and appropriate for this client and family?
◆ Were the family strengths considered when determining the learning objectives and teaching methods?
◆ If this session were to be repeated, which strategies or tools could be used?

Evaluation must always consider what the client and family believe they need to know, as well as what the nurse considers essential. It is also important for the nurse to recognize when the learning needs of the client, family, or caregiver are beyond the educational preparation of the nurse so that a referral to appropriate resources can be made.

Documentation

Documentation of teaching is essential (1) as a legal record, (2) as communication of teaching and learning to other health care professionals, and (3) for determination of eligibility for care needed and for reimbursement of care provided. The following parts of the teaching process should be documented:

◆ Assessment of the learner's readiness, need, and life experiences
◆ Identification of learning needs and barriers to successful learning
◆ Plan for teaching and learning outcomes
◆ Content taught
◆ Teaching techniques used

◆ Evaluation of teaching and learning, including learner response and recommendations for the next step

Methods of documentation vary, but the trend is toward the use of clinical pathways that outline teaching needs by diagnosis or procedure and include learning outcomes, content, methods, and strategies for teaching. An additional component of documentation is confidentiality. Community-Based Nursing Care Guidelines 6-1 displays guidelines for maintaining client confidentiality.

Barriers to Successful Teaching

It is helpful to be aware of some of the potential obstacles to successful teaching. Conditions and barriers to successful teaching differ between the acute care setting and community setting. Likewise there may be barriers to successful teaching that differ between community-based settings. In the next section barriers to successful teaching are presented and followed by characteristics of successful teaching.

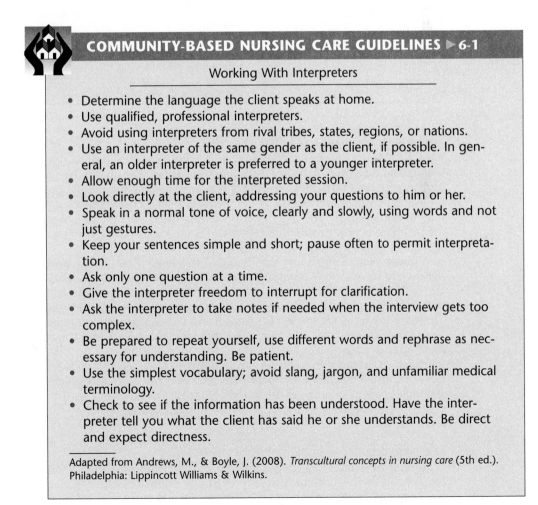

COMMUNITY-BASED NURSING CARE GUIDELINES ▶ 6-1

Working With Interpreters

- Determine the language the client speaks at home.
- Use qualified, professional interpreters.
- Avoid using interpreters from rival tribes, states, regions, or nations.
- Use an interpreter of the same gender as the client, if possible. In general, an older interpreter is preferred to a younger interpreter.
- Allow enough time for the interpreted session.
- Look directly at the client, addressing your questions to him or her.
- Speak in a normal tone of voice, clearly and slowly, using words and not just gestures.
- Keep your sentences simple and short; pause often to permit interpretation.
- Ask only one question at a time.
- Give the interpreter freedom to interrupt for clarification.
- Ask the interpreter to take notes if needed when the interview gets too complex.
- Be prepared to repeat yourself, use different words and rephrase as necessary for understanding. Be patient.
- Use the simplest vocabulary; avoid slang, jargon, and unfamiliar medical terminology.
- Check to see if the information has been understood. Have the interpreter tell you what the client has said he or she understands. Be direct and expect directness.

Adapted from Andrews, M., & Boyle, J. (2008). *Transcultural concepts in nursing care* (5th ed.). Philadelphia: Lippincott Williams & Wilkins.

TABLE 6-3	Combating Barriers to Successful Discharge Teaching
Barriers	**Sample Nursing Interventions**
Timing is not conducive to learning (client's physical or psychological conditions do not allow learning to occur)	Document client's lack of mastery of the material. Update physician or nurse practitioner on an ongoing basis to plan discharge. Refer for follow-up if learning is not adequate for safe self-care.
Past experiences impede perceived learning readiness or need.	Identify past experiences. Determine and clarify misconceptions. Determine if past experience will interrupt or enhance new learning.
Retention of information impeded by anxiety of going home or leaving security of health care environment.	See interventions for timing. Break learning into small, easily mastered segments. Use positive reinforcement and praise.
Cultural differences between nurse and client or family impede learning or understanding.	Work to build a trusting relationship with client and family. Show respect for the client's culture and incorporate it in discharge planning. Use resources to overcome a language barrier.
Lack of adherence	Establish trust. Identify reasons for lack of adherence. Clarity misinformation. Use formal and informal contracting.

BARRIERS TO DISCHARGE TEACHING

We have known for over a decade that discharge teaching does not always result in learning. In a questionnaire designed to evaluate the quality of discharge teaching, only one of five family caregivers reported feeling adequately prepared to care for the client at home (Leske & Pelczynski, 1999). Their retention of information may diminish due to the anxiety experienced with the client's homecoming. Time for teaching is now grossly limited in the acute care setting. Barriers to successful discharge teaching are shown in Table 6-3.

A major area of discharge teaching that has been identified as problematic is adherence to medications regime after discharge. Fifty percent of individuals over the age of 65 have multiple chronic conditions, with most routinely taking an average of two to six prescribed medications and concurrently use one to three medications. Therefore, there is great need for teaching in this age group (Bergman-Evans, 2006). Numerous studies have shown a high rate of nonadherence with the medication regimen after discharge from an inpatient setting resulting in re-hospitalization, clinic follow-up, or admission to home care. Comprehensive discharge teaching regarding medication management at home prevents or reduces this problem. Box 6-5 lists strategies to help clients get the full benefit from drug therapy. As the primary client educator, the nurse is in a vital position to promote adherence to prescribed treatment regimens.

BARRIERS TO SUCCESSFUL TEACHING IN THE HOME

A number of barriers to successful teaching in the home exist (Table 6-4). These barriers have the potential to interrupt the coordination of and consistency in teaching and communication with the care giving team.

A: Assessment	Completing a comprehensive medication assessment • Mental status assessment • Brown-bag assessment • Adherence • Assessment of medication-taking ability
I: Individualization	Partnering with clients to ensure individualization of the regiment
D: Documentation	Choosing appropriate documentation to assist with communication between client and provider(s)
E: Education	Providing accurate and ongoing education tailored to the age group and needs of the individual
S: Supervision	Continuing supervision of the medication regimen

Adapted from Bergman-Evans, B., (2006). AIDES to improving medication adherence in older adults. *Geriatric Nursing, 27*(3), 174–182.

TABLE 6-4   Combating Barriers to Successful Home Teaching

Barriers	Sample Nursing Interventions
Home Environment	
Examples: Home setting is nonstructured. Environment is the client and family's home turf. Equipment and setting are inadequate for teaching.	Involve client and family in all stages of planning. Build trusting relationship with client and family, maintaining respect for family's culture and values. Adapt the home environment to facilitate learning and compliance.
Nurse Caregiver	
Examples: Nurse has less control over the outcomes of the teaching. Nurse may have inadequate preparation for providing teaching in the home. Nurse must bring all the teaching supplies to the home. Nurse must coordinate client teaching among many providers. Nurse role shifts from client care manager to health care facilitator.	Approach the client with a nonjudgmental attitude. Acquire specific knowledge and skill in community-based care. Plan and organize ahead and bring all supplies. Facilitate communication and documentation among caregivers. Focus on enhancing client's self-care instead of providing care to the client.
Client/Family/Recipient of Teaching	
Examples: Wide variation in family members' ages and cognitive and developmental stages Lack of adherence unless client/family are involved in the teaching plan	Carefully assess learning need, learning readiness, and past learning experiences of all recipients of teaching. Involve family and client in all stages of planning and teaching.

Nursing students and novice home care nurses often express dismay over their diminished control of client behavior when providing care in settings other than the acute care setting. For instance, teaching in the home often requires adaptation to the particular home environment, where the client is in control. Further, the nurse is faced with accommodating the specific needs of the client and family within their own schedule and circumstances.

Another barrier relates to difficulty in coordinating client teaching among multiple providers. Often, many care providers are involved with the client's care. Other professionals may include other nurses, physical therapists, social workers, home health aides, nurse practitioners, and physicians. Each provider may teach a procedure, treatment, or process in a different way, confusing the client. It is difficult to maintain ongoing communication among multiple caregivers in several diverse settings.

Lack of time is a barrier to home care teaching. The time factor in acute care settings may prohibit teaching, and many home care referrals come from clinics or physicians' offices. As a result, the first teaching, in many cases, may be done in the home. Home care nurses are often pressed for time. It may be difficult for the home care nurse to feel teaching is ever complete or even adequate.

Successful Teaching Approaches

Discharge teaching in both home care and acute care settings must begin at admission. Every encounter the nurse has with the client or family is an opportunity to assess learning needs and teach to the identified needs. The first and most essential component of successful teaching in community-based settings is building a trusting relationship with the client and family. As trust builds, barriers are removed often resulting in enhanced learning and adherence to the prescribed regimen. Vigilant assessment of the family, its culture, and the community environment results in a comprehensive teaching plan. Joint planning leads to better adherence to treatment regimens because this process requires forming a partnership, building an alliance, and working together toward a shared goal. It takes time to build trust to initiate mutual planning, but this is the only way to individualize care.

Frequently, clients and family caregivers may only need reinforcement that the client is progressing normally in the recovery process. In these situations, the focus includes care for the caregiver as well as care for the client. Affirming the quality of care provided by the family caregiver by listening to the concerns and frustrations of the caregiver should be a priority of the nurse.

Anxiety has long been know to be a barrier to learning. When the client is on "home turf" and has more control of the environment and the situation, anxiety may be reduced (Fig. 6-3). On the other hand, often the discharge planning process in both home care and acute care creates high anxiety for the client and family. As part of the original and ongoing assessment process, the nurse assesses the learner's anxiety level. If the learner exhibits anxiety that is interrupting learning, the learning plan must be modified. Another way to reduce anxiety is to create lessons that include small "digestible" segments that build on information shared in previous teaching sessions.

In all settings, teaching is problematic if the nurse does not speak the same language as the client or if the client has sight, comprehension, or retention problems (see Community-Based Nursing Care Guidelines 6-2 and 6-3). There are several community-based guidelines that should be followed when providing

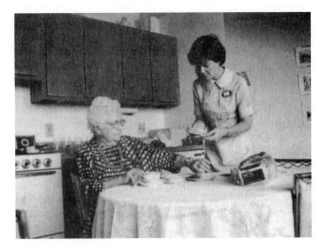

FIGURE 6-3. ▶ A teaching/learning experience in the home often is more successful because the client is in his or her own territory. The nurse is responsible for teaching and coordinating care.

health information to a client or family member who uses English as a second language:

- ◆ Listen carefully to what the client and family are telling you.
- ◆ Discuss one idea at a time, use simple, uncomplicated sentences, and use concrete examples to enhance learning.
- ◆ Determine the client's and family members' understanding of the illness being treated and the suggested treatment.
- ◆ Plan care with the client and family.
- ◆ Use materials printed in the client's or family members' first language, when possible. Or use materials written in simple straightforward English.
- ◆ Discuss the client's use of folk medicines and home remedies.
- ◆ Be aware of and bring to the client and families attention the contraindications for concurrent use of medications and folk medicines.

Successful health teaching also requires the nurse to function as the interdisciplinary team member who furnishes a link between the various agencies providing care. In the community, coordinating communication among many care providers is even more important to ensure consistency in teaching and reinforcement of learning and enhances continuity of care.

Some form of follow-up to provide a link between care providers in the community is essential. This may be either in the form of a phone call, letter, home visit or clinic visit. According to numerous studies, these strategies enhance continuity of care. Meticulous documentation is an essential component of a successful discharge teaching program.

Behaviorally oriented client education, which emphasizes a change of environment to facilitate client self-care, is the most successful method for improving the clinical course of chronic disease. In addition, behavioral education contributes to care that is more easily managed in the home. For example, when teaching about home safety, rearranging furniture so that it is in the field of vision for a client with hemianopsia is a behavioral-oriented strategy. This strategy encourages ambulation, and facilitates self-care while protecting client safety but must be accomplished within the context of the client and family's value system. Another example of successful behaviorally oriented health education is seen in Research in Community-Based Nursing Care 6-1.

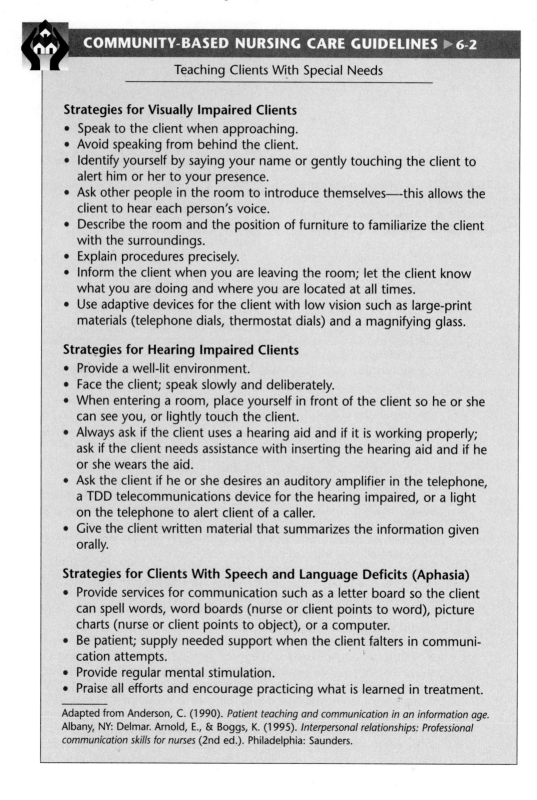

COMMUNITY-BASED NURSING CARE GUIDELINES ▷ 6-2

Teaching Clients With Special Needs

Strategies for Visually Impaired Clients
- Speak to the client when approaching.
- Avoid speaking from behind the client.
- Identify yourself by saying your name or gently touching the client to alert him or her to your presence.
- Ask other people in the room to introduce themselves—-this allows the client to hear each person's voice.
- Describe the room and the position of furniture to familiarize the client with the surroundings.
- Explain procedures precisely.
- Inform the client when you are leaving the room; let the client know what you are doing and where you are located at all times.
- Use adaptive devices for the client with low vision such as large-print materials (telephone dials, thermostat dials) and a magnifying glass.

Strategies for Hearing Impaired Clients
- Provide a well-lit environment.
- Face the client; speak slowly and deliberately.
- When entering a room, place yourself in front of the client so he or she can see you, or lightly touch the client.
- Always ask if the client uses a hearing aid and if it is working properly; ask if the client needs assistance with inserting the hearing aid and if he or she wears the aid.
- Ask the client if he or she desires an auditory amplifier in the telephone, a TDD telecommunications device for the hearing impaired, or a light on the telephone to alert client of a caller.
- Give the client written material that summarizes the information given orally.

Strategies for Clients With Speech and Language Deficits (Aphasia)
- Provide services for communication such as a letter board so the client can spell words, word boards (nurse or client points to word), picture charts (nurse or client points to object), or a computer.
- Be patient; supply needed support when the client falters in communication attempts.
- Provide regular mental stimulation.
- Praise all efforts and encourage practicing what is learned in treatment.

Adapted from Anderson, C. (1990). *Patient teaching and communication in an information age.* Albany, NY: Delmar. Arnold, E., & Boggs, K. (1995). *Interpersonal relationships: Professional communication skills for nurses* (2nd ed.). Philadelphia: Saunders.

COMMUNITY-BASED NURSING CARE GUIDELINES ▶ 6-3

Confidentiality

- Maintain confidentiality in consultation, teaching, and writing.
- Ensure privacy before engaging in a discussion of content to be entered into the record.
- Release information only with written consent.
- Use professional judgment regarding confidentiality when the information may be harmful to the client's health or well-being.
- Use professional judgment when deciding how to maintain the privacy of a minor. Be aware of your state's legal ramifications of the parent's or guardian's right to know.

RESEARCH IN COMMUNITY-BASED NURSING CARE ▶ 6-1

Evaluating the Effects of an Educational Symposium on Knowledge, Impact, and Self-Management of Older African Americans Living With Osteoarthritis

The aim of this study was to determine the influence of a 1-day educational symposium on knowledge, impact, and self-management of older African Americans living with osteoarthritis (OA). Participants were African American adults, age 60 or over who had OA and lived independently in the community. The participants were recruited at a 1-day educational symposium held at a nonprofit senior service. Each participant completed a demographic and background information, six-question investigator-developed knowledge test, the short form of the Arthritis Impact Measurement Scale (AIMS), and a Summary of Arthritis Management Methods (SAMMS) the day of the workshop. The knowledge test was completed both at the beginning and end of the day. The AIMS and SAMMS were administered a second time 3 months after the symposium. The results indicate that this symposium was effective in increasing participants' knowledge of OA, improving self-management, and decreasing the impact of OA on the daily function.

It is estimated that 70% to 85% of individuals over the age of 55 have OA. The result of this research is consistent with other work that supports the effectiveness of behaviorally oriented self-care education for chronically ill people. Health care education is a critical component of health care for older people.

Taylor, L. F., Kee, C. C., King, S. V., & Lawrence, F. (2004). Evaluating the effects of an educational symposium on knowledge, impact and self-management of older African Americans living with osteoarthritis. *Journal of Community Health Nursing, 21*(4),229–238.

Successful Teaching Techniques

The nurse needs to be familiar with a variety of teaching techniques and feel competent to choose which technique is most suitable for the circumstance. For example, demonstration of a new skill is used to change behavior, whereas videotapes are used to increase knowledge. Video use supplements one-on-one and group teaching. Videos can be viewed several times by anyone with access to a videotape player. Many acute care settings use closed-circuit television to display successful teaching programs and to reinforce learning. Before discharge, the client as well as the family or caregiver may watch programs several times if reinforcement is necessary. The videotape can be used the same way in the home.

Successful teaching strategies include demonstrating and return demonstration of a skill with opportunity for hands on practice in addition to telling the client about the procedure. Regardless of the setting, much teaching occurs while the nurse is providing client care—taking blood pressure or a temperature, giving a bath, examining a newborn or infant, weighing the client, and changing wound dressings. Client education seldom is the formal process one experiences in a classroom. Weaving teaching into all nursing activities saves time and allows the nurse to repeat the teaching several times.

Actual equipment and objects can be used for effective teaching, including the catheter, tubing, port, monitor, or other devices. Picture cards can be made to illustrate each item in a procedure. Photos can be made of each key step or diagrams can be drawn for the cards. Quizzes can be developed with short statements related to the procedure in true or false categories. The nurse can design posters with information the client needs to learn. Work sheets can be developed to use with a videotape or audiotape.

A new teaching technique for health education is the use of Web sites on the Internet. For example, one innovative program provides presurgical preparation for adolescent clients prior to tonsillectomy and adenoidectomy. Interactive content provides preparation without the client having to leave the home (O'Conner-Von, 2001). This method could be used for any type of teaching for clients who are computer literate and have access to a computer at home, school, or the public library.

Teaching the Challenging Client

Rather than refer to challenging clients who do not follow treatment regimes as noncompliant, it is more helpful to frame this issue as lack of adherence. Noncompliance suggests a one-sided expectation, while adherence is defined as "being connected or associated by contract, giving support or loyalty to: or a steady or faithful attachment" (Webster, 2002).

When the teaching plan is unsuccessful due to lack of adherence to the treatment plan, special teaching strategies are used. When the nurse and the client are partners in care they use a mutual process to plan and implement care. These strategies may incorporate the concepts of concordance, adherence, and partnering (Huffman, 2005). Concordance is an agreement between the nurse and the client about whether, when, and how treatments occur. Again this term suggests an agreement that respects the beliefs and wishes of both parties.

It is important to ascertain *why* the client is not following the prescribed treatment. Common reasons clients do not follow treatment regimens stem from lack of information, lack of skill, lack of client value for the treatment, and lack of self-efficacy. It is not uncommon for individuals to not follow a treatment plan because of anxiety or fear. Before any teaching occurs, the nurse must address the anxiety or fear of the learner. Learning needs stemming from lack of information or skills are easily met by identifying and providing knowledge and opportunities to practice skills.

A simple problem-solving technique that can be used is to ask the client about his or her perception of progress made with the teaching plan. Once the barrier to learning is identified, the nurse and client in partnership can tailor interventions accordingly. Barriers may come from client factors, home environment, and the teaching plan itself.

CLIENT FACTORS

Client factors may include lack of knowledge, skill, or self-efficacy. In other cases fear or lack of valuing the treatment plan will produce lack of adherence. Regardless, each factor may require a different approach to resolve the lack of adherence. It is important to first identify the cause as each factor calls for a different approach. Sometimes, nurses may interpret nonadherence as lack of knowledge when the client's behavior simply reflects the values and attitudes of the client and the client's community. Lack of adherence stemming from the client's attitudes and values, calls for a different approach in revising the plan than when adherence arises from lack of information. Lack of valuing the treatment may require modification of the teaching regimen to better fit the client's value system.

Likewise, lack of adherence may stem from the client's belief about their own self-efficacy or ability to perform to influence events that affect their life. Client's self-efficacy can be increased by:

◆ Setting realistic goals
◆ Using gentle persuasion to encourage the client to believe in his or her own ability to achieve goals
◆ Teaching easy management techniques first
◆ Use return demonstrations with immediate positive reinforcement
◆ Point out the client's incremental successes
◆ Helping the client reduce emotional responses to perceived threats and fears (Oliver, 2005).

Another strategy that may be helpful to address a specific health behavior involves a collaborative process in which the client chooses a goal, and the nurse and client negotiate a specific action plan to reach the goal. For example, if the client would like to stop smoking he or she may have an initial action plan of reducing the number of cigarettes consumed in a day from one pack to one half a pack by using nicotine gum. After a week the next step may be to start using a nicotine patch and only have one cigarette after each meal. Action plans have been shown clinically as a useful strategy to encourage behavior change for clients (Handley et al., 2006).

On the other hand, no individual is totally compliant. The nurse must use professional judgment to gauge what level of adherence to treatment is acceptable while continuously revising the teaching plan.

THE HOME ENVIRONMENT

The home environment may impede adherence to treatment regimen. Behaviorally oriented client education, which emphasizes the change of the environment in which the client does self-care, is often the most successful strategy. Changing the home environment is credited with improving the clinical course of clients instructed in the home. Careful assessment of the home environment allows the nurse to identify and modify problematic issues and enhance learning outcomes. These interventions may be as simple as providing better light for a teaching session by opening the drapes, moving a lamp, or replacing a burned-out light bulb.

THE TEACHING PLAN

As previously mentioned, effective teaching requires sound interpersonal skills and a nonjudgmental attitude is essential. Concordance is important to effective teaching. The nurse and the client can establish concordance at the first visit and each subsequent visit by contracting at the beginning of a therapeutic relationship about whether, when, and how treatments occur. Concordance may prevent some lack of adherence to the treatment plan from the outset. Most agencies have formal contracts such as a "Bill of Rights" or "Client Responsibilities." Review and implementation of the content of these standards on the first visit is one way to encourage adherence.

CLIENT SITUATIONS IN PRACTICE

◆ Teaching in the Home Setting

Assessment

Katie is the home care nurse assigned to care for Ina, a 76-year-old widow recently diagnosed with insulin-dependent diabetes. On Friday, November 1, Ina visited the clinic with complaints of polyuria, polydipsia, and polyphagia. Her blood sugar was 456 mg/dL. The clinic educator saw her on November 1 and charted the following on the referral form:

Client stated, "I have not slept well for 2 weeks because I have to get up so often to go to the bathroom." After the initial teaching session, which covered the basics of the diabetic diet and the action of insulin, the client was unable to demonstrate retention of knowledge or skills from any of the topics covered.

Recommendation to home care: Client requires diabetic teaching in the areas of following a diabetic diet, drawing up insulin, giving injections, and monitoring blood sugar. Client will receive insulin in the clinic until the home visit on Tuesday to teach about injections.

Reimbursement: This client requires teaching to manage home treatment of insulin-dependent diabetes diagnosed on 11/1. This teaching meets the criteria of Section 205.13 of Medicare Guidelines for Coverage of Services Revision 222.

On Tuesday, November 5, Katie visits Ina at home. Ina greets Katie at the door with the statement, "When I was at the clinic on Friday, I was so nervous about all of the things they were telling me, but I am more relaxed today. I talked to my friend Richard who is a diabetic and manages really well. When my granddaughter Karen was a little girl, I gave her shots and got along just fine."

Ina's home is dark so Katie asks if she can open the drapes and move two chairs closer to the window before they start to talk. They sit down by the window and Katie begins visiting with Ina in an attempt to begin developing a trusting relationship. Katie learns that Ina has some knowledge about diabetes from talking to her friend Richard, and Ina has also asked her son Mark, who is a nurse, to pick up some pamphlets about diabetes at the hospital.

Ina states that she learns best by doing. She does not drive but states that her son will be able to pick up her medication and syringes, or she can take the bus to the pharmacy. Katie notices a magnifying glass on the table and a large-print book on a bookshelf. Katie asks Ina about her vision. Ina responds that she has had three cataract surgeries and has difficulty reading, so she frequently uses the magnifying glass.

Katie concludes that Ina perceives a need to learn and is ready to learn. Katie also believes that Ina's past experiences will enhance her learning, not impede it. Concerned about Ina's restricted vision, Katie makes a note to continue to assess this aspect. At this point, Katie completes the learning assessment guide, as shown in Assessment Tools 6-2.

Identification of Learning Need

Katie and Ina conclude that Ina's overall learning need is as follows:

- *Risk for Injury related to lack of knowledge regarding diabetic self-care*

For this visit, Katie identifies the following priority need:

- *Risk for Injury related to client's lack of knowledge and inability to manage diabetes for the next 24 hours until the home visit the next day, as manifested by visual impairment*

Planning

Katie and Ina decide upon the following learning objectives for today:

1. Cognitive objective: Client will state when insulin is given and how much to draw up by the end of the visit on 11/5.
2. Psychomotor objective: Client will identify three sites for subcutaneous injection of insulin and demonstrate proper technique for injection by the end of the visit on 11/5.
3. Affective objective: Client will state that she is comfortable injecting insulin by the end of the visit on 11/5.

Implementation

1. Cognitive objective: Client will state when insulin is given and how much to draw up by the end of the visit on 11/5.

Together Katie and Ina review the written material on insulin, when it is given, and how much to draw up. Katie proceeds at a slow pace as she teaches, repeats the information frequently, and does not rush Ina. The teaching sheet is on white, non-glossy paper with bold, black print. After the teaching session, Ina states, "Insulin should be given before meals and as the schedule states. I am to give myself insulin according to the schedule." Katie leaves a videotape that covers the information in the teaching session.

2. Psychomotor objective: Client will identify three sites for subcutaneous injection of insulin and demonstrate proper technique for injection by the end of the visit on 11/5.

Katie demonstrates injecting the insulin into a model and identifies three sites for subcutaneous injection. Then Ina injects into the model. Katie draws up the insulin as ordered before dinner and Ina injects herself at 5:00. Ina is unable to see the numbers on the syringe.

Evaluation

Learning objectives 1 and 2 met: Ina identifies three sites for injection and injects herself correctly. Teaching focused on the most important problem for this client, the plan was collaborative, and reinforcement was provided with a videotape. The learner had the opportunity for hands-on practice, and a variety of teaching methods were used.

Implementation

3. Affective objective: Client will state that she is comfortable injecting insulin by the end of the visit on 11/5.

Ina discusses her feelings with Katie regarding the teaching session. Katie asks her if she feels comfortable giving herself an injection, and she says, "No, but I think it will come." Katie leaves a short videotape on injecting insulin for Ina to review before the next visit.

Evaluation

Learning objective #3 met at this time.

Teaching: Katie encourages Ina by stating how well she has done the first time handling the syringe. Katie tells Ina specifically what she did well: she did not hesitate before putting in the needle, she found a correct site, and she charted it accurately on the flow sheet. However, she is unable to identify the correct number of units on the syringe. She notes this need and adds an objective to address this issue to the list of the next lesson's objectives.

Assessment and Planning for the Next Teaching Session

Katie noted Ina's problems with her eyesight in the initial assessment, suggesting that Ina might have difficulty drawing up insulin with a syringe. Katie discussed her concern with Ina and asked to come back the next day. She also asked Ina if there was a friend or family member who might be available to assist with her care. Ina responded that her son Mark had indicated that he was willing to help with the injections. Katie requested that Ina contact Mark and ask that he be present at the next home visit.

Identification of Learning Need

Together, Katie and Ina decided on the following learning need for the home visit the next day:

• *Risk for Injury related to client's lack of knowledge and inability to read the calibrations on the syringe, as manifested by client's statement, "I have to use the magnifying glass to see print. I can't see the numbers on the syringes. Is it okay if I just estimate?"*

Planning

Katie and Ina decided that the learning objectives for tomorrow would be as follows:

1. Cognitive objective: Client will state when insulin is given, how much to draw up, and how to use the Magni-Guide syringe.
2. Psychomotor objective: Client will demonstrate how to draw up an accurate amount of insulin with the Magni-Guide syringe.
3. Affective objective: Client will state that she feels confident in her ability to draw up an accurate amount of insulin.

As Katie leaves Ina's home, Ina hugs her and says, "Thanks for all your help today. You have helped me so much!"

ASSESSMENT TOOLS 6-2

Sample Learning Assessment Guide

Client name *Ina*

Health condition requiring health education *Insulin-dependent diabetes*

diagnosed on November 1, 2007.

Primary caregiver *Home care nurse, client, and Mark*

Learner *Ina*   Relationship to client _____

Age *76*   Gender *Female*   Occupation *Retired legal secretary*

Developmental stages and implications for learner

Psychosocial Stage *The client is in the integrity versus ego despair stage. She*

describes her life as follows:

"I have been blessed. I have 10 wonderful children, 25 grand, and 10 great-grandchildren.

I loved my work after my kids grew up. My husband and I had a good relationship."

Cognitive stage *no evidence of cognitive impairment*

Language *speaks English, visual impairment, stoled " I was writing a novel about*

Ireland until I started to have problems with my eyes."

How does the caregiver or client feel about the responsibilities of self-care?
States she is more relaxed than 11/1 when diagnosed.

Describe any disabilities or limitations of the learner (including sensory
disabilities)

Visual impairment and statement "I am afraid that I will not be able to see the numbers

on the syringes."

Disabilities *arthritis in left knee and left hip*

Describe any preexisting health conditions of the learner
Client has had multiple cataract surgeries and has visual impairment.

List sociocultural factors that may impede learning *None*

State learner behaviors that indicate motivation to learn

Client stated she was more relaxed about her diagnosis, asked her son to get her information

about diabetes, contacted a friend with diabetes.

Can the learner read and comprehend at the reading level required by task?
Yes, but may not have visual acuity to see the colibrations on the syringe.

(continued)

ASSESSMENT TOOLS 6-2

Sample Learning Assessment Guide (*Continued*)

Does the learner show an ability to problem solve at a level that provides safe care in the home?

Client has managed health problems in her home with her granddaughter's illness 10 years ago.

Is the home environment conducive to the learning required by the care?

Home is very dark with poor lighting.

If not, what modifications are necessary? *Need better lighting in the kitchen.*

If the learner is not able to carry out the care, are other caregivers available for backup support? *yes*

If so, please name. *Mark (son), Karen (granddaughter), Richard (friend)*

Phone number *555-5555*

Address *3400 Belmont, White Kitty Lake, PA*

What other support is available for the client and caregiver? *Client has ten children, three of whom live in the area. Client is active in her church, which has a parish nurse and a befriender program.*

There is a support group for newly diagnosed diabetics, which meets at a hospital near client's home. Client lives on the bus line with service to the clinic, hospital, and church.

CONCLUSIONS

In the current health care system, health teaching has become an essential role for the nurse in community-based settings. Client, family, and staff satisfaction is improved if teaching results are positive. Quality instruction leads to more efficient use of resources. Good teaching assists clients and families to achieve independence in self-care. Interdisciplinary communication augment teaching efficacy. Comprehensive assessment of the client and family safeguards accurate identification of learning needs. Collaborative planning preserves successful learning outcomes because clients and families are more likely to learn when they have had input in the process. Learning to avoid or navigate barriers and incorporate characteristics of successful teaching enhances teaching in community-based nursing.

What's on the Web

Centers for Disease Control and Prevention (CDC)
Internet address:
http://www.cdc.gov (Home page for CDC)
This site offers abundant resources about topics related to disease prevention and health promotion.

Health Topics A–Z
Internet address:
http://www.cdc.gov/publications.htm
You can find information on any health topic on the Health Topics A–Z site. This CDC site offers an unlimited number of publications, software, and other products for teaching or research.

About CDC
Internet address:
http://www.cdc.gov/aboutcdc.htm
This site outlines all of the components of the CDC and the centers to assist you to find teaching materials for various topics.

Consumer Health Information Corporation (CHIP)
Internet address:
http://www.consumer-health.com/
This site provides patient education on a variety of topics from a variety of perspectives. They provide information for pharmaceutical companies, health care providers, and consumers.

Healthfinders
Internet address:
http://www.healthfinder.gov/
This is your guide to reliable health information with three versions of the site, one for consumers and professional health providers, one for children, and one in Spanish. Each site includes a health library, health topics, information about health care providers, and a directory of healthfinder organizations.

Health Literacy
Internet address:
http://nnlm.gov/outreach/consumer/hlthlit.html
The national Network of Libraries of Medicine provides this credible site on health literacy. The resources on the site include skills needed for health literacy, research, a list of organizations and programs, and a bibliography and webliography.

Mayo Clinic
Internet address: http://www.mayo.edu
This site has reliable information for a healthier life. You can find information quickly on the A–Z index of various conditions. You can also ask a specialist any questions that you may have about your client's conditions. There are timely topics, as well as slides on various subjects—lots of materials to use as you teach in community-based settings.

References and Bibliography

Anderson, C. (1990). *Patient teaching and communication in an information age.* Albany, NY: Delmar.

Arnold, E., & Boggs, K. (1995). *Interpersonal relationships: Professional communication skills for nurses* (2nd ed). Philadelphia: Saunders.

Andrus, M. R., & Roth, M. T. (2002). Health literacy: A review. *Pharmacotherapy, 22*(3), 282-302.

American Public Health Association. (2004). Disparities in health literacy. Retrieved on August 18, 2006, from http://www.medscape.com/

Bergman-Evans, B. (2006). AIDES to improving medication adherence in older adults. *Geriatric Nursing, 27*(3), 174–182.

Carpenito, L. J. (2006). *Nursing diagnosis: Application to clinical practice* (11th ed.). Philadelphia: Lippincott Williams & Wilkins.

Consumer Health Information Corporation (CHIP). (2006). Preventing home medication errors. Retrieved August 17, 2006, from http://www.consumer-health.com/media_center/caregivers_need.htm

Handley, M., MacGregor, K., Schillinger, D., et al. (2006). Using action plans to help primary care patients adopt healthy behaviors; A descriptive study. *Journal of the American Board of Family Medicine, 19*(3), 224-231.

Huffman, M. (2005). Homecare today: A case study in home health disease management. *Home Healthcare Nurse, 23*(10), 636–638.

Jarvis, C. (1996). *Physical examination of health assessment* (2nd ed.). Philadelphia: Saunders.

Knox, A. B. (1986). *Helping adults learn.* San Francisco: Jossey-Bass.

Leske, J. S., & Pelczynski, S. A. (1999). Caregiver satisfaction with preparation for discharge in a decreased-length-of-stay cardiac surgery program. *Journal of Cardiovascular Nursing, 14*(1), 35–43.

London, F. (1999). A nurse's guide to patient and family education. Philadelphia: Lippincott Williams & Wilkins.

Magoon, L. (2002). Hospital extra: Parents and medication errors. *American Journal of Nursing, 102*(9), 24A–24C.

Medicare Guidelines for Coverage of Services Revision 222, Section 205.13

Minnesota Department of Health. Division of Community Health Services. Public Health Nursing Section. (2001). *Public health nursing interventions: Application for public health nursing practice.* Minneapolis, Minnesota: Author.

O'Conner-Von, S. (2001). *Preparation of adolescents for outpatient surgery: A comparison of methods.* Unpublished doctoral dissertation. Rush University of Chicago, Illinois.

Oliver, M. (2005). Reaching positive outcomes by assessing teaching patients self-efficacy. *Home Healthcare Nurse, 23*(9), 559–562.

Pawlak, R. (2006). Economic considerations of health literacy. *Nursing Economics, 23*(4), 173-180.

Stanley, M., & Beare, P. (1999). *Gerontological nursing: A health promotion/protection approach* (2nd ed). Philadelphia: Davis.

Stone, J., Wyman, J., & Salisbury, S. (1999). *Gerontological nursing: A health promotion/protection approach* (2nd ed). Philadelphia: Davis.

Taylor, C., Lillis, C., & LeMone, P. (2006). *Fundamentals of nursing: The art and science of nursing care* (p. 486). Philadelphia: Lippincott, Williams & Wilkins.

Taylor, L. F., Kee, C. C., King, S. V., & Lawrence, F. (2004). Evaluating the effects of an educational symposium on knowledge, impact and self-management of older African Americans living with osteoarthritis. *Journal of Community Health Nursing, 21*(4), 229–238.

U.S. Department of Health and Human Services. (2000). Healthy people 2010 (Conference edition, Vols. 1–2). Washington, DC: Author.

Webster Online Dictionary. Retrieved on October 28, 2007, from http://www.merriam-webster.com

LEARNING ▼ ACTIVITIES

◆ **JOURNALING ACTIVITY 6-1**

1. In your clinical journal, discuss a situation you observed or were the caretaker for someone who had several teaching needs. Outline the process used to assess, plan, and teach the client and family members.
2. Using theory from this chapter, identify what was successful and what was not successful related to teaching and learning for this client and family.
3. What would you do differently from what was done if you are in a similar situation in the future? From this experience, what did you learn about yourself and teaching clients and families?

◆ CLIENT CARE ACTIVITY 6-2

Jennifer is a nurse working on a postpartum unit. She is caring for Joan, a 35-year-old primipara (normal spontaneous vaginal delivery [NSVD]), who delivered a boy yesterday and is going home at noon today. Joan states she has been working full time since she graduated from law school. She is the youngest of three siblings. She and her husband Tim took prenatal classes, and she describes him as being very excited about the baby. You observe Tim trying unsuccessfully to diaper the baby when you are in the room doing postpartum checks on Joan.

Jennifer interviewed Joan and Tim to determine their learning needs. They both tell Jennifer that they are wondering about having their baby circumcised. They wonder about the advantages and disadvantages of the procedure; how to take care of the surgical site after the procedure on their son and when they return home; and how to keep the area clean and free from stool. Prior to the teaching session, Joan has had pain medication and placed ice on her perineum. Both parents have good eye contact and relaxed postures as Jennifer interviewed them.

1. Determine the behaviors that show that Joan and Tim are ready to learn.
2. List the factors Jennifer should assess regarding Joan and Tim's readiness to learn.
3. Recognize what indicates to Jennifer that Joan and Tim show a need to learn.
4. Examine Joan and Tim's prior experience and knowledge base related to the topic.
5. Identify Joan and Tim's learning need in each domain: cognitive, affective, and psychomotor.
6. State one learning outcome for Joan and Tim for each learning need.
7. Discuss how the principles of community-based care apply to the learning needs of Joan and Tim.

◆ CLIENT CARE ACTIVITY 6-3

Hazel is a 65-year-old woman whose husband is blind and was recently diagnosed with early signs of dementia. Shannon is doing preadmission teaching with Hazel, who is scheduled for outpatient surgery tomorrow morning. Shannon knows it is important to assess Hazel's readiness to learn. If Hazel is thinking about her husband's care during the time she is preparing for surgery, she may not hear Shannon tell her that she should not drive or make important decisions for at least 24 hours after receiving general anesthesia.

Explain how Shannon will assess Hazel's readiness to learn. What questions would she ask?

◆ PRACTICAL APPLICATION ACTIVITY 6-4

Volunteer to teach a health-related class at a local elementary, middle, or high school. Ask the school nurse or the class teacher to recommend a topic, or go to the class and survey the students to find out what topics they would like to learn about. Use the content in this chapter to plan and develop the class. After you teach the students, use some of the following questions to evaluate your class.

- Were the objectives met? If not, why not?
- How do you know that students learned what you planned to teach?
- Did the timing of the teaching impede or enhance learning?
- Were the students satisfied with the outcome? If not, what would provide satisfaction?

- Did the teaching focus on the most important problem for the students?
- Was the plan collaborative?
- Was there reinforcement?
- Was the environment appropriate? If not, how was it modified?
- Was the equipment adequate?
- Were you prepared?
- Did you use a variety of teaching methods?
- Did learners have the opportunity for hands-on practice?
- Was the session structured to reduce anxiety and enhance learning?
- Was the teaching plan realistic?
- Were the learning objectives, teaching plan, and methods realistic and appropriate for students?
- If this session were to be repeated, what other strategies or tools could be used?

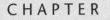
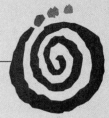

CHAPTER 7

Continuity of Care: Discharge Planning and Case Management

ROBERTA HUNT

LEARNING OBJECTIVES

1. Define continuity of care.
2. Define case management.
3. Discuss the implications of admission, discharge, and transfer.
4. Identify the relationships between discharge planning, case management, and continuity of care.
5. Relate community resources and the referral process to continuity of care.
6. Discuss nursing skills and competencies needed in the nurse case manager's and discharge planner's roles in community-based settings.
7. Determine how family, culture, and prevention influence health planning for continuity.
8. List common barriers that interrupt continuity.

KEY TERMS

case finding
case management
client advocacy
collaboration
consultation
continuity of care
coordinated care

delegation
discharge planning
managed care skills
referral and follow-up
screening
transferring
unlicensed assistive personnel

CHAPTER TOPICS

◆ Significance of Continuity of Care
◆ Entering and Exiting the Health Care System
◆ Discharge Planning
◆ Nurse Case Manager
◆ Nursing Skills and Competencies in Continuity of Care
◆ Barriers to Successful Continuity of Care
◆ Successful Continuity of Care
◆ Conclusions

THE NURSE SPEAKS

While working as a staff nurse in the hospital I was involved with a patient's acute care and symptom management, but after their discharge from the hospital, I would often wonder how the patient and their family were doing. The last few years I have had the privilege to work as a home hospice nurse; this has given me the opportunity (and time) to sit and talk with patients and their families about many different things. I am always interested to hear stories about nurses that have been instrumental in a patient's care and how a nurse's compassion and interaction with a person can provide greater comfort and dignity during challenging and emotional times. When I hear a story of the impact a nurse has had on a patient (and/or family), I have used this opportunity, when possible, to follow up with the nurse(s) to let them know how much their care is appreciated. I do my best to find out the nurse's name and work station and send them a thank you note for the care they provide. With a patient's permission, I will include a brief update on how patient and family are doing. I end the note asking the nurse to save the letter and reread it whenever he/she has a difficult shift as a reminder of the important work they do every day and the difference they make in the lives they touch.

—DENISE SILL-CLAUSEN, RN, BSN, PHN, Alinna Home Care, Hospice &
Palliative Care, Minneapolis, MN

Nurses have been involved in continuity of care since the late 1880s. The origins date back to the turn of the century, when nurses staffed settlement houses. An article by Tahan (1998, p. 56) describes a system of cards used by nurses at the settlement houses, which stated that the duties of the staff were to ". . . list family needs, establish a mechanism for follow-up, facilitate the delivery of services and ensure that families were connected with appropriate resources." In 1906, both Massachusetts General Hospital in Boston and Bellevue Hospital in New York City designated a nurse to tend to the needs of those patients about to be discharged.

This same focus on a continuum of care was used to facilitate the return of discharged World War II soldiers to civilian life (Lyon, 1993). Other examples are seen in the case management model used with clients with long-term rehabilitation needs. Recently, interest in discharge planning was renewed with the concern about escalating medical costs and need for improving continuity of care. Currently, nurses are involved with continuity of care, both in discharge planning and case management, more than ever as health care reform continues.

Clients are increasingly seen by a large variety of providers in an array of organizations and agencies, raising concerns about fragmentation of care. Future reforms in improving continuity of care concentrate on the use of inpatient facilities for briefer, more intense care as well as cost-containment efforts to deliver care at the lowest cost with more efficiency. All of this has resulted in expanded community-based care with an emphasis on primary, preventive care delivered with a continuum of care: Nurses will play an important role in shaping this reform. Currently, the best example of a large health care system in the United

States that has integrated the principles of continuity of care is the Veteran's Administration (Krugman, 2006).

Continuity of care is described as ongoing health care planning and referral that create a bridge between health care providers and health care settings. The nurse, as the case manager, is often the profession assigned or expected to ascertain the quality of the health plan. In this chapter, continuity of care is presented as facilitating entrance into, exit out of, and transfer within the health care system. Examples are given to show how case management enhances continuity. The concepts of community resources and referral are discussed. The chapter ends with a section on skills and competencies the nurse needs to improve continuity of care, a discussion of barriers to continuity, and examples of programs that have been successful in enhancing continuity.

SIGNIFICANCE OF CONTINUITY OF CARE

Continuity of care is described as the coordination of activities involving clients, providers, and (if applicable) payers to promote the delivery of health care. This is the process by which a client's ongoing health care needs are assessed, planned for, coordinated, and met without disruption. Some may view it as a method to control health care cost or ration care. Clients may view it as promoting their right to make choices about health care services.

Continuity of care is achieved when all appropriate care and treatment interventions are provided in a planned, coordinated, and consistent manner by staff working across professional/agency boundaries and through the required period of time. Most often continuity of care is only accomplished by integrating both formal and informal care. Formal care comprises what are commonly considered health care providers such as nurses, nurse aides, physical therapists, occupational therapists, and social workers. Informal care is the care that family, neighbors, friends, volunteers, and other nonprofessionals may provide for the individual with a health condition.

Continuity of care requires a strong organizational structure to prevent the client from getting "lost" in the system. Nurses must provide a leadership role in determining how and where the best care can be provided for a client and then ensuring that the client receives that care. This leadership is provided by care coordination through formal and informal nursing case management. Continuity is achieved by thoroughly assessing the client's needs and support, participating in multidisciplinary planning and intervention, and using appropriate resources, follow-up, and evaluation. Successful attainment of continuity of care is essential to ensure safe and quality health care and is promoted through successful planning and effective referral. Client and family satisfaction plays an important role in this process. Is there no component of client safety and satisfaction in continuity? Nurses play a vital role in promoting continuity in community-based settings.

ENTERING AND EXITING THE HEALTH CARE SYSTEM

Most often discharge planning is thought of as occurring between hospital and home but principles of continuity apply to transitions of care between any community settings. Discharge from a community-based setting requires the same or

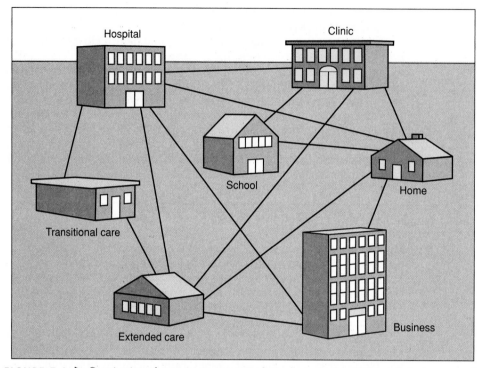

FIGURE 7-1. ▶ Continuity of care in community-based nursing is like a web between and among settings.

possibly greater level of attention than from acute care facilities. If discharge instructions for a client in ambulatory surgery are clearly explained, then successful follow-up, fewer complications, and good recovery are more likely. Likewise, if the nurse in the clinic provides the client with a clear, succinct explanation for care at home, recovery will be enhanced. If the home health care nurse of a pediatric client communicates with the school nurse about daily treatment needs, continuity will be improved and complications and added costs avoided.

Unlike in the past, when clients typically went from an acute care setting to home, clients today enter the health care system in various ways. They may be referred from a clinic visit to home care, from school to a physician's office, from home care to an acute care setting, or from adult day care to an extended care facility. Figure 7-1 illustrates the flow of continuity of care.

Clients may be transferred several times from one community-based setting to another. For example, Juan falls in the bathroom in his home and breaks his hip. He enters the system through the emergency department (ED) and is transferred to the operating room and then to the orthopedic unit in the hospital. After discharge from the hospital, he stays in a transitional facility for follow-up physical therapy and skilled nursing care. Then he is moved to assisted living for 4 months. After being transferred to three different services in the hospital and being discharged from four different agencies, he is back in his own home 6 months after the fall.

Admission

Admission occurs at whatever point an individual enters the health care system. Each new setting involves a new admission. No matter what the setting, the client and family enter with apprehension. Each new facility, unit, or agency presents strange surroundings and new people. Client and family anxiety levels may be high. What may be a routine admission to the nurse is seldom routine for a client. The nurse's confidence, competence, and concern are essential in putting the client and family at ease. The nurse's attitude may exert great influence on the course of care.

Apprehension may be lessened by the following nursing actions:

◆ Establishing rapport
◆ Indicating sincere concern for the client and family
◆ Defining the purpose and expectations of this admission
◆ Aiding the client in understanding how to participate as fully as possible in care-related decisions
◆ Clarifying the nursing role in relation to the client's health care needs
◆ Including the family in explanations, unless the client indicates otherwise
◆ Explaining equipment and procedures
◆ Explaining equipment to be used when calling for assistance
◆ Documenting the admission process

Admission procedures for entering any system share similarities. Examples of admission procedures in various health care facilities are summarized in Table 7-1.

TABLE 7-1 Overview of Admission to Various Health Care Facilities	
Facility	**Possible Admission Procedures**
Acute care setting	Introduction; orientation to room and equipment; complete nursing history, vital signs, and other physical assessment
Emergency department	Introduction; ABCs (airway, breathing, and circulation); vital signs; focused assessment for acute problems; orientation to surroundings
Clinic or physician's office	Introduction; exploration of reason for seeking medical care and focused assessment of that problem; vital signs
Nursing home	Introduction; review of written or verbal report from transferring agency; nursing history and assessment focusing on functional abilities; orientation to new surroundings
Hospice	Introduction; review of referral; nursing history and assessment focusing on pain control, functional abilities, coping, and support; wishes concerning terminal care and death (e.g., living will); orientation to procedures and care
Psychiatric facility	Introduction; mental health evaluation, including history, mood state, suicide risk, use of drugs, support system
Home visit	Introduction; review of referral and client's medical and nursing problems, home environment, caretaker and family support, community resources

Source: Craven, R. F., & Hirnle, C. J. (2007). *Fundamentals of nursing: Human health and function* (5th ed). Philadelphia: Lippincott Williams & Wilkins.

An admission form is always completed on entry into any health care service. Depending on the client's condition and the reason for admission, the length of the form varies. Insurance information, consent forms, and other forms are included in the admission paperwork.

During admission, it is reassuring if the nurse explains to the client and family members how they can participate in decision-making and care planning. The nurse may say, "The nutritionist will be here to talk to you this afternoon. He will discuss your food preferences. Unless the physician or nurse tells you differently, you may also eat any food brought from home. Perhaps your spouse will want to cook your favorite dish."

Admission may be as anxiety-provoking for the family as for the client. The nurse supports the family by giving the location of waiting rooms, rest rooms, public telephones, the nurses' station or offices, and other areas of interest, such as vending machines or cafeterias if the client is in an inpatient facility. If the client is being admitted for day surgery, the nurse may explain where the family can wait, who will bring a report, and when they can expect it. In many cases, comforting the family is as important as calming the client. For home care, the nurse will provide the family with information about the purpose of the visits and frequency, what other professionals will be providing additional service such as physical therapy or occupational therapy, and the overall plan of care.

Transferring

Sometimes the term discharge is used when client **transferring** is taking place. A client typically is transferred within the same institution, most often from the ED to the acute care setting or intensive care unit. Another type of transfer is when the client leaves the ED by ambulance to be transferred to another acute care facility or transitional hospital. For example, Nhu is a 60-year-old woman who is admitted to the ED at a small community hospital after a fall in her apartment. After examination, it is discovered that although she has no physical injuries her blood alcohol is 0.28. Her daughter and son confer with the nurse practitioner and decide to transfer her to an inpatient substance abuse program in a nearby community. She is in the inpatient program for 4 weeks and is then discharged to an outpatient substance abuse facility. After 4 months, she returns to her apartment but continues to go to Alcoholics Anonymous (AA) meetings in her community twice a week. In community-based health care, clients may be transferred from one setting to another.

DISCHARGE PLANNING

Discharge planning is an accepted nursing intervention aimed at the prevention of problems after discharge. These problems range from prolonged recovery to re-hospitalization, all of which add to the cost of care. Discharge planning ensures continuity of care by a systematic process of coordinating various aspects of care at the time the client is discharged from a facility or program. This planning involves many individuals who make assessments, collaborate with the client and family, plan, and then communicate the critical information to the organization or individual who will assume responsibility for the client's health care needs after discharge. The process, when it works well, is dynamic, interactive, and client centered. However there is a great deal of evidence that

RESEARCH IN COMMUNITY-BASED NURSING CARE ▶ 7-1

From Emergency Department to Home

Individuals over 65 discharged home directly from the emergency department are a vulnerable group. This study explored the management of the older person following care in an emergency department (ED) in preparation for discharge home by identifying the attitudes of staff in the ED and primary care sector. Two hundred and twenty-two medical and nursing staff in both the ED and primary care clinics completed a survey of both open and closed questions. Data were analyzed using SPSS for Windows while the qualitative data were content analyzed for themes. Many who completed the survey reported the level of communication between the ED and the primary care areas as unsatisfactory, with confusion regarding follow-up care and location of support for older people on discharge. Hospital staff indicated a higher level of satisfaction with communication between settings. Staff in both settings supported the inclusion of a discharge liaison nurse in the ED. This research suggests that staff in the ED and primary care setting see a need of multidisciplinary approach to developing referral guidelines, staff training, and a comprehensive dissemination of information between settings to improve continuity of care for the older person.

Dunnion, M. E., & Kelly, B. (2005). From emergency department to home. *Journal of Clinical Nursing, 14, 776–785.*

continuity through discharge planning is not adequate (Research in Community-Based Nursing Care 7-1).

The inception of Medicare in 1966 promoted discharge planning as an essential component of client care as Social Security legislation in the 1960s and 1970s provided coverage for hospital, physician, and other health care costs. Discharge planning became a central event as a method to reduce costs, lower hospital readmission rates, and provide the client with posthospital care options. The concept of discharge planning, beginning with admission to a hospital or ambulatory care setting, became even more critical with the advent of the diagnosis-related group (DRG) system.

Discharge planning is not limited to the physical transfer of the client, nor does it focus only on physical needs. It is much more. It is a process of early assessment of anticipated, individual client needs centered on concern for the total well-being of the client and family. It involves the client, family, and all caregivers in interactive communication during the entire planning process. It also requires ongoing interdisciplinary collaboration among many health care providers (Figure 7-2). This results in mutual agreement and appropriate options for meeting health care needs through a thorough and up-to-date review of all of the resource alternatives.

Ongoing nursing assessment of future client needs is mandated by accreditation agencies. The Joint Commission, formerly known as the Joint Commission on the

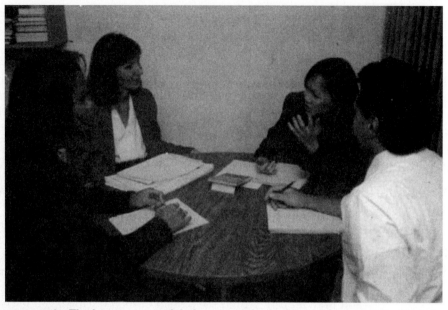

FIGURE 7-2. ▶ The key to successful planning is the exchange of information among those concerned about the client's care.

Accreditation of Healthcare Organizations (JCAHO), requires that the discharge plan should be initiated at admission as part of the nursing care plan.

Discharge planning creates bridges between settings, as shown in Figure 7-1. If the discharge plan is carefully thought out and based on collaboration among the nurse, physician, other health care providers, the client, and family, then the bridge will be strong and the transition between settings smooth. On the other hand, if the discharge plan is nonexistent or haphazardly thrown together, the transition will be bumpy with resulting complications, readmissions to various care facilities, or unnecessary stress, all interrupting the client's recovery. Consequently, poor continuity of care has the potential to result in disaster for the client and increased cost for the health care system. Discharge planning can be considered primary prevention in interrupting the development of complications following an exacerbation of a health condition.

NURSE CASE MANAGER

Case management, also known as care management or care coordination, is a complex concept with many definitions. This often leads to confusion about what is the correct or best definition. Case management will be defined in this book as activities that optimize the self-care capacities of clients and families by coordinating services. Although numerous definitions of case management exist, the goals in the last decade have remained constant. Typically the aim of case management is to achieve a balance between quality and cost of care. Quality is improved by emphasizing the importance of health promotion and disease prevention and increased continuity of care. Costs of care is decreased through empowering clients and families to maximize self-care to prevent unnecessary or lengthy inpatient care and multidisciplinary collaborative practice and **coordinated care** (Lee, Mackenzie, Dudley-Brown, & Chin, 1998).

Note how closely these goals parallel those of community-based nursing, which are to facilitate continuity and self-care in the context of the clients, family, culture, and community by considering the principles of disease prevention, health promotion, and collaboration.

Case management improves outcomes for the client and family. First of all, case management facilitates the provision of information about health benefits, service parameters, the disease process, and plan of treatment for clients and families. Successful case management involves the client in the decisions and actions of self-care. Case management allows for realistic evaluation in cases where there is low adherence to treatment plans. Finally, case managers facilitate consistency of care across the continuum of care.

There are several case management models used in community-based care. Community-based case management assists clients and families to access appropriate services for independent functioning. This model is used across a wide range of target populations. For example, a community may offer case management for those with chronic and persistent mental illness. Or case management for teenage Hmong girls at risk for dropping out of school, prostitution, drug use, or gang activity may be offered in another community. Home health care management offers the chronically ill services in the home setting. Chapter 11 provides numerous examples of this model at work. Similarly, hospice case management coordinates care and comfort of the dying and their families.

In some settings, a case manager's only role is to manage a number of cases, whereas in other settings the nurse has many roles, with case manager being one. For example, a nurse working in an ED may function as a staff nurse and also call clients for follow-up the day after their ED visit. A home care nurse may be the client's case manager responsible for coordinating care, as well as the direct care provider and health educator. The ways this role is operationalized differ by geographic area, provider, payment restriction, and setting. One model of interdisciplinary case management is seen in Research in Community-Based Nursing Care 7-2.

The role of the case manager is often viewed as that of a gatekeeper. Often the manager is a broker for services. For example, Margaret, an occupational health nurse who served worker's compensation clients, described her role as "interpreting the insurance company's medical information and working with health care providers to find the most efficient means of helping people return to the workplace." Other nurse case managers describe their roles as "assessing and evaluating delivery systems and benefit criteria . . . making sure that resources are available . . . stretching the dollar . . . client advocacy . . . and making sure the client and family are fully involved in the decision and care."

Thus, case management is a term with many definitions and implementation models. The nurse is often considered the best professional to act as a case manager for clients in all health care settings. In community-based care, case management is the vehicle to care coordination and continuity of care. Case management in community-based settings reflects a commitment to facilitate self-care in the context of the client's family, culture, and community.

RESEARCH IN COMMUNITY-BASED NURSING CARE ▶ 7-2

Dedicated Case Manager–Social Worker
Team Care for Trauma Patients

Injured clients admitted to Dartmouth-Hitchcock Medical Center receive coordinated care from arrival in the emergency department (ED) through discharge by a social worker and nurse case manager. A holistic approach is used to ensure that the client and family have the support and information they need at discharge. Both professionals attend trauma service rounds once a week and, in turn, update the rest of the case management team on psychosocial and financial issues that may be barriers to discharge. Many of the clients are 18 to 40 years of age, with a history of high-risk behavior, with over 40% uninsured. Because of the comorbidity of substance abuse and injury in this unit, coordinating the care of these clients is challenging. Support begins at admission when a member of the team meets the family as soon as they arrive. If family members are from out of town they are given information about the hospital and community such as where the hospital cafeteria is or the names and location of nearby hotels. The nurse or social worker may assist the family to contact other family and friends about the injured family member. Case management activities involve troubleshooting, determining the client needs, assisting with insurance and billing questions, and identifying what should be happening to facilitate a speedy and safe discharge.

Dedicated CM-SW team care for trauma patients. (2006). *Hospital Case Management,* *14*(9), 133–134, 139. Retrieved on September 8, 2006, from CINAHL PLUS with Full Text database.

NURSING SKILLS AND COMPETENCIES IN CONTINUITY OF CARE

To enhance continuity, the nurse must develop nursing expertise in anticipating the needs of clients and their families related to continuity and intervene accordingly. Discharge planning and case management are the primary roles for nurses related to continuity of care in community-based care. However, terminology is not consistent with titles varying from continuity-of-care nurse, discharge-planning nurse, or case manager given for a position with the same role responsibilities. Even within the same community one agency may use the term continuity of care nurse while another agency will have a role with identical responsibilities and give the title of that position nurse case manager. To add to the confusion, there is no universal level of educational preparation required for any of these roles. In this chapter the two primary roles of the nurse in continuity care will be discussed as those of discharge planner and case manager.

The Discharge Planning Nurse

Discharge planning follows the nursing process, beginning with assessment at the first encounter, as the nurse needs to know the client's plans and expectations for managing care. Planning and setting goals focus on both client and family needs and abilities. Written and verbal instructions about the medication regimen, treatment, and follow-up are provided to the client and family. They also need to be educated about any signs and symptoms that may indicate problems or complications with the condition and who to contact if these should occur. At this point, the client and family must have the opportunity to discuss any concerns or questions regarding care and recovery. The intervention phase of the nursing process involves identifying needed resources and making appropriate referrals. Important telephone numbers, names, and community services should be given in writing to the client and family and explained thoroughly.

The Nurse Case Manager

As discussed, the structure and scope of the role of the nurse care manager varies. In some situations case managers function across the continuum of care following and coordinating care whatever service the client and family are receiving. In other situations a case manager role is provided by each provider service so that a client may have a case manager in the hospital; long-term care facility; home care agency; or hospice service. A case manager may assist with financial arrangements, contact vendors and arrange for equipment, make referrals to home health care agencies, make appointments with health care providers, conduct pre-discharge teaching, and follow-up with arrangements for additional referrals as indicated.

Assessment

The nurse is often the first link in the continuity of care through the discharge planning process. In some settings, social workers may have the primary responsibility for discharge planning; however, nurses frequently coordinate and communicate the discharge plan. This may involve the nurse asking questions, making sure the client is satisfied with the information given, and questioning any inconsistencies. Without clear verbal and written communication among all participants, the plan may be unsuccessful.

Assessment of client discharge planning needs must begin on admission to the facility or at a preadmission. The nurse uses his or her skills to identify and anticipate the client's specific needs and the services that will be needed after discharge. Assessments may be conducted by different disciplines (e.g., the nurse, someone from the financial department, a physician, and a social worker) when the client enters the health care environment. The initial assessment identifies acute problems and needs. It must include a discussion with the client and family about what they perceive is their health care needs.

In all care coordination ongoing assessment monitors the client's response to treatment; seeks the client and family's input regarding their desires, needs, and resources; and initiates the coordination of the multidisciplinary team. The essential elements of assessment for a client include health and personal data, client and family knowledge, financial and support needs, and environmental data.

The nurse must concentrate on careful assessment of the client, identifying needs as early as possible. As soon as a client is admitted, the nurse assesses him or her for discharge needs. With each client encounter, the nurse discusses the discharge and asks the following questions: "When you are discharged . . ."

◆ If you are not able to care for yourself, who is available to be a family or friend caregiver?
◆ What it the willingness and ability level of your designated caregiver? (Adapted from: Zink, 2005)

The nurse, along with the client, is in the best possible position to clearly identify the client's needs related to care coordination. Because the nurse provides direct care and treatment for the client, the nurse is often in the unique position to observe responses to care. Clients at risk for inadequate self-care should be identified early. The information gained about the client's ability to provide self-care after discharge is critical to planning for discharge. Assessing needs, communicating with others, and involving the client and family on an ongoing basis contribute to a realistic strategy. If the client has special care needs after discharge, the trusting relationship established between nurse and client is essential to the next step of client and family teaching. The nurse can provide answers to the following questions:

◆ Will the family need changes in routine?
◆ Will the family be able to provide all of the care needed?
◆ Do they need home health care assistance?
◆ What are the family's resources and limitations?

A thorough collection of information is needed to plan effectively for continuity of care, but it is not always easily obtained. The client's successful recovery and return to optimal health often depend on collecting the right information during the assessment phase of planning. Nurses need to have multiple skills to facilitate this collection of information, interpret, confirm, and plan adequately.

Increasingly, the benefit of assessing populations who are at high risk for recidivism has been recognized. Because elderly clients are more likely to return to inpatient care than any other category of clients, many of the tools designed for this type of assessment are intended for them. Further, because of the shift in demographics with an increasing percentage of the population being over age 60, the cost–benefit value of this type of assessment is being investigated (Lagoe, Dauley-Altwarg, Mnich, & Winks, 2006).

One such tool is the Blaylock Risk Assessment Screening Score (BRASS) index. This may be used by the nurse at the bedside to gather comprehensive initial and ongoing data. The aim of the BRASS index is to identify, after hospital admission, elderly clients who are at risk for a prolonged hospital stay. Early identification of people who will have intense discharge needs may prevent or reduce postdischarge problems.

The BRASS index is shown in Figure 7-3. It contains 10 items, each judged by a nurse, using normal diagnostic procedures and questions at admission. The nurse goes through the questions, giving the client a score for every section. The Risk Factor Index at the bottom of the page indicates the client's need for discharge planning and resource planning. Research in Community-Based Nursing Care 7-3 presents research on the BRASS index.

Blaylock Discharge Planning Risk Assessment Screen

Circle all that apply and total. Refer to the Risk Factor Index*

Age
0 = 55 years or less
1 = 56 to 64 years
(2)= 65 to 79 years
3 = 80 + years

Living Situation/Social Support
0 = Lives only with spouse
1 = Lives with family
2 = Lives alone with family support
(3)= Lives alone with friends' support
4 = Lives alone with no support
5 = Nursing home/residential care

Functional Status
0 = Independent in activities of daily living and instrumental activities of daily living
Dependent in:
1 = Eating/feeding
1 = Bathing/grooming
1 = Toileting
1 = Transferring
1 = Incontinent of bowel function
1 = Incontinent of bladder function
1 = Meal preparation
1 = Responsible for own medication administration
1 = Handling own finances
1 = Grocery shopping
(1)= Transportation

Cognition
(0)= Oriented
1 = Disoriented to some spheres some of the time†
2 = Disoriented to some spheres all of the time
3 = Disoriented to all spheres some of the time
4 = Disoriented to all spheres all of the time
5 = Comatose

Behavior Pattern
(0)= Appropriate
1 = Wandering
1 = Agitated
1 = Confused
1 = Other

Mobility
0 = Ambulatory
(1)= Ambulatory with mechanical assistance
2 = Ambulatory with human assistance
3 = Nonambulatory

Sensory Deficits
0 = None
(1)= Visual or hearing deficits
2 = Visual and hearing deficits

Number of Previous Admissions/Emergency Room Visits
0 = None in the last 3 months
(1)= One in the last 3 months
2 = Two in the last 3 months
3 = More than two in the last 3 months

Number of Active Medical Problems
(0)= Three medical problems
1 = Three to five medical problems
2 = More than five medical problems

Number of Drugs
0 = Fewer than three drugs
1 = Three to five drugs
(2)= More than five drugs

Total Score: __11__

*Risk Factor Index: Score of 10 = at risk for home care resources; score of 11 to 19 = at risk for extended discharge planning; score greater than 20 = at risk for placement other than home. If the patient's score is 10 or greater, refer the patient to the discharge planning coordinator or discharge planning team.
†Sphere = person, place, time, and self.
Copyright 1991 Ann Blaylock

FIGURE 7-3. ► Sample of the Blaylock Discharge Planning Risk Assessment Screen.

RESEARCH IN COMMUNITY-BASED NURSING CARE ▶ 7-3

Predictive Validity of the
Blaylock Risk Assessment Screening Score

Discharge planning is one of the most important nursing interventions related to ensuring continuity. The Blaylock Risk Assessment Screening Score (BRASS) index is a risk screening instrument that can be used at admission to identify clients in need of discharge planning. This research tested the predictive validity of the BRASS index in screening clients with postdischarge problems.

Five hundred and three elderly clients were screened at admission with the BRASS index. It was found that the higher the BRASS scores, the greater the difficulty after discharge in all domains. This study found that the BRASS index is a good predictor for identifying clients who are not candidates for discharge to home. It also accurately predicts clients who will have problems after discharge.

Mistiaen, P., Duijnhouwer, E., Prins-Hoekstra, A., Ros, W., & Blaylock, A. (1999). Predictive validity of the BRASS index in screening clients with post-discharge problems. *Journal of Advanced Nursing, 30*(5), 1050–1056.

An example of the role of the nurse in discharge planning and the use of the BRASS index is seen in the following Client Situations in Practice.

CLIENT SITUATIONS IN PRACTICE: DISCHARGE PLANNING

Margret Carolan is a 72-year-old retired woman who lives alone and has no family, but she has supportive friends from her church. She does not drive because of her poor vision. She has a history of type 2 diabetes mellitus and congestive heart failure. Currently, she takes insulin, aspirin (ASA), propranolol, potassium (K-Dur), and furosemide (Lasix) every day. Three months ago, Ms. Carolan was seen in the emergency department for a transient ischemic attack. She is admitted to ambulatory surgery for arthroscopic surgery on her left knee under general anesthesia. She is instructed not to bear weight on her operative knee for 24 hours and to arrange for physical therapy twice a week for 1 month.

Ms. Carolan's Blaylock Discharge Planning Risk Assessment score is 11 (see Fig. 7-3). She is alert and oriented and depends on assistance for her transportation needs. Her history indicates that because she has complex problems, careful discharge planning is required. The team collects further data on her health, her personal situation including her environment, any teaching she may require for ongoing care, her financial status, and support needs she may require at home.

Ms. Carolan's discharge plan includes teaching her the following: weight-bearing instructions for the first 24 hours, signs and symptoms of infection, wound care, analgesic use, dosage of insulin, and possible increased or decreased dosage need. Referrals for postdischarge physical therapy are made, and transportation to and from the outpatient therapy clinic is arranged. No identified needs for home health care are apparent at this time. If complications arise, a home health care agency will be contacted.

When Ms. Carolan leaves the surgery center the nurse may lose contact with the client. Other members of the multidisciplinary team assume responsibility for the client's ongoing needs and implementation of the discharge plan.

When Mrs. Carolan returns to the orthopedic clinic a month after surgery, she is assessed by a physician and nurse practitioner. They find her completely recovered from her surgery and refer her back to her primary clinic. No more specialist visits are necessary. The orthopedic surgeon sends a report to her primary provider stating all goals were met.

Nursing Diagnosis

Nursing diagnoses provide a record of identified needs and strengths. Another method of need and strength identification is through documentation systems such as clinical pathways or in the case of home care, the OASIS systems. OASIS is an assessment tool developed to measure outcomes of persons receiving home health care. The OASIS data provide a consistent format and standardized time points for documenting client care status. If using nursing diagnosis, the visiting nurse may note that the previous home care nurse has documented Parental Role Conflict as a need, the second nurse will be ready to pick up on communications occurring within the home. Or if the nurse in charge of discharge planning in the hospital identified Risk for Loneliness as a potential issue for a client this would be a clue the clinic nurse could use to direct follow-up. As medical records are increasingly becoming standardized between and among health care provider organizations the client's chart is shared with all pertinent members of the health care team.

Planning

The goal of health planning is to assist the client and family in the achievement of an optimal level of wellness. The key to successful planning is the exchange of information between the client, present caregivers (e.g., nurse, physician, social worker, respiratory therapist, physical therapist, occupational therapist, nutritionist, psychologist, speech therapist), and those responsible for the continuing care (e.g., family, support services, and caregivers). Planning is always a mutual process between health care providers, the client, and the family, and involves the following:

◆ Recognizing and using the resources and capacities of the client (and if appropriate) family
◆ Educating client and (if appropriate) family members about the options available and encouraging their participation in the decision-making process
◆ Assisting the client and (if appropriate) family to feel they have control over their own welfare and to identify resources that could help them in this process

Sociocultural factors can influence the planning phase. It is important for the nurse to identify and acknowledge issues that may influence the plan. These may include beliefs about the causes of illness and death and dying, language, nutrition practices, healing practices, and sexual orientation.

Economic factors can influence the planning phase depending on the health insurance status of the client. Those without insurance or those who are underinsured will need more assistance in identifying and accessing community resources compared to clients with comprehensive health insurance.

Frequent communication and coordination among the multidisciplinary team, client, and client's family facilitates reaching realistic expected outcomes in a well-designed discharge plan. This is accomplished through these actions:

◆ Consulting between the physician and the social worker or discharge planner
◆ Determining the client's prognosis
◆ Setting priorities
◆ Designing realistic time frames
◆ Determining responsibility
◆ Analyzing alternative resources for appropriateness and availability
◆ Exploring financial resources and burdens
◆ Involving and educating the family
◆ Setting appropriate and realistic expected outcomes
◆ Coordinating community resources

Articulation of the expected outcomes helps the multidisciplinary team know what is expected of the client and what the client expects of the team. When these outcomes have been agreed on by the client and family, all participants know the goals and can evaluate whether they have been met.

Implementation: Nursing Interventions to Promote Continuity

Approaches to promote continuity have remained relatively stable over the last one hundred years. Letters of Lillian Wald and Mary Brewster, both nurses who worked in the settlement houses in New York City at the turn of the century and interviews of nurses currently practicing portray the role of discharge planner or case manager similarly (Rodgers, 2000). Developing the nurse–client relationship and formulating outside connections in the community were described to be central elements to successful care coordination by nurses in the late 19th as well as the early 21st century.

Forming the Nurse–Client Relationship

As is true of nursing care in all settings, the nurse–client relationship is the central element in developing continuity of care. According to Rodgers' research several components work together to build the nurse–client relationship. In modern day this process is called **counseling,** as the nurse establishes a trusting relationship with the client and family to engage them at an emotional level in the process of planning (Minnesota Department of Health [MDH], 2001). Counseling may be woven into all elements of the plan. The initial aspect of counseling is establishing a nurse–client relationship through a pact in which the relationship becomes the foundation of care coordination (Fig. 7-4).

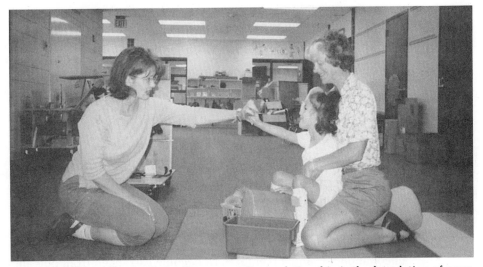

FIGURE 7-4. ▶ A strong and trusting nurse–client relationship is the foundation of coordinated care.

 I don't care what color you are, or where you come from or who you are or where you have been in your life, if you are my patient, I am going to do the very best that I can. I have a commitment. It's like when you walk into somebody's home and you form a bond with that person. It's like a pact that I'm going to be there for you until you die, and I'm going to take you through it, we're going to go through it together. (Rodgers, 2000, p. 303)

Another essential component in the nurse–client relationship is listening and being present. This concept has been mentioned several times throughout this book and is basic to good therapeutic communication. Sadly, these concepts are often missing in the relationship between the nurse and the client and bear repeating: Listening allows the nurse to assess the client's most immediate needs and is often a powerful nursing intervention. In some situations therapeutic presence may be the only intervention that provides comfort as seen below.

▶ Five years ago, my baby daughter died of SIDS. The nurse in the clinic just sat with me and let me cry. That was so helpful. I will always be thankful that she took the time to sit with me. (Julie, a nursing student)

Building trust is another strategy essential to developing the nurse client relationship.

Trust is built by:

◆ Cultivating the client's trust with the first contact.
◆ Establishing credibility with the client.
◆ Using an empathic, nonjudgmental approach.
◆ Guarding the client's privacy.
◆ Expecting testing behavior from clients.
◆ Learning to trust the client.
◆ Persevering with the nurse–client relationship (Wendt, 1996).

Another aspect of the nurse–client relationship related to continuity care is that the nurse must be being willing to persist in all situations, even those that appear impossible to resolve. This level of persistence may seem almost impossible with some of the complex individuals and families we care for in community settings. An example is seen in the following.

> George is one of the more difficult clients I have ever cared for. He is 80 years old with very brittle diabetes. His wife died last year. She was the one who could drive, cook, and check his blood sugar. His daughter said she would help by dropping by with a
> ▶ meal every day. He refused Meals On Wheels, says that welfare is for old people, and will only eat what his daughter brings for him. Now his daughter is in the hospital having a spinal fusion, so I don't think he is eating. I am trying to problem solve with him about alternatives, hoping we will be able to uncover an option he is comfortable with before he ends up back in the hospital. (Denise, a home health care nurse)

The last theme seen in the letters and interviews common to the quest for continuity is seen in the nurse–client relationship when the family is absent. It is not uncommon for family members to become estranged from one another or unable or unwilling to assist one another during illness. In some situations, when an individual has a chronic illness over a long period of time, everyone is exhausted from managing the work of the illness. In other cases, estrangement may have continued for many years. The nurses role calls for creative perseverance in problem solving.

> Ernest has no family or social support. He has three children, but they all live on the West Coast. Ernest and his wife separated 15 years ago because of his substance abuse. When we called to see if she would be able to assist with his care, she gave the
> ▶ nurse an earful! His family has been totally unwilling to assist with his care. Consequently, his discharge was delayed for a long period of time. Eventually we found a neighbor who was willing to get groceries for him and accompany him on the bus to his medical appointments. A home care nurse visited him three times a week for 6 months. (Phyllis, a home care nurse)

In all situations, the nurse–client relationship remains at the center of all interventions. Likewise, as clients move from one care setting or care provider to another the relationship remains the consistent element to care. The interdisciplinary team must plan intervention strategies carefully, considering how the changes affect the client and the family. Clients and family members will probably feel anxious about the change. This is especially true if they have been hurried through an acute care setting or if discharge plans were discussed only on admission when the client's acute condition prohibited them from fully participating. Being sensitive to the client's needs while planning care will help to reduce anxiety and increase the client's participation and acceptance of care transitions.

Assisting the Individual and Family

Some nursing interventions that enhance continuity focus on specific actions that assist the client to achieve the highest possible level of functioning and wellness. The interventions, which achieve coordinated care, involve screening, counseling, consultation, collaboration, case finding, and health teaching. Before describing each of these stages, it is important to note that these are not necessarily linear

---

◆ **BOX 7-1** Steps in Consultation ◆

1. Establish a trusting relationship with the client and family.
2. Clarify the client's perception of the problem, causes, and anticipated results.
3. Assess all issues in a mutual process with the client.
   • Determine the impact the issue has on the client's experience.
   • Identify everyone involved in the issue and how they are affected.
   • Determine how the client and family's attitudes, beliefs, and behaviors may be contributing to the issues.
   • Explore environmental aspects.
   • Identify strengths and barriers for the client and family.
   • Anticipate what may be gained or lost by solving or addressing the issue.
   • Consider how a solution might affect the client and family.
4. Through mutual planning, the nurse and client perform the following functions:
   • Identify the desired outcome.
   • Consider the advantages and disadvantages of each.
   • Support the client as they choose the preferred option.
5. Determine support essential to facilitate implementing the plan.
6. Evaluate the process and outcome.

Adapted from Minnesota Department of Health, Section of Public Health Nursing. (2001). *Public health nursing interventions II. Basic steps to the consultation intervention.* Minneapolis: Author.

---

or discrete actions. Although screening may be used throughout it is more likely to be used in the early stages of discharge planning while counseling and consultation are commonly used all the way through the planning process yet each intervention contributes to continuity of care.

Screening identifies individuals with unrecognized health risk factors or asymptomatic diseases (MDH, 2001). In discharge planning, one example of screening is using the BRASS index described earlier. Another example of screening could be when a case manager completes a fall risk assessment with a client who is high risk for falling and is living alone.

Through **consultation** the nurse seeks information and generates solutions to problems or issues through interactive problem solving with the client or family to enhance care coordination (MDH, 2001). Consultation is an interactive problem-solving process between the nurse and the client. From a list of alternative options generated by the nurse and client, the client selects those most appropriate for the situation (Box 7-1). As is discussed throughout this book, nursing interventions are mutually determined, implemented, and evaluated in community-based care.

Collaboration commits two or more individuals or agencies to achieve a common goal of promoting and protecting the health of another. The first and foremost collaboration is between the nurse and the client. Fostering or enabling the

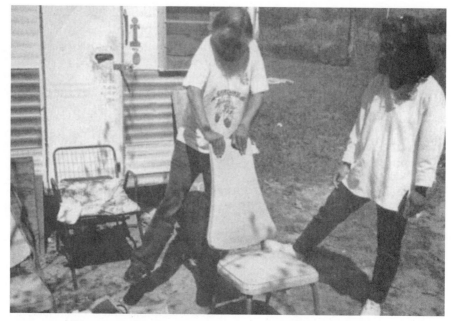

FIGURE 7-5. ▶ A community-based nurse teaches a Native American elder range-of-motion exercises outside his rural home. She is providing prevention and promotion strategies in her continuity of care of her client.

client to experience more of a sense of control is necessary to forging the nurse–client collaborative relationship. . . . From the first chapter, this text has emphasized mutual care planning and self-care. The ultimate in successful nursing care is the plan that leads the client to his/her highest achievable level of self-care.

Health teaching communicates information and skills that change knowledge, attitudes, values, beliefs, behaviors, and practices of individuals and families (MDH, 2001). Successful health education depends on the nurse to competently assess the client's ability to manage daily activities in the home, judge the client and family's compliance with the therapeutic regimen, assess the client's knowledge of self-care, and coordinate the team members. Teaching skills are important and may include both prevention and promotion strategies (Fig. 7-5). Health teaching is covered in detail in Chapter 6.

Case finding is a set of activities used by the nurse working in community settings that identifies clients who are not currently receiving health care but could benefit from such care (MDH, 2001). The nurse, of all members of the interdisciplinary team, usually has the most contact with the client and family. This contact allows the nurse to assess and identify client service needs that, if addressed, would enhance care coordination or case management. In some cases, this may be a simple process, with the nurse making one contact or giving the client one suggested referral. Case finding happens in every setting where care is provided, and it requires an open attitude and skillful assessment by the nurse.

Forming Outside Connections With the Community

Developing community connections is also essential to providing effective care coordination in community-based setting. The nurse's knowledge about the community is key to provide comprehensive, coordinated care. In addition, the nurse must know the client, the client's family and culture, and the broader community in which they live. To make appropriate referrals to ensure continuity, the nurse must know what services are available. For these outside connections to be accessed, the client and family first must know about the service and then must be willing to accept help.

> ▶ I had been making home visits to a client after the birth of her twins. She was about to be evicted from her home. Her relationship with the father of her babies was volatile. He was not living with her and not supportive. Every visit, she talked about the lack of progress she had made in finding a place to live. "Nobody will take someone with five kids," she would say over and over again. "I am going to be homeless with my kids," she exclaimed. In our community, there is virtually no low-cost housing. We had explored every option available to her, with no success. One day, when I went to make my weekly home visit and weigh the twins, she didn't answer the door. I could hear the kids inside and knew she must be home. I knocked and waited. She finally opened the door. Both of her eyes were black and blue, and her face was bruised and swollen. She looked down at the floor and shamefully said, "He beat me up in front of the kids. I am never going to see him again, but I have no place to go." I knew about special housing available in our county for families experiencing domestic violence. I explained to her that she would have to go to a shelter for domestic abuse, but from there she could get into the housing program. Her mother helped her pack up her kids, and she moved to the shelter the next day. (Mary, a senior nursing student)

Working With Others Within the Community: Collaboration and Delegation

Collaboration requires developing knowledge of other health care providers. This consists of becoming informed about the availability, scope, services, and referral mechanisms for various providers. Health care providers include, but are not limited to, physicians, dentists, ophthalmologists, therapists (such as occupational and physical), alternative care practitioners (such as chiropractors and acupuncturists), home health care agencies, outpatient clinics, diagnostic screening programs, and health education programs. Each health care provider has a role in ensuring continuity (Table 7-2).

When an intervention involves a multidisciplinary team, it is critical for the goals and plans to be structured and organized. However, it must also be flexible enough to allow for change as the client progresses toward health. If revisions to the plan are deemed necessary, the changes must be documented. For example, physical therapy for an older client with arthritis may be most effective in the afternoon, when the nurse is scheduled to visit. After discussing this with the client and the physical therapist, the nurse changes her visits for medication instruction to the morning to enhance the effectiveness of the physical therapy.

It takes a team effort to care for a client well, and the team leader is often the nurse. The nurse must take the following steps of coordinating multiple disciplines to facilitate continuity of care:

TABLE 7-2 Health Care Providers Used in Discharge Referrals	
Health Care Provider	**Role**
Home health nurse	Provides assessments, direct care, client teaching and support; coordinates services; evaluates outcomes
Home health aide	Provides hygiene care, cooking, supervision, and companionship
Social worker	Assists in finding and connecting with community resources or financial resources; provides counseling and support
Physical therapist	Assists with restoring mobility, strengthens muscle groups, teaches ambulation with new devices
Occupational therapist	Helps clients adjust to limitations by teaching new vocational skills or better ways to perform activities of daily living
Nutritionist	Teaches clients about meal planning and diet restrictions
Speech therapist	Assists clients to communicate better and works with clients who have swallowing problems
Respiratory therapist	Provides home follow-up for clients with respiratory problems including assessment, oxygen administration, and home ventilator care

Craven, R. F., & Hirnle, C. J. (2007). *Fundamentals of nursing: Human health and function* (5th ed.). Philadelphia: Lippincott Williams & Wilkins.

◆ Notify all disciplines involved when there is a change in the client's health status.

◆ Coordinate visits with the client to avoid two professionals visiting at the same time and tiring the client.

◆ Integrate services to provide maximum benefit to the client; for example, have the physical therapist measure blood pressure when visiting the home to ambulate the client.

◆ Problem solve jointly with other team members and include the client when appropriate.

Delegation is a critical competency for the 21st century nurse and a key intervention in successful case management. Delegation is the process for a nurse to direct another person to perform nursing tasks and activities and is a legal concept used to empower one person to act for another (National Council of State Boards of Nursing [NCSBN], 2006). **Unlicensed assistive personnel** (UAP) are any unlicensed workers, regardless of title, to whom nursing tasks are delegated (NCSBN, 2006). As more UAP are providing care to individuals in community settings, the case manager becomes central to the issues related to delegation.

According to the NCSBN (2006), all decisions related to delegation of nursing activities must be based on the fundamental principle of protection of the health, safety, and welfare of the public. Licensed nurses have the ultimate accountability for the management and provision of nursing care, including all delegated decisions and tasks. This accountability is outlined in the Five Rights of Delegation, shown in Box 7-2.

Managed care is an organized system of health care that carefully plans and monitors the use of health care services so that standards are met while costs are minimized. Many health maintenance organizations (HMOs) and insurance

---

◆ **BOX 7-2**   The Five Rights of Delegation ◆

1. The right task
2. Under the right circumstances
3. To the right person
4. With the right directions and communication; and
5. Under the right supervision and evaluation.

National Council of State Boards of Nursing. (2006). Joint Statement on Delegation from the American Nurses Association (ANA) and the National Council of State Boards of Nursing (NCSBN). Retrieved on September 12, 2006, from http://www.ncsbn.org/regulation/uap_delegation_documents.

---

companies use managed care. Preferred provider organizations (PPOs) are another form of a managed care organization. An increasing segment of the population receives health care through managed care. Box 7-3 lists **managed care skills** needed for nurses to work effectively in a managed care environment.

Often a nurse is the person responsible for evaluating what care is necessary. Sometimes this puts the nurse in the difficult position of seeing firsthand the needs of the client but discovering that coverage limitations of the managed care contract prohibits the provision of the needed care. Sometimes, this is the point where the nurse acts as an advocate for the client to secure the service.

◆ **BOX 7-3**   Skills Needed by Nurses in a Managed Care Environment ◆

- Negotiation skills
- Delegation skills
- Ability to analyze care in terms of cost and benefit
- Ability to understand the process of care provision across the continuum
- Ability to look at and predict outcomes
- Ability to collect and evaluate outcome data
- Business understanding, or ability to understand and use financial data
- Advocacy skills
- Assessment skills
- Ethical decision-making skills
- Collaboration skills

Kersbergen, A. L. (2000). Managed care. Shifts health care from an altruistic model to a business framework. *Nursing and Health Care Perspectives, 21*(2), 81–83.

COMMUNITY-BASED NURSING CARE GUIDELINES ▶ 7-1

Steps in the Referral Process

1. Establish the need for referral.
2. Set objectives for the referral.
3. Explore the resources that are available.
4. Have the client make decisions concerning the referral.
5. Make the referral to the selected service.
6. Supply the agency with needed information.
7. Support the client and family in pursuing the referral.

Referral and Follow-up

Referral and follow-up is the process by which nurses in all settings assist individuals and families in identifying and accessing community resources to prevent, promote, or maintain health (MDH, 2001). Obviously, just knowing what resources are present in the community is only the first step. For example, when caring for a client who has just had a knee replacement, the nurse learns that the client lives alone and does not have friends or family living nearby. It will be difficult for the client to cook for several weeks. Giving the client the telephone number for Meals On Wheels is one nursing intervention. In addition, the client is concerned about getting to the grocery store. There is a grocery delivery service that has a reduced rate for senior citizens. A second intervention is giving the client the name and telephone number of the service. Community-Based Nursing Care Guidelines 7-1 lists the steps in the referral process.

Referrals must consider the client's resources as well as the community's resources. A community with many resources can help support the client and family through a recovery period or can help families in their health promotion. The community with few resources will be inefficient in its support of citizens who require assistance with health care needs. To facilitate continuity of care when referring clients to an acute care setting, home, or community, the nurse must be aware of the various types of individuals and organizations available as community resources. Box 7-4 lists resources that can be used for the ill or older population of the community. Resources include physicians, hospital centers, clinics and nursing centers, specialized care centers, and long-term care facilities. School nurses and occupational nurses are resources, as are various agencies and organizations. Resources may include a range of health-related services, from drug and alcohol treatment programs to safety education to preventable injuries. Each resource exists to provide services to meet particular needs. The nurse must know what these resources are and their eligibility requirements.

Community resources can be characterized as either health care providers or supportive care providers. Health care providers include all health care settings, health departments, community service agencies, and private practice physicians. Support care providers include psychological services, churches, and self-help groups. Supportive care providers, or support services, are services that help people avoid problems or solve problems that interfere with their self-care and well-being. The primary service offered may not necessarily be health related and may

◆ **B O X　7-4** Community Resources for Elderly and Ill Clients ◆

Transportation Difficulty
- Provisions for older people offered by states and city services through reduced bus fares, taxi vouchers, and van services
- Volunteer organizations: Red Cross, Salvation Army, senior citizen centers and nonprofits, church organizations for emergency or occasional transportation

Prevention of Home Injuries
- Telephone checkup services through local hospitals, local services or friends, neighbors, or relatives
- Postal alert: register with local senior center; sticker on mailbox alerts letter carrier to check for accumulation of mail
- Private services paid for hourly
- Aide services by the Visiting Nurse Association
- Medicaid and Medicare provisions for home aides, which are limited to strict eligibility requirements
- Student help (inexpensive helpers) solicited by posting notices on bulletin boards at colleges and allied health schools
- Home sharing with another person who is willing to provide this kind of assistance in exchange for room and board

Nursing Care or Physical Therapy
- Visiting nurse services provided through Medicare, Medicaid, or other health insurance (must be ordered by a physician)
- Home health services through private providers listed in the phone book; also nonprofit providers, Medicare and Medicaid reimbursement for authorized services

Shopping, Cooking, and Meal Planning
- Home-delivered meals delivered by Meals On Wheels or church organizations once a week, with sliding fees
- Meals served at senior centers, churches, schools, and other locations
- Cooperative arrangements with neighbors to exchange a service for meals, food shopping, and other tasks

Social Isolation
- Senior centers or community education programs that provide social opportunities, classes, volunteer opportunities, and outings
- Church-sponsored clubs with social activities, volunteer opportunities, and outings
- Support groups for widows, stroke victims, and general support
- Adult day care with social interaction, classes, discussion groups, outings, and exercise

(continued)

◆ B O X 7-4 Community Resources for Elderly and Ill Clients (*Continued*) ◆

Need for Assistance With Home Management
- Homemaker services for those meeting income eligibility criteria
- Service exchanges with neighbors and friends (e.g., baby-sitting exchanged for housework help)
- Home helpers hired through agencies or through employment listings at senior centers, schools, etc.
- Help with housework in exchange for home sharing by renting out a room or portion of the home for reduced rent

Financial Issues
- Power of attorney given to a friend or relative for handling financial matters
- Joint checking account with friend or relative to facilitate paying bills
- Financial assistance available from the American Red Cross, Salvation Army, church groups, senior centers, or other organizations

Legal Assistance
- AARP legal services
- Legal aid or other lawyer referral services offered by the county or state bar association
- Other city/county aging services, hot lines for information and assistance in phone book

---

be more difficult to identify as compared to services directly related to health care needs. Support services are not always obvious to clients or their families, but acquiring information about them is an important piece of continuing care.

The ideal circumstance is to have the client and family participate in the referral process so they are involved in decision making and can choose the providers or organizations they prefer. The nurse, however, may be in the best position to determine needs. For example, Suzie, a juvenile diabetic, is having trouble regulating her glucose levels. She asks you, "What can I eat?" Her mother says, "Sometimes I'm confused about what she can eat." Her father states, "We've been having problems with our car lately. We can't drive all the way across town to talk to someone about this." The nurse makes a referral to a dietitian located near the family's home to help determine the source of the glucose level variances and to initiate nutritional planning with Suzie and her family. Often there are multiple referrals to make for a client, and the nurse acts as coordinator among members of this expanding team.

Barriers to Successful Referrals
Because of rising health care costs, the health plan is often driven by the client's financial resources rather than by what services the client needs. An example is a client who needs home visits for assistance with activities of daily living (ADL), meal

preparation, household chores, transportation, and physical therapy. The client's insurance pays only for physical therapy. This requires that the nurse, client, and client's support person, physician, and multidisciplinary team (e.g., social worker, physical therapist) set priorities based on what the client can afford and explore alternative ways to meet the additional needs. Alternatives might be Meals On Wheels, volunteer transportation, family participation, or church visitation.

Health care organizations must now find additional funds in the form of voluntary donations and state and federal programs. The same is true for many individuals who join HMOs or rely on government-funded health care such as Medicare and Medicaid. Insurance plans, HMOs, and government-funded programs provide a variety of coverage plans. Many do not cover preventive care, psychiatric treatment, outpatient support services, and medications. All third-party payers limit the amount of service for which payment is made (e.g., number of home health care visits).

The nurse may need to assist clients in learning about their insurance coverage in order to create a plan of care that the payer will cover. Most health care plans employ case managers who understand health care needs and subsequently make decisions, based on diagnosis and need, about services that will be authorized for payment. Sometimes the authorization or denial of payment for service conflicts with decisions made by the health care team. This interdisciplinary team may have to revise the plan, based not necessarily on what is felt to be best for the client but on what is optimal given the client's financial and social resources. For example, insurance companies will not pay for home health care that consists solely of a home health aide making daily visits for the client's personal care. The client must need the skilled services of an RN or physical or occupational therapist before the payer will pay for personal care needs. If the client cannot pay out of pocket for personal care, the team must reevaluate the client to determine if there are skilled nursing needs that could qualify the client for authorization of payment by the insurance carrier. The nurse is an important player when resource availability is dictated not necessarily by need but by payment source.

Other barriers to successful use of community resources may stem from the client's prior experiences with community agencies. If a client has not had a good experience with a referral in the past, he or she may be hesitant to use this type of service again. The same is true for a client's perception of a particular agency or organization. The nurse must acknowledge the client's feelings and opinions about past experiences. The nurse may find that the client lacked information about the organization and a different approach is all that is necessary. Perhaps the client's complaints about the organization are justified, in which case it may be in the client's best interest to find an alternative provider.

A common barrier to follow-up in using health care services is accessibility. Many communities do not have public transportation. Hospitals, clinics, and other health care services are closing, especially in rural areas, and many rural communities are left with no local health care services. This loss requires clients to travel long distances to reach health care services. Conversely, a city-dwelling client who may not own a car might have difficulty getting to a suburban clinic. The nurse must get information from the client about access to transportation before making a referral. This is especially important with low-income clients, urban clients, and those living in rural areas.

In the following situation, the nurse listens carefully to the family and client to determine their priorities and identifies a community-based service for referral. As a result of a thoughtfully developed referral, Amy, a young teen recently diagnosed with diabetes, is able to manage self care for her chronic condition early in the disease process.

CLIENT SITUATIONS IN PRACTICE

◆ Supporting the Client and Family in the Referral Process

Amy is a 14-year-old Native-American girl admitted to the acute care setting with type 1 diabetes mellitus. She is afraid and does not want to face the realities of her new diagnosis. She tells the physician, "I don't want anything to do with this diet and stuff! I just want to go home, hang out with my friends, and eat what I want." The physician asks the nurse to explore this statement and Amy's general feelings about her diagnosis. Amy, her mother and father, and the nurse sit down in the conference area. As the discussion proceeds, the nurse discovers that Amy is afraid that she won't ever be able to eat out with her friends. Amy's mother says, "She loves fry bread, but she can't ever eat that again, right? What am I supposed to cook for her, anyway?"

At this point, the nurse suggests the diabetes education classes at the hospital clinic. Amy's father responds, "I don't want to go back to that clinic where there are only White people." The nurse makes several telephone calls, trying to identify a resource for a teenager with a new diagnosis of diabetes who follows a traditional Native-American diet and whose family prefers a caretaker who is Native American. The nurse identifies the International Diabetes Clinic, which has a clientele and staff of many different nationalities. He also learns that there is a support group for Native-American teens with diabetes at the American Indian Center near the family's home.

The nurse visits Amy's home. He gives Amy and her parents a pamphlet about managing diabetes and discusses setting an appointment with the International Diabetes Clinic. The nurse tells Amy about the support group at the neighborhood American Indian Center. He gives Amy the name of the nurse at the American Indian Center and encourages her to call and check out the support group.

Advocacy

Sometimes our health care system is characterized as uncaring, impersonal, and fragmented. Clients become frustrated, often feeling devalued and unable to cope with the system. **Client advocacy** is defined as intervening for or acting on behalf of the client to provide the highest quality health care obtainable (MDH, 2001). A community-based nurse acts as an advocate for the client and family, providing information to the client to help ensure uninterrupted care. In many situations, the client is vulnerable, which often results in the nurse contacting a community service, other caregivers, or a physician on the client's behalf.

For example, a school nurse notices that a 13-year-old child often comes to the nurse's office on Monday mornings complaining of a stomach ache. When the girl comes in for the third week in a row, the nurse asks her, "Tell me about your weekend." The child starts crying and says, "My dad doesn't live with us anymore. My mom drinks beer and yells at me." The nurse and the child discuss the child's feelings and fears about her family situation. Then the nurse explains to the child that with her permission, she would like to talk to the school counselor about their conversation, to learn about some groups that may help her. Second, the nurse tells the child that she would like to call her mom and talk to the two of them about her stomach aches. In this situation, the nurse is acting as an advocate for the child, with the goal of facilitating self-care in the context of the student's family. The nurse is collaborating with other professionals to enhance care. Steps of Advocacy are seen in Box 7-5.

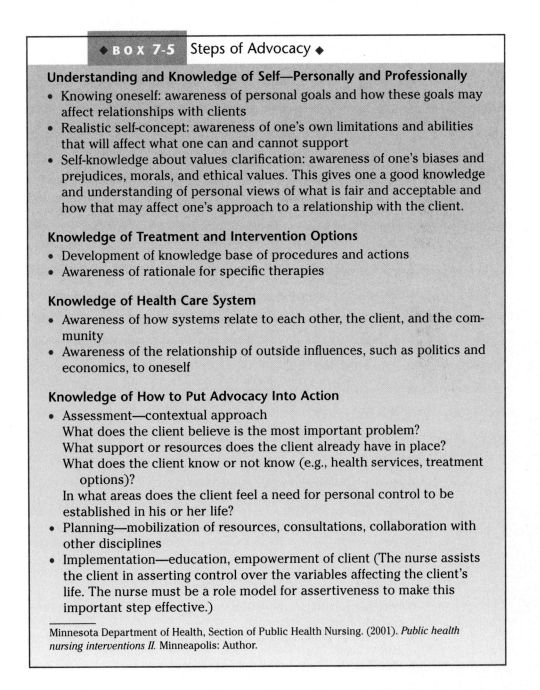

◆ **B O X 7-5** Steps of Advocacy ◆

Understanding and Knowledge of Self—Personally and Professionally
- Knowing oneself: awareness of personal goals and how these goals may affect relationships with clients
- Realistic self-concept: awareness of one's own limitations and abilities that will affect what one can and cannot support
- Self-knowledge about values clarification: awareness of one's biases and prejudices, morals, and ethical values. This gives one a good knowledge and understanding of personal views of what is fair and acceptable and how that may affect one's approach to a relationship with the client.

Knowledge of Treatment and Intervention Options
- Development of knowledge base of procedures and actions
- Awareness of rationale for specific therapies

Knowledge of Health Care System
- Awareness of how systems relate to each other, the client, and the community
- Awareness of the relationship of outside influences, such as politics and economics, to oneself

Knowledge of How to Put Advocacy Into Action
- Assessment—contextual approach
  What does the client believe is the most important problem?
  What support or resources does the client already have in place?
  What does the client know or not know (e.g., health services, treatment options)?
  In what areas does the client feel a need for personal control to be established in his or her life?
- Planning—mobilization of resources, consultations, collaboration with other disciplines
- Implementation—education, empowerment of client (The nurse assists the client in asserting control over the variables affecting the client's life. The nurse must be a role model for assertiveness to make this important step effective.)

Minnesota Department of Health, Section of Public Health Nursing. (2001). *Public health nursing interventions II*. Minneapolis: Author.

The role of the advocate involves informing clients about the nature of their health problems and the choices they have in seeking to resolve or alter their health care needs. This role is activated whenever clients are unable to take responsibility for their own health care, lack knowledge or skill, or do not have the financial or emotional basis from which to act. The advocacy role is also one of support after clients have been informed, made choices, and need to implement these choices. Clients have an inherent right to make their own decisions and to take responsibility for those decisions. The nurse lends support and respect for clients, whether or not the nurse agrees with their decisions.

To advocate for clients, the nurse must consider all aspects of the clients' lives.

Advocacy is often used with vulnerable populations who have a weak voice within a system. Some people, because of age, cognitive abilities, lack of sophistication, or other factors need assistance in speaking for themselves. Clarification of a do-not-resuscitate order on behalf of an elderly client who is unaware of the need to explicitly state his or her preference is one example of a nurse acting as a client advocate. The expertise and competence of nurses can also be used in supporting the needs and views of their clients and their clients' families. Nurses can be advocates for clients who feel they have been excluded from participation in health care decisions or who have little trust in the health care system or political representatives. Advocates also work to change the system by revealing gaps, opportunities, injustices, and inadequacies. Advocacy may be accomplished by engaging in some of the following activities:

♦ Empowering each client and family member they care for who experiences disparities in health care
♦ Discussing disparities in their communities with colleagues
♦ Writing about disparities for hospital, clinic, or professional organization newsletters
♦ Writing letters to, or calling and making an appointment to speak to, local or state politicians to describe evidence of health disparities that they encounter

Community-based nurses are well situated to act as an advocate for the individual and families given their knowledge of clients' needs and understanding of local services.

Evaluation

Evaluation is the measurement of the outcomes or results of implementing the discharge plan. This involves gathering data on the client's response to interventions. Data can be collected from the client, family, physician, and referral sources. The major purpose of evaluation is to see if goals were reached. Evaluation is ongoing; reviews are made to determine if needs were met, if problems were resolved, and if the plan needs to be revised. Evaluation continues as the client moves from one setting to another.

In evaluating the effectiveness of continuity of care, it is essential to consider these points:

♦ Whether health planning was initiated when the client first obtained health care services
♦ If discharge planning was discussed with the client and family at the beginning of care
♦ Whether the client and family participated in early planning for ongoing care

◆ If there was interdisciplinary planning with all involved professionals
◆ If the care being provided to the client was empathic, based on mutual trust and cultural sensitivity
◆ If the client and family believe they had all the information they needed
◆ Whether the client felt prepared for self-care at home
◆ Whether the client and family believe they had the resources needed for self-care
◆ If there is new information that suggests the plan should be revised

Evaluation is effective only if there is a plan with goals established by the client, family, and interdisciplinary team. The evaluation process is more meaningful if the expected outcomes are written in a clear, measurable way. Judgment skills are necessary when comparing real outcomes with expected outcomes. If the client's behavior matches the desired outcomes, the goal has been met. If the goals are not met, then the nurse must examine the reasons for the shortfall.

Unmet goals may be caused by inadequate data collection, incorrect identification of need, unrealistic planning, or poor implementation. The client's living situation or physical condition may have changed. New, previously unidentified needs may require additional care or services. Some services may no longer be necessary, or the client may be ready for discharge. Whatever the conclusion, after evaluation, the appropriate members of the interdisciplinary team along with the client and family must reassess and plan for the continuing needs of the client.

Documentation

A written plan of care that incorporates elements of continuity is an essential tool to guide and document communication and coordination among team members. Although collection and evaluation of data for case management are often done in varying degrees of formality (e.g., interviews, physical examinations, questionnaires), communication is better served if the recording of such data is kept formal and organized. Use of well-constructed and consistently used planning documents across the continuum of care becomes vital to the success of coordination of disciplines and, therefore, to effective planning. At the same time a plan must be current and dynamic to reflect the reality of the client and/or family at various points of time. For example, essential elements of discharge planning documentation include a record of: client and family teaching; emotional and mental status assessment and a statement directly related to the client's and family caregiver's ability to manage care after discharge; appropriateness and safety of housing; availability of transportation; availability, accessibility, and affordability of community resources needed; equipment, supplies, and medication needed; and a written follow-up plan of care (Smith, 2006).

The competencies necessary for community-based care have been discussed. Competent care begins with an ability to understand what promotes and what inhibits self-care, as well as using the techniques of establishing trust, making appropriate referrals, advocating, consulting, and collaborating to facilitate self-care. People living with a chronic condition often require a great deal of assistance with health promotion to help maximize continuity and improve the quality of their lives. Because chronic diseases are the major cause of morbidity and mortality in developed countries, nurses are increasingly involved with illness prevention and health promotion. Community-based nursing occurs within the context of the client's community. The nurse is responsible for identifying resources and constraints or limitations for care that exist within the client's community. Collaboration and advocacy are important aspects of ensuring continuity of care. All combined these elements contribute to continuity in community-based care.

BARRIERS TO SUCCESSFUL CONTINUITY OF CARE

The nurse must be aware of barriers that may adversely affect continuity. These blocks may result from social factors, family matters, communication difficulties, or cultural differences. The health care system itself poses many barriers to continuity of care.

Social Factors

Attitude of the Health Care Worker

The health care worker's attitudes and biases can affect whether the client and family will use available resources. Clients are quick to sense bias and judgment. For example, a prenatal clinic for low-income women may have no place for small children to wait while their mothers are examined. In fact, the mothers are discouraged from bringing their children to the clinic when they have appointments. The women sense this judgment, but most of them cannot afford child care. Consequently, they do not follow through on essential prenatal care, resulting in interrupted continuity.

Client Motivation

The client may not follow through on a suggested referral if there are more pressing matters at hand. When people are ill, they are often concerned only with meeting basic needs and not with meeting more involved goals, such as belonging or self-esteem. Consequently, when clients are asked to make decisions about their higher needs, their motivation may be diminished because all their energy is going toward getting their basic health care needs met. Client priorities can explain why preventive health care services, for instance, may not be considered a priority when the client has difficulty just feeding and clothing the family. The nurse must be aware of the client's priorities. The nurse must first assist with meeting the needs the client sees as a priority before progressing.

Lack of Knowledge

When clients do not understand the need for a service, they may avoid using that service. Understanding the reason for a referral to an outside organization, as well as understanding the consequences of not following through, increases the likelihood of client compliance. This can be true in the case of prenatal care for the adolescent who is pregnant for the first time. She may know she "should" go to the clinic for checkups during pregnancy, but she may not know why. If the adolescent understands the purpose of prenatal care and the consequences of not receiving care, she is more likely to follow-up with a referral to the antenatal clinic.

Family Barriers

Being involved in decisions about care after discharge and receiving relevant self-care information are important to clients and families as they move from one setting to another. It may be helpful to realize that family involvement may either enhance or interrupt continuity. Whatever the contributing factor affecting family involvement, be it family stress, family functioning, or financial resources, the nurse plays an important role in assisting the client and family in the problem solving process.

Communication Barriers

Poor communication about recovery information is often attributed to language problems and hearing limitations. In general, health care providers expect client compliance, respect, and cooperation. Communication barriers can occur when the client does not speak English. They also occur when there is a cultural difference significant enough to prohibit communication (e.g., reading and comprehension) or to create misunderstandings because of factors such as the age of the client, sexual orientation, or use of nonverbal communication. A client may be offended and not listen to instructions or refuse referrals to community providers if the nurse does not practice culturally sensitive communication techniques. Increasing age brings hearing limitations, impaired eyesight, and memory loss, which can interfere with communication and retention of information.

Transcultural Barriers

A prominent barrier, although not always the most obvious, may be the cultural barrier that exists between the provider and client. It may be difficult for the nurse to withhold judgment and accept the client or family of another culture. In the opinion of the nurse, clients from a different culture may ask "too many" questions, exhibit defensive behavior, lack deference to the recognized authority figure (e.g., nurses and other health care providers), or have different perceptions of their role in the discharge planning and referral process. Chapter 3 focuses on cultural care and the necessary transcultural nursing skills and competencies required of nurses in community settings.

Health Care System Barriers

Reimbursement

Health care services are costly in the United States, and not everyone has health insurance. Consequently, many people do not seek health care services because they cannot afford them. This is often the case with the "working poor," who are often underinsured or uninsured, or with those who are on medical assistance and may not qualify for needed services. At times it is difficult to find services in the community that will fill a client's needs within financial resources. Gaps in care often result from reimbursement requirements in the form of burdensome and confusing documentation regulations. The health care worker may be left feeling apathetic toward planning and referral when services are available only when there is a source of payment. Problem solving must occur to remove or work with these constraints.

In situations where the number of clinic or home visits is limited the nurse must be prepared to act as a client advocate and justify continued care beyond the certification period determined by the client insurance coverage or Medicare or Medicaid. In the case of Medicare the nurse may document the following: If the client has made no progress toward goals, what are the chances of goals being achieved during an extended period? The nurse must also document any acute changes of condition that prevented achievement of the goals or if the chronic condition may prevent achievement of goals from ever occurring (Zink, 2005).

Failed Systems

Sometimes systems within the health care setting create barriers to successful continuity. The primary health care team may unintentionally interrupt continuity in several different ways. First, insufficient staff may create delays. Lack of time to address continuity needs is another barrier to continuity. Third, if staff communication is poor, delays may result.

Caregivers and services outside of the primary health care team may create delays. For example, laboratory test results may not be ready on time, or transport may not be provided during prescribed time lines. These delays are often not within the control of the primary health care team. Sometimes a lack of services may create lack of continuity when parameters for access are too stringent.

SUCCESSFUL CONTINUITY OF CARE

Several current studies show that clients benefit from nursing follow-up after discharge from the hospital. One study found that when nurse practitioners (NPs) provided follow-up care with clients with hypercholesterolemia who had undergone coronary artery bypass grafting or percutaneous coronary surgical intervention, their cholesterol level was lower and their diet and exercise improved when compared to clients who did not receive follow-up nursing care. The NPs spent an average of 4.5 hours per client over the year. After one year, 65% of those receiving nurse follow-up had reduced their cholesterol to desirable levels, compared with 35% of clients who did not receive nurse follow-up (Allen et al., 2002). Nursing follow-up also proved effective for women with abusive partners to take protective measures against future abuse. In a randomized case-control study, the group with the nursing intervention adopted substantially more safety behaviors than those in the control group as measured 6 months after the intervention (McFarlane et al., 2002).

An intensive case management program in Chester, PA, assists children and adults with serious mental illness to manage their self-care, avoid hospitalization and remain in the community. This program began in 1987 after a woman with a serious mental illness shot and killed people at a shopping mall. Prior to the murders the woman made numerous visits to several psychiatric agencies but did not receive the care she desperately needed. The shooting was the impetus for developing the intensive case management program. Individuals with the most seriously illness and need frequent assistance are assigned an intensive case manager while those individuals requiring less assistance work with resource coordinators. Clients in the program complete a self-assessment scale every 6 months, identifying where they believe they have improved and areas where they still need assistance. The case managers make regular home visits to all clients and often accompany clients to clinic visits or to other community resources. This program is successful because the clients and family members develop a trusting relationship with their case manager and know that he or she is their advocate and has their best interest in mind (Critical Path Network, 2006).

Hip fractures represent a major health problem with the older population. This condition frequently results in care in several settings (e.g., the hospital, transitional/subacute hospital, and assisted living or long-term care facility). Watters and Moran (2006) describe a protocol to improve the continuity of care of clients with hip fractures from admission in the emergency department to a planned discharge. The protocol was developed on the basis of established evidence of best practice. The protocol provided interdisciplinary holistic care and case management and incorporated client and family teaching at the time of admission. A clinical nurse specialist was responsible for coordinating the protocol from the

RESEARCH IN COMMUNITY-BASED NURSING CARE ▶ 7-4

Effect of a Standardized Case Management Telephone Intervention by Nurses on Resource Use in Clients With Chronic Heart Failure

Although it is believed that case management promotes continuity of care and decreased hospitalization rates, few case control studies have tested this approach. This study assessed the effectiveness of a standardized case management intervention, using telephone calls to decrease resource use in clients with chronic heart failure. Clients were identified while hospitalized and assigned to either the treatment group or the control group. For 6 months the treatment group received telephone case management by a nurse using a support software program. The nurse called them 5 days after discharge and more or less frequently depending on the symptoms they reported. Case managers also spoke to family members, other professionals (e.g., physicians, dietitians, social workers, and physical therapists), and individuals from community agencies in the course of case management. Printed educational materials were mailed to those in the treatment group on a monthly basis. Those in the treatment group, who received standardized telephone calls from an RN case manager, required significantly fewer resources over the 6 months of the study. Significant cost savings were demonstrated with this intervention. The cost of acute care for each client in the usual care group was $2,186, while the average cost per client in the intervention group was only $1,192. This difference computes to about $1,000 less per client over the 6 months of the study. This savings is more than twice the cost of the intervention, which was $443 per patient for the 6-month case management intervention. It is important to note that few other investigators have scientifically tested an intervention of this type with chronically ill populations despite the fact that telephone case management is used widely in disease management programs across the country.

Source: Riegel, B., Carlson, B., Kopp, Z., LePetri, Glaser, D., & Unger, A. (2002). Effect of a standardized nurse case-management telephone intervention on resource use in patients with chronic heart failure. *Archives of Internal Medicine, 162*(6), 705–712.

emergency department to discharge. In the first 17 months of the program hospital costs were reduced by more than $200,000 with the average length of stay dropping from 11 days to 6.5 days (Watters & Moran, 2006).

A community-based geriatric case management program for frail elderly citizens is another example of successful continuity of care. Duke (2005) reported on the outcomes of this program where nurse and social work case managers worked together to provide a combination of traditional hands-on care as well as high technology distance–based health care through a tele-health unit. Depending on the needs of the individual, interventions included case management of medical and social conditions, telemedicine assessment for medically compromised clients, and utilization of hospice and promotion for acceptance of end-of-life decision making. On a monthly basis the nurse case manager also provided education about specific health care issues for assisted living staff members, and residents and their family members. The outcomes prove this model to be cost-effective while improving quality of life for enrollees (Duke, 2005).

The role of the nurse as a case manager in the care of individuals with chronic illness is evolving. One example is seen in the management of heart failure. Nearly 5 million individuals in the United States now require heart failure management, with an estimated half million new cases diagnosed each year (Rasmusson et al., 2005). Mortality remains high for these individuals, with over 50% dying within 5 years of diagnosis. Specialized nurses are well positioned to improve the delivery of heart failure care. Currently many centers successfully use nurse specialists to provide specialized heart failure care. The author suggests expanding the use of specialized nurses for this growing need (Rasmusson et al., 2005). Another example of the role of the nurse case manager is found in Research in Community-Based Nursing Care 7-4.

CLIENT SITUATIONS IN PRACTICE

◆ Case Management

Steve, age 40, and Barb, age 37, are a couple with three children: Brook, 15, Jane, 13, and Jack, 11. Both parents are professionals. Steve works at the Veterans Administration, where he is in charge of the information systems, and Barb is a professor at a small liberal arts college. Because Steve has a family history of colon cancer (his paternal grandfather died of colon cancer at age 41 and his father and uncle had surgery for colon cancer at ages 65 and 60, respectively), he was advised to have a colonoscopy at age 40. One month after his 40th birthday, Steve scheduled a test. He was diagnosed with colon cancer 3 days after the test, on Christmas Eve day. He has no symptoms. Because of the size of the tumor, Steve's physician recommends he have the surgery at a large medical center 200 miles from Steve's home. Two days after Christmas, he has a colon resection without a colostomy at Methodist Hospital. At that time, it is determined that the cancer is class C2 according to Dukes classification system (or stage 4 with the other commonly used classification). Although he was a candidate for a colostomy, he and Barb decided they wanted to try the more conservative approach, with the option of a colostomy later, if necessary.

Barb has been with Steve throughout his hospital stay while their three children have been home, 200 miles away, staying with Barb's elderly mother. It is 14 days after the operation, and he is to return home the day after tomorrow. He will begin chemotherapy at the rural hospital close to his home next week.

- *You are a staff nurse caring for Steve in the hospital. What strategies to ensure continuity of care would you use, starting from the first day?*
  The first step in care management is establishing a relationship with the client and family by listening and talking. By doing this, you hope to build trust.

  By now you would have established a very open relationship with Barb and Steve. You ask Barb and Steve how they anticipate the homecoming will go when they arrive home. Barb says, "We have both really missed the kids. I really want to have a normal life again—sleep in my own bed and make breakfast for everyone. Just normal stuff."
  Steve says, "I can't wait to get out of here. But I am worried about the chemo. We had one conversation with the nurse at the clinic, and she said that we have to have the chemo in the morning. I have most of my meetings at work in the morning and would rather do the chemo in the afternoon."

- *How could you, as a staff nurse, respond to this comment?*
  To help give some control back to the client, you might encourage him to call the clinic that day and explore whether chemotherapy could be scheduled at a time more convenient for his work schedule.

Nurse in the Outpatient Setting

You are working in a clinic as an oncology nurse, providing chemotherapy for Steve. This is the third week of his treatment, and you have established a relationship with both Barb and Steve. During Steve's visit, you ask them how things are going. Barb tells you, "Awful. Brook was picked up for shoplifting, and her grades are dropping in school." You note that Steve is unusually quiet and does not make eye contact with you. You ask, "Steve, you look down today. Are you doing okay?"
"It feels like it is all coming apart. I can't keep up at work, the kids are having trouble . . .," Steve shares.
"He won't listen to me about resting. And he's throwing up all the time. That medication you gave him doesn't work," Barb reports.

- *What are some interventions you could use at this point in your care of Steve and his family?*
  Possible interventions include the following:

  Using the steps of the referral process to find some community resources to support the family with the issues the family is facing, including the daughter's shoplifting and falling grades
  Advocating for the client by calling the oncology nurse practitioner or physician to identify additional antiemetics that may be helpful in controlling the nausea and vomiting
  Contacting a social worker (with the family's approval) to begin to collaborate and problem solve regarding the family's issues and stress

Ten months later, Steve has completed chemotherapy and radiation therapy. Because of the intensity of the radiology treatment, he has developed interrupted bowel function. He has been to the clinic and the ED several times in the past weeks with severe cramps. You receive a call late in the afternoon from Barb. She states that the medication given at the last clinic visit is not helping; Steve has been throwing up all day, has severe abdominal cramps, and has a temperature of 103°F. You tell them to go to the local ED.

At the ED, Steve is diagnosed with a bladder and kidney infection and bowel obstruction, and he is admitted to the hospital. A complete workup is performed while he is in the hospital, and liver cancer is discovered throughout his liver, with lesions in the brain as well. He is discharged home unable to eat, with a central line and hyperal for total parenteral nutrition.

Home Care Nurse

You are Steve's home care nurse. On the first home visit, his functional capacity for ADLs is clearly impaired. He is homebound and needs a home health care aide to help him bathe and shave. Barb is working two jobs to try to make ends meet. The plan is for the home health aide to come every other day, with you coming once a day to start the hyperal. Two months later, at one of your visits, Steve says, "The home aide says he can do the hyperal and clean the site on the days when he is here. Then you don't have to come every day."

- *Can you delegate the administration of hyperal to the home health aide?*
  According to the Five Rights of Delegation from the NCSBN (Box 7–2), this task may not be delegated for the following reasons:
  The CNA is not the right person for the task. Assessment may be needed. The RN would not be immediately available for assistance or direct supervision.
  Steve's condition continues to deteriorate over the next month. Steve and the family has changed the subject every time you have brought up the subject of palliative care or hospice care in the last few weeks. As you are getting ready to leave after a visit, Barb abruptly asks you, "Do you think that Steve is going to die soon?"

- *You sit down with Barb and ask her, "Are you wondering about the benefits of palliative or hospice care?" She indicates that she is feeling like she is no longer able to handle his deteriorating condition without more assistance. You conclude that Barb and Steve may be ready to talk about hospice care. How do you proceed?*
  Using the steps for consultation in Box 7-1, you determine the family's needs. Through mutual problem solving, you determine if and when the family is ready to meet with the hospice nurse. At that time, you contact her for the family and arrange for her to visit.

CONCLUSIONS

This chapter has taken a broad look at continuity of care. Discharge planning has been described as a significant process that ensures continuity of care by coordinating various aspects of a client's care beginning with admission through transition from one health care setting to another. Nurses on all levels are care managers for some parts of their jobs. Coordination of activities involving the clients, providers, and payers is essential in providing continued care. Identification of current and future needs leads to implementation of the referral process and continued care. Essential to quality health care is a strong, ongoing health care plan that includes appropriate use of resources and effective referrals. Barriers to effective discharge planning include social, family, communication, health care system, and community resources issues. The care manager in community-based settings always encourages self-care with a preventive focus that is provided within the context of the client's community while following the principles of collaboration to achieve continuity.

What's on the Web

American Healthways
Internet address: http://www.
americanhealthways.com/whatwedo.aspx
Healthways business is to keep, or move,
as many people as possible to the healthy
side of the health/care continuum. For
consumers, Healthways is a trusted
resource, which leads to healthier
behaviors. For physicians, Healthways is
an extension of their office staffs, helping
ensure patient compliance with their
treatment plans. For health plans,
employers and government agencies,
Healthways provides programs that help
reduce risk and lower costs.

Improving Chronic Illness Care
Internet address: http://www.improving
chroniccare.org/change/index.html
Due to the increasing percentage of the
population who develops chronic conditions, many managed care and integrated
delivery systems have taken a great
interest in correcting the many deficiencies in current management of diseases
such as diabetes, heart disease, depression, asthma, and others. The deficiencies of lack of coordinate care and follow-
up, as well as many clients being
inadequately educated to manage their
conditions, call for a model for managing
chronic conditions. This model for managing chronic conditions is the subject of

this Web site. There are many resources
on this site.

Case Management Society of America
8201 Cantrell Road, Suite 230
Little Rock, AR 72227
Telephone: (501) 225-2229
Fax: (501) 221-9068
Internet address: http://www.cmsa.org
This site offers educational opportunities,
both CEU (continuing education units) and
case management credential courses. It
also provides extensive information on
case management.

Case Management Resource Guide
Internet address: http://www.cmrg.com/
This site has a comprehensive, online
directory of health care organizations. It
also contains an extensive case manager
resource guide.

National Council of State Boards of
Nursing (NCSBN) Delegation Resource
Folder
Internet address: http://www.ncsbn.org
The NCSBN has produced an excellent
resource on delegation, which serves as
the major reference for information on
delegation. The council's material is contained in the delegation resource folder and
can be found on the council's Web site by
entering "delegation" in the search box.

References and Bibliography

Allen, J. K., Blumenthal, R. S., Margolis, S.,
et al. (2002). Nurse case management of
hypercholesterolemia in patients with coronary heart disease: Results of a randomized
clinical trial. *American Heart Journal, 144*(4),
678–686.
Blaylock, A., & Cason, C. L. (1992). Discharge
planning: Predicting patient's needs. *Journal of Gerontological Nursing, 18*(7), 5–10.
Craven, R. F., & Hirnle, C. J. (2007). *Fundamentals of nursing: Human health and
function* (5th ed.). Philadelphia: Lippincott
Williams & Wilkins.
Critical path network: Case managers help
mentally ill avoid hospitalization and

remain in the community. (2006). *Hospital
Case Management, 14*(6), 87–88.
Duke, C. (2005). The Frail Elderly Community–Based Case Management Project. *Geriatric Nursing, 26*(2), 122–127.
Dedicated CM-SW team care for trauma
patients. (2006). *Hospital Case Management, 14*(9), 133–134, 139.
Dunnion, M. E., & Kelly, B. (2005). From
emergency department to home. *Journal of
Clinical Nursing, 14,* 776–785.
Kersbergen, A. L. (2000). Managed care. Shifts
health care from an altruistic model to a
business framework. *Nursing and Health
Care Perspectives, 21*(2), 81–83.

Kesby, S. (2002). Nursing care and collaborative practice. *Journal of Clinical Nursing, 11*(3), 357–366. Retrieved January 19, 2003, from the CINAHL database.

Krugman, P. (2006). Health care confidential. *New York Times.* Retrieved April 9, 2007, from http://select.nytimes.com/2006/01/27/opinion/27krugman.html?_r=1&oref=slogin

Lagoe, R., Dauley-Altwarg, J., Munich, S., & Winks, L. (2005). A community-wide program to improve the efficiency of care between nursing homes and hospitals. *Topics in Advanced Practice Nursing eJournal, 5*(2). Retrieved on September 9, 2006, from http://www.medscape.com/viewarticle/503748

Lee, D. T., Mackenzie, A. E., Dudley-Brown, S., & Chin, T. M. (1998). Case management: A review of the definitions and practice. *Journal of Advanced Nursing, 27,* 933–939.

Lyon, J. C. (1993). Modules of nursing care delivery and case management: Clarification of terms. *Nursing Economics, 11*(3), 163–178.

McFarlane, J., Malecha, A., Gist, J., et al. (2002). An intervention to increase safety behaviors of abused women: Results of a randomized clinical trial. *Nursing Research, 51*(6), 347–354.

Minnesota Department of Health, Section of Public Health Nursing. (2001). *Public health nursing interventions II.* Minneapolis: Author.

Mistiaen, P., Duijnhouwer, E., Prins-Hoekstra, A., Ros, W., & Blaylock, A. (1999). Predictive validity of the BRASS index in screening patients with post-discharge problems. *Journal of Advanced Nursing, 30*(5), 1050–1056.

National Council of State Boards of Nursing. (2006). The Delegation Resource Folder [Data file]. Retrieved on September 17, 2006, from http://www.ncsbn.org/files/delegation.asp

National Council of State Boards of Nursing. (2006). Joint Statement on Delegation from the American Nurses Association (ANA) and the National Council of State Boards of Nursing (NCSBN). Retrieved on September 12, 2006, from *https://www.ncsbn.org/index.htm*

Powell, S. (2000). *Case management: A practical guide to success in managed care* (2nd ed.). Philadelphia: Lippincott Williams & Wilkins.

Rasmusson, K., Hall, J. Vesty, J., et al. (2005). Managing the heart failure epidemic: The evolving role of nurse specialist. *Topics in Advanced Practice Nursing eJournal, 5*(4). Retrieved on September 14, 2006, from http://www.medscape.com/viewpublication/

Riegel, B., Carlson, B., Kopp, Z., et al. (2002). Effect of a standardized nurse case-management telephone intervention on resource use in patients with chronic heart failure. *Archives of Internal Medicine, 162*(6), 705–712.

Rodgers, B. (2000). Coordination of care: The lived experience of the visiting nurse. *Home Healthcare Nurse, 18*(5), 301–307.

Smith, L. S., (2006). Documenting discharge planning. Chart Smart. *Nursing, 36*(5), 18.

Tahan, H. A. (1998). Case management: A heritage more than a century old. *Nursing Case Management, 3*(2), 55–60.

Watters, C. L., & Moran, W. P. (2006). Hip fractures–a joint effort. *Orthopaedic Nursing, 25*(3), 157–165.

Wendt, D. (1996). Building trust during the initial home visit. In R. Hunt (Ed.), *Readings in community-based nursing* (pp. 154–160). Philadelphia: Lippincott Williams & Wilkins.

Zink, M. R. (2005). Episodic case management in home care. *Home Healthcare Nurse, 23*(10), 655–662.

LEARNING ▼ ACTIVITIES

◆ JOURNALING ACTIVITY 7-1

1. In your clinical journal, describe a situation you observed in which a client or family experienced difficulty because of lack of continuity. If you were the nurse in charge, what would you have done differently?
2. In your clinical journal, relate a situation in which you observed a client who received effective continuity of care in discharge planning. What made the care effective?
3. In your clinical journal, describe a situation you have observed in clinical where a client received effective case management. What made the care effective?
4. In your clinical journal, describe a situation where you observed or initiated two of the following intervention strategies. Discuss what happened.

   Health teaching
   Screening
   Counseling
   Referral and follow-up
   Consultation
   Collaboration
   Advocacy

5. List any barriers you have noticed that have interrupted continuity for a client you have cared for in clinical setting. Discuss what happened and what you would do differently. Identify any system's issues that you think did not address the barriers (e.g., chart forms such as discharge forms, admission forms, unit policies).

◆ CLIENT CARE ACTIVITY 7-2

Mr. Heaney, a 66-year-old man, is admitted for a total knee replacement. He has had continuous pain in his left knee for the past 2 years secondary to osteoarthritis. Five years ago he had coronary bypass surgery and has limited sight. His wife of 45 years died just 2 months ago, and he has remained alone in their two-story home. He has visited the ED four times with cardiac symptoms in the last month related to not taking his cardiac medications regularly. Only one of their six children lives in the area. On postoperative day 1 he begins physical therapy. His left leg is in a continuous passive motion device when he is in bed. The plan is to discharge him on postoperative day 2 with outpatient physical therapy, the use of the continuous passive motion device at home, and continuation of oral analgesics for pain. He will use a walker for ambulation for at least 2 weeks and will continue to take the four cardiac drugs that he has been taking for the last 5 years. He appears to be slightly confused during the discharge planning conference when the discussion about his continuing care is discussed.

1. Describe your role as the primary nurse in Mr. Heaney's discharge planning.
2. Explain why you are in a position to coordinate continuity of care.
3. Identify the risks Mr. Heaney may have after discharge. Use the Blaylock Discharge Planning Risk Assessment Screen (Fig.7–3) to assess for risks.
4. Propose recommendations for his living situation and home care.
5. List agencies, facilities, or individuals you would recommend for Mr. Heaney's continuing care and give your reasons.

◆ CLIENT CARE ACTIVITY 7-3

You are a home health care nurse responsible for the care of 15 clients. It's Monday morning, and you are reviewing your phone messages as well as looking over the charts of the clients you are scheduled to visit in the next 2 days. How will you rearrange home visits for the next 2 days based on the following information?

SCHEDULED VISITS FOR MONDAY AFTERNOON AND TUESDAY

MONDAY

1:00 Mr. Carmody—routine visit to monitor symptoms of congestive heart failure
2:30 Mrs. Gothie—routine follow-up visit after hip replacement and discharge from acute care last Wednesday, and your last visit was Friday
4:00 Mrs. Violet—monthly blood draw for lithium levels

TUESDAY

9:00 Mr. Perlmutter—scheduled to discharge from the hospital Monday night after open heart surgery; assessment visit and blood draw
10:30 Mr. Sund—follow-up visit for knee replacement surgery; discharged from the hospital last Thursday, and your last visit was Friday
1:00 Mr. Vang—reinforcement teaching for care of a leg wound
2:30 Mrs. O'Conner—follow-up visit for assessment after scheduled discharge from the hospital on Monday evening; administration of IV antibiotic medication

PHONE MESSAGES ON MONDAY AT 8:00 AM

Mr. Vang called you this morning and said that he ran out of dressings on Friday. He was upset and stated that the sore on his leg looked redder, and there was some sticky green stuff dripping off of it.
Mrs. Sund called and said her husband had so much pain in his knee over the weekend that he could not sleep. She said he also has pain in the back of his calf, it is red, and it hurts if he flexes his foot.

◆ PRACTICAL APPLICATION ACTIVITY 7-4

Observe a nurse doing routine discharge planning with a client in the hospital, ED, or clinic. How did the nurse assess the following with the client or the client's family? (This could be done either through questions on the discharge form or additional questions the nurse asks.)

If you were the nurse, what would you have done differently from or in addition to the activities of the nurse you observed?

◆ CRITICAL THINKING ACTIVITY 7-5

List at least three barriers you have observed in your clinical setting that hinder effective case management. Discuss what could be done differently to enhance case management and continuity in these situations.

◆ **CRITICAL THINKING ACTIVITY 7-6**

Ask the nurse manager in the settings where you do clinical work about strategies used on his or her unit to ensure continuity of care. If the nurse manager indicates that he or she is not satisfied with continuity of care on the unit, ask what could be done to improve it. Volunteer to do a project to assist the head nurse to explore his or her concerns. If the nurse manager asks for suggestions of projects, offer to complete a literature review of best practice continuity of care programs in the specialty area of the unit.

COMMUNITY-BASED NURSING ACROSS THE LIFE SPAN

I n Chapter 2, you learned that although the U.S. health care system is the most expensive in the world, the United States lags behind other nations in key health indicators. This unit uses the recommendations from Healthy People 2010 (http://www.healthypeople.gov/) to outline the role that the nurse must play in improving the nation's health. All three chapters in this unit address the broad goals outlined in Healthy People 2010 to eliminate health disparity and increase quality and years of healthy life.

Each chapter begins with a discussion of the goals of Healthy People 2010, as well as the major causes of mortality and morbidity for each age group. Nursing assessments and interventions follow. Chapter 8 discusses health promotion and disease prevention for maternal/infant populations, children, and adolescents. Chapter 9 outlines health promotion and disease prevention for adults, and Chapter 10 focuses on elderly adults.

The content of each chapter is organized around the leading causes of mortality for each group. Disease prevention and health promotion strategies that address these causes are highlighted. Based on numerous sources, these strategies are intended for the practicing nurse to use to teach clients about health promotion and disease prevention. Unit III also contains numerous Web site and organization addresses, as well as resources related to health promotion and disease prevention for clients across the life span.

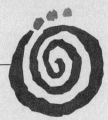

8

Health Promotion and Disease Prevention for Maternal/Infant Populations, Children, and Adolescents

ROBERTA HUNT

LEARNING OBJECTIVES

1. Identify the major causes of death for maternal/infant populations, children, and adolescents.
2. Discuss the major diseases and threats to health for maternal/infant populations, children, and adolescents.
3. Summarize the major health issues for maternal/infant populations, children, and adolescents.
4. Identify nursing roles at each level of prevention for major health issues.
5. Compose a list of nursing interventions for the major health issues for maternal/infant populations, children, and adolescents.
6. Determine health needs for maternal/infant populations, children, and adolescents for which a nurse could be an advocate.

KEY TERMS

Denver Developmental Screening
  Test (DDST)
fetal alcohol syndrome (FAS)
infant mortality rate
lead poisoning

low birth weight (LBW)
morbidity
mortality
neural tube defects (NTDs)
sudden infant death syndrome (SIDS)

CHAPTER TOPICS

◆ Significance of Health Promotion and Disease Prevention
◆ Eliminating Disparity in Health Care
◆ Maternal/Infant Populations
◆ Preschool-Age Children
◆ School-Age Children
◆ Adolescence
◆ Conclusions

THE NURSE SPEAKS

For over 10 years, I worked as a school nurse at a large high school in a small Midwestern town. One day, a 15-year-old student named Jennifer came into my office. She was obviously pregnant. She told me that she was going to the doctor the next day to find out if she was pregnant. She didn't think that she was, but wanted to find out for sure. I asked her if she could feel any kicking, and she said she could. I asked her if she could feel kicking when she held her hand on her stomach, and she said she could. When she left my office she said that she would let me know what the doctor said.

Several days later, she returned to see me and said that she had had an exam and was indeed pregnant and due in 1 month. I asked about the possibility of finding a prenatal class for her, but she wasn't interested. Although I saw her several times before her baby was born, she remained detached and uninterested in the baby or learning about the impending delivery. I was very concerned about Jennifer and her baby. I wondered if she would attach to the baby and thought that this family was at risk for lack of early bonding and attachment. I knew that babies born to young teen moms were at higher risk for child abuse and neglect than infants born to older women.

A month after her baby was born, I called Jennifer and asked if I could come to see her. She was living with her parents. She agreed to a home visit the next week. When I entered the home, Jennifer was holding her daughter and sitting at the kitchen table with her father. I sat down and explained that I was the school nurse and did home visits with some of the students from the high school. I kept things casual and at first we talked about general things. Then Jennifer began to talk about when she would be returning to school, when she hoped to graduate, and the classes she would be taking. Jennifer's mother came in as we were talking and stated, "The baby is sleeping all night now. Jennifer is a great mom. I am working the evening shift now, so I will take care of the baby when Jennifer is in school."

All the time we were talking, I was quietly observing Jennifer with her baby daughter. She was holding her close but with a relaxed posture. She frequently looked at the baby, and when the baby woke up Jennifer looked into her sleepy eyes and said softly said, "Hi Tiffany. Did you have a good nap?" Then she fed Tiffany a bottle. As she was feeding her, Jennifer was watching Tiffany's face. As soon as the baby started to act like she wanted to stop feeding, Jennifer would take the bottle out of her mouth. She said, "Tiffany likes to just drink a little and then be burped and rest."

I left Jennifer's home confident that with the support of her parents, Tiffany would be well cared for and Jennifer would be able to finish high school. My concern about her nonchalance about being pregnant and the birth of her baby did not appear to have interfered with her attaching to her baby. I was relieved that despite the lack of prenatal care and preparation, this family had all the basics to care for this newborn.

—ASHLEY MOORE, RN, PHN, St. Paul, Minnesota

SIGNIFICANCE OF HEALTH PROMOTION AND DISEASE PREVENTION

Crucial issues of health and health care are different today from what they were in the early part of the 20th century. Public health efforts have increased the life span of the average person, thanks to universal access to clean water, sanitation, and immunization and the development of effective medications, particularly antibiotics. Our focus as health care providers has changed from combating infectious diseases to addressing chronic conditions and unintentional injuries.

Health promotion is typically defined as a primary disease prevention strategy. It is commonly interchanged with terms such as health education and disease prevention. Often health promotion is discussed as the epitome of empowerment in that it is a process that enables people to use health as a resource for their lives. Health promotion is most often discussed as a strategy for an already healthy individual or population, but it applies to those with health conditions as well. Disease prevention is just as it states: preventing a disease from occurring. It also includes injury prevention, which will be foundational to the discussion in this and the following three chapters.

Recommendations from Healthy People 2010 form the foundation for all health promotion and disease prevention nursing actions. These recommendations are based on the primary causes of death, or **mortality**, rates and the rates of illness or injury, or **morbidity**, rates. The Healthy People 2010 report is based on mortality and morbidity statistics that represent the primary causes of death and illnesses and injuries experienced by the people living in the United States.

Most diseases and deaths result from preventable causes. The negative impact of many conditions can be minimized by early identification and intervention. This chapter addresses health promotion and disease prevention for pregnant women, infants, children, and adolescents.

ELIMINATING DISPARITY IN HEALTH CARE

One of the major goals of Healthy People 2010 is to eliminate health disparities. Health disparities exist by gender, race or ethnicity, education, income, disability, rural living localities, and sexual orientation. Infant mortality (IM) is a significant indicator of such disparities. In 2002, IM was 7.0 per 1,000 live births for all infants in the United States, compared with IM rates of 13.9 among African Americans, 8.6 for American Indians, 5.6 for Hispanics, and 5.8 for White, non-Hispanics. Of greater significance is the finding that, although IM rates have declined within all racial groups in the last 20 years, the proportional discrepancy between Blacks and Whites remains largely unchanged (The National Center for Health Statistics, 2006). The infant mortality rate rose to 7.22 in 2004 (United Health Foundation, 2006). Comparisons between races and infant mortality rates can be seen in Figure 8-1.

Disparity by ethnicity is believed to result from complex interactions among genetic variations, environmental factors, and specific health behaviors. Income and education underlie many health disparities in the United States. Income and education are intrinsically related; people with the worst health status are among

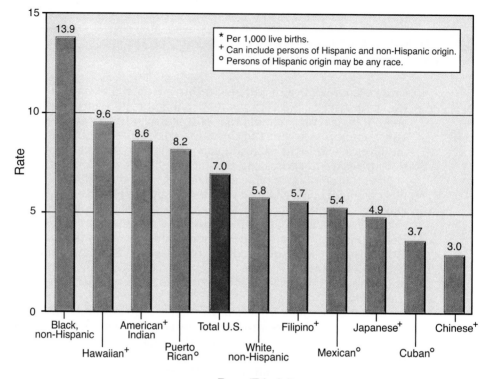

FIGURE 8-1. ▶ Infant mortality rates by selected racial/ethnic populations. *Source:* Mathews, R., Meneacker, F., & MacDorman, M. (2005). *Infant mortality statistics from 2002.* Retrieved on September 25, 2006, from http://www.cdc.gov/nchs/data/nvsr/nvsr53/nvsr53_10.pdf.

those with the highest poverty rates and least education. Income inequality in the United States has increased over the past 3 decades.

The percentage of all children living in poverty has increased in the last 5 years. In 2003, 18% of all children ages 0 to 17 lived in poverty. The poverty rate was higher for Black and Hispanic children in single family households as compared to White, non-Hispanic children in single family households (Federal Interagency Forum on Child and Family Statistics, 2005). The U.S. child poverty rate is the highest of the top 15 richest nations (Fig. 8-2). While the poverty rate for the elderly has dropped from 35% in 1959 to 10% today, the rate for children has only decreased from 26% to 18% (Fig. 8-3).

Poverty limits children's access to equal opportunities for growing up healthy. Low income communities are more likely to only have small convenience stores, liquor stores, and fast food where the selection and quality of fresh foods are limited. For decades having access to primary health care providers has been a problem. Of the 70 million rural Americans, more than 20 million have inadequate access to health care services in their communities. Low-income children are more likely to live in substandard housing where they are often exposed to structural hazards. In addition they are more likely as compared to children living in middle or upper income families to have lead

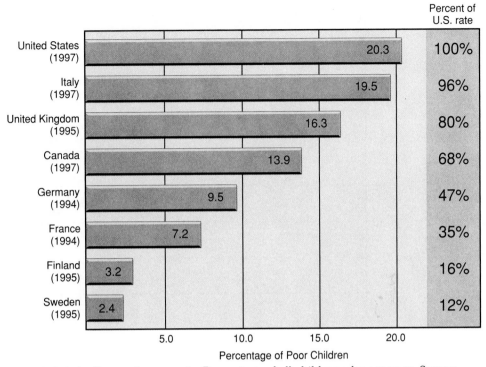

FIGURE 8-2. ▶ Comparing poverty: Percentage of all children who are poor. *Source: Rainwater, L., & Smeeding, T. (2003). Poor kids in rich nations.* New York: Russell Sage Foundation.

poisoning and asthma as a result. Designing communities so that all children have access to fresh food, primary health care, safe housing, and an environment free from pollution is vital to improving all children's long-term health (Equal Opportunities, 2006).

MATERNAL/INFANT POPULATIONS

Florence Nightingale wrote in 1894 that "money would be better spent in maintaining health in infancy and childhood than in building hospitals to cure disease" (Monteiro, 1985, p. 185). The same philosophy holds true today. The health of infants and children has farther-reaching implications than that of other population groups. The health of mothers, infants, and children is of critical importance as a predictor of the health of the next generation. The Maternal and Child Health Bureau (MCHB, 2006a) is charged with creating a society where children are wanted and born with optimal health, receive quality care, and are nurtured lovingly and sensitively as they mature into healthy, productive adults. Healthy People 2010 8-1 lists the Healthy People 2010 objectives for maternal and infant health.

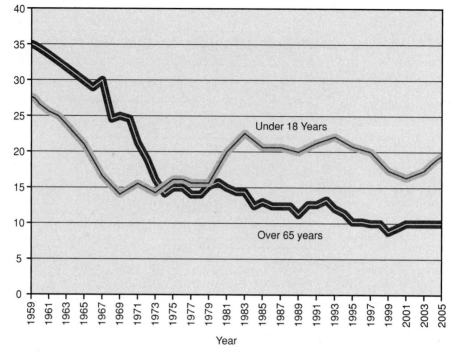

FIGURE 8-3. ▶ Poverty rates for children and the elderly, 1959-2004. *Source:* U.S Census Bureau, Historical Poverty Table. Retrieved on September 25, 2006, from http://www. census.gov/hhes/www/poverty/histpov/histpovtb.html.

▶ **HEALTHY PEOPLE 2010 ▶ 8-1**

Objectives for Maternal and Infant Health

Reduce fetal and infant deaths.

Increase proportion of pregnant women who receive early and adequate prenatal care.

Increase the proportion of pregnant women who attend a series of prepared childbirth classes.

Reduce preterm births.

Reduce the occurrence of spina bifida and other neural tube defects.

Increase abstinence from alcohol, cigarettes, and illicit drugs among pregnant women.

Increase the percentage of healthy full-term infants who are put down to sleep on their backs.

Increase the proportion of mothers who breast-feed their babies.

U.S. Department of Health and Human Services. (2000b). Maternal, infant, and child health. In *Healthy People 2010. National health promotion and disease prevention objectives.* Washington, DC: U.S. Government Printing Office.

Infant death is a critical indicator of the health of a population because it reflects the overall state of maternal health, as well as the quality and access of primary health available to pregnant women and infants. The **infant mortality rate** is the number of infants (ages birth to 1 year) who die out of every 1,000 live births. Although the 1980s and 1990s saw steady declines in the infant mortality rate in the United States, 27th among industrialized nations, it remains among the highest in the industrialized world at 7 per 1,000 births (Kids Count, 2006). Healthy People 2010 established the aggressive goal in 2000 to reduce the infant mortality rate to 4.5 deaths per 1,000 live births by 2010 but the rate has increased since 2000 (Kochanek & Martin, 2005).

Prenatal Care

The United States is the only industrialized nation in which not all pregnant women receive prenatal care. The percentage of U.S. mothers receiving early prenatal care (in the first trimester of pregnancy) varies substantially among racial and ethnic groups, from 76% for Black and Hispanic mothers to 89% for White mothers (MCHB, 2006b).

Every nurse in every setting should encourage pregnant women to begin prenatal care in the first trimester. Some of the topics that are important for the nurse to assess and intervene accordingly in home visits to pregnant women are those that Healthy People 2010 has deemed the leading causes of infant mortality: low birth weight, birth, and congenital anomalies.

Home visitation, where nurses can provide prenatal care and reduce the probability of low-birth-weight infants, helps lower the infant mortality rate. There is a large body of research that demonstrates the efficacy of home visiting for improving maternal-infant outcomes (Dawley & Beam, 2005; Kitzman et al., 2000). Home visiting women prior to and after birth to improve birth and newborn outcomes began in the early 20th century in the United States. Maternal/child home visiting continues as a model that is used throughout the globe. Today the Nurse Family Partnership has been replicated in 20 states at 250 program sites that serve over 13,000 families a year. This program improves newborn and child outcomes by positively influencing maternal role attainment and significantly decreasing maternal smoking and other substance abuse, child abuse and neglect, and children's emergency room visits (Dawley & Beam, 2005).

Low Birth Weight
The most important challenge facing women's and children's health in the United States is premature birth. **Low birth weight (LBW)**, or weight less than 2,500 g or 5.5 lb, is the leading cause of preventable neonatal death. This is included under disorders related to premature birth listed in Table 8-1. In the last 2 decades the United States has seen a steady increase in premature births with 1 in 9 infants born prematurely each year (Cole, 2006). LBW is associated with long-term disabilities, such as cerebral palsy, autism, mental retardation, vision and hearing impairment, and other developmental disabilities. LBW is also the main reason premature infants require care in neonatal intensive care units. It does not take a complicated cost analysis to conclude that it is much more expensive to care for a newborn in an intensive care unit than it would have been to provide prenatal care for the infant's mother. Technological advances have been made in the care of premature infants but have resulted in enormous financial, emotional, and social costs. In 2005 preterm births cost at least $26 billion a year (Institute of Medicine, 2006).

TABLE 8-1	Leading Causes of Death by Age Group, United States, 2004	
Age	**Cause of Death**	**Number of Deaths**
Younger than 1 y	Congenital anomalies	5622
	Disorders related to premature birth	4642
	Sudden infant death syndrome	2246
1–4 y	Unintentional injuries	1641
	Congenital anomalies	569
	Cancer	399
5–9 y	Unintentional injuries	1126
	Cancer	526
	Congenital anomalies	205
10–14 y	Unintentional injuries	1540
	Cancer	493
	Suicide	283
15–24 y	Unintentional injuries	15,449
	Homicide	5085
	Suicide	4316

Office of Statistics and Programming, National Center for Injury Prevention and Control, Centers for Disease Control and Prevention. (2006). Retrieved on September 21, 2006, from http://www.cdc.gov/ncipc/default.htm.

The consequences of preterm birth over the child's lifetime can be significant and often call for a broad range of services and social support. The emotional stress to the child and family are frequently considerable. The Institute of Medicine has made several recommendations for a national policy toward preventing and managing premature births. To prepare parents for a possible premature birth, prenatal preparation including preconception risk assessment and prenatal counseling is imperative. The primary intervention to prevent LBW is early initiation of prenatal care. Care in the neonatal intensive care units should be guided by policies that support and permit development of parental involvement from the moment of birth (Institute of Medicine, 2006). In the transition from hospital to home, health care providers should encourage home health nurses to become acquainted with the families in the hospital before discharge. Discharge teaching should prepare the parents to be comfortable using any equipment that the infant will need at home. A 24-hour hotline should be available for parents to obtain advice and reassurance.

Neural Tube Defects

Approximately 50% of all **neural tube defects (NTDs)** may be prevented with adequate consumption of folic acid in the first trimester of pregnancy. Currently, the U.S. Public Health Service recommends that all women of childbearing age consume 400 micrograms (mcg or μg) of folic acid daily. For women who are pregnant, 800 mcg per day is recommended (Federal Drug Administration, 1999).

Smoking

Smoking during pregnancy is the single most preventable cause of illness and death among mothers and infants. A pregnant woman who smokes is 1.5 to 3.5 times more likely to have a LBW infant (CDC, 2006a). Between 12% and 22% of

RESEARCH IN COMMUNITY-BASED NURSING CARE ▶ 8-1

Nurse-Delivered Smoking Relapse Prevention Program for New Mothers

For decades pregnancy has been recognized as a time of unique opportunity for smoking cessation, with 18% to 22% of women quitting smoking once they become pregnant. Nurses are often the best health care providers to promote smoking cessation programs. This study evaluated the acceptability of an evidence-based intervention using home health nurses to provide smoking relapse prevention skills to new mothers. Participants were women who had delivered a normal newborn and quit smoking during pregnancy, were smoke free for 7 days, and had saliva levels that indicated negligible cigarette consumption or minor exposure to second-hand smoke. Women who participated in this program were more than twice as likely to remain smoke free at both 3 and 6 months postpartum.

Groner, J., French, G., Ahijevych, K., & Wewers, M. E., (2005). Process evaluation of a nurse-delivered smoking relapse prevention program for new mothers. *Journal of Community Health Nursing, 22*(3), 157–167.

women smoke during pregnancy. Up to 25% of women who smoke before pregnancy stop before their first antenatal visit. However, the rest continue to smoke throughout the pregnancy (CDC, 2006b). Smoking cessation programs have been shown to be effective in reducing smoking rates. Nurses are often the best health care providers to promote smoking cessation programs to help their clients quit, especially when the client is pregnant (Groner, French, Ahijevych, & Wewers, 2005). Research in Community-Based Nursing Care 8-1 presents an example of research relating to a successful smoking cessation program for pregnant women. Smoking cessation program can be found on the Internet sites listed at the end of this chapter in What's on the Web. Postpartum resumption of smoking is discouraged due to the detrimental impact of passive smoke on infants and children.

Alcohol and Drug Use
Moderate to heavy alcohol use by women during pregnancy has been associated with many severe adverse effects, including **fetal alcohol syndrome (FAS)** or fetal alcohol effect and other developmental delays. FAS is recognized as the leading cause of mental retardation among women who consume alcohol during pregnancy. Infants and children with FAS have characteristic facial and associated physical features attributed to excessive ingestion of alcohol by the mother during pregnancy. It is the nurse's responsibility to discuss alcohol and drug use with the client in an open and nonjudgmental manner. Currently, it is recommended that women do not consume any alcohol during pregnancy. A tool kit called *Drinking and Reproductive Health,* from the American College of Obstetricians and Gynecologists, which nurses can use to assist pregnant women to stop drinking, can be found at http://www.acog.org/departments/healthIssues/FASDToolKit.pdf.

Newborn Care

The Child Health Guide: Put Prevention into Practice (Agency for Healthcare Research and Quality, 2004) is an excellent tool for monitoring infant and child health. It is available online at http://www.ahrq.gov/ppip/childguide/childguide.pdf. Request a copy via e-mail at ahrqpubs@ahrq.gov or a free copy can be ordered by calling (800) 358–9295. It provides parents with explanations of child preventive care and a convenient place to keep records of health care visits, growth, and immunizations. It recommends checkups at 3 weeks; 2, 4, 6, 9, 12, 15, and 18 months; and 2, 3, 4, 5, 6, 8, 10, 12, 14, 16, and 18 years with a pediatric nurse practitioner or physician. Bright Futures Family Tip Sheets can be downloaded from the Bright Futures Web site (http://www.brightfutures.org/TipSheets). It contains health supervision guidelines and information, including developmental charts for children, ranging from newborn through adolescence.

Screening

All newborns should have blood tests in the hospital for phenylketonuria (PKU), thyroid disease, and sickle cell disease. The current recommendation is that all newborns should be screened for hearing impairment before they leave the hospital. In 2006, the American Optometric Association recommend that newborns have an eye examination in the first year of life (Huggins, 2006). The parents should be encouraged to ask the nurse practitioner or physician if they are unsure whether these tests were done for their infant.

All infants' growth should be monitored and plotted on a growth chart outlining the developmental status of the infant. Charts are available from the Department of Health and Human Services (DHHS) in French and Spanish at http://www.cdc.gov/growthcharts. More information about this Web site is found at the end of this chapter. To reduce mortality and morbidity, both the parent and the nurse must be diligent in following preventive measures for normal-risk infants. In all community-based settings, the nurse can assist the parent in following basic prevention recommendations for children. Figure 8-4 outlines current recommendations for clinical preventive services for normal-risk children.

Immunizations

Fifty years ago, many children died from what today are preventable childhood diseases. Smallpox has been eradicated, poliomyelitis has been eliminated from the Western hemisphere, and cases of measles and chickenpox in the United States are at a record low. All of this progress has been made possible by the immunizations covered in Figure 8-4. The National Commission on Prevention priorities has identified childhood immunizations as one of the most effective and cost-effective clinical preventive services (Teutsch, 2006). However, only if the number of vaccinated children and adults remains high will immunization programs continue to be effective.

Immunizations are considered primary prevention because they prevent the occurrence of a disease. It is imperative that all children be immunized according to recommended standards. Immunizations should begin at birth and continue as recommended in Figure 8-4. Once a year, consult Every Child by Two at http://www.ecbt.org/ or the CDC at http://www.ecbt.org for updates.

Nutrition

Breast milk is widely acknowledged to be the most complete form of nutrition for infants (see Community-Based Teaching 8-1). The range of benefits includes
(*text continues on page 256*)

Recommended Immunization Schedule for Persons Aged 0–6 Years—UNITED STATES • 2007

Vaccine ▼ Age ▶	Birth	1 month	2 months	4 months	6 months	12 months	15 months	18 months	19–23 months	2–3 years	4–6 years
Hepatitis B[1]	HepB	HepB		see footnote 1		HepB			HepB Series		
Rotavirus[2]			Rota	Rota	Rota						
Diphtheria, Tetanus, Pertussis[3]			DTaP	DTaP	DTaP		DTaP				DTaP
Haemophilus influenzae type b[4]			Hib	Hib	*Hib*[4]	Hib		Hib			
Pneumococcal[5]			PCV	PCV	PCV	PCV				PCV / PPV	
Inactivated Poliovirus			IPV	IPV		IPV					IPV
Influenza[6]						Influenza (Yearly)					
Measles, Mumps, Rubella[7]						MMR					MMR
Varicella[8]						Varicella					Varicella
Hepatitis A[9]						HepA (2 doses)				HepA Series	
Meningococcal[10]										MPSV4	

- Range of recommended ages
- Catch-up immunization
- Certain high-risk groups

This schedule indicates the recommended ages for routine administration of currently licensed childhood vaccines, as of December 1, 2006, for children aged 0–6 years. Additional information is available at http://www.cdc.gov/nip/recs/child-schedule.htm. Any dose not administered at the recommended age should be administered at any subsequent visit, when indicated and feasible. Additional vaccines may be licensed and recommended during the year. Licensed combination vaccines may be used whenever any components of the combination are indicated and other components of the vaccine are not contraindicated and if approved by the Food and Drug Administration for that dose of the series. Providers should consult the respective Advisory Committee on Immunization Practices statement for detailed recommendations. Clinically significant adverse events that follow immunization should be reported to the Vaccine Adverse Event Reporting System (VAERS). Guidance about how to obtain and complete a VAERS form is available at http://www.vaers.hhs.gov or by telephone, 800-822-7967.

1. **Hepatitis B vaccine (HepB).** *(Minimum age: birth)*
   At birth:
   - Administer monovalent HepB to all newborns before hospital discharge.
   - If mother is hepatitis surface antigen (HBsAg)-positive, administer HepB and 0.5 mL of hepatitis B immune globulin (HBIG) within 12 hours of birth.
   - If mother's HBsAg status is unknown, administer HepB within 12 hours of birth. Determine the HBsAg status as soon as possible and if HBsAg-positive, administer HBIG (no later than age 1 week).
   - If mother is HBsAg-negative, the birth dose can only be delayed with physician's order and mother's negative HBsAg laboratory report documented in the infant's medical record.
   After the birth dose:
   - The HepB series should be completed with either monovalent HepB or a combination vaccine containing HepB. The second dose should be administered at age 1–2 months. The final dose should be administered at age ≥24 weeks. Infants born to HBsAg-positive mothers should be tested for HBsAg and antibody to HBsAg after completion of ≥3 doses of a licensed HepB series, at age 9–18 months (generally at the next well-child visit).
   4-month dose:
   - It is permissible to administer 4 doses of HepB when combination vaccines are administered after the birth dose. If monovalent HepB is used for doses after the birth dose, a dose at age 4 months is not needed.

2. **Rotavirus vaccine (Rota).** *(Minimum age: 6 weeks)*
   - Administer the first dose at age 6–12 weeks. Do not start the series later than age 12 weeks.
   - Administer the final dose in the series by age 32 weeks. Do not administer a dose later than age 32 weeks.
   - Data on safety and efficacy outside of these age ranges are insufficient.

3. **Diphtheria and tetanus toxoids and acellular pertussis vaccine (DTaP).** *(Minimum age: 6 weeks)*
   - The fourth dose of DTaP may be administered as early as age 12 months, provided 6 months have elapsed since the third dose.
   - Administer the final dose in the series at age 4–6 years.

4. ***Haemophilus influenzae* type b conjugate vaccine (Hib).** *(Minimum age: 6 weeks)*
   - If PRP-OMP (PedvaxHIB® or ComVax® [Merck]) is administered at ages 2 and 4 months, a dose at age 6 months is not required.
   - TriHiBit® (DTaP/Hib) combination products should not be used for primary immunization but can be used as boosters following any Hib vaccine in children aged ≥12 months.

5. **Pneumococcal vaccine.** *(Minimum age: 6 weeks for pneumococcal conjugate vaccine [PCV]; 2 years for pneumococcal polysaccharide vaccine [PPV])*
   - Administer PCV at ages 24–59 months in certain high-risk groups. Administer PPV to children aged ≥2 years in certain high-risk groups. See *MMWR* 2000;49(No. RR-9):1–35.

6. **Influenza vaccine.** *(Minimum age: 6 months for trivalent inactivated influenza vaccine [TIV]; 5 years for live, attenuated influenza vaccine [LAIV])*
   - All children aged 6–59 months and close contacts of all children aged 0–59 months are recommended to receive influenza vaccine.
   - Influenza vaccine is recommended annually for children aged ≥59 months with certain risk factors, health-care workers, and other persons (including household members) in close contact with persons in groups at high risk. See *MMWR* 2006;55(No. RR-10):1–41.
   - For healthy persons aged 5–49 years, LAIV may be used as an alternative to TIV.
   - Children receiving TIV should receive 0.25 mL if aged 6–35 months or 0.5 mL if aged ≥3 years.
   - Children aged <9 years who are receiving influenza vaccine for the first time should receive 2 doses (separated by ≥4 weeks for TIV and ≥6 weeks for LAIV).

7. **Measles, mumps, and rubella vaccine (MMR).** *(Minimum age: 12 months)*
   - Administer the second dose of MMR at age 4–6 years. MMR may be administered before age 4–6 years, provided ≥4 weeks have elapsed since the first dose and both doses are administered at age ≥12 months.

8. **Varicella vaccine.** *(Minimum age: 12 months)*
   - Administer the second dose of varicella vaccine at age 4–6 years. Varicella vaccine may be administered before age 4–6 years, provided that ≥3 months have elapsed since the first dose and both doses are administered at age ≥12 months. If second dose was administered ≥28 days following the first dose, the second dose does not need to be repeated.

9. **Hepatitis A vaccine (HepA).** *(Minimum age: 12 months)*
   - HepA is recommended for all children aged 1 year (i.e., aged 12–23 months). The 2 doses in the series should be administered at least 6 months apart.
   - Children not fully vaccinated by age 2 years can be vaccinated at subsequent visits.
   - HepA is recommended for certain other groups of children, including in areas where vaccination programs target older children. See *MMWR* 2006;55(No. RR-7):1–23.

10. **Meningococcal polysaccharide vaccine (MPSV4).** *(Minimum age: 2 years)*
    - Administer MPSV4 to children aged 2–10 years with terminal complement deficiencies or anatomic or functional asplenia and certain other high-risk groups. See *MMWR* 2005;54(No. RR-7):1–21.

The Recommended Immunization Schedules for Persons Aged 0–18 Years are approved by the Advisory Committee on Immunization Practices (http://www.cdc.gov/nip/acip), the American Academy of Pediatrics (http://www.aap.org), and the American Academy of Family Physicians (http://www.aafp.org).

SAFER • HEALTHIER • PEOPLE™

CS103164

FIGURE 8-4. ▶ Clinical preventive services for normal-risk children. *Source:* Centers for Disease Control (2007) http://www.cdc.gov/vaccines/recs/schedules/downloads/child/2007/child-schedule-color-press.pdf

Recommended Immunization Schedule for Persons Aged 7–18 Years—UNITED STATES • 2007

Vaccine ▼ / Age ▶	7–10 years	11–12 YEARS	13–14 years	15 years	16–18 years
Tetanus, Diphtheria, Pertussis[1]	see footnote 1	Tdap	Tdap		
Human Papillomavirus[2]	see footnote 2	HPV (3 doses)	HPV Series		
Meningococcal[3]	MPSV4	MCV4		MCV4[3] / MCV4	
Pneumococcal[4]		PPV			
Influenza[5]		Influenza (Yearly)			
Hepatitis A[6]		HepA Series			
Hepatitis B[7]		HepB Series			
Inactivated Poliovirus[8]		IPV Series			
Measles, Mumps, Rubella[9]		MMR Series			
Varicella[10]		Varicella Series			

Legend:
- Range of recommended ages
- Catch-up immunization
- Certain high-risk groups

This schedule indicates the recommended ages for routine administration of currently licensed childhood vaccines, as of December 1, 2006, for children aged 7–18 years. Additional information is available at **http://www.cdc.gov/nip/recs/child-schedule.htm.** Any dose not administered at the recommended age should be administered at any subsequent visit, when indicated and feasible. Additional vaccines may be licensed and recommended during the year. Licensed combination vaccines may be used whenever any components of the combination are indicated and other components of the vaccine are not contraindicated and if approved by the Food and Drug Administration for that dose of the series. Providers should consult the respective Advisory Committee on Immunization Practices statement for detailed recommendations. Clinically significant adverse events that follow immunization should be reported to the Vaccine Adverse Event Reporting System (VAERS). Guidance about how to obtain and complete a VAERS form is available at **http://www.vaers.hhs.gov** or by telephone, **800-822-7967.**

1. Tetanus and diphtheria toxoids and acellular pertussis vaccine (Tdap).
(Minimum age: 10 years for BOOSTRIX® and 11 years for ADACEL™)
- Administer at age 11–12 years for those who have completed the recommended childhood DTP/DTaP vaccination series and have not received a tetanus and diphtheria toxoids vaccine (Td) booster dose.
- Adolescents aged 13–18 years who missed the 11–12 year Td/Tdap booster dose should also receive a single dose of Tdap if they have completed the recommended childhood DTP/DTaP vaccination series.

2. Human papillomavirus vaccine (HPV). *(Minimum age: 9 years)*
- Administer the first dose of the HPV vaccine series to females at age 11–12 years.
- Administer the second dose 2 months after the first dose and the third dose 6 months after the first dose.
- Administer the HPV vaccine series to females at age 13–18 years if not previously vaccinated.

3. Meningococcal vaccine. *(Minimum age: 11 years for meningococcal conjugate vaccine [MCV4]; 2 years for meningococcal polysaccharide vaccine [MPSV4])*
- Administer MCV4 at age 11–12 years and to previously unvaccinated adolescents at high school entry (at approximately age 15 years).
- Administer MCV4 to previously unvaccinated college freshmen living in dormitories; MPSV4 is an acceptable alternative.
- Vaccination against invasive meningococcal disease is recommended for children and adolescents aged ≥2 years with terminal complement deficiencies or anatomic or functional asplenia and certain other high-risk groups. See *MMWR* 2005;54(No. RR-7):1–21. Use MPSV4 for children aged 2–10 years and MCV4 or MPSV4 for older children.

4. Pneumococcal polysaccharide vaccine (PPV). *(Minimum age: 2 years)*
- Administer for certain high-risk groups. See *MMWR* 1997;46(No. RR-8):1–24, and *MMWR* 2000;49(No. RR-9):1–35.

5. Influenza vaccine. *(Minimum age: 6 months for trivalent inactivated influenza vaccine [TIV]; 5 years for live, attenuated influenza vaccine [LAIV])*
- Influenza vaccine is recommended annually for persons with certain risk factors, health-care workers, and other persons (including household members) in close contact with persons in groups at high risk. See *MMWR* 2006;55 (No. RR-10):1–41.
- For healthy persons aged 5–49 years, LAIV may be used as an alternative to TIV.
- Children aged <9 years who are receiving influenza vaccine for the first time should receive 2 doses (separated by ≥4 weeks for TIV and ≥6 weeks for LAIV).

6. Hepatitis A vaccine (HepA). *(Minimum age: 12 months)*
- The 2 doses in the series should be administered at least 6 months apart.
- HepA is recommended for certain other groups of children, including in areas where vaccination programs target older children. See *MMWR* 2006;55 (No. RR-7):1–23.

7. Hepatitis B vaccine (HepB). *(Minimum age: birth)*
- Administer the 3-dose series to those who were not previously vaccinated.
- A 2-dose series of Recombivax HB® is licensed for children aged 11–15 years.

8. Inactivated poliovirus vaccine (IPV). *(Minimum age: 6 weeks)*
- For children who received an all-IPV or all-oral poliovirus (OPV) series, a fourth dose is not necessary if the third dose was administered at age ≥4 years.
- If both OPV and IPV were administered as part of a series, a total of 4 doses should be administered, regardless of the child's current age.

9. Measles, mumps, and rubella vaccine (MMR). *(Minimum age: 12 months)*
- If not previously vaccinated, administer 2 doses of MMR during any visit, with ≥4 weeks between the doses.

10. Varicella vaccine. *(Minimum age: 12 months)*
- Administer 2 doses of varicella vaccine to persons without evidence of immunity.
- Administer 2 doses of varicella vaccine to persons aged <13 years at least 3 months apart. Do not repeat the second dose, if administered ≥28 days after the first dose.
- Administer 2 doses of varicella vaccine to persons aged ≥13 years at least 4 weeks apart.

The Recommended Immunization Schedules for Persons Aged 0–18 Years are approved by the Advisory Committee on Immunization Practices (http://www.cdc.gov/nip/acip), the American Academy of Pediatrics (http://www.aap.org), and the American Academy of Family Physicians (http://www.aafp.org).

SAFER • HEALTHIER • PEOPLE™

CS100131

FIGURE 8-4. ▶ *Continued*

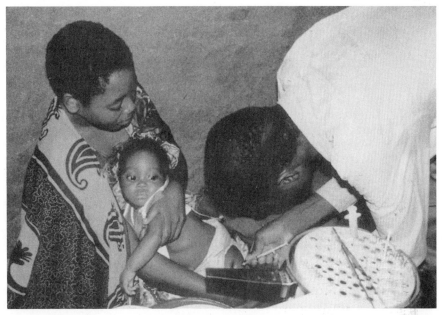

FIGURE 8-5. ▶ It is imperative that all children be immunized according to recommended standards.

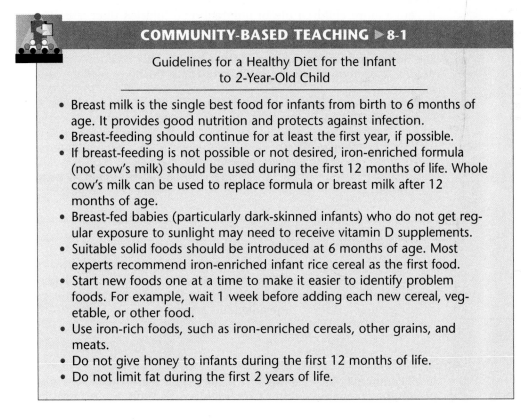

COMMUNITY-BASED TEACHING ▶ 8-1

Guidelines for a Healthy Diet for the Infant to 2-Year-Old Child

- Breast milk is the single best food for infants from birth to 6 months of age. It provides good nutrition and protects against infection.
- Breast-feeding should continue for at least the first year, if possible.
- If breast-feeding is not possible or not desired, iron-enriched formula (not cow's milk) should be used during the first 12 months of life. Whole cow's milk can be used to replace formula or breast milk after 12 months of age.
- Breast-fed babies (particularly dark-skinned infants) who do not get regular exposure to sunlight may need to receive vitamin D supplements.
- Suitable solid foods should be introduced at 6 months of age. Most experts recommend iron-enriched infant rice cereal as the first food.
- Start new foods one at a time to make it easier to identify problem foods. For example, wait 1 week before adding each new cereal, vegetable, or other food.
- Use iron-rich foods, such as iron-enriched cereals, other grains, and meats.
- Do not give honey to infants during the first 12 months of life.
- Do not limit fat during the first 2 years of life.

health, growth, immunity, and development. Breast-fed infants have decreased rates of diarrhea, respiratory infections, and ear infections (Hale, 2007). Breast-feeding has long-term benefits in that children who are ever breast fed are 15% to 25% less likely to become overweight, and those breast fed for 6 or more months are 20% to 40% less likely. Breast-feeding improves maternal health by reducing postpartum bleeding, promoting return to pre-pregnancy weight, and reducing the risks of breast cancer and osteoporosis long after the postpartum period. The American Academy of Pediatrics (AAP) considers breast-feeding to be the ideal method of feeding and nurturing infants.

As with any teaching, consider the developmental stage, cognitive abilities, and culture of the client when initiating breast-feeding teaching. Teenage mothers are more interested in knowing that breast-feeding is easy, saves time, and will enhance weight loss so they can fit into their pre-pregnancy clothes sooner. Older mothers are typically more interested in the long-term benefits to their babies. The La Leche League is a wonderful resource for information on breast-feeding (http://www.llli.org). Infant formula marketing can discourage breast-feeding, especially among low-income mothers (Arias, 2006). Infants who are breast-fed tend to gain weight more slowing compared to formula-fed infants and formula has been associated with the increase in obese infants (U.S. Babies Getting Fatter, 2006). Encouraging new mothers to breast-feed is a simple intervention that can have a strong and lasting effect on the health of the mother and baby, second only to early prenatal care.

Safety
Because more children die of unintentional injuries than any other cause, it is important to counsel parents on home safety (see Community-Based Teaching 8-2). The primary issue related to safety of the infant is sleeping positioning. Parents should put newborns to sleep on their backs. This position dramatically reduces deaths from **sudden infant death syndrome (SIDS)**, a leading cause of death in infants.

Parents should never smoke in the home if they have an infant or small child. Nor should a child or infant be in any environment where there is secondhand smoke. Secondhand smoke is known to be a risk factor for SIDS in infants, and asthma and other respiratory conditions and otitis media in infants and children. More information for parents on reducing the risk of SIDS is available from the National Institute of Child Health and Human Development at http://www.nichd.nih.gov/sids/.

PRESCHOOL-AGE CHILDREN

Healthy People 2010 objectives for child health are listed in Healthy People 2010 8-2. The leading cause of death in children ages 4 to 20 is motor vehicle traffic crashes. Among children ages 1 to 4 years, the leading injury-related causes of death are motor vehicle crashes, drowning, and fires and burns. These deaths are, for the most part, preventable.

Screening

In all community-based settings, the nurse can assist the parent in following basic prevention recommendations for children to reduce mortality and morbidity.

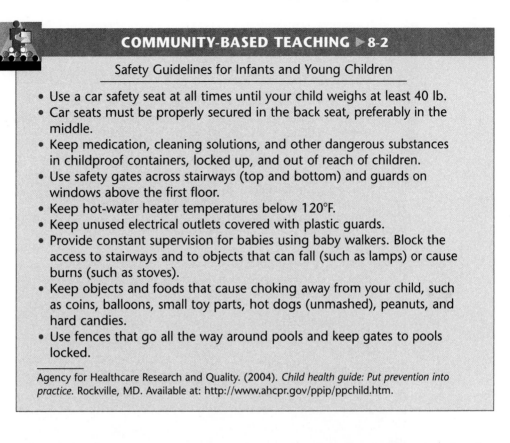

COMMUNITY-BASED TEACHING ▶ 8-2

Safety Guidelines for Infants and Young Children

- Use a car safety seat at all times until your child weighs at least 40 lb.
- Car seats must be properly secured in the back seat, preferably in the middle.
- Keep medication, cleaning solutions, and other dangerous substances in childproof containers, locked up, and out of reach of children.
- Use safety gates across stairways (top and bottom) and guards on windows above the first floor.
- Keep hot-water heater temperatures below 120°F.
- Keep unused electrical outlets covered with plastic guards.
- Provide constant supervision for babies using baby walkers. Block the access to stairways and to objects that can fall (such as lamps) or cause burns (such as stoves).
- Keep objects and foods that cause choking away from your child, such as coins, balloons, small toy parts, hot dogs (unmashed), peanuts, and hard candies.
- Use fences that go all the way around pools and keep gates to pools locked.

Agency for Healthcare Research and Quality. (2004). *Child health guide: Put prevention into practice.* Rockville, MD. Available at: http://www.ahcpr.gov/ppip/ppchild.htm.

Figure 8-4 outlines current recommendations for clinical preventive services for normal-risk children. All young children's growth should be monitored and plotted on a growth chart.

Periodic screening benefits all children. Most screening programs are developed and run by nurses in community-based settings. Preschool screening, which typically includes vision, hearing, height and weight, immunization status, and developmental screening, is an important preventive intervention. The cost of preschool screening is minimal when compared with the cost of undetected deficits that result in hardship and monetary costs to the child, parents, and society. The earlier a condition is identified, the greater the chances of lessening or eliminating the long-term effects.

The most widely used tool to assess development is the **Denver Developmental Screening Test (DDST)**. It is used to screen children from 1 month to 6 years, covering the topics of gross motor skills, fine motor skills, language development, and personal/social development. This easy-to-administer screening tool has the potential to identify developmental issues early for prompt intervention. The AAP recognized over a decade ago that screening and early identification leads to more effective therapy for children with developmental disabilities (AAP, 1995). The DDST is an excellent example of secondary prevention.

Lead Screening
Lead has been present in our environment since industrialization. Children are particularly sensitive to the toxic effects of lead. Most often, **lead poisoning** is

▶ **HEALTHY PEOPLE 2010** ▶ **8-2**

Objectives for Child Health

Reduce the rate of child deaths (ages 1–4 years).

Reduce or eliminate indigenous cases of vaccine-preventable disease.

Reduce iron deficiency among young children and females of childbearing age.

Increase the proportion of persons ages 2 years and older who consume at least two daily servings of fruit.

Increase the proportion of persons ages 2 years and older who consume at least three daily servings of vegetables.

Reduce the proportion of children and adolescents who have dental caries in their primary or permanent teeth.

Increase the proportion of children and adolescents who view television 2 hours or less per day.

Increase the proportion of the nation's public and private schools that provide access to their physical activity spaces and facilities for all persons outside of normal school hours (before and after the school day, on weekends, and during summer and other vacations).

Increase the proportion of preschool children ages 5 years and under who receive vision and hearing screening.

Sources: U.S. Department of Health and Human Services. (2000b). Maternal, infant, and child health. In *Healthy People 2010. National health promotion and disease prevention objectives*. Washington, DC: U.S. Government Printing Office.

U.S. Department of Health and Human Services. (2002). Preventing infant mortality [Fact sheet]. Retrieved January 21, 2003, from http://hhs.gov/news/pres/2002pres/infant.html

silent, with the individual having no symptoms until systemic damage has occurred. Decreased stature or growth, decreased intelligence, impaired neurobehavioral development, and adverse effects on the central nervous system, kidneys, and hematopoietic system are some of the common symptoms. Three percent of all Black children compared to 1.3% of all White children had lead blood levels above safe levels in 2005. More than half of occupied, privately owned housing built before 1980 contains lead-based paint. In general, screening and assessment for lead poisoning should focus on children younger than 24 months and should begin at 12 months because these ages are the most vulnerable (CDC, 2005a). Assessment of high-dose lead exposure should take place at birth.

Vision and Hearing Screening

Vision and hearing screening should be performed at 3 or 4 years of age and repeated once a year. Screening should be done earlier or more frequently than recommended if any of the following warning signs of visual or hearing impairment is present:

◆ Inward- or outward-turning eyes
◆ Squinting

◆ Headaches
◆ Decline in quality of schoolwork
◆ Blurred or double vision
◆ Hold objects close to eyes to see
◆ Poor response to noise or voice
◆ Hear some sounds but not others
◆ Slow language and speech development
◆ Abnormal sounding speech (Centers for Disease Control, 2006a)

Immunizations

Immunizations are important preventive health measures for the preschool child. The current recommended immunization schedule for children and adolescents is found in Figure 8-4. In 2006, the FDA licensed the first vaccine developed to prevent human papillomavirus (HPV) and cervical cancer. The Advisory Committee on Immunization Practices recommends the use of this vaccine in females ages 9 to 26 with the ideal age of administration between 11 to 12 years of age and administered before onset of sexual activity (CDC, 2006).

Nutrition

Nutritional status should be assessed. Infants and toddlers should be tested for anemia starting at 9 months of age. Hematocrit and hemoglobin screening should take place by 9 months if any of the following factors are present:

◆ Low socioeconomic status
◆ Birth weight less than 1,500 g
◆ Whole milk given before 6 months of age (not recommended)
◆ Low-iron formula given (not recommended)
◆ Low intake of iron-rich foods (not recommended)

Safety

Injury is the leading cause of death in young children. Many of the dangers for young children are in the home (see Community-Based Teaching 8-3). In most states, the law requires that infants and children be restrained in a safety seat when riding in a car, and parents who are not compliant may be fined. Table 8-2 provides information on general child seat use for infants to 12 year olds.

Other Preventive Health Measures

Child abuse is a serious concern in the United States, where more than 906,000 children are victims of abuse and neglect each year. Of these, approximately 1,500 fatalities resulted from child abuse or neglect (CDC, National Center for Injury Prevention and Control, 2006). Even when an adult's account of how a child is injured seems plausible, it is imperative that the nurse reassess the situation for possible child abuse. See Community-Based Teaching 8-4 for ways to prevent child abuse. Infants and children of all ages should be protected from the harmful effects of the sun. As the most common type of cancer in the United States, skin cancer is a significant public health issue. Anyone can get skin cancer, but individuals with

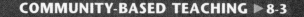

COMMUNITY-BASED TEACHING ▶ 8-3

Safety Guidelines for Parents of Children of All Ages

- Use smoke detectors in your home. Change the batteries every year and check once a month to see that they work.
- If you have a gun in your home, make sure that the gun and ammunition are locked up separately and kept out of children's reach.
- Never drive after drinking alcohol.
- Use car safety belts at all times.
- Teach your child traffic safety. Children under 9 years of age need supervision when crossing streets.
- Teach your children how and when to call 911.
- Learn basic lifesaving skills (cardiopulmonary resuscitation [CPR]).
- Post the telephone number of the poison control center near your telephone. Also, be sure to check the expiration date on the bottle of ipecac to make sure it is still good.

Agency for Healthcare Research and Quality. (2000). *Child health guide: Put prevention into practice.* Rockville, MD. Retrieved on May 18, 2003 at: http://www.ahcpr.gov/ppip/ppchild.htm

---

certain risk factors are particularly vulnerable. Some risks for skin cancer are the following (CDC, National Center for Chronic Disease Prevention and Health Promotion [NCCDPHP], 2006b):

- ◆ Lighter natural skin color
- ◆ Skin that burns, freckles, gets red easily, or becomes painful in the sun
- ◆ Blue or green eyes
- ◆ Blond or red hair
- ◆ Certain types of and a large number of moles
- ◆ Family history of skin cancer
- ◆ Personal history of skin cancer
- ◆ Exposure to the sun through work and play
- ◆ A history of sunburns early in life

Epidemiologic studies suggest that skin cancers can be prevented if children, adolescents, and adults are protected from ultraviolet (UV) radiation. At the end of the chapter in What's on the Web there is a web site where you can read more about community prevention strategies. Disease Control recommends five options for individuals and families to protect from sun exposure:

- ◆ Seek shade especially during midday
- ◆ Cover up with clothing to protect exposed skin
- ◆ Get a hat with a wide brim
- ◆ Grab shades
- ◆ Put on sunscreen

TABLE 8-2	General Child Seat Use Information		
	Buckle Everyone—Children Age 12 and Under in Back Seat!		
	Age/Weight	**Seat Type/Seat Position**	**Usage Tips**
Infants	Birth to at least 1 year and at least 20 lbs.	Infant-only seat/rear-facing or convertible seat/used rearfacing. *Seats should be secured to the vehicle by the safety belts or by the LATCH system.*	• Never use in a front seat where an air bag is present. • Tightly install child seat in rear seat, facing the rear. • Child seat should recline at approximately a 45 degree angle. • Harness straps/slots at or below shoulder level (lower set of slots for most convertible child safety seats). • Harness straps snug on child; harness clip at armpit level.
	Less than 1 year/ 20–35 lbs.	Convertible seat/used rear-facing (select one recommended for heavier infants). *Seats should be secured to the vehicle by the safety belts or by the LATCH system.*	• Never use in a front seat where an air bag is present. • Tightly install child seat in rear seat, facing the rear. • Child seat should recline at approximately a 45 degree angle. • Harness straps/slots at or below shoulder level (lower set of slots for most convertible child safety seats). • Harness straps snug on child; harness clip at armpit level.
Preschoolers/ toddler	1 to 4 years/at least 20 lbs. to approximately 40 lbs.	Convertible seat/forward-facing or forward-facing only or high back booster/harness. *Seats should be secured to the vehicle by the safety belts or by the LATCH system.*	• Tightly install child seat in rear seat, facing forward. • Harness straps/slots at or above child's shoulders (usually top set of slots for convertible child safety seats). • Harness straps snug on child; harness clip at armpit level.
Young children	4 to at least 8 years/unless they are 4'9'' (57'') tall.	Belt-positioning booster (no back, only) or high back belt-positioning booster. *NEVER use with lap-only belts—belt-positioning boosters are always used with lap AND shoulder belts.*	• Booster used with adult lap and shoulder belt in rear seat. • Shoulder belt should rest snugly across chest, rests on shoulder; and should NEVER be placed under the arm or behind the back. • Lap-belt should rest low, across the lap/upper thigh area—not across the stomach.

Source: National Highway Traffic Safety Administration (2006). Retrieved on Sept. 22, 2006, from www.nhtsa.dot.gov.

COMMUNITY-BASED TEACHING ▶ 8-4

Child Maltreatment Prevention Strategies

For Parents

- One key way to prevent child maltreatment is for nurses to assist parents to develop nurturing parenting skills and build positive relationships with their children. Through health teaching, modeling, and counseling the nurse can encourage nurturing parental behaviors such as:
  - Giving physical signs of affection such as hugs
  - Developing self-esteem in their children
  - Recognizing and understanding their children's feelings
  - Engaging in empathetic communication with their children
  - Learning alternative methods to shaking, hitting, or spanking
- Notify the parent that if they are afraid they might harm their child, to get help by calling someone and asking for help. Suggest talking with a friend or relative, other parents, clergy, or health care providers. Encourage parents to take time for themselves. The National Child Abuse Hotline number is (800) 422–4453.

For Communities

To help prevent child maltreatment, community resources and services to support families should be available and accessible. This can be accomplished by the nurse:

- Encouraging volunteer efforts at organizations that provide family support services.
- Collaborating with or sponsoring organizations such as sports teams and local businesses to communicate prevention messages.
- Community organizing by working with prevention organizations and local media to develop community strategies that support parents and prevent abuse.
- Health education to teach children, parents, and educators preventions strategies that can help keep children safe.
- Participate in policy development by engaging local legislators in increasing child maltreatment prevention efforts.

Adapted from: Centers for Disease Control and Prevention. National Center for Injury Prevention and Control. (2006a). *Child maltreatment: Prevention strategies.* Retrieved on September 22, 2006, from http://www.cdc.gov/ncipc/factsheets/cmprevention.htm

Poor nutrition and dental hygiene contribute to dental caries. Dental caries represent the single most common chronic disease of childhood, occurring five times as frequently as asthma, the second most common chronic condition among children. Unless identified and addressed early, caries are irreversible. Less than 19% of all children receive sealant to prevent caries. Poor children have nearly 12 times more restricted activity days because of dental-related illness than children from higher-income families. Pain and suffering due to untreated tooth decay can lead to difficulties eating, speaking, and attending to learning (CDC, 2006c).

Asthma is the second most common chronic condition in children, affecting 12% of children ages 0 to 17. In the last 20 years the prevalence of asthma in children has increased by over 75%. In 1 year, asthma accounts for 12.7 million physician visits, 1.9 million emergency department visits, and almost 500,000 hospitalizations (Krisberg, 2006). Both the immediate environment and the quality of the air in the home contribute to children developing asthma. In many sections of the United States, poor air quality and air pollution endanger the respiratory health of children and exacerbate symptoms in children who have asthma. Because respiratory diseases send more American children to the hospital than any other illness there is ample opportunity for disease prevention and health promotion (Respiratory diseases, 2006). Nurses play a vital role in assisting children and parents in managing the symptoms of asthma.

Handwashing is a simple and effective disease-prevention measure (Fig. 8-6). It is important to teach children handwashing skills. To explore different curriculum for teaching children about how, when, and why to wash hands see Web sites listed in What's on the Web at the end of the chapter.

As with all assessments, the effectiveness lies in the strength of the questions asked. There are many resources that include general interview and developmental surveillance questions for children of all ages and their parents at http://www.brightfutures.org/.

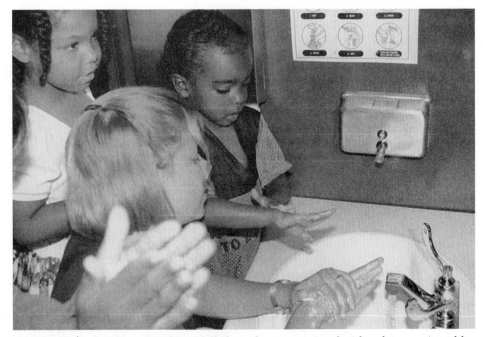

FIGURE 8-6. ▶ Good handwashing skills have been associated with a decrease in colds and influenza.

SCHOOL-AGE CHILDREN

The leading cause of death for all children between ages 5 and 14 years is motor vehicle accidents. Factors that contribute to these fatalities include drunk drivers and unrestrained children. Pedestrian deaths account for 25% of all motor vehicle-related deaths sustained by children (CDC, 2005).

Middle childhood is when the foundations of a healthy lifestyle are formed and when health promotion programs are likely to have the greatest impact. Healthy People 2010 8-3 presents Healthy People 2010 objectives for middle childhood.

HEALTHY PEOPLE 2010 ▶ 8-3

Objectives for School-Age Children and Adolescents

Reduce the rate of child (ages 5–9 years), adolescent, and young adult deaths.

Reduce coronary heart disease deaths.

Reduce or eliminate indigenous cases of vaccine-preventable disease.

Reduce the suicide rate.

Reduce iron deficiency among young children and females of childbearing age.

Reduce the proportion of children and adolescents who are overweight or obese.

Increase the proportion of persons ages 2 years and older who consume at least two daily servings of fruit.

Increase the proportion of persons ages 2 years and older who consume at least three daily servings of vegetables.

Reduce the proportion of children and adolescents who have had dental caries in their primary or permanent teeth.

Increase the proportion of adolescents who engage in moderate physical activity for at least 30 minutes on 5 or more of the previous 7 days.

Increase the proportion of adolescents who engage in vigorous physical activity that promotes cardiorespiratory fitness 3 or more days per week for 20 or more minutes per occasion.

Increase the proportion of children and adolescents who view television 2 hours or less per day.

Increase the proportion of the nation's public and private schools that provide access to their physical activity spaces and facilities for all persons outside of normal school hours (before and after the school day, on weekends, and during summer and other vacations).

Reduce the proportion of adolescents and young adults with *Chlamydia trachomatis* infections.

Reduce tobacco use by adolescents.

U.S. Department of Health and Human Services. (2000b). Maternal, infant, and child health. In *Healthy People 2010. National health promotion and disease prevention objectives.* Washington, DC: U.S. Government Printing Office.

Screening

The growth rate of children slows somewhat in the middle childhood years. Children's readiness for school depends on their experiences in the first 5 years of life. Nurses should assess the achievement of the child and provide guidance to the family on anticipated tasks. See the Bright Futures Web site for information on developmental tasks.

At age 5, screening should include vision and hearing, blood pressure, risk for lead exposure (with blood draw if deemed necessary), blood cholesterol, and developmental screening. Weight and height should also be assessed.

Safety

The most important topic to cover with all families with children is safety, and the one intervention that prevents the most loss of life and injury is using appropriate restraints when riding in an automobile. In 2004, about 28% of all children ages 4 to 7 and 39% of those ages 8 to 14 killed in motor vehicle crashes were unrestrained (National Center for Statistics and Analysis, 2005).

Seatbelt laws vary from state to state. In some states, children are required to be in a booster seat until they are over 70 lb., while other states require them to ride in a booster seat until they are 80 lb. Contact your jurisdiction's department of motor vehicles for the seatbelt law in your state. At this time, air bags are not safe for children younger than 13 years and can cause fatalities. Until passenger vehicles are equipped with air bags that are safe and effective for children, those younger than 13 years should not ride in a front passenger seat that is equipped with an air bag (National Highway Transportation Safety Association, 2006).

Another important safety intervention is the use of a bike helmet. Bicycling is a popular activity in the United States. About half a million people are injured in bike mishaps each year. Of these injuries, head injury is the most common cause of death and serious disability. The use of a bike helmet is effective in preventing head injury. Community programs to increase bike helmet use can reduce the incidence of head injury among bicycle riders.

Prevention of Chronic Conditions

There is significant data that many children in the United States are not adopting healthy lifestyle behavior, as obesity rates have doubled among children and teens since 1980. Among children and adolescents, annual hospital costs related to obesity were four times as much in the early 2000s as in the early 1980s. Because there is a strong relationship between obesity in childhood and the development of chronic illness in adulthood, there are numerous initiatives to prevent obesity in childhood. These initiatives for children focus on increasing physical activity, increasing daily intake of fruits and vegetables, and reducing fat intake, and ensuring that children get adequate sleep every night. As the child enters middle childhood, even more emphasis should be placed on secondary prevention, which allows early intervention for health conditions that may develop into chronic conditions in adulthood. The primary contributors to chronic conditions that can be addressed are weight, nutrition, and physical activity level.

Nutrition and Weight

Overweight and obesity are increasing among children and adolescents in the United States. The rate of overweight among children ages 6 to 17 years has more than doubled in the past 30 years, with most of the increase since the late 1970s. Eighteen percent of those between 6 and 17 are seriously overweight (National Center for Health Statistics, 2007). Obesity puts individuals at risk for elevated blood cholesterol and high blood pressure, which are in turn associated with heart disease and stroke, two leading causes of death in adulthood. Being overweight in childhood and adolescence has been associated with increased adult morbidity. Disease prevention and health promotion activities that decrease the incidence of obesity are directed at improving nutrition and increasing physical activity levels. Inadequate sleep is also associated with being overweight. Suggested number of hours of sleep for various age groups are seen in Table 8-3.

Reviewing basic information about the recommended intake by food groups with parent and child is an important intervention in helping families improve their nutrition and avoid overweight and obesity. Because children cannot change their exercise and eating habits by themselves, they need the help and support of their families. There is an excellent program that you can access on the internet and use to assist families to revise their eating and activity habit to facilitate weight loss. A Web site listed at the end of this chapter that may be helpful to use with families is Childhood Obesity at http://www.ahcpr.gov/child/dvdobesity.htm.

Physical Activity

Many states have eliminated physical education programs and after-school sports programs. Physical education programs are determined by state, but only one state follows the American Heart Association recommendation of daily physical education from kindergarten through 12th grade. These changes have had an impact on the daily reported activity of children. Further, children participate in more sedentary activities after school, such as watching television and playing computer games, than children did 10 years ago. Healthy People 2010 recommends children watch less than 2 hours of television a day.

TABLE 8-3	How Much Sleep Is Enough for My Child?
Age	**Suggested Number of Hours per Night**
Newborn	Generally sleep or drowse for 16 to 20 hours a day, divided about equally between night and day. Longest sleep is generally about 4–5 hours.
6–12 months	May nap about 3 hours during the day and sleep about 11 hours at night.
1 to 3 years	Most toddlers sleep about 10 to 13 hours.
Preschoolers	Most sleep about 10 to 12 hours a night. If they are not napping during the day they may benefit from quiet time.
School-age children	Most children 6–9 need 10 hours of sleep a night.
	Most children 10-12 need a little over 9 hours a night.
Teens	Adolescents need about 8 to 9.5 hours of sleep per night (note they need more sleep as compared to 10 to 12 years olds).

Adapted from: KidsHealth. How much sleep is enough for my child? Retrieved on September 23, 2006, from http://www.kidshealth.org/PageManager.jsp?dn=KidsHealth&lic=1&ps=107&cat_id=190&article_set=10233.

Discussing the need for daily physical activity is an important strategy for nurses in community-based settings. Children should be encouraged to participate in activities that provide an aerobic component, such as riding bikes every day (wearing a helmet, of course), walking instead of riding in a car from place to place, and playing outside everyday. Swimming, playing organized or unorganized sports, or doing physical activities as a family are other ways to increase a child's activity level.

Pointing out the benefits of exercise may also help parents encourage children to be more physically active. Helping parents understand the relationship between activity and normal weight, future health, and the threat of developing chronic disease are a few of the strategies the nurse can use to help parents understand the importance of structuring family life and the child's life to include physical activity. There is an excellent Web site (listed at the end of the chapter) related to physical activity called Fitness for Kids: Getting your children off the couch. It can be found at http://www.mayoclinic.com/health/fitness/fl00030.

ADOLESCENCE

Adolescence is one of the most dynamic stages of human development. It is accompanied by dramatic physical, cognitive, social, and emotional changes that present both opportunities and challenges for the adolescent, the family, and the broader community. Nurses must be sensitive to the dynamic nature of this stage as well as the increasing need for independence balanced with dependence. Further, as adolescents progress through the teen years, they become increasingly able to make their own health care decisions, and they want to make these choices.

Almost half of all deaths among adolescents age 16 to 20 are from unintentional injuries. The majority (78%) of the total mortality in this age group can be attributed to preventable causes.

Teens are far less likely to use seatbelts than any other age group (National Center for Statistics and Analysis, 2006). Alcohol is involved in about 25% of adolescent fatalities and 50% of all adolescent drowning (National Center for Injury Prevention and Control [NCIP], 2006). Suicide is the third leading cause of death among those aged 15 to 24. As with the 15- to 19-year-old group, 76% of the deaths in this age group can be attributed to preventable causes (NCIPC, 2006). At this time, most of the new human immunodeficiency virus (HIV) infections occur each year among those between ages 13 and 21 years.

The latest National Youth Risk Behavior Survey reported that high school students responded that 84% rode bicycles without a helmet, 18% carried a weapon, and 17% had attempted suicide in the 12 months preceding the survey. Twenty-three percent smoked cigarettes, 43% had at least one drink of alcohol, and 25% had 5 or more drinks of alcohol on at least one occasion during the 30 days preceding the survey (MMWR, 2006).

The survey reported that of the 47% of teens who had had sexual intercourse during their lifetime, 62% used a condom during the last intercourse. As far as dietary behaviors, 16% were overweight, 79% ate five or more servings of fruits and vegetables during the 7 days preceding the survey, and 4.5% took laxatives or vomited to lose weight during the 30 days preceding the survey. As far as physical activity, 68% did vigorous physical activity for at least 20 minutes on 3 or more of the 7 days preceding the survey, and 54% were enrolled in physical education class with 33% attending physical education class daily.

When results from 2005 are compared with results from 1999, 1995, and 1991 surveys, although the percentage of students who appear to be getting the message to buckle up has increased; those who *never* buckle up decreased from 29% to 18%. The percentage of students who report current alcohol use has declined dramatically from 51% in 1991 to 43% in 2005. In 1991, 54% of youth responded ever having intercourse compared to 47% in 2005. In addition, 62% of sexually active students used a condom during last sexual intercourse compared to 46% in 1991. These changes are encouraging as they show that persistent efforts to get young people to adopt healthier behaviors can achieve positive results (CDC, 2006b).

When different ethnic groups are compared, Black students, when compared to White and Hispanic high school students are least likely to use tobacco, alcohol, cocaine, and other drugs but most likely to report sexual risk behaviors and sedentary behaviors. White students are the least likely to report physical fighting, sexual risk behaviors, and being overweight but more likely to smoke cigarettes and binge drink. Hispanic students are more likely than other students to report attempted suicide and use drugs like cocaine, heroin, and methamphetamines (CDC, 2006b).

Healthy People 2010 objectives for school-age children and adolescents are shown in Healthy People 2010 8-3.

Screening

Recommendations for screening in early and later adolescence are found in the Bright Futures guidelines. Some other areas for screening adolescent clients include questions concerning smoking, alcohol and drug use, sexual activity, and injury prevention behaviors. Teens' behaviors often place them at risk for serious injury, sexually transmitted diseases (STDs), and chronic diseases. Bright Futures provides excellent developmental surveillance questions that address these issues. It is also important to keep developmental tasks in mind when assessing health issues and planning health promotion and disease prevention activities.

Because such a large proportion of deaths in this age group are preventable, safety should be the number one priority for health promotion and injury prevention. However, because of the nature of the adolescent client, this is a formidable challenge.

Prevention of Chronic Conditions

Smoking Cessation
Several excellent resources on the Internet address smoking cessation. Some are very colorful, specifically designed by teens for teens. One site is http://www.cdc.gov/tobacco/tips4youth.htm. Others are found at the end of the chapter.

See Community-Based Teaching 8-5 for community-based teaching strategies for adolescents who want to know more about the dangers of tobacco.

Nutrition
Teaching teens about nutrition is challenging (Fig. 8-7). Bright Futures in Practice: Nutrition is an excellent resource for nutrition information for infancy through adolescence. This resource is available through http://www.brightfutures.org/.

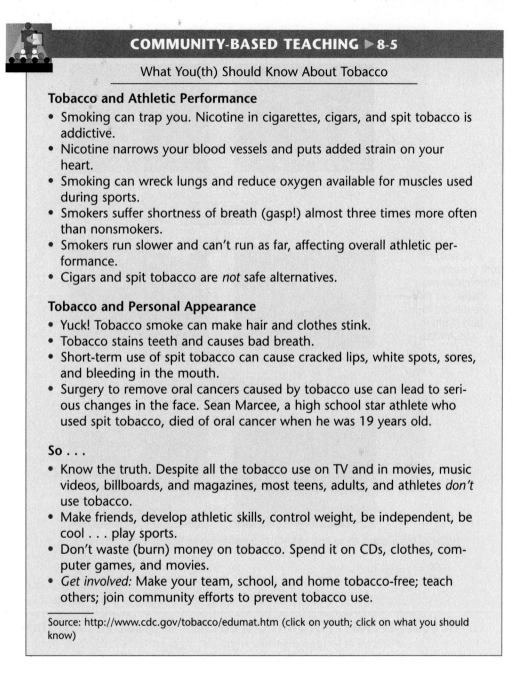

COMMUNITY-BASED TEACHING ▶ 8-5

What You(th) Should Know About Tobacco

Tobacco and Athletic Performance

- Smoking can trap you. Nicotine in cigarettes, cigars, and spit tobacco is addictive.
- Nicotine narrows your blood vessels and puts added strain on your heart.
- Smoking can wreck lungs and reduce oxygen available for muscles used during sports.
- Smokers suffer shortness of breath (gasp!) almost three times more often than nonsmokers.
- Smokers run slower and can't run as far, affecting overall athletic performance.
- Cigars and spit tobacco are *not* safe alternatives.

Tobacco and Personal Appearance

- Yuck! Tobacco smoke can make hair and clothes stink.
- Tobacco stains teeth and causes bad breath.
- Short-term use of spit tobacco can cause cracked lips, white spots, sores, and bleeding in the mouth.
- Surgery to remove oral cancers caused by tobacco use can lead to serious changes in the face. Sean Marcee, a high school star athlete who used spit tobacco, died of oral cancer when he was 19 years old.

So . . .

- Know the truth. Despite all the tobacco use on TV and in movies, music videos, billboards, and magazines, most teens, adults, and athletes *don't* use tobacco.
- Make friends, develop athletic skills, control weight, be independent, be cool . . . play sports.
- Don't waste (burn) money on tobacco. Spend it on CDs, clothes, computer games, and movies.
- *Get involved:* Make your team, school, and home tobacco-free; teach others; join community efforts to prevent tobacco use.

Source: http://www.cdc.gov/tobacco/edumat.htm (click on youth; click on what you should know)

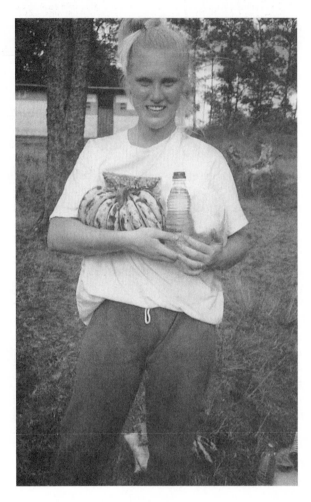

FIGURE 8-7. ▶ Suggestions for teaching adolescents about nutrition include instilling a sense of pride in identifying and choosing healthy meals and snacks.

Physical Activity

Nearly half of American youths ages 12 to 21 years are not vigorously active on a regular basis. Adolescents and young adults benefit from physical activity, particularly considering 14% of all adolescents are overweight. Moderate amounts of daily physical activity are recommended for people of all ages. This amount can be obtained in longer sessions of moderately intense activities, such as brisk walking for 30 minutes, or in shorter sessions of more intense activities, such as jogging or playing soccer or basketball for 15 to 20 minutes. Physical activity helps build and maintain healthy bones, muscles, and joints; controls weight; builds lean muscle; and reduces fat. Most importantly, physical activity prevents or delays the development of high blood pressure, helps reduce blood pressure in some adolescents with hypertension, and prevents the development of type 2 diabetes. Again there are resources for health education of parents and teens on the Bright Futures Web site.

Health Promotion

Sexual Health Promotion

The incidence of STDs has skyrocketed, and most new HIV infections occur in people between 13 and 21 years of age. Teens exhibit high behavioral risks for acquiring most STDs. Teenagers and young adults are more likely than other age groups to have multiple sex partners, to engage in unprotected sex, and (for young women) to choose sexual partners older than themselves. As part of holistic care, nurses in community-based settings should always assess sexuality. When discussing the topic of sexuality, take an open, frank, direct, and nonjudgmental approach. Talking openly and frankly with young teens about the benefits and risks of being sexually active may allow teens, especially girls, to understand that being sexually active is a choice. Early age of first coitus is a well-established risk factor for STDs because there is greater opportunity for exposure to pathogens. Early coitus is also associated with later high-risk cognitive, affective, and behavioral choices. Opportunities to interact with caring adults outside of their families, self-esteem building, and empowerment activities contribute to delay of first intercourse.

Other primary prevention strategies to promote sexual health include comprehensive sex education beginning in primary school. Abstinence is a highly positive choice for both sexes until they are ready to deal with the responsibility of being sexually active. However, it is not realistic as a sole strategy. The emphasis must be that sexual health promotion is for life and that contraception is useless if not practiced consistently. Use of condoms should be emphasized.

Some sexuality health promotion programs use a more dramatic approach, with speakers who are HIV-positive or have acquired immunodeficiency syndrome (AIDS). These speakers tell their stories to teen groups, often with great success. Nurses can develop audiovisual aids (e.g., diagrams, pictures, computer-assisted instruction, PowerPoint presentations, and videos) to make sex education unforgettable. Nurses can explore with teens the differences between the facts of physiology and untrue but fervently held beliefs. Helping teens understand the relationship between substance abuse and STDs is another important issue to address. Peer education is a program model that is highly successful and inexpensive to implement.

Nurses can play a critical role in the improvement of sexual health counseling by using a direct and frank approach in interactions with individual teens, parents, groups, and peers. Nurses in community-based settings can have enormous impact on sexual health promotion by acting as a positive role model for sexual health and being involved in issues related to sexual health.

Suicide and Violence Prevention

Suicide is a complex problem that can, in some cases, be prevented by early recognition and treatment of mental disorders. Most people who kill themselves have mental or substance abuse disorders. Thus, early identification and treatment of these disorders is paramount in the prevention of suicide.

Violence is a critical public health issue in the United States. In 2004, homicide was the fifth leading cause of death for children ages 10 to 14, and the second leading cause of death for youth 15 to 24. Violence among adolescents is a critical public health issue in the United States.

Health Promotion and Disease Prevention Activities With Teens

When teaching teens about health, it is particularly important to base the teaching on what the teen already knows about the subject. It is also helpful to determine what the teen wants to learn about and begin with these topics. Cognitively, many teens are not able to conceptualize or hypothesize. This, coupled with the fact that teens tend to be egocentric, complicates determining the best teaching modalities to reach the teen population. Successful disease prevention and health promotion activities for teens incorporate these considerations. Thus, it is most effective when teaching teens about physical activity or nutrition to talk about the immediate, particular, personal impacts in areas of importance to them.

For instance, a teenage girl who is overweight may respond to information on nutrition with the incentive of losing weight so she can wear the latest clothing styles. A boy may respond to the suggestion to increase physical activity in his daily life if the nurse talks about the benefits of belonging to a team or being a sports hero. When taught about smoking cessation, teens respond to the idea that if they smoke, they are less desirable to kiss, or that their hands, clothes, and hair will smell, but not to the notion that smoking increases the chances of developing lung cancer when they are older adults. Nor do teens respond to the idea that if they are not physically fit and well nourished there is an increased chance that they will develop heart disease, diabetes, stroke, and cancer. Most teens are developmentally unable to value such notions.

CONCLUSIONS

The primary issues involved in health promotion and disease prevention, based on Healthy People 2010, have been discussed from infancy through adolescence. Providing early prenatal care would eliminate many health conditions for newborn babies, save precious health care dollars, and improve the quality of life for countless infants. During infancy and childhood, periodic screening allows for early identification and intervention of common and preventable conditions. Helping young children and teens value and adopt healthy lifestyle choices by improving nutrition, increasing physical activity, and following basic safety recommendations is an important contribution nurses in community-based settings can make. Advocating and participating in activities related to these issues in their own communities is another way nurses can contribute to the health of children. Lastly, being vocal and involved in public policy issues such as gun control and allocation of health care dollars for public health, as well as supporting political candidates who value public health, are all ways that nurses can improve the health of the nation's children.

What's on the Web

American Social Health Association (ASHA)
P.O. Box 13827
Research Triangle Park, NC 27709
Internet address:
http://www.iwannaknow.org
This site is a part of the American Social Health Association. It is designed for teens and provides answers to questions about teen sexual health and STDs. Many resources are available on this site.

Body Mass Index: About BMI for Children and Teens
Internet Address:
http://www.cdc.gov/nccdphp/dnpa/bmi/childrens_BMI/about_childrens_BMI.htm
This site (from the CDC) describes the concept of BMI and how it can be used with children and teens. It is a very helpful resource when intervening with overweight and obese children and teens.

Bright Futures
Internet address:
http://www.brightfutures.org
This Web site provides information about preventive and health promotion needs of infants, children, adolescents, families, and communities. A number of publications, including handouts in Spanish, can be downloaded or ordered through the site. The Family Tip Sheets are an excellent resource when working with families with children and adolescents (found at http://www.brightfutures.org/TipSheets/). These materials are written in family–friendly language and may be used by families and children as well as professionals in a range of disciplines including health, education, and child care. The companion Referral Tool and Locating Community-Based Services for Children and Families are tailored to help providers and families connect with the service they need.

CDC Growth Charts
Internet address:
http://www.cdc.gov/growthcharts/
This site includes growth charts as well as educational materials to prepare professionals to use and interpret the growth charts. The World Health Organization (WHO) child growth standards are also on this site.

CDC Tobacco Information and Prevention Source
Internet address:
http://www.cdc.gov/tobacco/edumat.htm
OR
http://www.cdc.gov/prc/tested-interventions/adoptable-interventions/not-on-tobacco-smoking-cessation.htm
These pages have numerous resources listed for various audiences. For Teens look under the section for Parents, Educators, and Youth Group Leaders for health teaching resources to be used with individuals, families, and groups.

Child Health Guide: Put Prevention into Practice
Internet address:
http://www.ahrq.gov/ppip/childguide/child guide.pdf

The Child Health Guide: Put Prevention into Practice (Agency for Healthcare Research and Quality, 2004) is an excellent tool for monitoring infant and child health. It is available online, or request a copy via e-mail at ahrqpubs@ahrq.gov or a free copy can be ordered by calling (800) 358–9295. The guide is also available in Spanish.

Childhood Obesity
Internet address:
http://www.ahcpr.gov/child/dvdobesity.htm
This site describes a free interactive DVD; one developed for children and families and one for clinicians to prevent and treat childhood obesity and overweight.

Childhood Obesity: Make Weight Loss a Family Affair
Internet address:
http://www.mayoclinic.com/print/childhood-obesity/FL00058
This site has many tips about weight loss for children and teens and ways to change family behaviors to adopt healthier eating. There are also numerous tools that children and family can use to facilitate weight loss.

Children's Resources/Health and Human Services for Kids
Internet address: http://www.hhs.gov/kids/
This is the first site to check out when looking for health teaching materials or Web sites to use with any age child. There are numerous materials for health professionals and educators to use on an exhaustive list of health topics.

Community Preventive Services
Internet address:
http://www.thecommunityguide.org/index.html
This site is helpful for identifying and planning programs and interventions to improve the health of your community. There is also a section for public health professionals.

Healthfinder
Internet address:
http://www.healthfinder.gov

Healthfinder is a search engine for consumer health education material, maintained by the U.S. Department of Health and Human Services. Resources for many of the topics covered in the chapter can be found on this site.

Handwashing
Healthy Child Care
Internet address:
http://www.healthychild.net
The Medicine Chest on this site has a section on teaching children of all ages the benefits of regular hand washing. Some of the different programs are summarized and there is a list of additional internet resources at the end of the site.

Healthy People 2010
Internet address:
http://www.health.gov/healthypeople
This document outlines the nationwide health promotion and disease prevention initiative designed to improve health for all people in the United States.

Fitness for Kids: Getting your children off the couch
Internet address:
http://www.mayoclinic.com/health/fitness/fl00030
Children love to play and be physically active but without encouragement, they may opt to sit around. This Web site gives parents tips how to help kids stay active.

La Leche League
1400 North Meacham Road
Schaumburg, IL 60173-4808
Telephone: (847) 519-7730
Internet address:http://www.llli.org
This Web site provides information on breast-feeding, online discussion groups, and listings of local groups.

Media Smart Youth
Internet address:
http://www.nichd.nih.gov/msy/
This is an interactive after-school program for children ages 11 to 13. it is designed to teach them about the relationship between the media and health especially in the areas of nutrition and physical activity.

National Asthma Control Program
Internet address:
http://www.cdc.gov/asthma/interventions/children.htm
Asthma is a serious and growing health problem, with the asthma rate rising more rapidly in preschool-age children than in any other group. Client education is imperative for effective management of asthma. This is one of many Web sites offering health education about asthma. On the last page of this Web site you will find a comprehensive list of organizations offering information on pediatric asthma as well as best practice programs. If you find that there is a need for an asthma education program in your community this is the Web site for you. Also check out http://www.cdc.gov/asthma/basics.htm for slides and materials to use with parents.

National Immunization Program
Internet address:
http://www.cdc.gov/nip/publications/
Parents often have questions about vaccinations. Unfortunately, information is sometimes published that is inaccurate or can be misleading when taken out of context. This site helps provide accurate information about immunizations.

National Institute of Child Health and Human Development
Internet address:
http://www.nichd.nih.gov
This site is an excellent resource for health education information for nurses to use with parents and families. It includes research about the health status of children.

Tips4Youth Web page
Internet address:
http://www.cdc.gov/tobacco/tips4youth.htm
This page compiles sites listing smoking cessation programs geared toward children and teens.

The Women, Infants, and Children (WIC) Program
Internet address:
http://www.fns.usda.gov/wic/
The WIC Program saves lives and improves the health of nutritional at-risk

women, infants, and children. Numerous studies prove that the WIC Program is one of the nation's most successful and cost-effective nutrition intervention programs. Since its beginning in 1974, the WIC Program has earned the reputation of being one of the most successful federally funded nutrition programs in the United States. All nurses working in community-based settings benefit from knowing about the WIC Program and sharing that information with the clients they serve.

References and Bibliography

_____ (2006). U.S. Babies Getting Fatter. Health Day. Retrieved on September 22, 2006, from http://www.nlm.nih.gov/melineplus/print/news/fullstory_37151.html

Agency for Healthcare Research and Quality. (2004). *Child health guide: Put prevention into practice.* Rockville, MD. Retrieved on September 20, 2006, from http://www.ahrq.gov/ppip/childguide/childguide.pdf

American Academy of Pediatrics, Committee on Practice and Ambulatory Medicine. (1995). Recommendations for pediatric health care. *Pediatrics, 96*(2 Pt 1), 373–374.

American College of Obstetricians and Gynecologists. (2006). *Drinking and reproductive health: A fetal alcohol spectrum disorders prevention tool kit.* Retrieved on April 11, 2007, from http://www.acog.org/departments/healthIssues/FASDToolKit.pdf

Arias, D. (2006). Infant formula marketing can discourage U.S. breastfeeding: Low income moms are at higher risk. *The Nation's Health, 36*(3).

Centers for Disease Control and Prevention. (2006). *HPV and HPV vaccine: Information for healthcare providers.* Retrieved on April 14, 2007, from http://www.cdc.gov/std/hpv/STDFact-HPV-vaccine-hcp.htm

Centers for Disease Control and Prevention. (2006). Youth risk behavior surveillance—United States, 2005. *MMWR, 55*(No. SS-5). Retrieved on September 24, 2006, from http://www.cdc.gov/mmwr/PDF/SS/SS5505.pdf

Centers for Disease Control and Prevention. Chronic Disease Prevention. (2006a). Preventing chronic diseases: Investing wisely in health. Preventing smoking during pregnancy. Retrieved on September 20, 2006, from http://www.cdc.gov/nccdphp/publications/factsheets/Prevention/pdf/smoking.pdf

Centers for Disease Control and Prevention. Chronic Disease Prevention and Health Promotion. (2006b). The health consequences of smoking on pregnancy. Retrieved on September 26, 2007, from http://www.cdc.gov/tobacco/health_effects/pregnancy.htm

Centers for Disease Control and Prevention. Chronic Disease Prevention (2006c). Preventing dental caries. Retrieved on September 23, 2006, from http://www.cdc.gov/nccdphp/publications/factsheets/Prevention/oh.htm

Centers for Disease Control and Prevention. National Center on Birth Defects and Developmental Disabilities. (2006a). *Learn the signs. Act early. Vision loss fact sheet.* Retrieved on September 22, 2006, from http://www.cdc.gov/ncbddd/autism/Actearly/vision_loss.html

Centers for Disease Control and Prevention. National Center for Chronic Disease Prevention and Health Promotion, Division of Cancer Prevention and Control. (2006b). 2006 Fact Sheet: Skin cancer primary prevention and education initiatives. Retrieved September 23, 2006, from http://www.cdc.gov/cancer/nscpep/about2004.htm

Centers for Disease Control and Prevention. National Center for Environmental Health. (2005a). Childhood lead poisoning fact sheet. Retrieved on September 21, 2006, from http://www.cdc.gov/nceh/publications/factsheets/ChildhoodLeadPoisoning.pdf

Centers for Disease Control and Prevention. National Center for Injury Prevention and Control. (2005). Injury Center. *International Walk to School Week.* Retrieved on September 23, 2006, from http://www.cdc.gov/ncipc/duip/spotlite/walk_to_school.htm

Centers for Disease Control and Prevention. National Center for Injury Prevention and Control. (2006). *Child maltreatment: Prevention strategies.* Retrieved on September 22, 2006, from http://www.cdc.gov/ncipc/factsheets/cmprevention.htm

Centers for Disease Control and Prevention. National Center for Injury Prevention and

Control. (2006b). Media Relations. *Fewer high school students engage in health risk behaviors; racial and ethnic differences persist.* Retrieved on September 24, 2006, from http://www.cdc.gov/od/oc/Media/pressrel/r060608.htm

Cole, F. S. (2006). Preventing and managing premature births: Toward a national policy. *Medscape Public Health and Prevention, 4*(1). Retrieved on September 19, 2006, from http://www.medscape.com/viewarticle/533712

Dawley, K., & Beam, R. (2005). "My nurse taught me how to have a healthy baby and be a good mother;" Nurse home visiting with pregnant women 1888 to 2005. *Nursing Clinics of North America, 40*(4), 803–815.

Equal Opportunities. (2006). American Public Health Association. Retrieved on September 25, 2006, from http://www.apha.org/nphw/2006/pg_kickoff_tuesday.htm

Federal Drug Administration. (1999). How folate can help prevent birth defects. Retrieved on April 14, 2007, from http://www.cfsan.fda.gov/~dms/fdafolic.html

Federal Interagency Forum on Child and Family Statistics, 2005. (2005). *America's children: Key national indicators of well-being, 2002.* Washington, DC: U.S. Government Printing Office.

Fox, M. (2006). *Preterm births have risen in the US, but fewer newborns die.* Reuters. Retrieved on September 19, 2006, from http://www.medscape.com/viewarticle/540903_print.

Groner, J., French, G., Ahijevych, K., & Wewers, M. E. (2005). Process evaluation of a nurse-delivered smoking relapse prevention program for new mothers. *Journal of Community Health Nursing, 22*(3), 157–167.

Hale, R. (2007). Infant nutrition and the benefits of breastfeeding. *British Journal of Midwifery, 15*(6): 368–371.

Huggins, C., (2006). Early screening spots vision problems in infants. Retrieved on September 20, 2006, from http://www.hlm.nih.gov/medlineplus/news/fullstory_35187.html

Institute of Medicine. (2006). Preterm birth: Causes, consequences, and prevention. Report Brief. Retrieved on September 19, 2006, from http://www.iom.edu/CMS/3740/25471/35813/35975.aspx

Kids Count Data Book. (2006). Annie E. Casey Foundation: Baltimore, MD.

Kitzman, H., Olds, D. L., Sidora, K., et al. (2000). Enduring effects of nurse home visitation on maternal life course: A 3-year follow-up of a randomized trial. *JAMA, 283*(15), 1983–1989.

Kochanek, K. D., & Martin, J. A. (2005). National Center for Health Statistics. *Supplemental analyses of recent trends in infant mortality.* Retrieved on September 18, 2006, from http://www.cdc.gov/nchs/products/pubs/pubd/hestats/infantmort/infantmort.htm

Krisberg, K. (2006). Poor air quality, pollution endangers health of children. *The Nation's Health, 36*(2). Retrieved on September 25, 2006, from http://www.mescape.com/viewarticle/523845_print

10MMWR Weekly Report. (2005). Youth Risk Behavior Surveillance Volume 55, Number SS5. Retrieved on October 30, 2007, from http://www.cdc.gov/mmwr/PDF/ss/ss5505.pdf. Also available at http://www.cdc.gov/mmwr/mmwr/ss.html? or http://www.cdc.gov/mmwr/preview/mmwrhtml/ss5505al.htm?s_cid=ss5505al_e

Maternal and Child Health Bureau [MCHB]. (2006a). Fact Sheet. Retrieved on September 18, 2006, from http://mchb.hrsa.gov/about/default.htm

Maternal and Child Health Bureau. (2006b). *Women's Health USA, 2005.* (2005). Retrieved on September 18, 2006, from http://mchb.hrsa.gov/whusa-05/pages/0426ap.htm

Mathews, R., Meneacker, F., MacDorman, M. (2005). Infant mortality statistics from 2002. Retrieved on September 25, 2006, from http://www.cdc.gov/nchs/data/nvsr/nvsr53_10.pdf

Monteiro, L. A. (1985). Florence Nightingale on public health nursing. *American Journal of Public Health, 75*(2), 181–186.

National Center for Disease Statistics. (2005). QuickStats: Infant mortality rates, by selected racial/ethnic populations–United States, 2002. *MMWR, 54*(05), 126. Retrieved on September 18, 2006, from http://www.cdc.gov/mmwr/preview/mmwrhtml/mm5405a5.htm

National Center for Statistics and Analysis. (2003). Traffic safety facts. Retrieved on September 23, 2006, from www-nrd.nhtsa.dot.gov/pdf/nrd-30/NCSA/TSF2003/809762.pdf from http://www.cdc.gov/nchs/products/[pubs/pubd/hestats/overwght00.htm

National Highway Traffic Safety Administration (2006). *General Child Seat Use Information.* Retrieved from http://www.nhtsa.dot.gov

National Center for Health Statistics. (2007). Prevalence of overweight among children and adolescents: United States, 2003–2004. Retrieved on October 30, 2007, from http://www.cdc.gov/nchs/products/pubs/pubd/hestats/overweight/overweight_child_03.htm

National Highway Traffic Safety Administration (U.S.) Department of Transportation. (2006). *Advanced frontal air bags.* Retrieved on September 23, 2006, from http://www.nhtsa.dot.gov/cars/testing/ncap/airbags/pages/FAQsAdvFrontABs.htm

Rainwater, L., & Smeeding, T. (2003). Poor Kids in Rich Nations. New York: Russell Sage Foundation. Retrieved on August 29, 2006.

Respiratory diseases send more American children to hospital than any other illness. (2006). *Medscape Business of Medicine,* 7(1). Retrieved on September 25, 2006, from http://www.medscape.com/viewarticle/529958_print

Teutsch, R. (2006). Cost effectiveness of prevention. Medscape Public Health & Prevention.

Retrieved on September 21, 2006, from http://www.medscape.com/viewarticle/540199

United Health Foundation. (2006). America's Health Rankings: A Call to Action for People and Their Communities. Retrieved on September 18, 2006, from http://www.unitedhealthfoundation.org/ahr2006.html

U.S Census Bureau, Historical Poverty Table. Retrieved on September 25, 2006, from http://www.census.gov/hhes/poverty/histpov/hstpov3.html

U.S. Department of Health and Human Services. (2000b). Maternal, infant, and child health. In *Healthy People 2010. National health promotion and disease prevention objectives.* Washington, DC: U.S. Government Printing Office.

U.S. Department of Health and Human Services, Health Resources and Services Administration, Maternal and Child Health Bureau. (2002). Child health USA 2002. Washington, DC: Government Printing Office.

LEARNING ▼ ACTIVITIES

◆ JOURNALING ACTIVITY 9-1

1. In your clinical journal, describe a situation you have encountered when doing health screening or health promotion activities.
   - What did you learn from this experience?
   - How will you practice differently based on this experience?
2. In your clinical journal, describe a situation in which you have observed infants or children not receiving the disease prevention or health promotion services that they needed.
   - How could or would you like to advocate for this issue when you begin to practice as an RN?
   - What could you do now?

◆ CLIENT CARE ACTIVITY 9-2

You are working as a community-based nurse making home visits to pregnant teens through the clinic where you are employed. The school nurse calls the clinic and requests that a home visit be made to Shantrell, who has shared with the school nurse that she is pregnant. She has been to your clinic for health care but has not had prenatal care. All you know is that Shantrell is 16 years old, pregnant, and no longer going to school.

When you drive to the client's home, you notice that the house is very old, with old cars and debris in the yard.

- What else do you assess as you drive through the neighborhood?

You knock on the door. You notice that the paint is peeling on the outside of the house, and it looks like it hasn't been painted in a long time. Your client, Shantrell, comes to the door. You greet her, tell her your name, the name of the clinic you work for, and why you are visiting. During the first part of the visit, you spend some time getting to know Shantrell.

- What could you use for a guide for interview questions?

You learn that Shantrell found out she was pregnant 1 month ago, and she is now 3 months pregnant. She has not come into the clinic because she thought that she only needed to see the doctor the month before the baby was born.

- What would you want to screen for?
- What topics would you want to address during the rest of the visit?
- What other questions would you ask?
- What will be your number-one priority?
- What do you hope to screen for and teach about in the next visit?

◆ CLIENT CARE ACTIVITY 9-3

Shantrell has given birth to a baby girl weighing 7 lb., 6 oz. She named the baby Precious. Both mom and baby did well during and after delivery. The baby is crying when you arrive for the visit. Shantrell picks up the baby, holds her close, and quietly talks to her.

- What does this tell you about Shantrell's ability to comfort the newborn?
- What do you do at this point?

Shantrell says she is breast-feeding Precious because "Remember we talked about it and I thought I didn't want to do it. You told me that if I breast-feed my baby, I will lose my big tummy and look slimmer faster." You ask how the feeding is going, and she states, "Good. When I am at school, my mom gives her a bottle of milk."

- What screening would you do at every visit?
- What special risks may this infant have?
- What would your priority be at this visit?

◆ PRACTICAL APPLICATION ACTIVITY 9-4

Contact the director of a day care center in a community where there is a high rate of low-income families or that serves low-income families. These families are likely to have limited access to well child care and health care. Talk to the day care director about the health teaching that he or she sees as important to the kids and parents they serve. Develop a class or classes according to the director's request. One idea is to use the hand-washing curricula listed in What's on the Web. (Some of these curricula are in Spanish and Hmong as well as English.) Another approach is to develop a teaching sheet according to the topics that the day care staff members identify as important for them. Check the Bright Futures Web site for teaching materials once you decide on a topic.

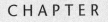
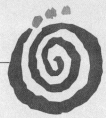

9

Health Promotion and Disease Prevention for Adults

ROBERTA HUNT

LEARNING OBJECTIVES

1. Identify the leading causes of death for adults.
2. Discuss the major diseases and threats to health for adults.
3. Summarize the primary health issues for adults.
4. Identify nursing roles for each level of prevention for primary health issues for adults.
5. Compose a list of nursing interventions for the primary health issues for adults.
6. Determine health needs for adults for which a nurse could be an advocate.

KEY TERMS

health indicator
moderate physical activity
obese
overweight

CHAPTER TOPICS

- ◆ Health Status of Adults
- ◆ Eliminating Disparity in Health Care
- ◆ Health Screening for Adults
- ◆ Interventions for Leading Health Indicators
- ◆ Conclusions

THE NURSE SPEAKS

My first job working as a staff nurse was on the oncology unit for a large teaching hospital in New York. Many of our patients did not have insurance. One day I floated to a general medical–surgical unit, where I took care of a 50-year-old woman named Linda who was admitted for cholecystitis. It was a quiet day on the unit, so as I was doing my morning assessment, I took some time to talk to her. She told me that her husband was disabled and that they had four children. Although she worked full time as a nurse's aide, to get family insurance, she had to pay $800 a month, and they could not afford to pay such a large premium. Consequently, no one in her family was insured except her husband. Her younger sister passed away the year before from breast cancer. She told me "that it was my third sister who has died of breast cancer. Two of my mother's sisters and my grandma died of breast cancer." We talked about the importance of yearly mammography for women over 50, particularly if they have a family history of breast cancer. She said she was aware of the need for the screening but had never had mammography because she could not afford to pay $900 for the test. I told her about the National Breast and Cervical Cancer Early Detection Program (NBCCEDP) and gave her the number to call. She told me she would contact them and make an appointment.

Three months later I saw Linda on the oncology unit. She had contacted the NBCCEDP and had mammography. She was in the hospital for surgery for early-stage breast cancer. I never appreciated the importance of early screening and detection so much as I did that day.

—SUSAN LARSON, RN, Oncology Nurse, St. Paul, Minnesota

HEALTH STATUS OF ADULTS

The major causes of death in the United States (Table 9-1) often result from behaviors and lifestyle choices that contribute to injury, violence, and illness. Environmental factors, such as lack of access to quality health services, also contribute to the major causes of death. For the nurse, this underscores the importance of understanding and monitoring health behaviors, environmental factors, and community health systems. This chapter will assist the nurse to understand and learn to monitor health behaviors that affect health and contribute to the major causes of death and disability. Ultimately nursing interventions in community-based care are intended to encourage healthy behaviors.

Because the average person is living longer, more attention is now focused on preserving quality of life rather than simply extending length of life. Chief among the factors involving preserving quality of life is the prevention and treatment of musculoskeletal conditions. Demographic trends also indicate that people will need to continue to work to an older age. Nurses will increasingly be involved in efforts to decrease the adverse social and economic consequence of high rates of activity limitation and disability of older persons.

TABLE 9-1 Leading Causes of Death According to Age, United States, 2003	
Age	**Cause of Death**
25–44 years	Unintentional injuries
	Malignant neoplasms
	Diseases of heart
45–64 years	Malignant neoplasms
	Diseases of heart
	Unintentional injuries
65 years and over	Diseases of heart
	Malignant neoplasms
	Cerebrovascular diseases

Source: National Center for Health Statistics. (2005). *Chartbook on trends in the health of Americans.* Retrieved on October 31, 2007, from http://origin.cdc.gov/nchs/data/hus/hus05acc.pdf (p. 183).

Leading **health indicators** are shown in Healthy People 2010 9-1. These illuminate individual behavioral, physical, social, and environmental factors and health systems issues that affect the health of individuals. "The health indicators are intended to help everyone more easily understand the importance of health promotion and disease prevention and to encourage wide participation in improving health in the next decade" (U.S. Department of Health and Human Services [DHHS], 2000, p. 25).

ELIMINATING DISPARITY IN HEALTH CARE

The central goals of Healthy People 2010 (DHHS, 2000) are to increase quality and years of healthy life and to eliminate health disparities. Health disparities exist by gender, race or ethnicity, education, income, disability, rural living areas, and sexual orientation. Men have a life expectancy that is 6 years shorter than women's, and they have a higher rate of death for each of the 10 leading causes of death. Women have had an increasing rate of death from lung cancer in the past 20 years, whereas the men's rate has decreased.

Disparity by ethnicity is believed to result from complex interactions among genetic variations, environmental factors, and specific health behaviors. African

HEALTHY PEOPLE 2010 ▶ 9-1

Leading Health Indicators

1. Physical activity
2. Overweight and obesity
3. Tobacco use
4. Substance abuse
5. Responsible sexual behavior
6. Mental health
7. Injury violence
8. Environmental quality
9. Immunization
10. Access to health care

American men are twice as likely as Hispanic men to die of heart disease. Heart disease death rates are more than 29% higher for African Americans than for Whites. Black women have higher death rates than Whites due to heart disease, cancer, and stroke. Women are more likely than men to report having arthritis, asthma, autoimmune diseases, and depression. Asians and Pacific Islanders, on average, have health indicators that suggest they are one of the healthiest population groups in the United States. Blacks and Hispanics receive fewer mammograms, Pap smears, influenza vaccinations, and less prenatal care (Agency for Healthcare Research and Quality [AHRQ], 2005). Post-myocardial infarction (MI) care in women still lags behind that in men (Greenland, & Gulati, 2006).

Income and education underlie many health disparities in the United States. The two are intrinsically related; people with the worst health status are among those with the highest poverty rates and least education. Poverty disproportionately affects women. Income inequality in the United States has increased over the past 3 decades. Minorities are more likely to be uninsured and less likely to have a regular source of, or access to specialty care. Low income clients receive lower intensity hospital care and receive fewer cardiac procedures and have higher mortality following these procedures (AHRQ, 2005).

People with disabilities are identified as people who have activity limitations, people who need assistive devices, or people who perceive themselves as having a disability. Roughly 15% of the adult population reports some level of limitation in physical functioning. Many people with disabilities lack access to health services and medical care (DHHS, 2005).

Twenty-five percent of Americans live in rural localities. Those living in rural areas are less likely to use preventive screening services, exercise regularly, or wear seat belts, and are more likely to be uninsured. Compared to urban counterparts, residents in rural communities report fair or poor health more frequently, more often have chronic conditions such as diabetes, and die more frequently from heart disease (AHRQ, 2004).

Gay men and lesbians have health problems unique to their populations. Gay men are more likely than heterosexual men to have acquired human immunodeficiency virus (HIV) and other sexually transmitted diseases (STDs), and they are at an increased risk for substance abuse, depression, and suicide. In some parts of the United States, lesbian, gay men, bisexual individuals, and transgender people are reluctant to reveal their sexual orientation or gender identity to health care providers and will avoid health care settings because of lack of trust (Paxon, 2005).

HEALTH SCREENING FOR ADULTS

As with clients at other ages, health screening for adults is intended for primary, secondary, or tertiary prevention. Primary prevention to prevent the initial occurrence of a disease with an adult client could be immunization screening and recommendation of an annual flu shot. Secondary prevention could be screening for hypertension at a health fair or yearly mammography for women over 40 years of age. Tertiary prevention could be initiating an exercise program for an obese client who has type 2 diabetes. Screening is always intended to identify people who are at risk for developing a health condition so that appropriate intervention can be undertaken.

The nurse should encourage the client to actively practice prevention. One way to accomplish this is to use the *Pocket Guide to Good Health for Adults* available at no cost from AHRQ at http://www.ahcpr.gov, by calling (800) 358-9295, or email ahrqpubs@ahrq.gov. This resource is for clients to keep accurate information about their health, health treatments, and screenings and for the nurse to guide clients in identifying and planning health promotion and disease prevention activities. The guide contains information on screening as well as topics related to the leading health indicators. It also contains forms for record keeping essential for health promotion and disease prevention. There are questions throughout the guide to empower the client to take charge of his or her own health care.

The American College of Preventive Medicine has identified the most effective and cost effective clinical preventive services. Among the services that apply to the adults are aspirin to prevent heart disease; immunizations, screening, and counseling for tobacco use and problem drinking; screening for colorectal cancer, cervical cancer, vision impairment, blood pressure, and cholesterol; and pneumococcal and influenza immunizations (Teutsch, 2006).

General Screening

Major areas of adult health screening covered in the *Pocket Guide to Good Health for Adults* include blood pressure, cholesterol, weight, and immunizations. Maintaining a normal blood pressure protects people from heart disease, stroke, and kidney problems. It is recommended that all adults have their blood pressure checked regularly. Those with high blood pressure should work with their health care provider to lower it by changing their diet, losing weight, exercising, and if prescribed, taking medication.

Cholesterol should be checked in men from ages 35 to 65 years and women from ages 45 to 65. If it is within a normal range it should be checked every 5 years. If it is not there are many strategies to lowering it by changing diet, losing excess weight, and getting exercise. The client's knowledge about cholesterol and heart disease can be assessed by using quizzes available from the National Heart, Lung, and Blood Institute at http://nhlbisupport.com/chd1/how.htm. Weighing too much or too little can lead to health problems. Healthy diet and regular exercise are factors that contribute to weight loss. Assessment should include the evaluation of body mass index (BMI), waist circumference, and overall medical risk.

Immunization is cited as one of the greatest achievements of public health in the 20th century. Box 9-1 shows immunizations needed by adults. It is important to continue to increase the proportion of children who receive all vaccines, as well as the proportion of adults who are vaccinated annually against the flu.

Oral health care is also important for overall general health. Not only will proper oral care preserve teeth for a lifetime, but flossing every day contributes to a longer life (Community-Based Teaching 9-1). Poor oral hygiene and gum disease is associated with heart disease, diabetes, blood infection, and even low birth weight infants (Healthcare in the News, 2006).

Cancer Screening

Colorectal cancer is the second leading cause of death from cancer. If colorectal cancer is caught early, it can be treated. The risk of developing colorectal cancer increases with advancing age. Risk factors include inflammatory bowel disease and a family or personal history of colorectal cancer or polyps. Lack of regular physical activity, low fruit and vegetable intake, a low-fiber diet, obesity, and alcohol

---

◆ **BOX 9-1** Recommended Immunizations for Adults ◆

- Tetanus–diphtheria: every 10 years
- Measles-mumps-rubella (MMR): For women considering pregnancy, if born after 1956
- Pneumococcal (pneumonia): At about age 65 or before for those with a chronic condition.
- Influenza: Most people 50 or older need flu shot every year. If under 50 a flu shot is recommended for those who work with high-risk populations or live with someone who works with high-risk populations; or pregnant women after the first trimester; or for those who have a chronic condition, such as lung, heart, or kidney disease; diabetes; HIV; or cancer, may need both influenza and pneumococcal immunizations.
- Hepatitis B: For people who have contact with human blood or body fluids, have unprotected sex, or share needles during intravenous drug use. Health professionals should also consider hepatitis B immunization. Those who travel to areas where hepatitis B is common.

Agency for Healthcare Research and Quality. (2006). *The Pocket Guide to Good Health for Adults.*

---

consumption are other contributing factors. Reducing the number of deaths from colorectal cancer chiefly depends on detecting and removing precancerous colorectal polyps, as well as detecting and treating the cancer in its early stages. People 50 years and older should been screened regularly using a combination of the four recommended screening tests: fecal occult blood test, sigmoidoscopy, colonoscopy, or barium enema (Centers for Disease Control and Prevention [CDC], 2006c).

Regular mammography screening for women age 50 and older has been shown to reduce deaths from breast cancer (CDC, 2006). Some women may need to begin having mammograms earlier, depending on their health history. All women should have an annual Pap smear starting at age 18 or when they become sexually active. Those who have three or more normal annual tests may be tested less frequently, at the discretion of the nurse practitioner or physician.

The CDC National Breast and Cervical Cancer Early Detection Program provides free screening exams for all women throughout the United States. Consult the Web site at http://www.cdc.gov/cancer/nbccedp/ for more information or to find out where your client can get a free or low-cost mammogram and Pap test in your area.

COMMUNITY-BASED TEACHING ▶ 9-1

Basic Principles of Oral Health

- Visit your dentist regularly for checkups.
- Brush after meals.
- Use dental floss daily.
- Limit the intake of sweets, especially between meals.
- Do not smoke or chew tobacco products.

Prostate cancer is the most commonly diagnosed form of cancer, second to skin cancer, and is second to lung cancer as a cause of cancer-related death among men. The two most common tests used by physicians to detect prostate cancer are the digital rectal exam and the prostate-specific antigen (PSA). There is good evidence that PSA screening can detect early-stage prostate cancer; evidence is inconclusive about whether early detection improves health outcomes. The CDC does not recommend routine screening for prostate cancer because there is no scientific consensus on whether screening and treatment of early stage prostate cancer reduces mortality. The CDC does, however, support a man's right to discuss the pros and cons of prostate cancer screening and treatment with his doctor and his right to make his own decision about screening (CDC, 2006c).

Skin cancer is the most common form of cancer in the United States. More than 1 million new cases of skin cancer will be diagnosed each year. Exposure to the sun's ultraviolet rays appears to be the most important environmental factor in the development of skin cancer. Skin cancer can be prevented by following consistent sun-protective practices. Risk factors include the following:

◆ Light skin color, hair color, and eye color
◆ Family history of skin cancer
◆ Personal history of skin cancer
◆ Chronic exposure to the sun
◆ History of sunburns early in life
◆ Certain types and a large number of moles
◆ Freckles, which indicate sun sensitivity and sun damage (CDC, 2006e)

Numerous resources can be found at this CDC Web site: http://www.cdc.gov/HealthyYouth/skincancer/pdf/facts.pdf.

Screening for High-Risk Groups

Overall, African Americans are more likely to develop cancer than persons of any other racial or ethnic group (CDC, 2002e). In addition, the following conditions may require additional screening. If the client falls into any of these categories, he or she should discuss potential screening with a nurse practitioner or physician.

◆ Has diabetes, or is older than 40 and African American, or is older than 60 years of age—requires additional eye exams
◆ Has had intercourse without condoms, has had multiple partners, or has had an STD—may require screening for STDs
◆ Has injected illegal drugs or had a blood transfusion between 1978 and 1985—may need an HIV or hepatitis test
◆ Has a family member with diabetes, is overweight, or has had diabetes during pregnancy—may need a glucose test
◆ Is over age 65—needs a hearing test
◆ Now or in the past, has consumed a lot of alcohol, smoked, or chewed tobacco—may need a mouth exam
◆ Is male and over age 50—needs a prostate exam
◆ Male between ages 14 and 35 years, particularly if a testicle is abnormally small or not in the normal position—may need a testicular exam
◆ Has had a family member with skin cancer or has had a lot of sun exposure—may need a skin exam
◆ Has had radiation treatments of the upper body—may need a thyroid exam

◆ Has been exposed to tuberculosis; has recently moved from Asia, Africa, Central or South America, or the Pacific Islands; has kidney failure, diabetes, HIV, or alcoholism; or uses illegal drugs—may need a tuberculosis (purified protein derivative [PPD]) test

The Pocket Guide to Good Health for Adults (2003) is available at http://www. ahrq.gov/ppip/adguide/adguide.pdf

INTERVENTIONS FOR LEADING HEALTH INDICATORS

Evidence exists that some of the leading causes of death and disability in the United States–such as heart disease, cancer, stroke, some respiratory diseases, unintentional injuries, HIV, and acquired immunodeficiency syndrome (AIDS)–can often be prevented by making lifestyle changes. About two thirds of all mortalities and a great amount of morbidity, suffering, and rising health care costs among adults result from three causes. Heart disease and cancer are the leading causes of death in adults. Only three categories of behavior contribute enormously to these causes: tobacco use, dietary patterns, and physical inactivity (National Center for Health Statistics [NCHS], 2005). Staying physically active, eating right, and not smoking (or quitting if you do smoke) are the three most important strategies to better health (Fig. 9-1).

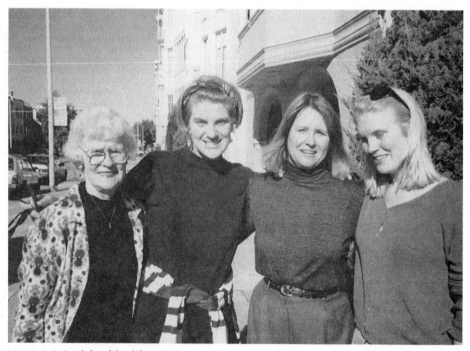

FIGURE 9-1. ▶ A healthy lifestyle incorporating physical activity, good nutrition, social support, and avoidance of activities that are detrimental to health can improve quality of life for adults of all ages.

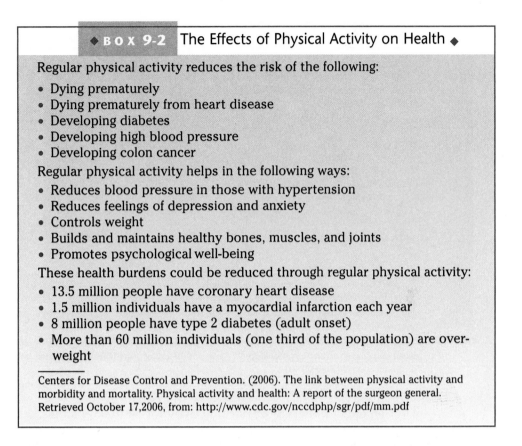

◆ **BOX 9-2** The Effects of Physical Activity on Health ◆

Regular physical activity reduces the risk of the following:

• Dying prematurely
• Dying prematurely from heart disease
• Developing diabetes
• Developing high blood pressure
• Developing colon cancer

Regular physical activity helps in the following ways:

• Reduces blood pressure in those with hypertension
• Reduces feelings of depression and anxiety
• Controls weight
• Builds and maintains healthy bones, muscles, and joints
• Promotes psychological well-being

These health burdens could be reduced through regular physical activity:

• 13.5 million people have coronary heart disease
• 1.5 million individuals have a myocardial infarction each year
• 8 million people have type 2 diabetes (adult onset)
• More than 60 million individuals (one third of the population) are overweight

Centers for Disease Control and Prevention. (2006). The link between physical activity and morbidity and mortality. Physical activity and health: A report of the surgeon general. Retrieved October 17,2006, from: http://www.cdc.gov/nccdphp/sgr/pdf/mm.pdf

Physical Activity

Engaging in regular physical activity on most days of the week reduces the risk of developing or dying from some of the leading causes of illness and death. Box 9-2 presents an overview of the relationship between physical activity and morbidity and mortality.

More than 65% of adults in the United States do not engage in recommended amounts of physical activity. Physical inactivity is more common among women than men, African American and Hispanic adults than White adults, older adults than younger adults, and less affluent people than more affluent people (NCHS, 2005).

"How much activity?" and "How do I start?" are two common questions clients ask regarding physical activity. Clients who have been sedentary or are obese may want to start by reducing sedentary time and gradually building physical activity into each day. A client may begin by gradually increasing daily activities such as taking the stairs or walking or swimming at a slow pace.

The need to avoid injury during physical activity is a high priority. Before beginning an exercise program all adults over 40 should speak to their physician or nurse practitioner. Walking is an ideal activity to increase physical activity because it is safe and accessible to most people. For those who have been physically inactive, a starting point can be walking 10 minutes, 3 days a week, building to 30 to 45 minutes of more intense walking and gradually increasing to most

TABLE 9-2 Examples of Moderate Amounts of Physical Activity*		
Common Chores	**Sporting Activities**	
Washing and waxing a car for 45–60 min	Playing volleyball for 45–60 min	Less Vigorous, More Time
Washing windows or floors for 45–60 min	Playing touch football for 45 min	
Gardening for 30–45 min	Walking 1¼ miles in 35 min (20 min/mile)	
Wheeling self in wheelchair for 30–40 min	Basketball (shooting baskets) for 30 min	↑
Pushing a stroller 1½ miles in 30 min	Bicycling 5 miles in 30 min	
Raking leaves for 30 min	Dancing fast (social) for 30 min	↓
Walking 2 miles in 30 min (15 min/mile)	Water aerobics for 30 min	
Shoveling snow for 15 min	Swimming laps for 20 min	
Stairwalking for 15 min	Basketball (playing a game) for 15–20 min	More Vigorous, Less Time
	Jumping rope for 15 min	
	Running 1½ miles in 15 min (10 min/mile)	

*A moderate amount of physical activity is roughly equivalent to physical activity that uses approximately 150 calories of energy per day, or 1,000 calories per week.

Some activities can be performed at various intensities; the suggested durations correspond to expected intensity of effort.

National Institutes of Health. (2000). *The practical guide: Identification, evaluation, and treatment of overweight and obesity in adults.* National Heart, Lung and Blood Institute Obesity Education Initiative. NIH Publication Number 00-4084.

if not all days. **Moderate physical activity** for 30 to 45 minutes, 3 to 5 days per week, is a reasonable initial goal. Most adults should be encouraged to set a long-term goal of 30 minutes or more of moderate-intensity physical activity on most, preferably all, days of the week. Table 9-2 shows examples of moderate amounts of physical activity achieved from both common chores and sporting activities.

With time, weight loss, and increased functional capacity, the client may want to engage in more strenuous activities. These include fitness walking, cycling, rowing, cross-country skiing, aerobic dancing, and jumping rope. If jogging is desired, the client's ability to jog must be assessed first. Competitive sports such as tennis, soccer, and volleyball provide enjoyable physical activity for some individuals, but again, care must be taken to avoid injury. There is no such thing as one "magic" exercise. Rather to get the greatest health and fitness benefits a mix of moderate and vigorous exercise as well as strength training is required (Mougois, 2006). Individuals who are not physically active cite many reasons for their inactivity. Box 9-3 provides some suggestions that nurses can follow to assist clients to overcome obstacles to regular activity.

Social support from family and friends has been consistently and positively related to regular exercise. Nurses who work closely with clients in community-based settings have ample opportunity to encourage moderate physical activity for 30 minutes a day for all adults.

Overweight and Obesity

Overweight and obesity are major contributors to many preventable causes of death, with a general rule that higher body weight is associated with higher death rates. The percent of the adult population that is overweight or obese has increased

---

◆ BOX 9-3 Counseling Strategies to Encourage More Physical Activity ◆

Excuse	Suggested Response
I don't have time to exercise.	Exercise does take time but think of all the time you spend watching TV. Many forms of exercise can be done while watching TV (riding a stationary bike, using hand weights).
I don't have the energy to be more active.	Once you are more active you will have more energy.
It's hard to remember to exercise.	Leave your sneakers near the door to remind you to walk, bring a change of clothes to work and head straight for exercise on the way home. Put a note on your calendar to remind you.

---

in the last 3 decades with more than 60% of the U.S. population overweight and half obese (Fig. 9-2). Being overweight or obese substantially raises the risk of illness from high blood pressure, high cholesterol, type 2 diabetes, heart disease and stroke, gallbladder disease, arthritis, sleep disturbances, and endometrial, breast, prostate, and colon cancers (NCHS, 2005).

The rate of obesity and overweight is on the increase. It continues to vary by race, gender, income, and age. Women from lower income households are more likely to be overweight. Obesity is more common among African American and Hispanic women

	NHANES II (1976-80) (n=11,207)	NHANES III (1988-94) (n=14,468)	NHANES (1999-2000) (n=3,603)	NHANES (2001-02) (n=3,916)	NHANES (2003-04) (n=3,756)
Overweight or obese (BMI greater than or equal to 25.0)	47.1	55.9	64.5	65.7	66.2
Obese (BMI greater than or equal to 30.0)	15.0	23.2	30.9	31.3	32.9

* Age-adjusted by the direct method to the year 2000 U.S. Bureau of the Census estimates using the age groups 20-39, 40-59, and 60-74 years.

** NHANES II did not include individuals over 74 years of age, thus trend estimates are based on age 20-74 years.

FIGURE 9-2. ▶ Age-adjusted prevalence of overweight and obesity among U.S. adults, ages 20 to 74. BMI, body mass index; NHANES, National Health and Nutrition Examination Survey. Source: National Center for Health Statistics. (2006). Prevalence of overweight and obesity among adults: United States, 2003-2004. Retrieved on October 20, 2006, from http://www.cdc.gov.mill1.sjlibrary.org/nchs/products/pubs/pubd/hestats/obese03_04/overwght_adult_03.htm

than among White women and more common among women compared to men. The prevalence of obesity among men increased significantly from 27% in 1999 to 31% in 2004, while that rate for women remained stable at 33% (NCHS, 2006). Despite the fact that 90% of Americans know that most of their fellow citizens are overweight, just 40% believe themselves to be too fat (Pew Research Center, 2006).

◆ **BOX 9-4** Calculating Body Mass Index and Waist Circumference ◆

You can calculate BMI as follows:

BMI = weight (kg) / height squared (m^2)

If pounds and inches are used, do the following:

BMI = weight (lb) × 703 ÷ height squared (inches^2)

Calculation Directions and Example

Here is a shortcut method for calculating BMI. (Example: for a person who is 5 feet 5 inches tall weighing 180 lbs)

1. Multiply weight (in pounds) by 703: 180 × 703 = 126,540
2. Multiply height (in inches) by height (in inches): 65 × 65 = 4,225
3. Divide the answer in step 1 by the answer in step 2 to get the BMI:
   126,540/4,225 = 29.9
   BMI = 29.9

Waist Circumference Measurement

To measure waist circumference, locate the upper hip bone and the top of the right iliac crest. Place a measuring tape in a horizontal plane around the abdomen at the level of the iliac crest. Before reading the tape measure, ensure that the tape is snug, but does not compress the skin, and is parallel to the floor. The measurement is made at the end of a normal expiration.

Measuring-Tape Position for Waist (Abdominal) (Circumference in Adults)

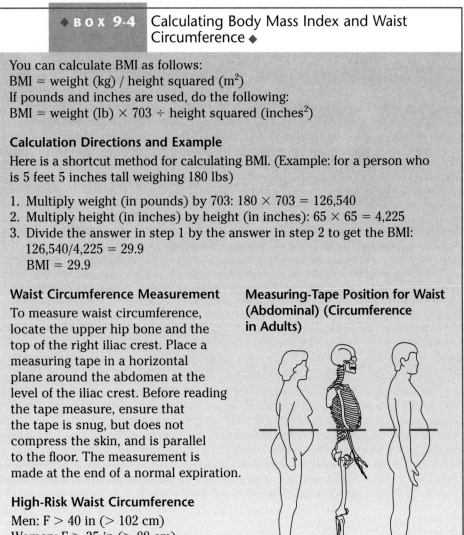

High-Risk Waist Circumference

Men: F > 40 in (> 102 cm)

Women: F > 35 in (> 88 cm)

National Institutes of Health, National Heart, Lung, and Blood Institute, Obesity Education Initiative. (1998). *The practical guide: Identification, evaluation, and treatment of overweight and obesity in adults.* Bethesda, MD: U.S. Department of Health and Human Services.

A person with a BMI between 25.0 and 29.9 is considered **overweight**. A person with a BMI of 30.0 or greater is considered **obese**. Box 9-4 shows how to calculate BMI and waist circumference. Table 9-3 provides a BMI estimation table.

Dietary therapy, physical activity, and behavioral therapy are the usual interventions for overweight and obesity. For the morbidly obese, pharmacotherapy and weight-loss surgery may be considered. A combination of diet modification, increased physical activity, and behavior therapy can be effective for most obese individuals. There are some simple behavior changes that promote weight loss. Eating a high-fiber diet improves health by lowing cholesterol and enhancing weight loss. There is a relationship between obesity and sleep with those individuals who get at least 7 hours of sleep are less likely to be overweight or obese. Therefore by addressing a variety of health habits the nurse can assist individuals to reach a normal weight. Of course it is important to address one issue at a time in small incremental steps. For example, encourage a client to go to bed 15 minutes earlier for a month. The next month, move the bedtime another 15 minutes earlier. Or encourage clients to add one piece of fruit per day to their diet for a month. After a month, advance to having two pieces of fruit a day.

Weight-loss therapy is not appropriate for some individuals, including most pregnant or lactating women, people with uncontrolled psychiatric illness, and those with serious illnesses that might be exacerbated by caloric restriction. Clients with active substance abuse or a history of anorexia nervosa or bulimia nervosa should receive care by a specialist.

It is recommended that health care providers first complete a behavioral assessment to determine a client's readiness for weight loss. This calls for the nurse to spend some time to assess the client's readiness for weight loss. The nurse should consider the following questions during this counseling session (NIH, 2000):

◆ Has the client sought weight loss on his or her own initiative?
◆ What events have led the client to seek weight loss now?
◆ What is the client's stress level and mood?
◆ Does the client have an eating disorder?
◆ Does the individual understand the requirement of treatment and believe that he or she can fulfill them?
◆ How much weight does the client expect to lose?
◆ What other benefits does he or she anticipate?

Next, a diet with a 500- to 1,000-calorie deficit should be planned. This usually means 1,000 to 1,200 calories for women and 1,200 to 1,600 calories for men. Sample diets for American, Asian, Southern, Mexican American, and lacto-ovo vegetarian clients are found in the appendices of the NIH *Practical Guide*, along with tips for weight loss, including methods of food preparation and how to choose food when dining away from home (NIH, 2000).

The nurse and client can plan and monitor the weight-loss program by using a weight and goal record. The client can keep a record of food consumption and physical activity each week by using a diet and activity-tracking sheet. Samples of these resources are found in the appendices of the *Practical Guide,* along with additional resources for healthy eating and physical activity. Through health education, nurses can help reduce the proportion of adults who are obese. All of these tools are available online at http://www.nhlbi.nih.gov/guidelines/obesity/prctgd_c.pdf.

TABLE 9-3	Body Mass Index Estimation																	
	Healthy Weight							Overweight						Obese				
BMI	19	20	21	22	23	24	25	26	27	28	29	30	31	32	33	34	35	36
Height (inches)	Body Weight (lbs.)																	
58	91	96	100	105	110	115	119	124	129	134	138	143	148	153	158	162	167	172
59	94	99	104	109	114	119	124	128	133	138	143	148	153	158	163	168	173	178
60	97	102	107	112	118	123	128	133	138	143	148	153	158	163	168	174	179	184
61	100	106	111	116	122	127	132	137	143	148	153	158	164	169	174	180	185	190
62	104	109	115	120	126	131	136	142	147	153	158	164	169	175	180	186	191	196
63	107	113	118	124	130	135	141	146	152	158	163	169	175	180	186	191	197	203
64	110	116	122	128	134	140	145	151	157	163	169	174	180	186	192	197	204	209
65	114	120	126	132	138	144	150	156	162	168	174	180	186	192	198	204	210	216
66	118	124	130	136	142	148	155	161	167	173	179	186	192	198	204	210	216	223
67	121	127	134	140	146	153	159	166	172	178	185	191	198	204	211	217	223	230
68	125	131	138	144	151	158	164	171	177	184	190	197	203	210	216	223	230	236
69	128	135	142	149	155	162	169	176	182	189	196	203	209	216	223	230	236	243
70	132	139	146	153	160	167	174	181	188	195	202	209	216	222	229	236	243	250
71	136	143	150	157	165	172	179	186	193	200	208	215	222	229	236	243	250	257
72	140	147	154	162	169	177	184	191	199	206	213	221	228	235	242	250	258	265
73	144	151	159	166	174	182	189	197	204	212	219	227	235	242	250	257	265	272
74	148	155	163	171	179	186	194	202	210	218	225	233	241	249	256	264	272	280
75	152	160	168	176	184	192	200	208	216	224	232	240	248	256	264	272	279	287
76	156	164	172	180	189	197	205	213	221	230	238	246	254	263	271	279	287	295

National Institutes of Health, National Heart, Lung, and Blood Institute, Obesity Education Initiative. (1998). *The practical guide: Identification, evaluation, and treatment of overweight and obesity in adults.* Bethesda, MD: U.S. Department of Health and Human Services.

Tobacco Use

Cigarette smoking, responsible for more than 440,000 deaths annually, continues to be the main preventable cause of disease and death in the United States (CDC, 2006). Smoking is a major risk factor for developing heart disease, stroke, lung cancer, and chronic lung disease. The percentage of adolescents who smoke decreased from 1990 to 2003, but is now on the increase. In 2004, 22% of teens smoked (Chartbook, 2005). Half of all adolescent smokers who continue to smoke in adulthood will die from smoking-related illness. Whites are more likely than African Americans and Hispanics to use tobacco.

The financial costs of smoking and smoking-related disease, including lost earnings and productivity, approach $175 billion per year. Stopping the use of tobacco is the most cost-effective method of preventing disease among adults. Each smoker who successfully quits smoking reduces future medical costs by an estimated $47 in the first year and $853 during the following 7 years (Preventing Chronic Diseases, 2005).

An integrative literature review of 29 studies was conducted to determine the effectiveness of nursing-delivered smoking cessation interventions. It was found that smokers who were offered advice by nursing professionals had an increased likelihood of quitting compared to smokers without such nursing interventions. This result reflected a significantly positive effect for smoking cessation interventions by nurses, especially in the hospital setting. The challenge to nurses is to

						Very Obese												
	37	38	39	40	41	42	43	44	45	46	47	48	49	50	51	52	53	54
Height (inches)						Body Weight (lbs.)												
58	177	181	186	191	196	201	205	210	215	220	224	229	234	239	244	248	253	258
59	183	188	193	198	203	208	212	217	222	227	232	237	242	247	252	257	262	267
60	189	194	199	204	209	215	220	225	230	235	240	245	250	255	261	266	271	276
61	195	201	206	211	217	222	227	232	238	243	248	254	259	264	269	275	280	285
62	202	207	213	218	224	229	235	240	246	251	256	262	267	273	278	284	289	295
63	208	214	220	225	231	237	242	248	254	259	265	270	278	282	287	293	299	304
64	215	221	227	232	238	244	250	256	262	267	273	279	285	291	296	302	308	314
65	222	228	234	240	246	252	258	264	270	276	282	288	294	300	306	312	318	324
66	229	235	241	247	253	260	266	272	278	284	291	297	303	309	315	322	328	334
67	236	242	249	255	261	268	274	280	287	293	299	306	312	319	325	331	338	344
68	243	249	256	262	269	276	282	289	295	302	308	315	322	328	335	341	348	354
69	250	257	263	270	277	284	291	297	304	311	318	324	331	338	345	351	358	365
70	257	264	271	278	285	292	299	306	313	320	327	334	341	348	355	362	369	376
71	265	272	279	286	293	301	308	315	322	329	338	343	351	358	365	372	379	386
72	272	279	287	294	302	309	316	324	331	338	346	353	361	368	375	383	390	397
73	280	288	295	302	310	318	325	333	340	348	355	363	371	378	386	393	401	408
74	287	295	303	311	319	326	334	342	350	358	365	373	381	389	396	404	412	420
75	295	303	311	319	327	335	343	351	359	367	375	383	391	399	407	415	423	431
76	304	312	320	328	336	344	353	361	369	377	385	394	402	410	418	426	435	443

incorporate smoking cessation interventions as part of standard practice so that the nurse discusses tobacco use with all clients, gives advice to quit, and uses behavioral counseling. Nurses interface with clients in numerous settings, allowing them to play an important role in reducing cigarette smoking by adults (Rice & Stead, 2006).

The community-based nurse should screen for tobacco use and encourage cessation with every client. Current guidelines for clinicians assisting clients with smoking cessation are shown in Community-Based Nursing Care Guidelines 9-1.

Alcohol and Substance Use and Abuse

There is a great deal of confusion about the benefits and detriments of alcohol consumption. In the last decade, some research suggested that moderate alcohol use might provide some protection from coronary artery disease. However, research has established that the pattern of drinking, or having a drink every day may provide health benefit, while drinking large quantities of alcohol at one sitting which is known to have a negative impact on health, is what determines the effects of alcohol on one's health (Mukamal et al., 2003). These findings are consistent with what we have known for some time—binge drinking creates health problems.

Many serious problems are associated with alcohol and illicit drug abuse. The financial costs of substance abuse are high, estimated at $276 billion per year (DHHS, 2000). Substance abuse is associated with child and spousal abuse, STDs,

---

COMMUNITY-BASED NURSING CARE GUIDELINES ▶ 9-1

Quick Reference Guide for Clinicians Treating
Tobacco Use and Dependence

Ask	Systematically identify all tobacco users at every visit.
Advise	Strongly urge all tobacco users to quit.
Assess	Determine willingness to make a quit attempt.
Assist	Aid the client in quitting.
Follow up	Ask clients if they still smoke. Give ex-smokers a pat on the back. Send cards or call clients soon after their visit and just before their original quit day.

Fiore, M., Bailey, W., Cohen, S., et al. (2000). *Quick reference guide for clinicians: Treating tobacco use and dependence.* Rockville, MD: U.S. Department of Health and Human Services, Public Health Service. Retrieved on October 18, 2006, from http://www.surgeongeneral.gov/tobacco/tobaqrg.pdf.

---

motor vehicle accidents, escalation of health care costs, low worker productivity, and homelessness. Alcohol abuse alone is associated with motor vehicle accidents, homicides, suicides, and drowning. Chronic alcohol use can lead to heart disease, cancer, liver disease, and pancreatitis (National Institute of Alcohol Abuse and Alcoholism [NIAAA], 2006).

For individuals over 18 years, 40% of men and 20% of women report drinking five or more alcoholic drinks on at least 1 day (binge drank) in the past year. Whites and Hispanics are more likely than African Americans to use alcohol. Whites are more likely than African Americans and Hispanics to use illicit drugs (NIAA, 2005).

Assessment and intervention with substance-related health issues is an important role for the nurse in community-based settings. The more direct, honest, and open the nurse is when addressing this issue, the more likely clients will be to view their own patterns of alcohol use as an important aspect of health promotion.

Box 9-5 gives an assessment for alcohol abuse. Teaching the client about avoiding substance abuse issues is the next step after assessment (see Community-Based Teaching 9-2 and Community-Based Nursing Care Guidelines 9-2).

Interventions targeted to groups and communities have demonstrated some efficacy in reducing substance abuse. School-based prevention programs directed toward altering perceived peer-group norms about alcohol use and helping develop skills in resisting peer pressure to drink are successful in reducing alcohol use among participants. Raising the minimum legal drinking age has reduced alcohol consumption, traffic accidents, and related fatalities among young persons younger than 21 years of age. Higher cost for alcohol is also associated with lower alcohol consumption and lowered adverse outcomes. In college settings, one-to-one motivational counseling has been effective in reducing alcohol-related problems. It is important that the nurse direct efforts to reduce the

---

◆ BOX 9-5   Quick Assessment for Alcohol Abuse ◆

A "yes" answer to any of the following questions may be a warning sign that the client has a drinking problem and should talk to a health care provider.

- Have you ever felt that you should cut down on your drinking?
- Have people annoyed you by criticizing your drinking?
- Have you ever felt bad or guilty about drinking?
- Have you ever had a drink first thing in the morning to steady your nerves or to get rid of a hangover?

Agency for Health Care Research and Quality (2006). *The Pocket Guide to Good Health for Adults.* Available at http:www.ahrq.gov/ppip/adguide/

---

proportion of adults using illicit drugs and engaging in binge drinking of alcoholic beverages.

Responsible Sexual Behavior

STDs remain a major public health challenge in the United States, with more than 19 million new infections each year, almost half among young adults ages 15 to 24 (CDC, 2004) Unprotected sex can result in unintended pregnancies and STDs, including HIV. About half of all new HIV infections in the United States are among individuals over 25 years of age, with the majority being infected through sexual behavior. Women bear the greatest burden of STDs, suffering more frequent and more serious

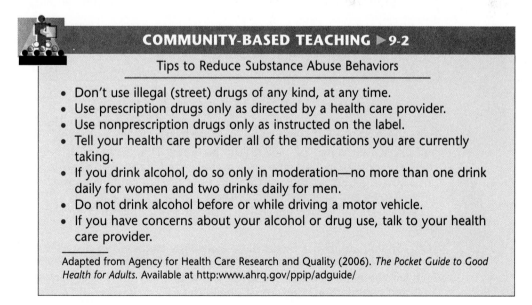

COMMUNITY-BASED TEACHING ▶ 9-2

Tips to Reduce Substance Abuse Behaviors

- Don't use illegal (street) drugs of any kind, at any time.
- Use prescription drugs only as directed by a health care provider.
- Use nonprescription drugs only as instructed on the label.
- Tell your health care provider all of the medications you are currently taking.
- If you drink alcohol, do so only in moderation—no more than one drink daily for women and two drinks daily for men.
- Do not drink alcohol before or while driving a motor vehicle.
- If you have concerns about your alcohol or drug use, talk to your health care provider.

Adapted from Agency for Health Care Research and Quality (2006). *The Pocket Guide to Good Health for Adults.* Available at http:www.ahrq.gov/ppip/adguide/

COMMUNITY-BASED NURSING CARE GUIDELINES ▸ 9-2

Guidelines for Alcohol and Substance Use Intervention

Ask

Ask clients if they use alcohol or other drugs, how much, and the frequency.

Ask about binge drinking (more than three drinks per occasion or seven drinks per week). Congratulate recovering alcoholics and drug users.

Ask clients the assessment questions in Box 9-5. Also ask about any adverse consequences they have experienced from their drinking.

Advise

State your conclusion.

Ask what benefits the clients would enjoy if they reduced alcohol or drug intake.

Prepare

Encourage client to set a date to quit drinking, attend Alcoholics Anonymous, or get counseling for concerns related to his or her substance use.

Negotiate a Drinking Goal

Consider referral for additional evaluation by an addiction specialist or mutual help group.

Follow up

Follow up by asking about progress. Be straightforward, matter of fact, and nonjudgmental. Praise and encourage any small steps taken. Continue to validate any effort. Acknowledge that change is difficult. Support an effort to cut down or abstain, while making your recommendation clear.

Adapted from *Helping Patients who Drink too Much: A Clinician's Guide.* (2005). National Institutes of Health. National Institute on Alcohol Abuse and Alcoholism. Retrieved on October 18, 2006, from http://pubs.niaaa.nih.gov/publications/practitioner/CliniciansGuide2005/guide_slideshow.htm.

complications than men. The highest rates are found among Blacks (51%); Whites (29%); and Hispanics (18%) (Trends in HIV/AIDS, 2005). Condoms, used correctly and consistently, can prevent STDs, including HIV. However, it is estimated that there are more than 250,000 people in the United States who are HIV-positive but do not know they are infected. The CDC now recommends screening all individuals ages 13 to 64 and yearly screening for people at high risk for HIV (CDC, 2006b).

Nurses should never hesitate to assess sexual health. Here are some simple questions:

◆ Are you afraid you might have a sexually transmitted disease?
◆ Do you have questions about tests or treatment?
◆ Do you need to find a doctor or clinic where you can get private, personal, and confidential care? You can call the CDC:

1-800-CDC-INFO
(1-800-232-4636)
TTY: 1-888-232-6348
In English and Spanish (*en Español*)

Health teaching is the most important disease prevention activity the nurse can use to address health issues related to sexual behavior. Again, sexuality must always be assessed, with teaching and interventions based on the client's knowledge base, concerns, and cultural sensitivities. As discussed in Chapter 8, young teens should be encouraged to delay the age of first intercourse. Teaching about the effectiveness of various contraceptive methods and providing condoms are interventions that have been shown again and again to be essential to sexual health promotion.

Mental Health

Twenty-six percent of the population is affected by mental illness during a given year, with depression as the most common disorder (Kessler, 2005). Mental health is not just the absence of illness but a "state of successful mental functioning, resulting in productivity, fulfilling relationships, and ability to adapt to change and cope with adversity" (DHHS, 2000, p. 37). Over a 12-month period, 60% of those with a mental disorder got no treatment at all. Improvements are needed to speed initiation of treatment as well as enhancing the quality and duration of treatment (Wang, 2005).

Adults and older adults have the highest rates of depression, with about 1 in 20 American adults experiencing major depression in a given year. Major depression affects twice as many women as men. Research suggests that for women menopausal transition is linked to new onset of depressive symptoms (Cohen, 2006). There is a high rate of depression among those with chronic conditions; one in three people who have survived a heart attack develop depression (National Institute of Mental Health [NIMH], 2006). Major depression is the leading cause of all disabilities and the cause of more than two thirds of suicides each year. Financial costs from lost work time are high. Unfortunately, there is still widespread misunderstanding about mental illness and associated stigmatization, which often prevents individuals with depression from getting professional help.

Depression affects daily functioning and, in some cases, incapacitates the individual. Depression is a common condition that is often not recognized by health care providers in the community (Brown, 2004). Home care nurses use the OASIS (outcome and assessment information set) method of assessment, which is discussed in Chapter 12. A modified version of the OASIS Depressive Symptoms Items is found in Box 9-6.

Depression is a treatable condition—medications and psychologic treatment are effective for most people suffering from depression. But to receive treatment, people with depression have to be identified and encouraged to seek help. An important role of the nurse in community-based care is to identify those experiencing depression and convince them to seek assistance early.

There is an urgent need for improving detection and treatment of depression and other mental illness as a means of reducing suicide (NIMH, 2003). At least 90% of people who commit suicide have had or are experiencing mental illness, a substance abuse disorder, or a combination; therefore, it is essential that health care professionals be diligent about screening and intervention when mental

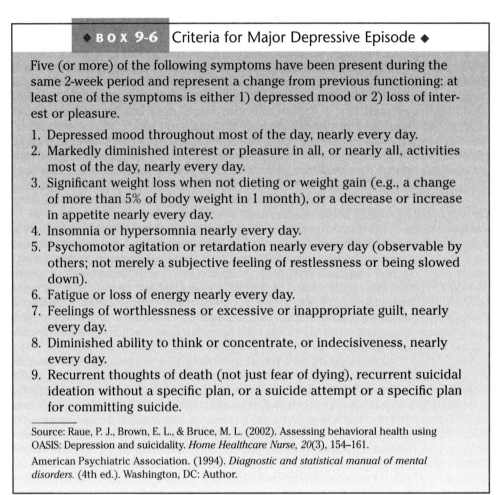

◆ **BOX 9-6**   Criteria for Major Depressive Episode ◆

Five (or more) of the following symptoms have been present during the same 2-week period and represent a change from previous functioning: at least one of the symptoms is either 1) depressed mood or 2) loss of interest or pleasure.

1. Depressed mood throughout most of the day, nearly every day.
2. Markedly diminished interest or pleasure in all, or nearly all, activities most of the day, nearly every day.
3. Significant weight loss when not dieting or weight gain (e.g., a change of more than 5% of body weight in 1 month), or a decrease or increase in appetite nearly every day.
4. Insomnia or hypersomnia nearly every day.
5. Psychomotor agitation or retardation nearly every day (observable by others; not merely a subjective feeling of restlessness or being slowed down).
6. Fatigue or loss of energy nearly every day.
7. Feelings of worthlessness or excessive or inappropriate guilt, nearly every day.
8. Diminished ability to think or concentrate, or indecisiveness, nearly every day.
9. Recurrent thoughts of death (not just fear of dying), recurrent suicidal ideation without a specific plan, or a suicide attempt or a specific plan for committing suicide.

Source: Raue, P. J., Brown, E. L., & Bruce, M. L. (2002). Assessing behavioral health using OASIS: Depression and suicidality. *Home Healthcare Nurse, 20*(3), 154–161.

American Psychiatric Association. (1994). *Diagnostic and statistical manual of mental disorders.* (4th ed.). Washington, DC: Author.

illness is suspected. Again, nurses should not be afraid to ask questions regarding mental health concerns and to refer clients accordingly. It is important that the proportion of adults with recognized depression who receive treatment continues to rise.

Injuries and Violence

Injury and violence are a serious threat to the health of American adults. Motor vehicle accidents are the most common cause of serious injury among adults. Nearly 40% of all traffic fatalities were related to alcohol use, with drivers between 21 and 24 years old having the highest intoxication rate. About 3 in 10 Americans will be involved in an alcohol-related crash in their lifetimes (National Center for Injury Prevention and Control [NCIPC], 2006).

COMMUNITY-BASED TEACHING ▶ 9-3

Recommendations for Preventing Injuries

- Always wear a seatbelt while in the car.
- Never drive after drinking alcohol.
- Always wear a safety helmet while riding a motorcycle or bicycle.
- Use smoke detectors in your home; check to make sure they work every month, and change the batteries every year.
- Keep the temperature of hot water less than 120°F, particularly if there are children or older adults living in your home.
- If you choose to keep a gun in your home, make sure that the gun and the ammunition are locked up separately and are out of the reach of children.
- Prevent falls by older adults by repairing slippery or uneven walking surfaces, improving poor lighting, and installing secure railings on all stairways.

Adapted from Agency for Health Care Research and Quality (2006). *The Pocket Guide to Good Health for Adults.* Available at http:www.ahrq.gov/ppip/adguide/

Certain types of injuries appear to affect some groups more frequently. Native Americans and Alaskan Natives have disproportionately high death rates from motor vehicle accidents, residential fires, and drowning. There are higher rates of death from unintentional injury among African Americans. In every age group, drowning rates are almost two to four times greater for males than females. Homicide is especially high among African American and Hispanic youths. Nurses must be involved in efforts to reduce death caused by motor vehicle accidents and homicide. Community-Based Teaching 9-3 provides recommendations for preventing injuries in general.

Injuries are among the leading causes of death for women in the United States. Many injuries to women result from violent acts; others are caused by unintentional events such as falls, motor vehicle accidents, burns, drowning, and poisonings. Some injuries affect women more frequently than men, with hip fractures and domestic violence being the most common.

Intentional injury, or physical assault, is a leading cause of injury to women, with more women than men experiencing intimate partner violence. Intimate partner violence is a major cause of violence-related injuries. One in three women injured during a physical assault or rape require medical care. Women are also more likely than men to be murdered in the context of intimate partner violence. From 1976 to 2002, about 11% of homicide victims were killed by an intimate partner (Fox & Zawitz, 2004).

The first and foremost responsibility of the nurse in cases where domestic abuse is suspected is to assess for domestic abuse. Nurses should never be afraid to ask the question, "Do you have any concerns about your personal safety?" In order to be comfortable with this type of assessment, the nurse should acquire basic information about domestic abuse as well as develop basic clinical skills for identifying and assessing domestic abuse. Next, the nurse must be familiar with resources within his or her own community for referral phone numbers and contact persons.

Environmental Quality

An estimated 25% of preventable illnesses worldwide can be attributed to poor environmental quality. Poor air quality, including both ozone (outside air) and tobacco smoke (inside air), is one of the prime contributors. In the United States, air pollution alone is estimated to contribute to 50,000 premature deaths and an estimated $40 billion to $50 billion in health-related costs annually. Incidence of asthma has been on the rise for the past few decades among adults and children.

It is important that the proportion of individuals exposed to poor air quality is reduced, as well as the proportion of nonsmokers exposed to secondhand smoke. One intervention involves teaching clients about the importance of maintaining smoke-free indoor air and the hazards of secondhand smoke. Second, the nurse can teach clients the threat that poor outdoor air quality poses for health and the importance of supporting political candidates and legislation that protect air quality. This topic is discussed in more detail in Chapter 15.

Immunizations

Immunization is cited as one of the greatest achievements of public health in the 20th century. It is important to continue to increase the proportion of children who receive all vaccines, as well as the proportion of adults who are vaccinated annually against the flu. Figure 9-3 summarizes recommended screening, immunization, and health promotion activities.

Access to Health Care

According to Healthy People 2010, access to quality care is important to eliminate health disparities and increase the quality and years of healthy lives for all Americans. One way to improve access is to improve the continuum of care. Until the 1980s, the proportion of people without health insurance gradually declined. Since the late 1980s, this proportion has increased to 25% of the population uninsured for part of the previous year. Half of all young adults ages 18 to 29 do not have health insurance (Rhoades, 2006). The variation in access to health care by race and ethnicity is seen in Figure 9-4.

Use of Complementary Therapies

Increasingly, the benefits of complementary and alternative modalities are seen in empirical research. These modalities are advantageous as primary, secondary, or tertiary prevention strategies. For instance, transcendental meditation improves blood pressure and insulin resistance (Paul-Labrador et al., 2006). This knowledge can be used in primary, secondary, and tertiary interventions with individuals at risk for developing type 2 diabetes or CHD. Acupuncture has been shown to be beneficial for hot flashes (Huang et al., 2006). Tai Chi improves balance and strength with individuals with type 2 diabetes, which leads to increased walking speed, which may in turn lead to greater participation in more rigorous physical activity (Orr et al., 2006).

Recommended Adult Immunization Schedule, by Vaccine and Age Group
UNITED STATES • OCTOBER 2006–SEPTEMBER 2007

Vaccine ▼ / Age group ▶	19–49 years	50–64 years	≥65 years
Tetanus, diphtheria, pertussis (Td/Tdap)[1],*	1-dose Td booster every 10 yrs // Substitute 1 dose of Tdap for Td		
Human papillomavirus (HPV)[2]	3 doses (females)		
Measles, mumps, rubella (MMR)[3],*	1 or 2 doses	1 dose	
Varicella[4],*	2 doses (0, 4–8 wks)	2 doses (0, 4–8 wks)	
Influenza[5],*	1 dose annually	1 dose annually	
Pneumococcal (polysaccharide)[6,7]	1–2 doses		1 dose
Hepatitis A[8],*	2 doses (0, 6–12 mos, or 0, 6–18 mos)		
Hepatitis B[9],*	3 doses (0, 1–2, 4–6 mos)		
Meningococcal[10]	1 or more doses		

*Covered by the Vaccine Injury Compensation Program. NOTE: These recommendations must be read with the footnotes (see reverse).

For all persons in this category who meet the age requirements and who lack evidence of immunity (e.g., lack documentation of vaccination or have no evidence of prior infection)

Recommended if some other risk factor is present (e.g., on the basis of medical, occupational, lifestyle, or other indications)

Recommended Adult Immunization Schedule, by Vaccine and Medical and Other Indications
UNITED STATES • OCTOBER 2006–SEPTEMBER 2007

Vaccine ▼ / Indication ▶	Pregnancy	Congenital immunodeficiency, leukemia, lymphoma, generalized malignancy, cerebrospinal fluid leaks; therapy with alkylating agents, antimetabolites, radiation, or high-dose, long-term corticosteroids	Diabetes, heart disease, chronic pulmonary disease, chronic alcoholism	Asplenia[11] (including elective splenectomy and terminal complement component deficiencies)	Chronic liver disease, recipients of clotting factor concentrates	Kidney failure, end-stage renal disease, recipients of hemodialysis	Human immunodeficiency virus (HIV) infection[3,11]	Healthcare workers
Tetanus, diphtheria, pertussis (Td/Tdap)[1],*	1-dose Td booster every 10 yrs // Substitute 1 dose of Tdap for Td							
Human papillomavirus (HPV)[2]	3 doses for females through age 26 yrs (0, 2, 6 mos)							
Measles, mumps, rubella (MMR)[3],*			1 or 2 doses					
Varicella[4],*			2 doses (0, 4–8 wks)					2 doses
Influenza[5],*	1 dose annually		1 dose annually		1 dose annually			
Pneumococcal (polysaccharide)[6,7]	1–2 doses		1–2 doses					1–2 doses
Hepatitis A[8],*	2 doses (0, 6–12 mos, or 0, 6–18 mos)			2 doses	2 doses (0, 6–12 mos, or 0, 6–18 mos)			
Hepatitis B[9],*	3 doses (0, 1–2, 4–6 mos)				3 doses (0, 1–2, 4–6 mos)			
Meningococcal[10]	1 dose			1 dose	1 dose			

*Covered by the Vaccine Injury Compensation Program. NOTE: These recommendations must be read with the footnotes (see reverse).

For all persons in this category who meet the age requirements and who lack evidence of immunity (e.g., lack documentation of vaccination or have no evidence of prior infection)

Recommended if some other risk factor is present (e.g., on the basis of medical, occupational, lifestyle, or other indications)

Contraindicated

Approved by
the Advisory Committee on Immunization Practices,
the American College of Obstetricians and Gynecologists,
the American Academy of Family Physicians,
and the American College of Physicians

DEPARTMENT OF HEALTH AND HUMAN SERVICES
CENTERS FOR DISEASE CONTROL AND PREVENTION

CDC

This schedule indicates the recommended age groups and medical indications for routine administration of currently licensed vaccines for persons aged ≥19 years, as of October 1, 2006. Licensed combination vaccines may be used whenever any components of the combination are indicated and when the vaccine's other components are not contraindicated. For detailed recommendations on all vaccines, including those used primarily for travelers or that are issued during the year, consult the manufacturers' package inserts and the complete statements from the Advisory Committee on Immunization Practices (www.cdc.gov/nip/publications/acip-list.htm).

Report all clinically significant postvaccination reactions to the Vaccine Adverse Event Reporting System (VAERS). Reporting forms and instructions on filing a VAERS report are available at www.vaers.hhs.gov or by telephone, 800-822-7967.

Information on how to file a Vaccine Injury Compensation Program claim is available at www.hrsa.gov/vaccinecompensation or by telephone, 800-338-2382. To file a claim for vaccine injury, contact the U.S. Court of Federal Claims, 717 Madison Place, N.W., Washington, D.C. 20005; telephone, 202-357-6400.

Additional information about the vaccines in this schedule and contraindications for vaccination is also available at www.cdc.gov/nip or from the CDC-INFO Contact Center at 800-CDC-INFO (800-232-4636) in English and Spanish, 24 hours a day, 7 days a week.

FIGURE 9-3. ▶ Recommended adult immunization schedules. Source: Centers for Disease Control and Prevention. (2006). Retrieved on October 20, 2006, from http://www.cdc.gov/vaccines/recs/schedules/downloads/adult/06-07/adult-schedule.pdf

Footnotes

Recommended Adult Immunization Schedule • UNITED STATES, OCTOBER 2006–SEPTEMBER 2007

1. **Tetanus, diphtheria, and acellular pertussis (Td/Tdap) vaccination.** Adults with uncertain histories of a complete primary vaccination series with diphtheria and tetanus toxoid–containing vaccines should begin or complete a primary vaccination series. A primary series for adults is 3 doses; administer the first 2 doses at least 4 weeks apart and the third dose 6–12 months after the second. Administer a booster dose to adults who have completed a primary series and if the last vaccination was received ≥10 years previously. Tdap or tetanus and diphtheria (Td) vaccine may be used; Tdap should replace a single dose of Td for adults aged <65 years who have not previously received a dose of Tdap (either in the primary series, as a booster, or for wound management). Only one of two Tdap products (Adacel® [sanofi pasteur]) is licensed for use in adults. If the person is pregnant and received the last Td vaccination ≥10 years previously, administer Td during the second or third trimester; if the person received the last Td vaccination in <10 years, administer Tdap during the immediate postpartum period. A one-time administration of 1 dose of Tdap with an interval as short as 2 years from a previous Td vaccination is recommended for postpartum women, close contacts of infants aged <12 months, and all healthcare workers with direct patient contact. In certain situations, Td can be deferred during pregnancy and Tdap substituted in the immediate postpartum period, or Tdap can be given instead of Td to a pregnant woman after an informed discussion with the woman (see www.cdc.gov/nip/publications/acip-list.htm). Consult the ACIP statement for recommendations for administering Td as prophylaxis in wound management (www.cdc.gov/mmwr/preview/mmwrhtml/00041645.htm).

2. **Human papillomavirus (HPV) vaccination.** HPV vaccination is recommended for all women aged ≤26 years who have not completed the vaccine series. Ideally, vaccine should be administered before potential exposure to HPV through sexual activity; however, women who are sexually active should still be vaccinated. Sexually active women who have not been infected with any of the HPV vaccine types receive the full benefit of the vaccination. Vaccination is less beneficial for women who have already been infected with one or more of the four HPV vaccine types. A complete series consists of 3 doses. The second dose should be administered 2 months after the first dose; the third dose should be administered 6 months after the first dose. Vaccination is not recommended during pregnancy. If a woman is found to be pregnant after initiating the vaccination series, the remainder of the 3-dose regimen should be delayed until after completion of the pregnancy.

3. **Measles, mumps, rubella (MMR) vaccination.** *Measles component:* adults born before 1957 can be considered immune to measles. Adults born during or after 1957 should receive ≥1 dose of MMR unless they have a medical contraindication, documentation of ≥1 dose, history of measles based on healthcare provider diagnosis, or laboratory evidence of immunity. A second dose of MMR is recommended for adults who 1) have been recently exposed to measles or in an outbreak setting; 2) have been previously vaccinated with killed measles vaccine; 3) have been vaccinated with an unknown type of measles vaccine during 1963–1967; 4) are students in postsecondary educational institutions; 5) work in ahealthcare facility; or 6) plan to travel internationally. Withhold MMR or other measles-containing vaccines from HIV-infected persons with severe immunosuppression.

   Mumps component: adults born before 1957 can generally be considered immune to mumps. Adults born during or after 1957 should receive 1 dose of MMR unless they have a medical contraindication, history of mumps based on healthcare provider diagnosis, or laboratory evidence of immunity. A second dose of MMR is recommended for adults who 1) are in an age group that is affected during a mumps outbreak; 2) are students in postsecondary educational institutions; 3) work in a healthcare facility; or 4) plan to travel internationally. For unvaccinated healthcare workers born before 1957 who do not have other evidence of mumps immunity, consider giving 1 dose on a routine basis and strongly consider giving a second dose during an outbreak. *Rubella component:* administer 1 dose of MMR vaccine to women whose rubella vaccination history is unreliable or who lack laboratory evidence of immunity. For women of childbearing age, regardless of birth year, routinely determine rubella immunity and counsel women regarding congenital rubella syndrome. Do not vaccinate women who are pregnant or who might become pregnant within 4 weeks of receiving vaccine. Women who do not have evidence of immunity should receive MMR vaccine upon completion or termination of pregnancy and before discharge from the healthcare facility.

4. **Varicella vaccination.** All adults without evidence of immunity to varicella should receive 2 doses of varicella vaccine. Special consideration should be given to those who 1) have close contact with persons at high risk for severe disease (e.g., healthcare workers and family contacts of immunocompromised persons) or 2) are at high risk for exposure or transmission (e.g., teachers of young children; child care employees; residents and staff members of institutional settings, including correctional institutions; college students; military personnel; adolescents and adults living in households with children; nonpregnant women of childbearing age; and international travelers). Evidence of immunity to varicella in adults includes any of the following: 1) documentation of 2 doses of varicella vaccine at least 4 weeks apart; 2) U.S.-born before 1980 (although for healthcare workers and pregnant women, birth before 1980 should not be considered evidence of immunity); 3) history of varicella based on diagnosis or verification of varicella by a healthcare provider (for a patient reporting a history of or presenting with an atypical case, a mild case, or both, healthcare providers should seek either an epidemiologic link with a typical varicella case or evidence of laboratory confirmation, if it was performed at the time of acute disease); 4) history of herpes zoster based on healthcare provider diagnosis; or 5) laboratory evidence of immunity or laboratory confirmation of disease. Do not vaccinate women who are pregnant or might become pregnant within 4 weeks of receiving the vaccine. Assess pregnant women for evidence of varicella immunity. Women who do not have evidence of immunity should receive dose 1 of varicella vaccine upon completion or termination of pregnancy and before discharge from the healthcare facility. Dose 2 should be administered 4–8 weeks after dose 1.

5. **Influenza vaccination.** *Medical indications:* chronic disorders of the cardiovascular or pulmonary systems, including asthma; chronic metabolic diseases, including diabetes mellitus, renal dysfunction, hemoglobinopathies, or immunosuppression (including immunosuppression caused by medications or HIV); any condition that compromises respiratory function or the handling of respiratory secretions or that can increase the risk of aspiration (e.g., cognitive dysfunction, spinal cord injury, or seizure disorder or other neuromuscular disorder); and pregnancy during the influenza season. No data exist on the risk for severe or complicated influenza disease among persons with asplenia; however, influenza is a risk factor for secondary bacterial infections that can cause severe disease among persons with asplenia. *Occupational indications:* healthcare workers and employees of long-term–care and assisted living facilities. *Other indications:* residents of nursing homes and other long-term–care and assisted living facilities; persons likely to transmit influenza to persons at high risk (e.g., in-home household contacts and caregivers of children aged 0–59 months, or persons of all ages with high-risk conditions); and anyone who would like to be vaccinated. Healthy, nonpregnant persons aged 5–49 years without high-risk medical conditions who are not contacts of severely immunocompromised persons in special care units can receive either intranasally administered influenza vaccine (FluMist®) or inactivated vaccine. Other persons should receive the inactivated vaccine.

6. **Pneumococcal polysaccharide vaccination.** *Medical indications:* chronic disorders of the pulmonary system (excluding asthma); cardiovascular diseases; diabetes mellitus; chronic liver diseases, including liver disease as a result of alcohol abuse (e.g., cirrhosis); chronic renal failure or nephrotic syndrome; functional or anatomic asplenia (e.g., sickle cell disease or splenectomy [if elective splenectomy is planned, vaccinate at least 2 weeks before surgery]); immunosuppressive conditions (e.g., congenital immunodeficiency, HIV infection [vaccinate as close to diagnosis as possible when CD4 cell counts are highest], leukemia, lymphoma, multiple myeloma, Hodgkin disease, generalized malignancy, or organ or bone marrow transplantation); chemotherapy with alkylating agents, antimetabolites, or high-dose, long-term corticosteroids; and cochlear implants. *Other indications:* Alaska Natives and certain American Indian populations and residents of nursing homes or other long-term–care facilities.

7. **Revaccination with pneumococcal polysaccharide vaccine.** One-time revaccination after 5 years for persons with chronic renal failure or nephrotic syndrome; functional or anatomic asplenia (e.g., sickle cell disease or splenectomy); immunosuppressive conditions (e.g., congenital immunodeficiency, HIV infection, leukemia, lymphoma, multiple myeloma, Hodgkin disease, generalized malignancy, or organ or bone marrow transplantation); or chemotherapy with alkylating agents, antimetabolites, or high-dose, long-term corticosteroids. For persons aged ≥65 years, one-time revaccination if they were vaccinated ≥5 years previously and were aged <65 years at the time of primary vaccination.

8. **Hepatitis A vaccination.** *Medical indications:* persons with chronic liver disease and persons who receive clotting factor concentrates. *Behavioral indications:* men who have sex with men and persons who use illegal drugs. *Occupational indications:* persons working with hepatitis A virus (HAV)–infected primates or with HAV in a research laboratory setting. *Other indications:* persons traveling to or working in countries that have high or intermediate endemicity of hepatitis A (a list of countries is available at www.cdc.gov/travel/diseases.htm) and any person who would like to obtain immunity. Current vaccines should be administered in a 2-dose schedule at either 0 and 6–12 months, or 0 and 6–18 months. If the combined hepatitis A and hepatitis B vaccine is used, administer 3 doses at 0, 1, and 6 months.

9. **Hepatitis B vaccination.** *Medical indications:* persons with end-stage renal disease, including patients receiving hemodialysis; persons seeking evaluation or treatment for a sexually transmitted disease (STD); persons with HIV infection; persons with chronic liver disease; and persons who receive clotting factor concentrates. *Occupational indications:* healthcare workers and public-safety workers who are exposed to blood or other potentially infectious body fluids. *Behavioral indications:* sexually active persons who are not in a long-term, mutually monogamous relationship (i.e., persons with >1 sex partner during the previous 6 months); current or recent injection-drug users; and men who have sex with men. *Other indications:* household contacts and sex partners of persons with chronic hepatitis B virus (HBV) infection; clients and staff members of institutions for persons with developmental disabilities; all clients of STD clinics; international travelers to countries with high or intermediate prevalence of chronic HBV infection (a list of countries is available at www.cdc.gov/travel/diseases.htm); and any adult seeking protection from HBV infection. Settings where hepatitis B vaccination is recommended for all adults: STD treatment facilities; HIV testing and treatment facilities; facilities providing drug-abuse treatment and prevention services; healthcare settings providing services for injection-drug users or men who have sex with men; correctional facilities; end-stage renal disease programs and facilities for chronic hemodialysis patients; and institutions and nonresidential daycare facilities for persons with developmental disabilities. *Special formulation indications:* for adult patients receiving hemodialysis and other immunocompromised adults, 1 dose of 40 μg/mL (Recombivax HB®) or 2 doses of 20 μg/mL (Engerix-B®).

10. **Meningococcal vaccination.** *Medical indications:* adults with anatomic or functional asplenia, or terminal complement component deficiencies. *Other indications:* first-year college students living in dormitories; microbiologists who are routinely exposed to isolates of *Neisseria meningitidis*; military recruits; and persons who travel to or live in countries in which meningococcal disease is hyperendemic or epidemic (e.g., the "meningitis belt" of sub-Saharan Africa during the dry season [December–June]), particularly if their contact with local populations will be prolonged. Vaccination is required by the government of Saudi Arabia for all travelers to Mecca during the annual Hajj. Meningococcal conjugate vaccine is preferred for adults with any of the preceding indications who are aged ≤55 years, although meningococcal polysaccharide vaccine (MPSV4) is an acceptable alternative. Revaccination after 5 years might be indicated for adults previously vaccinated with MPSV4 who remain at high risk for infection (e.g., persons residing in areas in which disease is epidemic).

11. **Selected conditions for which *Haemophilus influenzae* type b (Hib) vaccine may be used.** Hib conjugate vaccines are licensed for children aged 6 weeks–71 months. No efficacy data are available on which to base a recommendation concerning use of Hib vaccine for older children and adults with the chronic conditions associated with an increased risk for Hib disease. However, studies suggest good immunogenicity in patients who have sickle cell disease, leukemia, or HIV infection or who have had splenectomies; administering vaccine to these patients is not contraindicated.

Use of trade names and commercial sources is for identification only and does not imply endorsement by the U.S. Department of Health and Human Services.

FIGURE 9-3. ▶ *Continued*

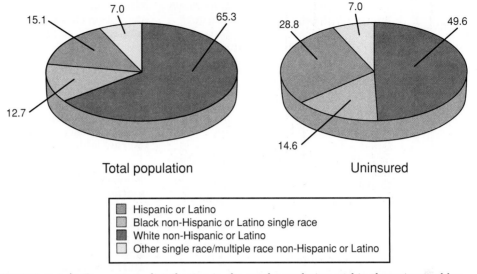

FIGURE 9-4. ▶ Percentage distribution in the total population and in the uninsured by race/ethnicity of people under age 65, in 2004.

Source: Rhoades, J. A. (2006). *The uninsured in America, 2004: Estimates for the U.S. civilian noninstitutionalized population under age 65.* Agency for Healthcare Research and Quality. Retrieved on October 19, 2006, from http://www.meps.ahrq.gov/mepsweb/data_files/publications/st83/stat83.pdf

CONCLUSIONS

Current critical issues of health and health care have changed dramatically in the past 100 years. Today, most diseases and deaths result from preventable causes. The nurse plays an essential role in early identification of and intervention in these conditions. Nurses can be successful in this charge by screening, particularly in high-risk groups. By identifying conditions early in their course, nurses can provide interventions that will substantially minimize the effects of these conditions. By following the health indicators identified by Healthy People 2010, nurses can help adults live longer and healthier lives.

What's on the Web

American Social Health Association (ASHA)
P.O. Box 13827
Research Triangle Park, NC 27709
Internet address: http://www.ashastd.org
The ASHA has been providing health information to the American public since 1914. They are recognized by the public, clients, providers, and policy makers for develop-

ing and delivering accurate, medically reliable information about STDs. Public and college health clinics across the United States order ASHA's educational pamphlets and books to give to clients and students. Community-based organizations depend on ASHA, too, to help communicate about risk, transmission, prevention, testing, and treatment.

The Pocket Guide to Good Health for Adults
Internet address: http://www.ahrq.gov/
ppip/adguide/
This online consumer guide from the
AHRQ explains preventive care for adults.
Print copies, available free of charge, can
be requested by calling (800) 358-9295 or
e-mail at ahrqpubs@ahrq.gov. The guide is
also available in Spanish.

Cookbooks
*Heart-Healthy Home Cooking African Ameri-
can Style*
Internet address: http://www.nhlbi.nih.
gov/health/public/heart/other/chdblack/
cooking.htm

Delicious Heart-Healthy Latino Recipes
(bilingual cookbook)
Internet address: http://www.nhlbi.nih.
gov/health/public/heart/other/sp_recip.htm
Print copies can be ordered for a small fee
by phone at (301) 892-8573

Obesity Education Initiative
Internet address: http://www.nhlbi.nih.
gov/about/oei/index.htm
This excellent Web site offers abundant
information for providers, clients, and
public educators related to obesity, produced by the National Heart, Lung, and
Blood Institute.

Resources for Alcoholism
Al-Anon Family Group Headquarters, Inc.
Internet address: http://www.al-anon.
alateen.org/
This Web site makes referrals to local Al-
Anon groups, which are support groups
for sponsors and other significant adults
in an alcoholic person's life.

Alcoholics Anonymous (AA) World
Services, Inc.
Internet address: http://www.aa.org

National Council on Alcoholism and Drug
Dependence (NCADD)
Internet address: http://www.ncadd.org
This Web site lists telephone numbers
of local NCADD affiliates that can
provide information on local treatment
resources and educational materials on
alcoholism.

National Institute on Alcohol Abuse and
Alcoholism (NIAAA)
Internet address: http://www.niaaa.nih.
gov
This site offers free publications on all
aspects of alcohol abuse and alcoholism,
with some in Spanish.

Resources for Cancer Screening
American Cancer Society
Internet address: http://www.cancer.org

National Cancer Institute
Internet address: http://www.nci.
nih.gov

National Cancer Institute Cervical Cancer
Information
Internet address: http://cancernet.nci.
nih.gov

National Cervical Cancer Coalition
Internet address: http://www.nccc-
online.org

Resources for Chronic Disease
Prevention
Internet address:
http://www.naccho.org/topics/HPDP/
chronicdisease/overview.cfm

Resources for Domestic Violence
National Domestic Violence Hotline
Hotline number: 1-800-799–SAFE (7233)
1-800-787-3224 (TTY)
Internet address: http://www.ndvh.org/
The Web site and hotline number provide
information for individuals experiencing
domestic abuse. The hotline is available
24 hours a day and 365 days a year. There
is a database of 4,000 shelters and services across the United States, Puerto
Rico, Alaska, Hawaii, and the U.S. Virgin
Islands. With just one contact, those
experiencing domestic violence can find
out about the options available in their
own community. Bilingual services are
available.

Resources for Smoking Cessation
American Lung Association
Tobacco Control

Internet address: http://www.lungusa.org/tobacco

National Center for Chronic Disease Prevention and Health Promotion
Chronic Disease Prevention: Risk Behaviors—Tobacco Use
Internet address: http://www.cdc.gov/tobacco/edumat.htm

Nursing Center for Tobacco Intervention
Internet address: http://www.con.ohio-state.edu/tobacco
This Web site is designed to increase nurse provider participation in the delivery of tobacco cessation interventions with all tobacco users. This site has excellent information as well as links to other sites with outstanding teaching materials for health education.

Quick Reference Guide for Clinicians: Treating Tobacco Use and Dependence
Internet address: http://www.surgeongeneral.gov/tobacco/tobaqrg.pdf
This guide summarizes the strategies for providing appropriate treatments for every client who could benefit from a smoking cessation program.

Virtual Office of the Surgeon General
Reducing Tobacco Use Report
Internet address: http://www.surgeongeneral.gov/tobacco/smokesum.htm.

Patient and Provider Education Materials for the Seasonal Flu
Internet address: http://www.cdc.gov/flu/professionals/patiented.htm

References and Bibliography

Agency for Healthcare Research and Quality. (2003). Assessing health care quality for minority and other disparity populations.

Agency for Healthcare Research and Quality. (2004). *Health care disparities in rural areas.* Retrieved on October 15, 2006, from http://www.ahrq.gov

Agency for Healthcare Research and Quality. (2005). *Fact sheet: Women's health care in the United States.* HRQ Publication No. 00–P041). Rockville, MD. Retrieved October 16, 2006, from http://www.ahrq.gov/

American Psychiatric Association. (1994). *Diagnostic and statistical manual of mental disorders.* (4th ed.) Washington, DC: Author.

Brown, E. L., Bruce, M. L., Faue, P., & Nassisi, P. (2004). How well do clinicians recognize depression in home care patients? *Home Healthcare Nurse, 22*(8), 569–571. Retrieved on October 30, 2007, from http://www.ahrq.gov/qual/qdisprep.pdf

Centers for Disease Control. (2006). Fact sheet: health effects of cigarette smoking. Retrieved on October 30, 2007, from http://www.cdc.gov/tobacco/data_statictics/Factsheets/health_effects.htm

Centers for Disease Control and Prevention. (2004). Reportable sexually transmitted disease in the United States, 2004. Retrieved on October 30, 2007, from http://www.cdc.gov/std/stats04/trends2004.htm

Centers for Disease Control and Prevention. (2006). Breast cancer. *Screening guidelines.* Retrieved on October 17, 2006, from http://www.cdc.gov/cancer/breast/basic_info/screening.htm

Centers for Disease Control and Prevention. (2006b). *CDC releases revised HIV testing recommendations in healthcare settings.* Retrieved on October 18, 2006, from http://www.cdc.gov/hiv/topics/testing/resources/factsheets/pdf/healthcare.pdf

Centers for Disease Control and Prevention. (2006c). Colorectal (colon) cancer. *Screening guidelines.* Retrieved on October 17, 2006, from http://www.cdc.gov/cancer/colorectal/basic_info/screening/guidelines.htm

Centers for Disease Control and Prevention. (2006d). Fact sheet 2006: Prostate cancer initiatives. Retrieved on October 17, 2006, from http://apps.nccd.cdc.gov/EmailForm/print_table.asp

Centers for Disease Control and Prevention. (2006e). *Skin cancer: preventing America's most common cancer fact sheet, 2002.* Retrieved on October 17, 2006, from http://www.cdc.gov/HealthyYouth/skincancer/pdf/facts.pdf

Cohen, L. S., Soares, C. N., Vitonis, A. F., et al. (2006). Risk for new onset of depression during the menopausal transition: The Harvard Study of moods and cycles. *Archives of General Psychiatry, 63,* 385–390.

Fiore, M., Bailey, W., Cohen, S., et al. (2000). *Quick reference guide for clinicians: Treating tobacco use and dependence.* Rockville, MD: U.S. Department of Health and Human Services, Public Health Service. Retrieved February 5, 2003, from http://www.surgeongeneral.gov/tobacco/tobaqrg.htm

Fox, J. A., & Zawitz, M. W. (2004). *Homicide trends in the United States.* Washington, DC: Department of Justice. Retrieved on October 19, 2006, from http://www.ojp.usdoj.gov/bjs/homicide/homtrnd.htm

Greenland, P., & Gulati, M. (2006). Improving outcomes for women with myocardial infarction. *Archives of Internal Medicine, 166,* 1162–1163.

Health Effects of Cigarette Smoking Fact Sheets, 2004.

Healthcare in the News. (2006). *Gum disease linked to chronic health conditions.* Retrieved on October 30, 2007, from http://www.stronghealth.com/encyclopedia/contents.cfm?pageid=P08637

Huang, M. I., Nir, Y., Chen, B., Schnyer, R., & Manber, R. (2006). A randomized controlled pilot study of acupuncture for postmenopausal hot flashes: Effect on nocturnal hot flashes and sleep quality. *Fertility and Sterility, 86*(3), 700–710.

Kessler, R. C., Berglund, P., Demler, O., et al. (2005). Lifetime prevalence and age-of-onset distributions of DSM-IV disorders in the National Comorbidity Survey Replication. *Archives of General Psychiatry, 62*(6), 593–602.

Mougios, V., Kazaki, M., Christoulas, K., et al., (2006). Does the intensity of an exercise programme modulate body composition changes? *International Journal of Sports Medicine, 27,* 178–181.

Mukamal, K. J., Conigrave, K. M., Mittleman, M. A., et al. (2003). Roles of drinking pattern and type of alcohol consumed in coronary heart disease in men. *New England Journal of Medicine, 348*(2), 109–118.

National Center for Health Statistics. (2005). *Chartbook on trends in the health of Americans.* Retrieved on October 30, 2007, from http://www.cdc.gov/nchs/pressroom/04news/hus04.htm

National Center for Injury Prevention and Control [NCIPC]. (2006). Injury prevention: Motor vehicle injuries. Retrieved on October 19, 2006, from http://www.cdc.gov/programs/injury 02.htm

National Institute of Alcohol Abuse and Alcoholism. (2006). Report to the Extramural Advisory Board, 2006, Division of Epidemiology and Prevention Research. Retrieved on October 18, 2006, from http://www.niaaa.nih.gov/NR/rdonlyres/802A4ECB-D680-4E8B-BF36-319D06412167/0/Briefing Book2.pdf

National Institute of Alcohol Abuse and Alcoholism. (2005). *Percent reporting heavy alcohol use in the past month by age group and demographic characteristics: NSDUH (NHSDA), 1994–2002.* Retrieved on October 18, 2006, from http://www.niaaa.nih.gov/Resources/DatabaseResources/QuickFacts/AlcoholConsumption/dkpat21.htm

National Institutes of Health, National Heart, Lung, and Blood Institute, Obesity Education Initiative. (1998). *The practical guide: Identification, evaluation, and treatment of overweight and obesity in adults.* Bethesda, MD: U.S. Department of Health and Human Services.

National Institutes of Health. (2000). *The practical guide: Identification, evaluation, and treatment of overweight and obesity in adults.* National Heart, Lung, and Blood Institute Obesity Education Initiative. NIH Publication Number 00-4084. Retrieved on October 17, 2006, from http://www.nhlbi.nih.gov/guidelines/obesity/prctgd_c.pdf

National Institute of Mental Health. (2003). *Older adults: Depression and suicide facts.* Retrieved on October 19, 2006, from http://www.nimh.nih.gov/publicat/elderlydepsuicide.cfm

National Institute of Mental Health. (2006). Depression and heart disease. Retrieved on October 30, 2007, from http://www.emoryhealthcare.org/departments/fuqua/patient_info/depheart.pdf

Orr, R., Tsang, R., Lam, P., et al. (2006). Mobility impairment in type 2 diabetes: association with muscle power and effect of Tai Chi intervention. *Diabetes Care, 29,* 2120–2122.

Paul-Labrador, M., Polk, D., Dwyer, J. H., et al. (2006). Effects of randomized controlled trail of transcendental meditation on components of the metabolic syndrome in subjects with coronary heart disease. *Archives of Internal Medicine, 166*(11), 1218–1224.

Paxon, S. (2005, March 2). Paper presented at national conference on chronic disease prevention and control. Retrieved on October 16, 2006, from http://www.cdc.gov/nchs/data/series/sr_10/sr10_232.pdf

Pew Research. (2006). *Americans see weight problems everywhere but in the mirror.* Retrieved on October 18, 2006, from http://pewresearch.org/assets/social/pdf/Obesity.pdf

Preventing Chronic Diseases: Fact Sheet. (2005). Centers for Disease Control. Retrieved on October 17, 2006, from http://www.cdc.gov/nccdphp/publications/factsheets/Prevention/pdf/tobacco.pdf

Raue, P. J., Brown, E. L., & Bruce, M. L. (2002). Assessing behavioral health using OASIS: Part 1: Depression and suicidality. *Home Healthcare Nurse, 20*(3), 154–161.

Rhoades, J. A. (2006). *The uninsured in America: 2004: Estimates for the U.S. Civilian Noninstitutionalized Population under Age 65.* Agency for Healthcare Research and Quality. Retrieved on October 19, 2006, from http://www.meps.ahrq.gov/mepsweb/data_files/publications/st83/stat83.pdf

Rice, V. H., & Stead, L. F. (2006). Nursing interventions for smoking cessation. Cochrane Database System Review, 1, CD001188.

Teutsch, S. (2006). Cost-effectiveness of prevention. Retrieved on October 20, 2006, from http://www.medscape.com/viewarticle/540199

Treating tobacco use and dependence [Fact sheet]. (2000, June). U.S. Public Health Service. Retrieved June 10, 2003, from http://www.surgeongeneral.gov/tobacco/smokfact.htm

Trends in HIV/AIDS–33 States, 2001–2004. (2005). *MMWR, 54*(45),1149–1153. Retrieved on October 18, 2006, from http://www.cdc.gov/mmwr/preview/mmwrhtml/mm5445a1.htm

U.S. Department of Health and Human Services. (2000). *Healthy people 2010. National health promotion and disease prevention objectives.* Washington, DC: U.S. Government Printing Office.

U.S. Department of Health and Human Services. (2005). Vital and health statistics. *Summary health statistics for U.S. adults: National health interview survey, 2005.* Series 10, Number 232. Retrieved on October 16, 2006, from http://www.cdc.gov/nchs/data/series/sr_10/sr10_232.pdf

Wang, P. S., Berglund, P., Olfson, M., et al. (2005). Failure and delay in initial treatment contact after first onset of mental disorders in National Comorbidity Survey Replication. *Archives of General Psychiatry 62*(6), 603–613.

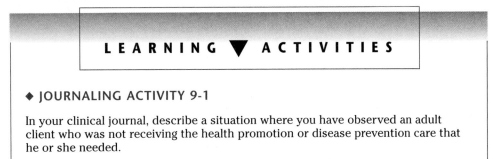

LEARNING ▼ ACTIVITIES

◆ JOURNALING ACTIVITY 9-1

In your clinical journal, describe a situation where you have observed an adult client who was not receiving the health promotion or disease prevention care that he or she needed.

- What intervention would the client have benefited from receiving?
- How would you advocate for these issues when you begin to practice as an RN?
- What could you do now?
- Do you see evidence that the current health care system values and provides prevention and health promotion care? Why do you think that this type of care is or is not valued or provided? What arguments would you make that health care should provide such an emphasis in care?

◆ JOURNALING ACTIVITY 9-2

1. In your clinical journal, describe a situation you have encountered when screening and doing health promotion and disease prevention teaching and planning with an adult client.

- What did you learn from this experience?
- How will you practice differently based on this experience?

◆ CLIENT CARE ACTIVITY 9-3

You are working as a home care nurse, caring for Richard, a 45-year-old client who has advanced chronic obstructive pulmonary disease (COPD) and is on oxygen constantly. Richard, a former smoker, has had several upper respiratory infections this winter, with one resulting in hospitalization for a week. Richard lives with his 25-year-old daughter and her husband, who are both teachers and heavy smokers.

- Which health indicators contribute to Richard's health status?
- What could you as the nurse for this family do to promote Richard's health?
- What community health interventions would you use?
- What steps will you take to address this issue?

◆ PRACTICAL APPLICATION ACTIVITY 9-4

In a community-based setting, survey the people there to identify their health promotion and disease prevention needs. With some of the people from the agency, either staff members and clients or both participating in the discussion, determine the best way to provide health promotion and disease prevention teaching and care. Use the resources in the chapter to develop teaching sheets and classes. What's on the Web has several great sites listed in Chapters 9 and 10.

◆ CRITICAL THINKING ACTIVITY 9-5

You are visiting with a family friend who asks you about your studies in nursing classes. You explain that you are studying about disease prevention and health promotion. The friend, who is 45 years old, says, "I am not sick. What would someone my age need to do to prevent disease?"

- What would be your response to his question?

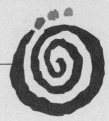

10

Health Promotion and Disease Prevention for Elderly Adults

ROBERTA HUNT

LEARNING OBJECTIVES

1. Identify the major causes of death for the elderly.
2. Discuss the major diseases and threats to the health of elderly adults.
3. Summarize the major health issues for older adults.
4. Identify nursing roles for each level of prevention for major health issues affecting elderly adults.
5. Compose a list of nursing interventions for the major health issues of older adults.
6. Determine health needs of the elderly for which a nurse could be an advocate.

KEY TERMS

life expectancy at birth
life expectancy at 65 or 85
medication safety

personal definition of health
polypharmacy

CHAPTER TOPICS

◆ **Health Status of Elderly Adults**
◆ **Health Screening in Elderly Adults**
◆ **Interventions for Leading Health Indicators**
◆ **Conclusions**

THE NURSE SPEAKS

Bea was unforgettable. She was a woman who had lived a hard life, which was reflected in her face and physical condition. She was short, thin, missing several teeth, and appeared older than her 73 years. Most remarkable was Bea's short vibrant red-orange hair, which spiked out in all directions. There were never any cards or flowers or visitors in Bea's room, but it was reported that her husband visited in the evening. Bea was not the kind of patient to inspire extra staff support, but Bea's continued presence on the unit and her weekly assignment to one of the students resulted in visits by almost all of the students each week. The students found her mysterious past, red hair, and one-of-a-kind smile hard to resist.

Spring break and on-campus activities had resulted in several weeks away from the unit. On our return, I was surprised to find Bea still on the unit. She had undergone additional major surgery and once again spent time in intensive care on mechanical ventilation. The staff noted that she was supposed to be up and walking, but when brought to a standing position, she would throw herself back on the bed, dead weight and hard to move despite her less than 100 pounds. The nursing staff felt I might be able to find a more interesting patient than Bea, so I assigned Bea to a student who had not yet cared for her. The next morning, I went in to check on the student and Bea. Bea still had that amazing red hair (which seemed a little more gray at the base), she was thinner (if that could be possible), she looked tired, and there was no smile. She was alone in a dark double room in the bed farthest from the door, a central line was infusing a variety of fluids, and she wore a nasal cannula for oxygen.

Two students were talking to Bea about their plans for the summer, beginning with a much-anticipated massage. I joined the conversation and agreed there was nothing more relaxing than a day at the spa. I asked Bea if she would like to have a spa day and suggested that if she did, she and the student plan it for the next day. Bea was noncommittal. In postconference, Bea's spa day was discussed. The next morning, each of the students asked me if Bea's student was going ahead with the spa day.

About 9 o'clock, I finally made it to Bea's room. I had brought my lavender essential oil and planned to demonstrate how to use the oil to provide a hand massage. The student noted that Bea was presently resting, having received a complete bath and a long massage. Prior to the bath, the student had suggested that Bea get up for a short walk. According to the student, and to the amazement of the staff, Bea popped out of bed and circled the unit, leaving the student struggling to keep up. No wonder Bea was resting. Around 10 o'clock, we got Bea up in a chair, wrapped her in a warm bath blanket obtained from preop, and washed her hair using the hair-wash-in-a-hat. Bea's hair looked great—soft, shiny, clean, and, of course, very red. A foot soak was prepared using a few drops of lavender essential oil. The aroma of lavender began to fill the room. The student asked Bea if she would like a hand massage, and Bea agreed after some convincing. As the student began the steps of the hand massage, using Jane Buckle's 'M' Technique and a 5% lavender essential oil solution, Bea closed her eyes and snuggled into her blanket. When it came to massaging the second hand, Bea was ready. The aroma of lavender now filled the room and wafted into the hall. The students started stopping by. They reminded Bea who they were and asked her how her spa day was going. The students told Bea how relaxed and comfortable she looked and expressed some envy.

Eventually Bea was returned to a fresh bed with the curtains pulled back. Staff walking by the door started stopping in, wondering what was going on. They told Bea she smelled great and so did her room. The student told the staff about Bea's spa day as she reported off. Each of the nursing staff commented that this was what they had gone into nursing for and never had the time to do. Staff members also observed that they had never seen Bea look so great. During postconference, Bea's student shared how excited the staff was about Bea's spa day. The staff noted she looked much better and were definitely impressed by her walk around the unit, the first in a long time. The social worker decided she wanted to see for herself what this was all about, so she went in to see Bea and asked her how her morning had gone. Bea stated, "This is the first time I have felt like a real person in a long time."

Now whether this change in Bea was due to the massage, the hair wash, the warm blanket, the essential oil, an increase in positive social interaction, or Bea's own self-determination, it is hard to know. I like to think that it was a holistic intervention plan focused on Bea, helping her and those about her find Bea, a woman with strength, a great smile, a mysterious past, and amazing hair.

—MARY KATHRYN MOBERG, MS, RN, Associate Professor, The College of St. Catherine

HEALTH STATUS OF ELDERLY ADULTS

Life expectancy at birth, as well as **life expectancy at ages 65 and 85**, has increased over time as death rates for many causes of death have declined. Life expectancy at birth is the number of years that a person born in that year can expect to live. Life expectancy at 65 or 85 is the number of years that a person who is 65 or 85 years old can expect to live. The leading causes of death for elderly adults are listed in Table 10-1. The largest decrease in mortality has been in death rates for heart disease and stroke; death rates for pneumonia and influenza have increased in the past 2 decades (Centers for Disease Control and Prevention [CDC], 2007).

The elderly population in the United States is growing. Life expectancies at ages 65 and 85 have increased over the past 50 years. People who live to age 65 can expect to live, on average, nearly 18 more years. Since 1900, the percentage of people 65 years and older has tripled. In 1994, about 1 in 8 Americans were elderly but about 1 in 5 would be elderly by the year 2030. In addition, the elderly population will continue to be more and more diverse (Hobbs, 2006). This growing segment

TABLE 10-1 Leading Causes of Death in Adults 65 Years and Older, United States, 2004	
Cause of Death	**Number**
Heart disease	533,302
Cancer	385,847
Stroke	130,538

Source: Centers for Disease Control and Prevention. (2006). Office of Statistics and Programming, National Center for Injury Prevention and Control. Retrieved on October 20, 2006, from http://webapp.cdc.gov/sasweb/ncipc/leadcaus10.html

of the population has health care needs that are different from those of other segments of the population. Of people older than 70 years, 80% have one or more chronic conditions.

Living arrangements of persons over 65 years of age show that as people age, they are more likely to live alone. Further, they are more likely to have difficulty performing one or more physical activities, activities of daily living (ADL), or instrumental activities of daily living (IADL). Figure 10-1 shows selected chronic conditions limiting activity for people older than 65. All of these factors have implications for the ability of the elderly to perform self-care and live independently while managing a chronic illness and the amount of nursing care this population may need as they age (Administration on Aging, 2005).

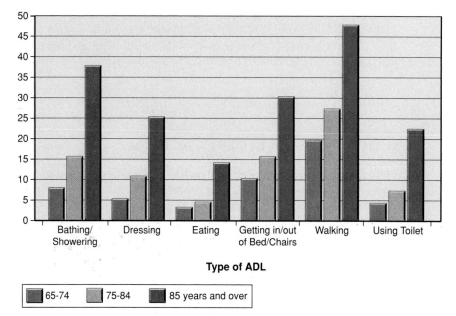

FIGURE 10-1. ▶ Percentage of persons with limitations in activities of daily living (ADL), by age group, in 2003. Source: Administration on Aging. *A profile of older Americans, 2005.* Retrieved on October 20, 2006, from http://www.aoa.gov/PROF/Statistics/profile/2005/2005profile.pdf.

HEALTH SCREENING IN ELDERLY ADULTS

As with clients at other ages, health screening for the elderly is intended for primary, secondary, or tertiary prevention. Primary prevention (to prevent the initial occurrence of a disease) with an elderly client could be immunization screening, recommendation of an annual flu shot, or a safety assessment of the home to identify areas where a fall could occur. Examples of secondary prevention are screening for hypertension and teaching breast self-examination to a group or an individual. Tertiary prevention could be initiating an exercise program for an elderly client who has heart disease or a home safety check to eliminate hazards that may result in falls. Screening is always performed so that people at risk for certain conditions can be identified, with interventions provided as appropriate.

One way to encourage the elderly client to put prevention into practice is to use *The Pocket Guide for Staying Healthy at 50+*. This guide is available online at http://www.ahcpr.gov/ppip/50plus/50plus.pdf, or it can be ordered free by calling (800) 358-9295 or email ahrqpubs@ahrq.gov. It includes recommendations about lifestyle choices that prevent certain chronic diseases, primary prevention screening, and immunizations. It is an excellent tool for guiding health promotion and disease prevention activities.

General Screening

All screening discussed for adults also applies to elderly adults. This section discusses screening that is particularly important for elderly adults. The American College of Preventive Medicine has identified the most effective and cost-effective clinical preventive services. Among the services that apply to the elderly are aspirin to prevent heart disease; screening and counseling for tobacco use and problem drinking; screening for colorectal cancer, cervical cancer, vision impairment, blood pressure, and cholesterol; and pneumococcal and influenza immunizations (Teutsch, 2006).

High blood pressure is more common in people over age 45, especially African Americans. Therefore, the elderly should have their blood pressure checked periodically, with the frequency determined by their nurse practitioner or physician. Cholesterol levels start to increase in middle-aged men, in women just before menopause, and in anyone who has just gained weight; cholesterol should be measured in people meeting these descriptions.

Heart disease is the leading cause of death for people over 65 years of age. Heart disease is the number-one killer of women, yet only 8% of women realize that it is a greater threat than cancer. Research in Community-Based Nursing Care 10-1 provides more information about the disparity of care and knowledge of the differences among heart disease in men as compared to women. Thirty-eight percent of women and 25% of men will die within 1 year of the first recognized heart attack, and 46% of female and 22% of male heart attack survivors will be disabled within 6 years. Women are almost twice as likely as men to die after bypass surgery (National Coalition of Women with Heart Disease, 2007).

As with other chronic conditions, the risk factors for developing heart disease should be identified and addressed in childhood (e.g., poor diet, lack of exercise, smoking, and weight gain). It is essential that every adult be aware of his or her own risk factors for heart disease.

RESEARCH IN COMMUNITY-BASED NURSING CARE ▶ 10-1

Women's Heart Disease: New Study Shows Differences

Despite the fact that cardiovascular disease is the leading cause of death in women, researchers are only beginning to understand that heart disease in women is screened for, measured, and treated differently compared to heart disease in men. This is an important discovery because recent statistics have shown that the rate of heart disease has declined in men but not in women. The WISE–short for Women's Ischemia Syndrome Evaluation–has discovered some of the differences between heart disease in men and in women. Rather than having disease that is characterized by obvious occlusion of coronary vessels, women tend to have small areas of build-up of plaque, causing microvascular disease not usually apparent on coronary angiogram. Consequently both risk factors and symptoms for coronary artery disease (CAD) differ between men and women. The risk factors that contribute to the development of heart disease include: metabolic syndrome, mental stress and depression, and smoking; all have a greater impact on women compared with men. Further, low levels of estrogen before menopause is a significant risk factor for developing microvascular disease. Women will often have some chest pain but it may not be the most prominent symptom. Rather, they may experience neck, shoulder, upper back, or abdominal discomfort; shortness of breath; nausea or vomiting; sweating; lightheadedness or dizziness; unusual fatigue. The symptoms are more subtle because there are smaller arteries involved. The WISE study concludes that angioplasty and stenting are not the best options for women with more diffuse plaque. Rather, there is a great need to control risk factors such as high blood pressure, high cholesterol, and glucose intolerance.

Mayo Clinic. (2006). *Women's heart disease: New study shows differences*. Retrieved on October 21, 2006, from http://www.mayoclinic.com/health/womens-heart-disease/HB00075.

Type 2 diabetes is more common in people over age 45, with one in five individuals over 65 developing diabetes. Screening for diabetes is recommended for people who have a family member with diabetes, those who are overweight, and those who have had diabetes during pregnancy. Type 2 diabetes is a risk factor for developing heart disease.

Hearing impairment is common in older adults: More than 35% of people over 65 and 50% of people over 75 have some degree of hearing loss. Hearing loss can lead to miscommunication, social withdrawal, confusion, depression, and reduction in functional status. Likewise, older adults have more vision problems such as glaucoma, cataracts, or macular degeneration. Older people are more likely than younger adults to suffer accidental injuries because of vision problems, making regular eye exams important.

Elderly individuals should also be screened for risk of osteoporosis, depression, alcohol abuse, and violence as discussed in Chapter 9.

The adult immunization schedule applies to elderly adults as well. However, the current recommendation is that everyone older than 50 years receives an annual flu shot and, if over 65, a pneumonia shot as well. Elderly people should be screened for tuberculosis (TB) if they have been in close contact with someone who has TB; have recently moved to the United States from Asia, Africa, Central or South America, or the Pacific Islands; have kidney failure, diabetes, or alcoholism; are positive for human immunodeficiency virus (HIV); or have injected or now inject illegal drugs. Making vaccinations more convenient is known to increase immunization rates among elderly and at-risk people. Nurses working in community-based settings are often the professionals who initiate this type of service.

Cancer Screening

Most breast cancer occurs in women older than 50, so mammography is recommended every 1 to 2 years after a woman reaches 50 years of age. Women should have a Pap test every 3 years except in the presence of genital warts, multiple sex partners, or an abnormal Pap test, in which case, testing should be done annually. Women over age 65 with a history of normal Pap smears or with a hysterectomy may stop having Pap tests after consulting with a nurse practitioner or physician.

Colon cancer is more common in the elderly than in younger adults. Starting at age 50, fecal occult blood testing should be done every year in combination with other screening tests as recommended by the health care provider.

Prostate cancer is most common in men over age 50, African Americans, and men with a family history of prostate cancer. Screening includes digital rectal examination and prostate-specific antigen blood testing. Other information on this topic is found in Chapter 9.

Additional Screening

Environmental screening with a home safety check is an essential component of health promotion and disease prevention for the elderly client. As discussed in Chapter 5, other screening that is important for elderly clients is hearing and vision screening, functional assessment, and cognition status. With all clients, it is important to screen for all leading health indicators. Refer to Healthy People 2010 9-1 in Chapter 9 for a list of the leading health indicators from Healthy People 2010. Interventions to address these indicators are covered in the next section.

INTERVENTIONS FOR LEADING HEALTH INDICATORS

Once screening has been done, conditions that put the client at risk are addressed. Many factors have contributed to the decline in mortality from heart disease and stroke. Some of these include changes in health behaviors, a decrease in smoking, improvements in nutrition, increases in the overall educational level of the older population, and innovations in medical technology.

Because the average person is living longer, more attention is now focused on preserving quality of life than on extending length of life. Most elderly people have one or more chronic conditions, and as a result of increased longevity, they will be

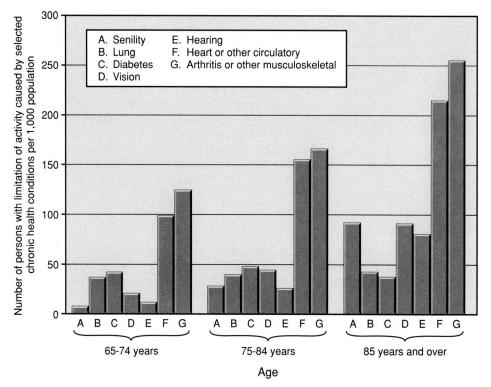

FIGURE 10-2. ▶ Limitations of activity caused by one or more chronic health conditions among adults, 2002–2003. *Chartbook on trends in the health of Americans.* (2002). Centers for Disease Control and Prevention, National Center for Health Statistics, National Health Interview Survey. (p. 53).

living longer with these conditions (Fig. 10-2). Nurses will be increasingly involved in efforts to decrease the adverse social and economic consequences of a high rate of activity limitation and disability of older persons. Thus, health promotion and disease prevention interventions for this segment of the population are important.

This shift in focus requires dispelling myths commonly held about the elderly, including seeing the elderly as sick and sedentary, sexless, and senile. Nurses can facilitate successful aging by considering the elderly client holistically, and they can maximize functioning by addressing physical and psychologic well-being, as well as competence in adaptation (Fig. 10-3).

Physical Activity

Older adults, both male and female, can obtain significant health benefits from a moderate amount of daily physical activity. Additional health benefits can be gained through even greater amounts of physical activity. Care should always be taken to avoid injury.

Previously sedentary older adults who begin physical activity programs should start with short intervals of moderate physical activity, from 5 to 10 minutes, and

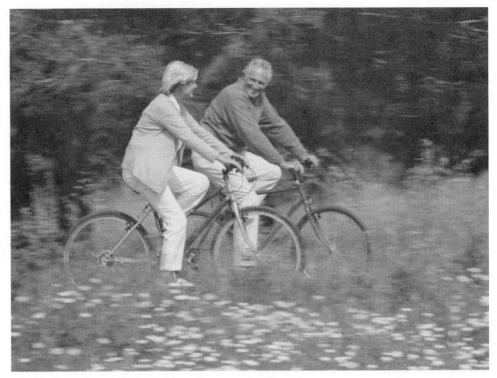

FIGURE 10-3. ► Using health promotion and disease prevention strategies can create a longer and healthier life. Used with permission from U.S. Administration on Aging, Department of Health and Human Services.

gradually build up to the desired amount. Benefits of physical activity include cardiorespiratory endurance and muscle strengthening. Stronger muscles reduce the risk of falling and improve the ability to perform routine tasks of daily life. Other benefits of physical activity include the following:

◆ Helps maintain the ability to live independently and reduces the risk of falling and fracturing bones
◆ Reduces the risk of dying from coronary heart disease and of developing high blood pressure, colon cancer, and diabetes
◆ Helps reduce blood pressure in some people with hypertension
◆ Helps people with chronic, disabling conditions improve their stamina and muscle strength
◆ Reduces symptoms of anxiety and depression and fosters improvements in mood and feelings of well-being
◆ Helps maintain healthy bones, muscles, and joints
◆ Helps control joint swelling and pain associated with arthritis (Agency for Healthcare Research and Quality [AHRQ] & Centers for Disease Control and Prevention, 2002).

Box 10-1 lists ways in which communities can promote physical activity for elderly adults.

> ◆ **B O X 10-1** What Communities Can Do to Promote Physical Activity in Elderly Adults ◆
>
> - Provide community-based physical activity programs that offer aerobic, strengthening, and flexibility components specifically designed for older adults.
> - Encourage mall and other indoor or protected locations to provide safe places for walking in any weather.
> - Ensure that facilities for physical activity accommodate and encourage participation by older adults.
> - Provide transportation for older adults to parks or facilities that provide physical activity programs.
> - Encourage health care providers to talk routinely to their older adult clients about incorporating physical activity into their lives.
> - Plan community activities that include opportunities for older adults to be physically active.
>
> ————
> Centers for Disease Control and Prevention. (1999). National Center for Chronic Disease Prevention and Health Promotion. *Physical activity and health: A report of the Surgeon General.* Available at: http://www.cdc.gov/nccdphp/sgr/olderad.htm.

Overweight and Obesity

Because no consensus exists regarding optimal weight for older persons, it is difficult to make recommendations regarding weight loss in the elderly. In the past, it was believed that lean body weight throughout life is optimal, but stability in weight after age 50 is also important. However, obesity has been tied to dozens of health problems: hypertension, diabetes, knee replacement surgery, heart failure, cholecystitis, pulmonary embolism, chronic fatigue, and insomnia (Patterson, Frank, Kristal, & White, 2004). This study highlights the urgent need for effective and practical public health approaches to preventing weight gain and treating obesity.

Tobacco Use

Smoking among adults has declined. However, because smoking remains the health indicator that is known to most negatively affect health, it is important to address the question of smoking with elderly clients and encourage them to quit. Community-Based Teaching 10-1 can be used for teaching older clients about the advantages of quitting at any age.

Substance Abuse

Not everyone who drinks regularly has a drinking problem. The questions in Box 9-5 in Chapter 9 can be used to help an elderly client recognize a drinking problem.

COMMUNITY-BASED TEACHING ▶ 10-1

Check Your Smoking I.Q.

If you or someone you know is an older smoker, you may think that there is no point in quitting now. Think again. By quitting smoking now, you will feel more in control and have fewer coughs and colds. On the other hand, with every cigarette you smoke, you increase your chances of having a heart attack, a stroke, or cancer. Need to think about this more? Take this older smokers' I.Q. quiz. Just answer "true"or "false" to each statement below.

True or False

1. ○ True ○ False   If you have smoked for most of your life, it's not worth stopping now.
2. ○ True ○ False   Older smokers who try to quit are more likely to stay off cigarettes.
3. ○ True ○ False   Smokers get tired and short of breath more easily than nonsmokers the same age.
4. ○ True ○ False   Smoking is a major risk factor for heart attack and stroke among adults 60 years of age and older.
5. ○ True ○ False   Quitting smoking can help those who have already had a heart attack.
6. ○ True ○ False   Most older smokers don't want to stop smoking.
7. ○ True ○ False   An older smoker is more likely to smoke more cigarettes than a younger smoker.
8. ○ True ○ False   Someone who has smoked for 30 to 40 years probably won't be able to quit smoking.
9. ○ True ○ False   Very few older adults smoke cigarettes.
10. ○ True ○ False   Lifelong smokers are more likely to die of diseases like emphysema and bronchitis than nonsmokers.

Answers

1. False.   Nonsense! You have every reason to quit now and quit for good—even if you've been smoking for years. Stopping smoking will help you live longer and feel better. You will reduce your risk of heart attack, stroke, and cancer; improve blood flow and lung function; and help stop diseases like emphysema and bronchitis from getting worse.
2. True.   Once they quit, older smokers are far more likely than younger smokers to stay away from cigarettes. Older smokers know more about both the short- and long-term health benefits of quitting.
3. True.   Smokers, especially those over 50 years old, are much more likely to get tired, feel short of breath, and cough more often. These symptoms can signal the start of bronchitis or emphysema, both of which are suffered more often by older smokers. Stopping smoking will help reduce these symptoms.

(continued)

COMMUNITY-BASED TEACHING ▶ 10-1

Check Your Smoking I.Q. *(Continued)*

4. True. Smoking is a major risk factor for four of the five leading causes of death including heart disease, stroke, cancer, and lung diseases like emphysema and bronchitis. For adults 60 and over, smoking is a major risk factor for six of the top 14 causes of death. Older male smokers are nearly twice as likely to die from stroke as older men who do not smoke. The odds are nearly as high for older female smokers. Cigarette smokers of any age have a 70% greater heart disease death rate than do nonsmokers.

5. True. The good news is that stopping smoking does help people who have suffered a heart attack. In fact, their chances of having another attack are smaller. In some cases, ex-smokers can cut their risk of another heart attack by half or more.

6. False. Most smokers would prefer to quit. In fact, in a recent study, 65% of older smokers said that they would like to stop. What keeps them from quitting? They are afraid of being irritable, nervous, and tense. Others are concerned about cravings for cigarettes. Most don't want to gain weight. Many think it's too late to quit— that quitting after so many years of smoking will not help. But this is not true.

7. True. Older smokers usually smoke more cigarettes than younger people. Plus, older smokers are more likely to smoke high-nicotine brands.

8. False. You may be surprised to learn that older smokers are actually more likely to succeed at quitting smoking. This is more true if they're already experiencing long-term smoking-related symptoms like shortness of breath, coughing, or chest pain. Older smokers who stop want to avoid further health problems, take control of their life, get rid of the smell of cigarettes, and save money.

9. False. One of five adults aged 50 or older smokes cigarettes. This is more than 11 million smokers, a fourth of the country's 43 million smokers! About 25% of the general U.S. population still smokes.

10. True. Smoking greatly increases the risk of dying from diseases like emphysema and bronchitis. In fact, over 80% of all deaths from these two diseases are directly due to smoking. The risk of dying from lung cancer is also a lot higher for smokers than nonsmokers: 22 times higher for males, 12 times higher for females.

National Heart, Lung, and Blood Institute.
Available at: http://www.nhlbi.nih.gov/health/public/lung/other/smoking.html.

Older problem drinkers have a good chance for recovery because once they decide to seek help they usually stay with treatment programs. Alcohol dependence is often not appreciated as relevant to the care of older adults. There is emerging evidence that reduction in alcohol use among older adults abusing alcohol can enhance health related quality of life. Because of the comorbidity of alcohol abuse and depression, it is important to screen for alcohol abuse in all cases where depression is suspected (Zisserson & Oslin, 2003). For additional information on substance abuse see Chapter 9.

Responsible Sexual Behavior

Understanding normal changes in sexual response is the first step to sexual health promotion. With aging, women may notice changes in the shape and flexibility of the vagina and a decrease in vaginal lubrication. This can be addressed by using a vaginal lubricant. Men may find that it takes longer to get an erection or that the erection may not be as firm or large as in earlier years. As men get older, impotence increases, with some chronic conditions contributing to this change (e.g., heart disease, hypertension, and diabetes). For many men, impotence can be managed and reversed. Many pharmaceutical options are available to enhance sexual enjoyment. Nurses and nurse practitioners are often the trusted member of the health team to whom a client may first direct his or her question about sexuality.

Having safe sex is imperative for people at all ages. In some areas of the country, the incidence of HIV among the elderly is on the rise. It is always essential that the nurse discuss the importance of safe sex, particularly regarding having sex with a new partner or multiple partners. Before having sex with a new partner, the client should be encouraged to be tested for sexually transmitted diseases (STDs) and talk to the new partner about doing the same.

Mental Health

Many issues related to mental health emerge as individuals age. The losses associated with aging, including loss of health, friends, and spouse, all contribute to the development of depression among the elderly (Fig. 10-4). Between 8% to 20% of older adults in the community and up to 37% in primary care settings suffer from depressive symptoms (CDC, 2007). Depression often occurs with other serious illnesses such as heart disease, diabetes, or cancer. Depression can and should be treated and there are many effective therapies available. Unfortunately, depression is commonly under-diagnosed and under treated in the older adult population. Interrupting depression in the elderly significantly extends life (Hyer, 2006).

Depression is one of the most common conditions associated with suicide in older adults. Older Americans are disproportionately likely to die by suicide. Although they make up 23% of the population, they account for 18% of all suicide deaths. The highest rate of suicide in the Unites States is found in White men age 85 and older, which is five times the national rate (National Institute of Mental Health, 2006).

Box 9-6 provides criteria for identifying depression. Once depression is identified, it can be treated successfully. Support groups, other talk therapy, antidepressant drugs, and electroconvulsive therapy are some forms of treatment that may be used for clients with depression.

Preparing for major changes in life, keeping and maintaining friendships, developing interests or hobbies, and keeping the mind and body active may help

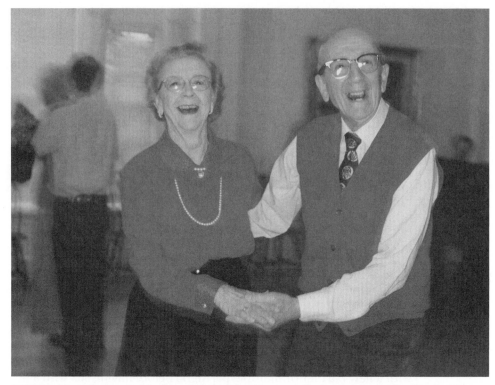

FIGURE 10-4. ▶ A satisfying marital relationship contributes to longevity. Used with permission from U.S. Administration on Aging, Department of Health and Human Services.

prevent depression. Being physically fit, eating a balanced diet, and following the nurse practitioner or physician's recommendations regarding medication can also minimize depression. Other suggestions for the client facing depression include the following:

◆ Accept the fact that help is needed.
◆ Consult a health care provider who has special training in mental health issues of the elderly.
◆ Do not be afraid of getting help because of the cost.

If the depressed older person will not seek help, friends or relatives can help by explaining how treatment may help the person feel better. Sometimes the family can arrange for the health care provider to call the family member or make a home visit to start the process. Community mental health centers offer treatment and often have resources.

Safety and Injury Prevention

Injuries are a leading cause of morbidity and mortality among the elderly. The primary causes of injury among this age group are motor vehicle accidents, falls, and mishaps. Risk factors related to injuries include polypharmacology, depression, vision and hearing impairments, and reduced reaction time.

Motor vehicle-related death rates for older adults are the highest of any age group. Per miles driven, drivers older than 75 years have higher rates of vehicle-related death than all other age groups except teenagers. Measures that could benefit older people as well as other age groups are increased use of public transportation and restricted driving privileges when circumstances warrant. For example, in some states, the length of the license term for older drivers has been reduced from 4 years to 2 years. In some states, physicians are required to report to the state's licensing agency cases of certain medical conditions that could affect a person's ability to drive.

Falls are recognized as a leading cause of injury and death among the elderly. In the United States, one of every three people 65 years and older falls each year. Half of those older than 75 who fracture a hip as a result of a fall die within 1 year of the incident (CDC, 2006). By 2020, the cost of fall injuries is expected to reach $32 billion. The general risk factors for falling include fall history, gait and balance impairment, the use of sedative and hypnotic medications, incontinence, difficulties in performing ADL, inactivity, visual impairment, home hazards, and reduced lower limb strength (Yuan & Kelly, 2006). The elderly are at increased risk for injury from falls because of the high incidence of osteoporosis in this age group. Prevention of fractures is related to increasing bone density and preventing falls. See Community-Based Teaching 10-2 for tips to prevent fractures in the elderly.

Polypharmacy, or the prescription of more than one medication, resulting in a complex medication regimen, is becoming more common. Elderly clients typically

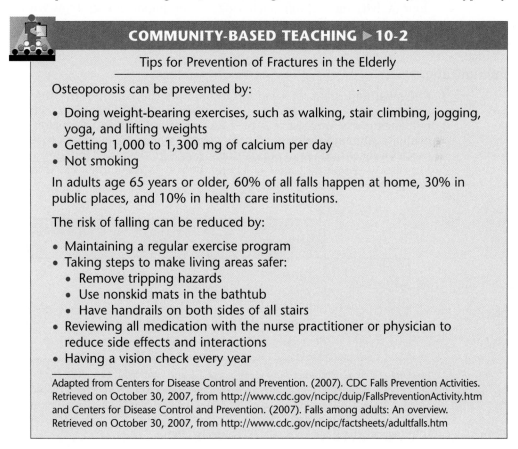

COMMUNITY-BASED TEACHING ▷ 10-2

Tips for Prevention of Fractures in the Elderly

Osteoporosis can be prevented by:

- Doing weight-bearing exercises, such as walking, stair climbing, jogging, yoga, and lifting weights
- Getting 1,000 to 1,300 mg of calcium per day
- Not smoking

In adults age 65 years or older, 60% of all falls happen at home, 30% in public places, and 10% in health care institutions.

The risk of falling can be reduced by:

- Maintaining a regular exercise program
- Taking steps to make living areas safer:
  - Remove tripping hazards
  - Use nonskid mats in the bathtub
  - Have handrails on both sides of all stairs
- Reviewing all medication with the nurse practitioner or physician to reduce side effects and interactions
- Having a vision check every year

Adapted from Centers for Disease Control and Prevention. (2007). CDC Falls Prevention Activities. Retrieved on October 30, 2007, from http://www.cdc.gov/ncipc/duip/FallsPreventionActivity.htm and Centers for Disease Control and Prevention. (2007). Falls among adults: An overview. Retrieved on October 30, 2007, from http://www.cdc.gov/ncipc/factsheets/adultfalls.htm

take more medications than other age groups. Medication errors are increasingly recognized as a potential for injury. Taking medication the wrong way or with other medications that cause harmful interactions can make the client worse rather than better. **Medication safety** should be practiced by all those taking a number of medications. Prescription Medicines and You (*Your Medication: Play It Safe. Patient Guide,* National Council on Patient Information and Education, 2004) is an excellent guide designed to help avoid medication errors and get the most from the medication. See What's on the Web for information on how to obtain a copy.

Environmental Quality

Because the elderly are more vulnerable to alterations in environmental conditions, poor air quality has a greater impact on this age group. As people age, their bodies are less able to compensate for the effects of all environmental hazards. The proportion of elderly individuals exposed to poor air quality, both second-hand smoke and other air pollution, must be reduced. Further, older adults benefit from reducing their own exposure to poor air quality. This can be accomplished by avoiding tobacco smoke, smoke from wood-burning stoves, mold, dust mites and cockroaches, and keeping pets out of sleeping areas. It is also important to check and clean furnace and heating units and fix water leaks promptly. Last of all monitoring the Air Quality Index (http://www.epa.gov/airnow) and avoiding outdoor activity on poor air quality days is an important strategy. With the elderly population increasing, maintaining air quality is even more essential to maintaining and improving the health of the nation.

Immunizations

The most important intervention to improve the health of the elderly related to immunizations is to increase the number of elderly people vaccinated against influenza every year. Nurses play an important role in organizing, staffing, and evaluating immunization clinics. As nurses, we have some work to do in this area, particularly with diverse populations. The recommended immunization schedule for elderly people is found in Figure 10-5. It is recommended that older adults receive a flu shot every year.

	Year	Not Hispanic or Latino		Hispanic or Latino
		White	Black	
			Percent	
Influenza	2003	68.6	47.8	45.4
	2004	67.3	45.7	54.6
Pneumococcal Disease	2003	54.6	37.0	31.0
	2004	60.9	38.6	33.7

FIGURE 10-5. ▶ Percentage of people age 65 and over who reported having been vaccinated against influenza and pneumococcal disease, by race and Hispanic origin. Source: Federal Interagency Forum on Aging Related Statistics. *Older Americans Update 2006: Key indicators of well-being* (p. 32). Retrieved on October 24, 2006, from http://www.agingstats.gov/update2006/default.htm.

Access to Health Care

Access to care is important to increase the quality and years of healthy life for all Americans. Elderly individuals may perceive that they do not have access because they have unfounded concerns about cost for services. They also may have limited mobility as a result of either a chronic condition or lack of transportation. Perhaps the elderly person has a limited ability to speak English or is distrustful of health care providers. These are all issues of access that may affect the client's health. The nurse must always assess the client's perception of access and intervene accordingly.

CONCLUSIONS

Life expectancy at birth, as well as at 65 and 85 years of age, has increased over the past decades. The elderly are growing in number and have special health needs. Because elderly people are living longer with more chronic conditions, attention is now focused on preserving their quality of life. Nurses can use the leading health indicators to illuminate individual behaviors and physical, social, and environmental factors that require intervention to prevent disease and promote health in the older segment of the population.

What's on the Web

AgePage: Depression: Don't Let the Blues Hang Around
Internet address: http://www.niapublications.org/engagepages/depression.asp
This document from the National Institute on Aging addresses depression as it relates to older people and provides a list of resources.

Alzheimer's Association
Internet address: http://www.alz.org
This site provides consumer and professional information, including a section dedicated to family caregivers and friends of people with Alzheimer's disease. Contains links to local chapters and other support groups and resources. Includes information in Spanish.

Diabetes Education
Centers for Disease Control and Prevention
Internet address:
http://www.cdc.gov/diabetes
Information about diabetes statistics and state programs can be found at this CDC site.

National Center for Health Statistics. (2005). *Chartbook on trends in the health of Americans.* Retrieved on October 17, 2006, from http://www.cdc.gov/nchs/data/hus/hus05.pdf
This resource from the CDC National Center for Health Statistics includes a special report on the aging population in the United States. It is updated every year so look for the most recent version.

Centers for Disease Control, National Center for Injury Prevention and Control.
Internet address:
http://www.cdc.gov/ncipc/

National Council on Aging
Internet address:
http://www.ncoa.org/index.cfm
This site provides information geared toward elderly people on topics including finances, housing, long-term care, rural aging, employment, health care, social security, senior centers, and end-of-life care.

National Institute of Diabetes and Digestive and Kidney Diseases
Internet address:
http://www2.niddk.nih.gov/
This National Institutes of Health (NIH) site provides information about research and recent advances related to diabetes.

National Diabetes Education Program
Internet address:
http://www.ndep.nih.gov/
Consumer information about diabetes is available through this organization supported by the National Institutes of Health (NIH), U.S. Department of Health and Human Services (DHHS), and the CDC.

Older Americans 2006: Key Indicators of Well-Being
Internet address: http://agingstats.gov/update2006/default.htm
This report of the Federal Interagency Forum on Aging-Related Statistics provides information on indicators that address the lives of the older population, including access to health care, home care, vaccinations, social activity, and dietary quality. It is updated yearly, so find the most recent version. There are slides, statistics and other resources related to older adult health on this site. Retrieved on October 30, 2007, from http://www.agingstats.gov/agingstasdotnet/main_site/default.aspx

The Pocket Guide for Staying Healthy at 50+.
Internet address:
http://www.ahcpr.gov/ppip/50plus/
This guide is available online at http://www.ahcpr.gov/ppip/50plus/50plus.pdf, or it can be ordered free by calling (800) 358-9295 or email ahrqpubs @ahrq.gov. Put Prevention Into Practice: Staying Healthy at 50+. This online consumer guide from the AHRQ explains preventive care for older adults. Print copies, available free of charge, can be requested by calling (800) 358-9295. The guide is also available in Spanish.

Resource Directory for Older People
Internet address:
http://www.aoa.gov/PRESS/publications/rd2006.pdf
This site features a list of organizations compiled by the Administration on Aging

and the National Institute on Aging. This resource is updated frequently so look for the latest version.

Your Medicine: Play It Safe Patient Guide
Internet address:
http://www.ahrq.gov/consumer/safemeds/safemeds.htm
This consumer guide from the National Council on Patient Information and Education and the AHRQ can be used as a teaching tool to facilitate medication safety. Print copies, available in six languages, can be ordered for a small fee at http://www.talkaboutrx.org/ or by calling (800) 358-9295.

You Can Do It: Steps to a Healthier Aging Campaign
AoA launched You Can! Steps to Healthier Aging as a social marketing campaign using the best marketing practices including message testing, behavior change theory and listening to the views of the target audience and Aging Network. You Can! Tool kits are available on the following internet site.

Internet address: http://www.aoa.gov/youcan/tools/introduction.asp

Potential Partners for Health Promotion Activities for the Elderly
American Association of Retired Persons
Internet address: http://www.aarp.org

American Council on Science and Health
Internet address: http://www.acsh.org

American Society on Aging
Internet address: http://www.asaging.org

Institute for Cancer Prevention
Internet address: http://www.ifcp.us

National Association for Home Care and Hospice
Internet address: http://www.nahc.org

National Health Policy Forum
Internet address: http://www.nhpf.org

National Wellness Institute
Internet address: http://www.nationalwellness.org

People's Medical Society
Internet address: http://www.peoplesmed.org

References and Bibliography

Administration on Aging. (2005). *A profile of older Americans: 2005.* Retrieved on October 20, 2006, from http://www.aoa.gov/ PROF/Statistics/profile/2005/2005profile.pdf

Agency for Healthcare Research and Quality and Centers for Disease Control and Prevention. (2002). *Physical activity and older Americans: Benefits and strategies.* Retrieved December 10, 2002, from http://www. ahcpr.gov/ppip/activity/htm

Agency for Healthcare Research and Quality and National Council on Patient Information and Education. (2003). *Your medicine: Play it safe* (AHRQ Publication No. 03-0019). Rockville, MD, and Washington, DC. Retrieved on October 23, 2006, from http://www.ahrq.gov/consumer/safemeds/ safemeds.pdf

Centers for Disease Control and Prevention. (1999). National Center for Chronic Disease Prevention and Health Promotion. *Physical activity and health: A report of the Surgeon General.* Available at http:// www.cdc.gov/nccdphp/sgr/olderad.htm

Centers for Disease Control and Prevention. (2000). *Falls and hip fractures among older adults.* National Center for Injury Prevention and Control. Available online at http:// www.cdc.gov/ncipc/factsheets/falls.htm

Centers for Disease Control and Prevention. (2007). Health information for older adults. Retrieved on October 30, 2007, from http://www.cdc.gov/aging/info.htm#3

Federal Interagency Forum on Aging Related Statistics. Older Americans update 2006: Key indicators of well-being (p. 32). Retrieved on October 24, 2006, from http://www. agingstats.gov/update2006/default.htm

Hobbs, F. (2006). *The elderly population.* United States Census Bureau. Retrieved on October 20, 2006, from http://www. census.gov/population/www/pop-profile/ elderpop.html

Hyer, R. (2006). Interrupting depression in the elderly significantly extends life. Retrieved on October 23, 2006, from http://www.medscape.com/ viewarticle/531875_print

Mayo Clinic. (2006). Women's heart disease: New study shows differences. Retrieved on October 21, 2006, from http://www. mayoclinic.com/health/womens-heart-disease/HB00075

National Center for Health Statistics. (2005). *Health, United States, 2005 with chartbook* on trends in the health of Americans. Retrieved on October 17, 2006, from http:// www.cdc.gov/nchs/data/hus/hus05.pdf

National Coalition for Women with Heart Disease. (2007). Women and heart disease fact sheet. Retrieved on October 30, 2007, from http://womenheart.org/information/ women_and_heart_disease_fact_sheet.asp

National Heart, Lung, and Blood Institute. Retrieved on October 30, 2007, from http://quitsmokingsupport.com/ whyquitsmoking.htm

National Institute of Mental Health. (2006). *Older adults: Depression and suicide facts.* Retrieved on October 23, 2006, from http://www.nimh.nih.gov/health/publications/older-adults-depression-and-suicide-facts.shtml

Patterson, R. E., Frank, L. L., Kristal, A. R., & White, E. (2004). A comprehensive examination of health conditions associated with obesity in older adults. *American Journal of Preventive Medicine, 27*(5), 385–390.

Teutsch, S. (2006). Cost-effectiveness of prevention. Retrieved on October 20, 2006, from http://www.medscape.com/viewarticle/ 540199

U.S. Department of Health and Human Services. (2000). Healthy people 2010. National health promotion disease prevention objectives. Washington, DC: U.S. Government Printing Office.

Yuan, J. R., & Kelly, J. (2006). Falls prevention , or "I think I can, I think I can": an ensemble approach to falls management. *Home Healthcare Nurse, 24*(2), 103–111.

Zisserson, R. N., & Oslin, D. W. (2003). Alcoholism and at-risk drinking in the older population. *Geriatric Times,*(IV), 5. Retrieved on October 23, 2006, from http://www. geriatrictimes.com/g031011.html

LEARNING ▼ ACTIVITIES

◆ JOURNALING ACTIVITY 10-1

In your clinical journal, describe a situation where you have observed an elderly client who was not receiving the health promotion or disease prevention care that he or she needed.

- What interventions did you think should have been pursued?
- How would or could you advocate for these issues when you begin to practice as an RN?

◆ JOURNALING ACTIVITY 10-2

1. In your clinical journal, describe a situation you have encountered when screening and doing health promotion and disease prevention teaching and planning with an elderly adult.

- What did you learn from this experience?
- How will you practice differently based on this experience?

◆ CLIENT CARE ACTIVITY 10-3

Roberta is a 62-year-old Black woman employed as a housekeeper in a hotel. She does not have health insurance. As you are completing *The Pocket Guide to Staying Healthy at 50+* you learn that she has not had a pelvic or breast examination in 10 years.

- What do you do?

Roberta says, "I used to be more active. I used to play basketball when I was a teenager, and now I can hardly walk up a flight of stairs. I would like to be more active and lose some weight. Would that help my high blood pressure?"

- What do you say and do?
- What resources do you use?

She tells you that she has smoked since she was 16 years old and has decided that she wants to quit.

- What do you say and do?
- What resources do you use?

◆ PRACTICAL APPLICATION ACTIVITY 10-4

You are working in a community clinic that serves many senior citizens from the surrounding area. Last year, you noted that in November through March, most of the clinic visits were for colds, influenza, sore throats, bronchitis, and pneumonia, in order of frequency. As you are reviewing the clinic records, you learn that 80% of the clinic visits resulting in hospitalization resulted from bronchitis, pneumonia, and influenza.

1. What clinic activities related to health promotion and disease prevention would you plan for the next year in the late fall?

2. How would you go about assessing and planning for the activities? (Consult Chapter 5 for some ideas.)

3. Develop a plan for the activities with a list of who would be involved in the planning, the goals and objectives of the plan, and a time line.

◆ PRACTICAL APPLICATION ACTIVITY 10-5

A local senior citizens center has contacted your instructor and asks that a team of students provide a health fair for the center's fall festival held in late October or early November.

- What would you like to know about this group before beginning this project?
- When forming a group to work on this task, whom would you invite to participate in planning the project?
- How would you involve the various community partners in the planning?
- What screening activities would you suggest?
- What other activities would be important to offer based on the time of the year and the typical health needs of the elderly?

SETTINGS FOR PRACTICE

T he settings and roles of the nurse have changed over time. In the late 1800s, a nurse was a woman in a black dress and a long black cape, carrying a black satchel, visiting homes to care for the sick. As health care shifted toward care of the ill in the hospital, the nurse was a woman dressed in a severely starched white uniform, white stockings, and a starched white cap, bending over the bed of a sick person.

Today, male and female nurses work in a wide variety of settings, taking on many roles. These settings are discussed in Chapter 11. The nurse working in the community is no longer recognizable by sex, uniform, or setting. Nurses are now involved in all levels of health care delivery. Nurses practice in corporations, neighborhood schools, day surgery centers, churches, long-term care facilities, and a variety of ambulatory clinics. Their clients may be well children or they may be older people, abused women, homeless families, prisoners, or drug addicts.

Increasingly, the home is becoming the focus for many nurses practicing in the current health care system. Agencies providing home care, the significance of home care, and the transfer of acute care nursing to home care nursing skills are discussed in Chapter 12. Barriers to successful home care and skills and competencies are also addressed. The first visit is described, along with safety issues and lay caretaker involvement. Chapter 13 provides an overview of specialized home health care nursing, where hospice care, pain management, wound care, disease management, and case management in the home setting will be covered.

In Chapter 14, the role of the mental health nurse in community-based settings will be outlined. This will include a discussion of the historical perspective, significance of community mental health, agencies and service available in community-based settings, and challenges to successful implementation of nursing care in these settings. The global community as a setting for practice in community care will be the focus of Chapter 15. This chapter will discuss the global nature of health, disparity, and natural and human created disasters. All nurses benefit from understanding the global nature of health, particularly when working with immigrants, refugees, and new Americans.

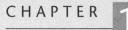

CHAPTER 11

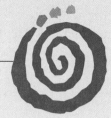

Practice Settings and Specialties

ROBERTA HUNT

LEARNING OBJECTIVES

1. Describe different settings in which nursing care is provided.
2. Identify three settings in which children receive nursing care and the services that these settings offer.
3. Identify three settings in which elderly clients receive nursing care and the services that these settings offer.
4. Compare the roles of the advanced practice nurse and the registered nurse.
5. Contrast the roles of the nurse in a school setting with the roles in the work setting.
6. Discuss the trends in settings for practice.

KEY TERMS

adult day care
adult foster care homes
advanced practice nurses
ambulatory care centers
assisted living facilities
boarding care homes
case manager
certified nurse midwife
clinical nurse specialist
day surgery centers
detoxification facilities
employee assistance
    programs

employee wellness
    programs
extended care facilities
home health care
homeless shelter
nurse practitioner
nursing-managed
    health centers
nursing centers
occupational health nurse
outpatient services
parish nursing
practice settings

rehabilitation center
residential center
retirement communities
school nurse
skilled nursing facilities
specialized care centers
subacute rehabilitation
    centers
transitional housing
wellness promotion
work-site health
    promotion

CHAPTER TOPICS

◆ **Practice Settings and Practice Opportunities**
◆ **Nursing Specialties**
◆ **Conclusions**

THE NURSE SPEAKS

We offered an ongoing "Faithfully Fit" exercise class at the church as part of the Parish Nurse program. It is an exercise class mostly for older, retired people. Afterwards, we meet at the church and have devotions. One of the regular participants brought her neighbors, Warren and Colette, who eventually became a big part of the class. They both grew up in another faith from ours but had not been to church for over 40 years. Warren had had three or four bouts of different kinds of cancer before this and about a year after joining the exercise class he came up with esophageal cancer. I brought a card the first day after we heard about this and we all signed the card in class. From there the class took over and we sent cards almost every day either to Warren or to Colette for support. They had three daughters who lived in Chicago, Madison (WI), and California and no family in the area. When he came home from the hospital he had a feeding tube. We started bringing supper for her every night. Some nights whoever brought it stayed with them and ate while some nights they just left the meal. He got well enough to come back to the class and, of course, this was really fun even though he was pretty weak. So we watched him get better and better. Then they moved into a condominium next to our church. They hadn't been there 2 weeks and she was diagnosed with lung cancer. This was almost a year after his diagnosis. Someone in the class coordinated rides and the food and we all participated and, of course, prayed for them. When they were too ill to come to the class they looked out from their condo onto our exercise class that was held in the church. They would wave at us. Then we did things like take Colette to coffee and Warren to the library to spend time with them. It was not just the parish nurse or the exercise group that was involved in this process by then but the whole neighborhood. The realtor that sold the house, her hairdresser, two of his work colleagues all began to help so it became a community thing. For me, that is what parish nursing is all about. It should start inside the church and move to outside the church into the community.

Anyway, they died in the spring within a few weeks of each other. Warren had hooked up with the priest from his own faith near the end of his life and had last rites. Colette would have none of that and she huffed around that apartment. Colette had a great deal of spirit and did not hesitant to express her opinions. Prior to All Saints Day, St. Cecelia sent us an invitation to their All Saints mass. It was a beautiful celebration and they listed all the people, either members or people with whom they had contact with for the prior year who had died. Warren and Colette were listed in the program. In the church there were beautiful rod iron candle holders with little candles in them, each labeled with the name of the person remembered in the service. Of course we could not see the names during the service. During the service one candle kept sputtering and was so noisy and finally went out. After the service they encouraged us to find the name of our loved one and see the candle. When we discovered that it was Colette's candle that was making all the ruckus, those of us there from our neighborhood laughed. She was speaking even after her death.

—LYNDA MORLOCK, RN, PHN, Former Parish Nurse,
St. Anthony Lutheran Church, St. Anthony, MN

The settings for health care delivery have undergone rapid and dramatic changes in the past decade. This is due, in part, to escalating health care costs. It is also attributable to the self-care movement. Reduced infant mortality, control of communicable diseases, and the aging of "baby boomers" have increased the number of people living to older age. Life span has also increased for those with specific chronic diseases, such as cystic fibrosis, sickle cell anemia, diabetes, and acquired immunodeficiency syndrome (AIDS), and for those who have been paralyzed by stroke or trauma.

These recent changes have made it possible for nurses to work in fields or specialization from an infinite number of choices. Unlike in the past, fewer than 60% of nurses currently work in hospital inpatient and outpatient departments, with more nurses working in community or public health and primary care settings. Employment of registered nurses is expected to grow faster than the average for all occupations through 2010, with many new jobs being created. Although there will always be a need for traditional hospital nurses, a large number of new nurses will be employed in home health, long-term care, and ambulatory care. Further, given the changes in health care delivery, it is expected that more nurses will work in nursing-based clinic practice, health maintenance organizations (HMOs), federal agencies, health planning agencies, prison and jails, insurance companies, and pharmaceutical and durable medical equipment companies. Technologic advances in client care, which allows a greater number of health problems to be treated, will drive this growth. Further, as discussed in Chapter 10, the number of older people, who typically have more health care needs than other segments of the population, is increasing (U. S. Census Bureau, 2006).

This chapter discusses the different settings for practice that a nurse may encounter. Schools of nursing are expanding placement for clinical training of their students well beyond what was typical 1 or 2 decades ago. However, no one school can cover all these settings within its curriculum. People entering nursing today must seek out ways of venturing into new and different settings by reading about, observing, and volunteering in some of these settings.

PRACTICE SETTINGS AND PRACTICE OPPORTUNITIES

With the increased emphasis on self-care, disease prevention, and health promotion, health care delivery is needed in settings other than traditional hospitals. Further, health care has had to extend to the underserved areas (e.g., to people who live in remote rural areas of the country).

As the need increases for local health care facilities that provide comprehensive services, the way the services are made available to consumers is changing. The growing number of nontraditional health care facilities reflects this trend. A glance at our social systems shows that almost every established institution provides some type of health care. Industrial plants, businesses, schools, prisons, churches, and civic groups provide varying degrees of care, usually with a focus on prevention. Although state laws govern the tasks nurses may perform, it is usually the work setting or the agency that determines day-to-day activities.

The number and type of **practice settings** for community-based nursing exceeds our capacity to examine in this book. However, an overview of a number of settings will be given. Further, it is difficult to place health care settings in precise categories; many of them overlap. For instance, a clinic may be located in a hospital, or some long-term care facilities may be specialized facilities. The

COMMUNITY-BASED NURSING CARE GUIDELINES ▷ 11-1

Sampling of Variety of Nursing Functions in Health Care Settings

Hospital: Acute Care

Serves as administrator or manager
Assesses and monitors client's health status
Provides direct care
Coordinates care of others
Teaches client and family
Provides support for family members
Makes referrals

Home Care

Assesses client, family, and culture
Assesses home and community environment
Develops relationship based on mutual trust
Contacts physician regarding client's condition
Plans, implements, and evaluates plan of care
Provides direct care
Coordinates care given by others
Teaches client and family
Provides support for family members
Makes referrals

Clinic (Ambulatory) Care

Makes health assessments
Assists primary care provider (may be primary care provider)
Provides direct care
Coordinates care given by others
Teaches client and family
Plans, implements, and evaluates the plan of care
Provides health promotion and disease prevention
Serves as a client advocate

Extended Care Facility

Serves as administrator
Coordinates care of others
Assesses client's condition
Develops treatment plans
Provides direct care
Maintains contact with the client's physician

(continued)

COMMUNITY-BASED NURSING CARE GUIDELINES ▷ 11-1

Sampling of Variety of Nursing Functions in Health Care Settings (*Continued*)

Residential Centers

Provides direct care
Provides health assessments
Provides health promotion and prevention
Provides counseling and support
Makes referrals
Collaborates with other health team members
Coordinates services

Schools and Industry

Conducts health screening
Completes health assessments
Provides first aid or initial emergency care
Provides health education
Provides health promotion and disease prevention
Provides counseling and support
Makes referrals

Pharmaceutical and Durable Medical Devices

Conducts research
Provides education about new medication and devices
Outreach
Provides consultation

Insurance Companies

Case management
Outreach
Provides counseling and consultation

categories in this section are arbitrary and were chosen for ease in identifying some of the settings and types of care that community-based nurses may provide (see Community-Based Nursing Guidelines 11-1).

Hospital Care

Hospitals remain the major site in which nurses practice. Most hospital nurses provide bedside care and carry out the delegated medical functions prescribed by physicians and independent nursing diagnosis. They may also supervise licensed practical nurses and aides. Typically, nurses are assigned to one specialty area within the hospital.

Technically, acute care nursing is community-based nursing because acute care nurses do take care of individuals and families in a specific community. They also perform the initial assessment to prepare the client for discharge from the hospital. Further, as discussed in Chapter 6 and 7 it is the hospital nurse who does most of the preliminary teaching of clients and caregivers for procedures to be done in the home. The nurse in the hospital often provides information about resources in the community vital for ongoing self care. This provides the crucial link to self care with a disease prevention focus within the context of the client's family, culture, and community.

Care in the Home: The Home Visiting Nurse

The home visiting nurse has worked in community-based care since the middle of the 19th century. Both occupational health nursing, and maternal and child care nursing originated in the home setting as well. Today home visiting nurses fall into two main categories, maternal/child visits and home health care.

Maternal and child visiting typically follows the basic premises of community-based care. In many industrialized nations, the home visiting nurse is central to promoting health and preventing disease in the maternal–child population. In fact, in the past few decades, various studies have demonstrated how home visits improve outcomes for high-risk pregnancies and at-risk infants. As discussed in Chapter 8, one of the goals of Healthy People 2010 (DHHS, 2000) is to reduce the rate of low-birth-weight infants. Pregnant teenagers receiving home visits from nurses deliver heavier babies than teenagers who are not visited by a nurse. Women who smoked before pregnancy who receive home visits are less likely to smoke during pregnancy than women without home visits, which decreases the risk of having a low-birth-weight infant. Numerous studies over the last 20 years have shown that postpartum home visits are associated with a decrease in recorded physical child abuse and neglect in the first 2 years of life, especially in unmarried teen mothers of low socioeconomic status (Olds, et al., 1986, 1988; Olds, Henderson, & Kitzman, 1994). Current research demonstrates enduring effects of nurse home visitation on maternal life course, evident in the rate of subsequent pregnancies, mean interval between the first and second birth, and mean number of months of welfare used (Kitzman, et al., 2000).

Unfortunately in the last decade the role of the home visiting nurse in maternal child care in the United States has been eroded by lack of funding. Consequently, there has been a dramatic reduction in services provided to low-income women. This is particularly tragic considering the increase in the rate of low-birth-weight infants. Home visiting is proven to be an effective means to enhance health outcomes, yet it is used relatively infrequently in the United States, compared with many other countries. The European Union, through the World Health Organization, is promoting the role of the maternal child home visiting nurse coined the "family nurse." As a result, countries widely using home visiting for maternal child care have lower infant mortality rates, low rates of low-birth-weight infants, and more extensive use of family planning compared to the United States. At the same time, the percentage of the nation expenditure on health care in these nations is less compared to the United States.

In addition to home health care and maternal child care there are other populations and roles for home visitors. Home visiting allows the nurse to establish a trusting relationship with the family and the child so that additional interventions may follow. Home visits with school children facilitate case finding as well as provide more intense assessment and intervention for children with chronic conditions. It enhances continuity of care for all populations with all conditions.

Home Care Nursing

Home health care is a growing area with service provided mainly through home visits. Nursing agencies can contract directly with clients, or with Medicare or private insurance plans to provide a selected number of visits to a particular client. Chapter 12 and 13 discuss home health care nursing in more depth. Most clients receiving home care are elderly individuals although service is provided to people across the life span. Currently, home visiting is most commonly seen with those recently hospitalized or those with chronic illnesses, primarily the elderly receiving home health care services.

Most seniors prefer to stay in their own homes and communities rather then enter long-term care or assisted living facilities. There are other community-based programs designed to lengthen the period of time that seniors are able to remain in their homes.

Block Nurse Program

This program is a community-based service that depends on professional and volunteer services of neighborhood residents to provide information, social and support services, skilled nursing care, and other assistance to the elderly to promote self-sufficiency and avoid nursing home placement. This can range from arranging for a neighborhood Boy Scout to do yard work, to contacting Meals on Wheels to deliver meals, to making a referral for transportation to medication appointments.

It is important to note that this program was developed by a group of nurses in 1982 who wanted to provide better care for the elderly living in their neighborhood. This concept depends on grassroots community interest and active commitment of service groups, churches, businesses, schools, colleges, and universities. Evaluation of data from over 2 decades ago demonstrated that $3 is saved for every $1 spent keeping the elderly at home and out of long-term care facilities, which are primarily funded by Medicare. In the 37 sites in Minnesota evaluated, $30 million was saved by preventing premature nursing home placement. This model has been duplicated throughout the United States with great success. The Block Nurse program provides skilled nursing, case management, and supervision of home health aides and homemakers, often with nursing students as the care providers. The Web page for further information is http://www.elderberry.org/index.asp.

Adult Day Care Centers/Adult Foster Care

Adult day care centers offer social, recreational, and therapeutic activities to seniors who are in need of supervision during the day. Nurses are frequently part of the professional staff and are responsible for health assessments and design and management of therapeutic regimens and medications. Often, physical care (e.g., bathing) takes place at the day care center. These vital organizations offer more personal attention and have a quieter atmosphere than most senior centers. In addition, they provide care for the dependent individual who cannot manage alone but is not in need of nursing home placement. Adult day care is not reimbursable through Medicare. However, Medicare does pay all costs in a licensed day care center with a medical model or an Alzheimer's environment if the senior qualifies financially (National Respite Network, 2006).

Adult foster care homes (AFCHs)—also known as board and care homes, or family care homes—are safe, small (usually fewer than six clients per home) residential sites that provide housing and protective oversight. Many AFCHs provide

TABLE 11-1 Resources for Community-Based Respite Care		
Resource	**Description**	**Contact Information**
Eldercare Locator	A federal government service for identifying resources for respite care	http://www.eldercare.gov OR 1-800-677-1116
The Family Caregiver Alliance	A San Francisco nonprofit that tracks respite programs	http://www.caregiver.org (under tab for public Policy & Research click on Caregiving across the states or call 1-800-445-8106)
Disease-specific groups	For many chronic illnesses here there may be advocacy groups. For example, Alzheimer's disease	http://www.census.gov/population/www/socdemo/age.html#older or call 1-800-272-3900 (TDD: 1-866-403-3073)
Professional care managers	For example, the National Association of Professional Geriatric Care Managers	http://www.caremanager.org (under the button Find a Care Manager)
State or local agencies on aging	Senior service, elder services, public or private agencies	Local phone book blue pages or yellow pages on internet

care to frail elderly adults and those with dementia. Nationwide, these facilities may be referred to by many names, including residential, adult, foster, family, boarding, or assisted living. Adult foster care homes are optional elements of state Medicaid programs. Therefore, states determine what services are covered, who may be eligible, and what services they receive. Locating adult foster care or day care centers can be facilitated by contacting the state department of health or social services. Table 11-1 provides suggestions for identifying resources within the community.

Parish Nursing

Parish nursing is "a health promotion and disease prevention role based on the care of the whole person which encompasses seven functions" (Solari-Twadell & McDermott, 1999, p. 3). These functions are those of integrator of faith and health, health educator, health counselor, referral agent, trainer of volunteers, developer of support groups, and health advocate. Parish nursing finds its historical roots in the late 1800s when nurses sent by religious organizations practiced in many rural mountainous areas of the Southeast.

Parish nurses may offer screening, health education, resource and referral services, counseling, consultation, outreach, collaboration, and case management to parishioners. According to one study, the most frequent nursing interventions of parish nurses are active listening, followed by the NANDA diagnoses of health-seeking behaviors, and potential for spiritual well-being (Weis, Schank, Coenen, & Matheus, 2002). Often, parish nurses reach out to vulnerable populations: older adults, single parents and their children, and grieving individuals. Many churches have nurses on their staffs. Others use volunteers. Clients view parish nursing as a useful, meaningful, and effective health intervention and setting. Parish nurses are a source of client empowerment and as a result have an important role in promoting self-care and self-advocacy (Weis, Schank, & Matheus, 2006).

Residential Care for the Elderly

Some older adults, particularly those with chronic conditions, may be very isolated living at home. Living arrangements for these individuals in a **residential center** may be a better option. Successful placement, however, requires research, client and family involvement, planning, and a focus on the client's maintaining control of his or her own life. There are multiple levels of residential living from which to choose.

Extended care facility residents were queried in a study about factors that influence the quality of care they receive. They responded that the most important aspect was their ability to retain control of their lives. To provide effective care, the nurse must be familiar with the resident's health problems and needs. Aging is a normal, irreversible process. Many of the problems of aging can be prevented by considering that the older adult's physical, emotional, social, and spiritual needs are complex and interrelated. These factors are important to any older adult living in any kind of residential setting.

Residential facilities provide a unique setting for community-based nursing because the nurse has a captive audience. Here the nurse can take advantage of the close proximity of the residents to do health teaching, health promotion, and disease prevention. By building trust through good relationships with the residents, nurses expand their roles to become counselors and advocates, providing direct support.

Retirement Communities

Designed for the functionally and socially independent, **retirement communities** provide a community living style for individuals who choose to live with other seniors. Accommodations include homes or apartments with supportive services provided by the retirement community.

Assisted Living Facilities

Geared toward the individual who has need for some assistance in daily activities (e.g., medications, meals, dressing, bathing), but who is able to function fairly independently, **assisted living facilities** generally house residents in bedrooms located in a homelike environment.

Extended Care Facilities and Skilled Nursing Facilities

More institutional in their design, with ongoing medical and nursing services and supervision, **extended care facilities** (also known as nursing homes) provide care for individuals who need ongoing daily care, generally for the rest of their lives. **Skilled nursing facilities** provide nursing, medical, and therapy services for elderly people requiring ongoing medical or rehabilitative services but not hospitalization. Most individuals stay for a few weeks in a skilled facility and are then discharged home or transferred into an extended care facility because they can no longer manage at home after an acute illness or injury or chronic condition. For guidelines for consumers choosing a nursing home, see Community-Based Nursing Care Guidelines 11-2.

For more than 2 decades, nursing research has demonstrated a link between lower nurse staffing levels in hospitals and adverse client outcome. In 2005, researchers published evidence that increased direct care by RNs improves outcomes for nursing home residents (Horn, 2005). More registered nurse direct care was associated with fewer pressure ulcers, hospitalizations, and urinary tract

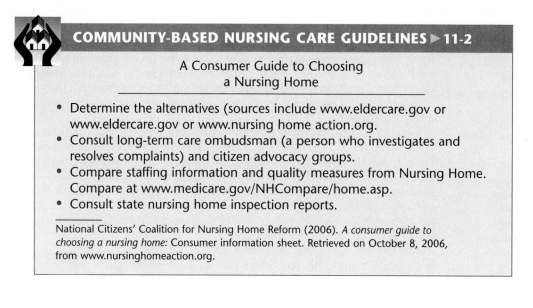

COMMUNITY-BASED NURSING CARE GUIDELINES ▶ 11-2

A Consumer Guide to Choosing a Nursing Home

- Determine the alternatives (sources include www.eldercare.gov or www.eldercare.gov or www.nursing home action.org.
- Consult long-term care ombudsman (a person who investigates and resolves complaints) and citizen advocacy groups.
- Compare staffing information and quality measures from Nursing Home. Compare at www.medicare.gov/NHCompare/home.asp.
- Consult state nursing home inspection reports.

National Citizens' Coalition for Nursing Home Reform (2006). *A consumer guide to choosing a nursing home:* Consumer information sheet. Retrieved on October 8, 2006, from www.nursinghomeaction.org.

infections (UTIs); decreased weight loss, catheterization, and deterioration in the ability to perform activities of daily living (ADL); and increased use of nutritional supplements. Better care translates to lower cost. There is an urgent need for additional research to confirm these findings. If future studies find similar relationships, it is likely that the same concern that has required high nurse-patient ratios in the hospital setting will be recommended for long-term care facilities. Further, this research highlights the importance of families inquiring about the number and resident/registered nurse ratio when assessing the quality care of a long-term care facility.

Subacute Rehabilitation Centers

Focused on the rehabilitation of individuals who have suffered an illness or accident, **subacute rehabilitation centers** provide longer term rehabilitative services, such as nursing and medical care, as well as physical, occupational, and speech therapy. Generally, length of stay in this type of facility is limited. Individuals are discharged when they have reached the rehabilitative goals or when they are no longer making progress. The following situation describes this setting.

CLIENT SITUATIONS IN PRACTICE

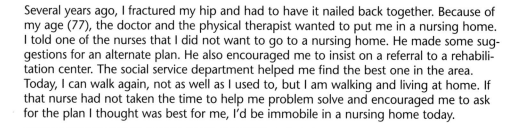

Several years ago, I fractured my hip and had to have it nailed back together. Because of my age (77), the doctor and the physical therapist wanted to put me in a nursing home. I told one of the nurses that I did not want to go to a nursing home. He made some suggestions for an alternate plan. He also encouraged me to insist on a referral to a rehabilitation center. The social service department helped me find the best one in the area. Today, I can walk again, not as well as I used to, but I am walking and living at home. If that nurse had not taken the time to help me problem solve and encouraged me to ask for the plan I thought was best for me, I'd be immobile in a nursing home today.

Boarding Care Homes

This type of facility provides personal custodial care for residents who are not able to live independently. **Boarding care homes** do not have nursing or medical supervision or care. Residents generally stay indefinitely.

Residential Care Across the Life Span

Residential programs provide health care services across the life span in the areas of chemical dependency treatment facilities, group homes for the mentally ill or developmentally delayed, halfway houses for recovery from addiction, detoxification units for safe withdrawal from alcohol or drugs, shelters for battered women, and hospices for the terminally ill. Nursing functions and roles vary with the type of residential program or facility; they may consist of direct caregiver, including delegated medical functions, **case manager,** health educator, discharge planner, counselor, collaborator, consultant, or advocate.

Shelters for Battered Women

Domestic violence crosses all social, economic, racial, and ethnic boundaries. Shelters have been built around the country to house battered women and their children. They provide a safe place where the women will have an advocate and easy access to counseling. The nurse functions primarily as advocate, case manager, health educator, and collaborator for the women and their children. Individual and group meetings with residents are part of the nurse's regular routine. The nurse who works with battered women must have good communication skills and must be aware of the resources available to meet the needs of these women and children. Box 11-1 describes one nurse's personal experience with domestic violence.

Homeless Shelters and Transitional Housing

The percentage of people in the United States who are homeless has been increasing since 1970. The fastest-growing segment is women and children, making up almost 40% of the homeless population in many cities in the United States (U.S. Conference of Mayors, 2006). Most of these families are single-parent, female-headed families with up to three children who are primarily preschoolers. There is an urgent need for transitional housing to facilitate the transition from crisis housing in homeless shelters to permanent stable housing. The homeless population has three to six times higher rates of physical illnesses than the general population and is twice as likely to suffer from mental illness. Further, the homeless have greater difficulty gaining access to health care than do poor families with homes (Morris & Strong, 2004). In addition, individuals without homes are exposed to nature's elements and to society's violence, placing them at increased risk for illness or injury. They also may be addicted to drugs and alcohol, have poor nutrition and hygiene, and live in overcrowded facilities. Children in homeless shelters have critical and chronic health needs while at the same time limited access to health care services (Yousey & Carr, 2005).

There is an urgent need for preventive approaches to alleviate homelessness and the health consequences that follow (Morris & Strong, 2004). In treating illnesses and injuries in the homeless population, the nurse may offer a variety of services, such as screening or health teaching. Assessing and completing immunization status of children who are homeless is an important primary prevention intervention. Screenings for skin conditions and evidence of early signs of chronic conditions

---

◆ **BOX 11-1** A Nurse's Personal Experience With Violence ◆

I was 9 years old when I walked into the bathroom and saw him beating her over the bathtub. I began screaming, leave her alone! He looked at me and kept on hitting her. At that moment I knew that I hated him. I promised myself that I would never allow a man to put his hands on me. Thirteen years later, I married a man who was just like my stepfather. Even though he did not physically abuse me, the words that came from his mouth were very poisonous. Each day he broke down my self-worth by telling me that I was a terrible mother, I did not love my children, and that I would be nothing without him.

I stayed with him for 12 years, isolated from my family and friends. I believed his lies even though I was an educated nurse. Finally, I gathered up enough strength to leave him. I packed my bags and my two children and left. We moved into a small apartment and I was so afraid because I did not know how I was going to make it on my own. Gradually I regained my self-esteem and self-confidence. I was able to return to school and obtained my MSN degree. It hasn't been easy, but with the support of my family and friends, I made it. In retrospect, I asked my 13-year-old son the other day, "If you could do one thing differently in your life what would it be?" He thought about it for a few moments and then he looked at me and said, "I wish you would have listened when I tried to tell you about daddy." Imagine that, my son observed the verbal abuse and chaos in the family, he tried to tell me about his father looking at other women, and printing pornography from the Internet, and I didn't listen. Imagine if I had listened!

It took a lot out of me to share this story because I had to confront the demons of my past. It is so important for us as nurses to be alert to the signs of domestic violence. When the opportunity presents itself we must be brave enough to ask the question: Do you feel safe at home? Not only must we be prepared to ask the question, we must also be able to provide the resources for obtaining help. So my message to women of all ages, ethnicity, and socio-economic background is that it is not OK for someone to abuse you. It is not OK for someone to demoralize you. You did not do anything wrong. You are just a victim. Seek help. Take care of yourself. Most importantly, be safe.

---

such as diabetes and hypertension are secondary prevention interventions. Another example is screening for normal development in children by using the Denver Developmental Screening Tool II to identify developmental delays. When the community-based nurse assists clients to follow up with existing health issues and access to care, such as obtaining medication for mental health conditions including depression, it is tertiary prevention. Nurses play an important role in the care of individuals and families who are homeless.

Camps

Camp programs for children and adults employ nurses in private, church, YWCA, YMCA, and Girl Scout and Boy Scout programs. Nurses may be employed as camp nurses in camps for children with chronic illnesses, such as asthma, seizure disorders, or AIDS. Camp nursing offers a unique setting to apply a variety of interventions, including health teaching, collaborating, counseling, and carrying out delegated medication functions.

Camp programs for children with chronic conditions have become more common. Serving children often precluded from having a camp experience, these camps are staffed with individuals who are familiar with the issues facing these individuals. These types of camps provide oversight and assistance for whatever needs children or teens may have. For instance at a camp for children with asthma, the nurse may assist the child with a nebulizer treatment or help them to decide when to use an inhaler. Significant improvements in children's symptoms control and life experiences are documented from attending an educational asthma camp (Hodges, 2005). Some of these camps also provide assistance with social, emotional, and self-care challenges facing the children related to the particular condition.

Rehabilitation Centers

A freestanding or hospital-associated **rehabilitation center** for drug dependency treatment or for physical or emotional rehabilitation is another setting for care. The goal of this type of facility is to help clients reach optimal health so they can become part of the productive community again. Rehabilitation centers often have a philosophy of improving quality of life and facilitating independent self-care to the client's full ability. An interdisciplinary health care team collaborates to plan and implement care. The role of the nurse frequently calls for interventions of direct care, teaching, and counseling.

Detoxification Facilities

Clients are admitted to **detoxification facilities** for the express purpose of detoxifying their bodies from chemicals. Medication administration and ongoing monitoring of the client's physical well-being from the day of admission are critical delegated medical functions to ensure the client's safety. Nurses are responsible for health assessment, identification of immediate physical needs, and referral to community organizations at the time of discharge.

Treatment Facilities for Addictions

Clients in treatment facilities for addictions usually do not require close monitoring for physiologic changes after the first 48 to 72 hours of the detoxification period. The goal of treatment is for clients to begin their own recovery process to allow them to return to the community as better functioning and productive members of society. Recovery is a lifelong commitment that clients must make to address their addiction. The nurse is responsible for health assessment, planning, and management of identified problems. Direct care is provided through medication administration and management of acute problems. In some programs the nurse acts as a case manager or counselor. A multidisciplinary approach is typically used, and the focus for discharge planning is the successful reentry of the client into society.

CLIENT SITUATIONS IN PRACTICE

◆ Role of the Nurse in a Residential Treatment Center for Teenagers

Jason is a nurse at a residential chemical dependency treatment program for male and female adolescents. Criteria for admission require that clients be between 11 and 17 years old, and diagnosed as chemically dependent or chronic substance abuse with legal consequences. The average length of the prescribed program is 30 to 45 days.

Jason has a small office close to the dormitory-style rooms where the clients stay. His responsibilities include the delegated medical functions of medication supervision and oversight of self-administration of medications, and obtaining health histories and assessments on each new admission. Other common interventions he is involved in are health education, disease prevention, health promotion, and collaboration with the other services in the facility during the treatment phase and for discharge planning. Another important role is that of formal and informal counselor. He enjoys working with adolescents who have varied emotional and physical problems.

It is important that the teens trust Jason and develop a therapeutic relationship with him. Establishing trust is always a challenge, but it is particularly so with teens who have addiction problems. Another challenge in this particular facility is that the population is co-ed. Sex education is imperative; as is problem solving about the many "attachments" the clients develop among each other. Jason states with a smile, "I just did not learn how to handle problems like this at nursing school. Some days, I really need to use every ounce of imagination I can muster." Jason reports both independence and challenge in his practice.

Ambulatory Care or Outpatient Services

Clinics

Clients who do not require inpatient care (in an acute setting) can receive treatment, care, and education on an outpatient basis. **Outpatient services**, also called **ambulatory care centers**, are rapidly expanding and are now provided by hospitals, HMOs, private and public hospitals, physicians' offices, community agencies, and public health departments (city, state, and federal). Services cover a broad range and include medical care, surgery, diagnostic tests, administration of medications (including intravenous therapy), physical therapy, kidney dialysis, counseling, birthing classes (Fig. 11-1), aerobics classes, well-child care, and health education for management of chronic illness.

Ambulatory care centers are located around the community for ease of access. They may be found in hospitals, low-income neighborhoods, and shopping malls. They may be provided in conjunction with a physician's practice and a managed care facility. Some settings, such as urgent care centers, offer walk-in, emergency care during extended hours when physicians' offices may be closed.

Some ambulatory clinics offer services to select groups or specific populations, for instance, community-based nurses practice in migrant camps (Fig. 11-2). Native American reservations, correctional facilities, and remote rural settings such as coal mining towns are other examples. Nurses can be an impetus for improved health and quality of life for a wide range of client populations.

FIGURE 11-1. ► Expectant
parents learn techniques to
promote relaxation and comfort during birth. Classes in
breast-feeding, infant care,
and child care are also provided by many maternity centers. (From Ricci, S. [2007.]
*Essentials of Maternity, New-
born, and Women's Health
Nursing.* Philadelphia: Lippincott Williams & Wilkins.)

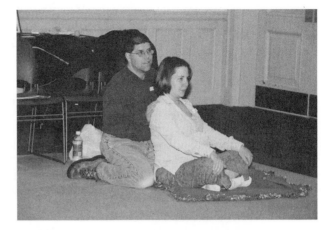

In some clinics, nurses have the primary role in conducting assessments and caring for clients who need health maintenance or health promotion. In some locations, nurse practitioners have established their own independent ambulatory services. Clinic nurses take on a variety of roles, depending on the medical specialty of the physician in charge and the type of clients served. For example, a nurse working in an HMO wound care clinic may care only for clients with private insurance. Community clinics may have a more heterogeneous population, with some clients insured and some uninsured. The clients' ability for self-care may

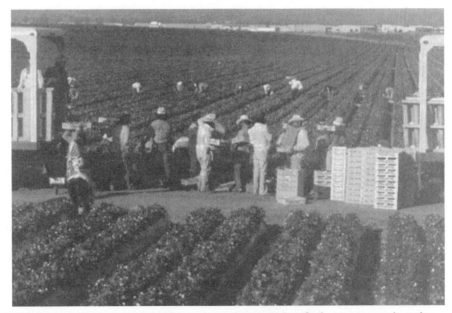

FIGURE 11-2. ► Experienced health care workers need to find ways to reach under-served people, such as these migrant workers. Migrant workers are defined by their common occupation and lifestyle, but they may cross various ethnic or racial lines.

vary between the two clinics, depending on the individual client, family and social support, and other resources. Further, continuity of care may vary depending on what the insurance coverage will pay for as well as the family and community support that is available for the client.

Physicians' Offices

Physicians in private and group practices, in primary care or specialties, employ nurses. These nurses prepare clients, perform some assessments and routine laboratory work, assist with examinations, administer injections and medications, change wound dressings, assist with minor surgery, and maintain records. In some cases they use telephone triage to direct clients to come to the clinic or emergency department immediately or type a simple intervention and call back the next day. Occasionally, physician offices will employ RNs to work as case managers.

Day Surgery Centers

Advanced technologies have influenced both the care of the client and the environment where care is provided. Minimally invasive procedures (e.g., laparoscopy, use of flexible endoscopes and lasers, and microwave therapies) now allow surgical procedures to be done in an ambulatory setting rather then in the hospital. Nurses working in **day surgery centers** have a range of duties: case management and delegated functions such as admission and assessment, preoperative and postoperative monitoring, and discharge planning and teaching. All of these responsibilities are compressed into a very short time frame, requiring a high level of skill.

Community Health Centers

For more than 3 decades, a network of federally subsidized community health centers has served as a major safety net provider for low-income Americans. Community health centers are private, nonprofit, community-based organizations. The number of community health centers more than doubled from 1,400 in 1990 to 3,745 in 2006. Community health centers provide services to over 15 million people, up from 5 million in 1990. Most clients have low incomes. While 29% of people nationwide are minorities, at least 63% of community health center clients are minorities. More than four in 10 community health center clients are uninsured, and one in three received coverage through Medicare (Health Resources and Services Administration, 2006b).

Working in community health centers provides rich transcultural opportunities, while at the same time provides challenges for the most experienced health care professionals. Working as an advocate to find ways to secure health care for the underserved has become increasingly taxing as the number and percentage of the citizens in the United States without access to health care continues to swell. Innovative nursing solutions to help develop appropriate services for uninsured Americans include working with community partners to develop programs and services and securing grants and new funding sources. There are also numerous opportunities to affiliate with community health centers in addition to being employed there. Nurses can volunteer to staff a free clinic; participate in outreach, such as launching campaigns on health education; and speak to neighborhood gatherings, community forums, and church groups. Working in this setting is often reported as being exciting and rewarding.

Specialized care centers provide health care for a specific population or group. Some of these are walk-in clinics; others provide residential care. Specialized care differs depending on the population served. For instance, a walk-in clinic may serve only teens or homeless teens.

Specialized clinics for individuals with cancer or human immunodeficiency virus (HIV) and AIDS are available in most cities. The clinics offer diagnosis, treatment, and care, including chemotherapy and are generally associated with a hospital or an HMO. Nurses provide direct client care, treatment, monitoring, and assistance with planning of interventions; they also attempt to minimize discomfort, manage pain, and maximize quality of life. The members of the multidisciplinary team collaborate closely. Nurses focus their time on care and support for the clients and families. Thus, the interventions of health teaching, counseling, collaborating, delegated medical functions, screening, and sometimes outreach are typical of this role.

Day Care Centers

Day centers for older adults were discussed at the beginning of this chapter. More commonly, day care centers provide services for infants, children, or disabled adults. Care may be provided for children while their parents work or after school before parents return from work. Some specialized day care centers provide care for children with minor illnesses when the parents must work. Other centers provide day care for children with chronic illnesses who cannot attend public school or, adults who because of physical, mental, or developmental disabilities, cannot find employment. Nurses usually serve on the staff, as the center manager or develop a business providing specialized day care.

Mental Health Services

Mental health centers may be connected to a hospital or may be independent agencies. They may be part of a network of other coordinated social and health care services. Treatment provided may be short-term or long-term care or crisis intervention. The nurse is commonly involved in assessment, health teaching, counseling, and delegated functions such as administration of medications. Knowledge of the community for referral is necessary. In some cases nurses function as case managers. Nurses may be involved in 24-hour hotline services. Generally mental health care is interdisciplinary, thus calling for the nurse to use collaboration skills. Clients may vary from mentally healthy people in a situational crisis to those with acute or chronic schizophrenia or Alzheimer's disease. Often the nurse acts as an advocate in various capacities.

Maternal and Well-Child Services

Maternal and well-child health care programs may be conducted at a specialized center. Prenatal and postnatal care may be provided in which assessment and education are the focus. Postnatal follow-ups are sometimes made by telephone or with home visits. The nurse may advise clients on exercise, nutrition, and family planning. These services are discussed in more detail in Chapter 8.

Nutrition Services

Nutrition centers may provide health teaching and counseling for mothers and children, older adults, and homeless or addicted clients. Government-sponsored Women, Infants, and Children (WIC) Programs help fortify the dietary intake of infants, children, and pregnant women. For decades the research has demonstrated that for every $1 spent on WIC, $3 is saved in the improved health status of the women and children receiving the food vouchers. Meals on Wheels and food pantries may be part of the program for older adults, homebound individuals, or clients and families living in poverty. Programs for adolescents with eating disorders, nutrition counseling for people with diabetes, and programs for the overweight client illustrates the variety of nutrition programs that can be offered in specialized clinics.

Senior Citizens Centers

Senior citizen health clinics, designed to provide health care for seniors, are found in senior high-rise buildings, neighborhood senior centers, and other locations where high concentrations of elderly citizens live. These clinics provide blood pressure screening, medication review, hospital discharge follow-up, basic nursing screening and assessment, and disease prevention and health promotion interventions. Some clinics offer home visits.

In this setting, the clinic nurse may identify older adults who are in need of companionship or friendship. In some community-based senior citizen clinics, volunteers provide friendship on a one-to-one basis. These types of programs demonstrate success by providing older adults with the opportunity to have support and friendship, which has been shown to reduce depression and the number of clinic visits.

Nursing Centers

Among the newer forms of community-based care are **nursing-managed health centers**. With more than 40 million Americans not having health insurance, countless undocumented workers, cuts in Medicaid funding and increase in health care spending, the need of a safety net has been intensified in the last decade (Hansen-Turton, 2005). Nurse-managed health centers are increasingly offering communities another option for access to high-quality primary care to those individual with limited access. Physician backup is available, and consultation is used as needed.

A nursing center is not only a setting; it is also a philosophy of care. A nursing center is managed by nurses in partnership with the community; they serve by shaping broader services offered to the community. Nursing centers bring nursing care directly to communities to help maximize the health of diverse populations, one of the two broad goals for Healthy People 2010 (U.S. DHHS, 2000). Nursing centers are the perfect design to meet this charge (Fig. 11-3).

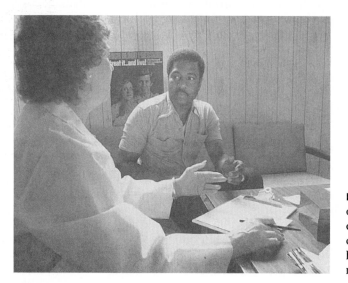

FIGURE 11-3. ▶ Nurses counsel men and women, children, and elderly clients in community health centers across the nation.

Most academic nursing centers focus on community health, outreach, and **wellness promotion,** and many operate out of schools of nursing, with faculty and students providing the services. As mentioned, they often provide services to the underserved, uninsured, and disadvantaged populations, including women and children, the homeless, and minorities. However, there are nursing centers that serve insured populations as well. See Box 11-2 for a description of the development and success of a community nursing center.

◆ **BOX 11-2** A Community Nursing Center for the Health Promotion of Senior Citizens ◆

Community Nursing Centers usually function as the first level of contact between members of vulnerable populations and health care. This cost-effective model offers direct access to nurses who offer holistic, client-centered health services. A community nursing center was developed in Chester, Pennsylvania in 1997 as a partnership between the faculty at Neumann College Division of Nursing and Health Sciences and Widener University School of Nursing, and the Health Advisor Committee of Chester. The intent of the collaboration was to determine health care needs of underserved senior citizens in this community and develop a system to meets these needs. The needs assessment identified health needs in the county as early cancer detection; expansion of support to the home for the frail elderly; expansion of support for chronic psychiatric, drug, and alcoholic clients; prevention of sexually transmitted diseases; provision of better health promotion for the public; and the reduction of premature cardiovascular deaths. From these needs the goals for the nursing center became:

• Identify the unmet health promotion needs of elderly men and women.
• Establish a nurse-managed center to provide health promotion activities, and research and placement of nursing students to focus on the health of elderly men and women.
• Provide culturally competent health promotion activities to the elderly residents.
• Promote relationships with existing health maintenance organizations to meet the health promotion needs of elderly men and women.

Students and faculty worked from the inception of the partnership to develop the program. Forms were developed to track the progress of the client, including an intake form, admission record, and nursing visit report. The faculty and undergraduate and graduate nursing students from both universities worked in the center to meet the identified needs and serve as an effective referral system to services within the community. From 1997 to 2001 over 400 clients were seen at the center. The evaluation data suggested that the center has had a positive impact on the health of those receiving nursing care at the center at the primary, secondary, and tertiary level of prevention.

Source: Newman, D. M., (2005). A community nursing center for the health promotion of senior citizens based on the Neuman systems model. *Nursing Education Perspectives, 26*(4), 221–223.

Research on nursing centers is limited, but studies document changes in client and family knowledge, attitudes, behavior, and health status; client satisfaction; cost-effectiveness; and quality of care (Research in Community-Based Nursing Care 11-1). Surveillance of health issues and nutrition were found to be the most common types of nursing interventions in nursing centers (Tagliareni, & King 2006). Several factors impede research on nursing centers, primarily lack

---

RESEARCH IN COMMUNITY-BASED NURSING CARE ▶ 11-1

Review of Studies of Whether Nurse Practitioners Working in Primary Care Provide Equivalent Care as Compared to Physicians

This was a systematic review of randomized controlled trials and prospective observational studies comparing nurse practitioners and physicians providing care at the first point of contact for clients with undifferentiated health problems in a primary care setting, which provided data on one or more of the following outcomes: patient satisfaction, health status, costs, and process of care. These studies were identified through Cochrane, MEDLINE, Embase, CINAHL, science citation index, database of abstracts of reviews of effectiveness, national research register, hand searches, and published bibliographies. Eleven trials and 23 observational studies were included in the review.

The review, which complied the data from the 34 studies, revealed the following:

- Clients were more satisfied with care by a nurse practitioner.
- No difference in health status was found.
- Nurse practitioners spent more time with clients and made more investigations than did physicians.
- No differences were found in prescriptions, return consultations, or referrals.
- Nurse practitioners seemed to provide a quality of care that is at least as good, and in some ways better, than doctors.

The researchers recommended that there should be an increased involvement of nurse practitioners in primary care. They also suggested that future research should explore the reasons that clients were more satisfied with nurse practitioner care than physician care. In addition, nurse practitioners and doctors did not necessarily work under similar circumstances or with similar pressures on their time, and this should be considered in future research. Further, research on nurse practitioners needs to be broadened to encompass a wider range of client groups with more complex psychosocial problems or chronic diseases.

Horrocks, S., Anderson, E., & Salisbury, C. (2002). Systematic review of whether nurse practitioners working in primary care can provide equivalent care to doctors. *BMJ, 324,* 819–823.

of resources, time, staff, and money. However, the need for research is acute. Current accurate data on the number of nursing centers, diversity of missions, economic status, quality, and other issues are not available (Mackey & McNiel, 2002).

Schools

In 1902, Lillian Wald placed a nurse, Lina Rogers, in a school setting in New York City as an experiment. The experiment, to determine if placing nurses in schools could reduce the spread of contagious diseases, proved to be successful. This was the beginning of the school nursing movement that has provided the backbone of nursing-related health promotion activity in the school setting. Today, schools of all kinds comprise a major sector of practice for community-based nursing: day care centers, preschools, elementary schools, secondary schools, colleges, and universities. Children seen by school nurses reflect the changing society of the nation, with different racial and ethnic backgrounds, varying socioeconomic backgrounds, and complex disabilities. Often school nurses are the most important source of health assessment, health education, and emergency care for the nation's children.

The **school nurse** focuses on the healthy, growing individual, or in some cases specializes in educational settings for the mentally or physically disabled. State laws determine if the school can provide emergency treatment for injuries, maintenance of health records, immunizations, referral for health and social services, physical assessments, and teaching (Fig. 11-4). One school nurse describes her position as follows:

> ▶ I am responsible for about 1,200 high school students. Our office is open daily, and we serve 50 to 60 students each day with such complaints as headaches, sore throats, and fever. The biggest change over the past few years has been the decrease in the number of high school-age single mothers we serve. A decade ago I developed a program for these young women that includes safe sex, birth control options, child care, and child health. The decrease in the pregnancy rate is related to this program. The best evaluation data from the program shows that only one of the young women who have completed the classes has had another unintended pregnancy. I would say I am nurse, mother, confidante, baby-sitter, first-aid giver, record keeper, and friend as a school nurse.

Many school nurses have become "drop-in" counselors. Often the school nurse is the one to whom a child or adolescent goes with personal questions and problems. These nurses use an established network of referrals for students' personal needs. A school nurse may refer to speech and hearing services, individual and family counseling, gay and lesbian support and youth groups, the department of social services, crisis drop-in centers, drug and alcohol programs, foster care, drop-in health clinics, and parents-in-training groups.

A school health program may include identification of communicable, chronic, and disabling diseases; immunizations; safety; and health education. School nursing requires competence in health teaching, delegated medical functions, collaboration, counseling, case finding, consultation, referral and follow-up, advocacy, and case management. Required educational preparation varies from that of a registered nurse to a nurse practitioner with a graduate degree. Most families in a community are already associated with the schools. Expansion

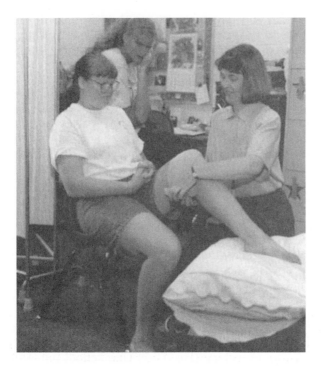

FIGURE 11-4. ▶ A school nurse assesses and treats an injured child. This is essential to a comprehensive school health program.

of school-based clinics into comprehensive neighborhood health and social service centers provides another opportunity for offering nursing care to people where they live.

There has been some criticism of the conventional health education function typical of school nurses in most school districts. This criticism is that it has little to do with health-promoting school projects and is not integrated with other community-based pediatric services. There are more and more calls for school nursing service to either re-evaluate its function and processes or to move to a broader primary health care practitioner role. Whitehead (2006) recommends that school nurses embrace the evolving broad-based health promotion concepts and move beyond a traditional reliance on the current limited health education role. Another trend is toward school-based health centers (SBHC) which are increasing in the United States. SBHC is a model that provides a nurse-managed clinic in a school. Most SBHCs offer primary care with a disease prevention/health promotion model but some include a nurse practitioner or physician's assistant operating a medical model (Scully & Hackbarth, 2005).

Occupational Health Nurse

Occupational health nursing began in 1895 when Ida M. Steward was hired by the Vermont Marble Company to visit mothers and infants, care for the ill at home, and curb communicable diseases. During the same time period, Margaret Sanger, PHN, was instrumental in advocating for the women factory workers in the lower East Side of Manhattan. This role was soon expanded to include disease and injury prevention and first aid in the work place.

Currently, the toll of workplace injuries and illness remains significant. Every year, almost 6,000 people die from work-related diseases (U.S. Department of Labor, 2006). Employers acknowledge that the health and well-being of employees are vital to morale and enhance the productivity of the company. Consequently, most companies provide health insurance, and many have developed programs to enhance health through the promotion of healthy lifestyles. This has spawned new language and a new focus for health care with programs such as **work-site health promotion, employee wellness programs,** and **employee assistance programs,** all of which focus on the health of employees. Healthy snacks and meals, exercise programs and facilities, and educational classes are all used by companies to promote health.

A survey of almost 6,000 occupational health nurses throughout the United States and Canada provides an interesting picture of occupational health nursing (Strasser, et al., 2006). First it shows that the educational level varies, with 36% having a diploma, 31% an associate degree, 29% a bachelor's degree, and 3% a master's degree. As far as time spent in various roles and activities: 27% was spent in direct care, 43% as a case manager, 14% as a health educator or counselor, and 9% as a consultant.

The focus of the **occupational health nurse** is on keeping employees healthy, preventing illness and accidents, providing assistance to the employee who is returning to work after an illness or injury, and ensuring a safe business or industrial environment. Given the expanding opportunities in this type of service nurses can market their expertise to employers. They can provide programs aimed at job-related safety, weight reduction, and addiction-free lifestyles as well as promote nutrition, exercise, smoking cessation, and family planning.

Disaster Nursing

Traditionally disaster nursing has been provided through the American Red Cross. Nurses have been central to the provision of services through the American Red Cross throughout the history of disaster nursing. Beginning with the 1880 Johnstown flood and the 1888 yellow fever epidemic, nurses have provided assistance during times of crisis. More than 30,000 nurses are involved in the American Red Cross in paid and volunteer positions. These activities consist of providing direct assistance in times of crisis, developing and teaching courses, and acting in management and supervisory roles. There are opportunities for both registered nurses and nursing students (American Red Cross, 2006).

There is renewed interest and appreciation for this type of nursing care following the attacks on the World Trade Center on September 11, 2001. Although we know more today about disaster nursing, terrorism, and bioterrorism preparedness than we did in September of 2001, some believe there is a need for additional education, training, and other preparation for all health care workers in anticipation of another terrorist event.

To be prepared, nurses benefit from first developing their own individual family and home disaster plan. They must understand medical management of those exposed to biological agents as well as how to protect themselves when treating victims. According to the Centers for Disease Control and Prevention (CDC, 2006), protection varies according to the agent. The CDC provides education for the appropriate precautions on its Web site: http://www.bt.cdc.gov/. There is additional discussion of disaster nursing in Chapter 15.

NURSING SPECIALTIES

Although all nurses need to be communicators, teachers, managers, and care providers, nurses may specialize in certain areas. A nurse's title may reflect his or her setting, such as school nurse, home care nurse, or occupational health nurse. Other titles may define the role the nurse plays in a setting, such as health educator, case manager, discharge planner, or continuity of care nurse. The nursing specialty may also be defined by level of education and completion of additional certification.

Specialties Requiring Registered Nurse License

Advanced practice nurses include nurse practitioners and clinical nurse specialists. The number of nurse practitioners and certified nurse midwives increased dramatically in the last 2 decades. In 2000 there were an estimated 95,000 nurse practitioners and 8,000 certified nurse midwives practicing in the United States, an increase of about 160% from the early 1990s. Over this time period these two professions have become more widely accepted by physicians, clients, and the general public as key members of the health care delivery team (National Center for Health Workforce Analysis Bureau of Health Professions [NCHWABHP], 2005). There are several underlying forces which have contributed to this dramatic change. First, the concerns about the rising cost of health care along with the growing recognition that advanced practice nurses provide cost-effective, high quality care. Second, consumers are better educated about health care diagnosis and treatment as more health information has become widely available to the general public. Third, is the trend that consumers play a more active role in the purchase of health services, the utilizations of services, and the choice of care providers. Fourth, the dramatic increases in the number of advanced practice nurses occurred as consumers are more open to practitioners, interventions, and approaches beyond the traditional ones. A fifth factor stems from the growing number of uninsured and underinsured people in need of health care and the increased demand for advanced practice nurses to work with underserved populations. Last of all, nurse practitioners are more commonly used instead of medical residents in primary care (Health Resources and Services Administration, 2006).

A **nurse practitioner** is a registered nurse who has graduated from a nurse practitioner program, and successfully completed the advanced practice licensing exam. Nurse practitioners first began to appear in the United States and Canada in the late 1960s. The core competencies of this level of practice are found in Box 11-3. Nurse practitioners may be generalists or may specialize in the care of particular types of clients. The most common include neonatal, pediatric, adult, geriatric, and family nurse practitioners and nurse midwives. They work in clinics, hospitals, and long-term care facilities, for public and private agencies, and in almost any setting providing health care. There are also nurse practitioners in medical specialty areas such as oncology, nephrology, and rheumatology.

Not only do nurse practitioners provide quality health care, but they do so at a fraction of the cost of physician care. For example, extended care facilities with nurse practitioners have been found to provide better care to residents (Intrator, et al. 2005). The proportion of nursing home facilities with nurse practitioners doubled from less than 10% to over 20% in the last decade. This trend may have a

---

◆ **BOX 11-3** Condensed Competencies From the National Organization of Nurse Practitioner Faculties ◆

- Health promotion and protection
- Disease prevention
- Teaching and coaching
- Critical thinking
- Role modeling
- Improving health outcomes
- Team collaboration
- Monitoring and ensuring quality care
- Cultural competence
- Interpersonal communication skills
- Assessment of all aspects of patient's health status
- Diagnosis of health states
- Planning care
- Implementing care safely and efficiently
- Evaluating care
- Consultation

Source: Rhoads, J., Ferguson, L. A., Langford, C. (2006). Measuring nurse practitioner productivity. *Dermatology Nursing, 18*(1), 32–38.

---

positive impact on both quality care and cost containment in nursing homes. Further, this suggests greater opportunities for geriatric nurse practitioners in the future.

A **certified nurse midwife** has provided care for women during normal pregnancy, labor, and delivery since the inception of the certification and accreditation process in the early 1970s. The certified nurse midwife practices in connection with a health care agency in which medical services are available if the client develops complications. In the United States, a nurse midwife is required by law to have a baccalaureate degree in nursing and a graduate degree from an accredited nurse midwife program, and he or she must pass the certification examination from the American College of Nurse Midwives. The number of certified nurse midwives more than doubled, from 3,000 to 8,000, in the last 10 years (National Center for Health Workforce Analysis, 2005).

A **clinical nurse specialist** can practice in acute care or community settings. First formally recognized as a nursing specialty in 1965, such positions today generally focus on a particular expertise (e.g., diabetes or oncology). As with nurse practitioners, the last 20 years has seen a substantial increase in the number of clinical nurse specialist (Jones, 2005). The specialist may develop and oversee a specialty program, act as a resource and consultant for other staff, and establish educational programs for the general public. Nurses have different degrees of autonomy and responsibility, depending on the setting. Educational and professional role requirements differ as well. Most states require the nurse to have a master's degree to be a clinical nurse specialist. National certification by professional associations may be available. The role of the clinical nurse specialist is evolving as the health care delivery system continues to be transformed (Jones, 2005).

CONCLUSIONS

Rapid and dramatic changes have occurred in health care delivery in the community. Today opportunities exist for men and women to assume many roles in different settings with a variety of clients. Because of the increasing elderly population, many nurses are entering the field of geriatric nursing, but many other opportunities exist for the practicing nurse. Such practice settings include, but are not limited to, the home, nursing centers, a variety of clinics and ambulatory care centers, specialized care centers, long-term care facilities, residential programs, schools, and industry. The nurse may specialize in primary care, as a case manager, clinical nurse specialist, or nurse practitioner. The dramatic expansion in the use of advanced practice nurses in the last 2 decades suggests that the importance of the role of the nurse in community-based settings will continue to expand in subsequent years. The principles of community-based care apply to all nursing roles in all settings. All of this points to the expanding opportunities our profession presents for each of us to develop an exciting and evolving career in nursing.

What's on the Web

Internet address: http://allnurses.com/
To find an exhaustive array of information on different specialty roles in nursing, consult allnurses.com and click on the Nursing Specialties category. This site provides access to resources for more than 50 nursing specialties, including but not limited to many community-based nursing roles, such as school, ambulatory care, parish, and correctional health nursing; telephone triage; intravenous therapy; and advanced practice nursing or nurse practitioner duties.

American Academy of Ambulatory Care Nursing
Telephone: (856) 256-2350
Toll-free: (800) AMB-NURS
Internet address: http://aaacn.inurse.com/
This organization advances and influences the art and science of ambulatory care nursing practice and health care delivery systems to improve the health of individuals and communities.

American Academy of Nurse Practitioners (AANP)
Telephone: (512) 442-4262

Internet address: http://www.aanp.org/
This organization promotes high standards of health care as delivered by nurse practitioners and acts as a forum to enhance the identity and continuity of nurse practitioners.

American Association of Occupational Health Nurses (AAOHN)
2920 Brandywine Road, Suite 100
Atlanta, GA 30341
Telephone: (770) 455-7757
Internet address: http://www.aaohn.org/
This site provides information about occupational health nursing and the professional organization. AAOHN's mission is to advance the profession of occupational and environmental health nursing as the authority on health, safety, productivity, and disability management for worker populations.

American Holistic Nurses Association (AHNA)
Telephone: (800) 278-2462
Internet address: http://www.ahna.org/
The mission of AHNA is to unite nurses in healing. AHNA serves as a bridge between

the traditional medical paradigm and universal complementary and alternative health practices. AHNA supports the concepts of holism: a state of harmony between body, mind and emotions, and spirit within an ever-changing environment.

American School Health Association (ASHA)
Internet address: http://www.ashaweb.org/
ASHA unites many school professionals who are committed to safeguarding the health of school-age children. The goals of the organization are to advocate for children and youth, represent all school health professionals, and promote professional education, public education, research, and service to children and youth. The Web site offers information about publications and conferences related to school health.

Healthy People 2010
Educational and Community-Based Programs

Internet address: http://www.healthypeople.gov/document/HTML/Volume1/07Ed.htm
This resource is one chapter in Healthy People 2010, which is full of information about various community-based settings (schools, work sites, and other community settings) and the opportunities for community-based programs. It outlines issues and trends in each setting, identifies disparity considerations as well as opportunities for health promotion and disease prevention programming. Goals and objectives for each setting are articulated.

Visiting Nurse Associations of America (VNAA)
Internet address:
http://www.vnaa.org/vnaa/gen/html~home.aspx
This Web site has information about visiting nurse agencies, conferences, and professional information, as well as caregiver information and home care resources.

References and Bibliography

American Red Cross. (2006). Nursing. Retrieved October 11, 2006, from http://www.redcross.org/services/nursing/0,1082,0_327_,00.html

Centers for Disease Control and Prevention. (2006). Emergency preparedness and response. Retrieved October 11, 2006, from http://www.bt.cdc.gov/

Hansen-Turton, T. (2005). The nurse-managed health center safety net: A policy solution to reducing health disparities. *Nursing Clinics of North America, 40*(4), 729–738.

Health Resources and Services Administration. (2006). Bureau of Health Professions. *A comparison of changes in the professional practice of nurse practitioners, physician assistants, and certified nurse midwives: 1992 and 2000.* Retrieved on September 29, 2006, from http://www.bhpr.hrsa.gov/healthworkforce/reports/scope/scope1-2.htm

Health Resources and Services Administration. (2006b). Primary care health centers. Retrieved on October 30, 2007, from http://bhpr.hrsa.gov/healthworkforce/reports/scope/scope1-2.htm

Hodges, B. (2005). Asthma camp. *Paediatric Nursing, 17*(6), 20–22.

Horn, S. D. (2005). RN staffing time and outcomes of long-stay nursing home residents: pressure ulcers and other adverse outcomes are less likely as RNs spend more time on direct patients care. *The American Journal of Nursing, 105*(11), 58–71.

Horrocks, S., Anderson, E., & Salisbury, C., (2002). Systematic review of whether nurse practitioners working in primary care can provide equivalent care to doctors. *BMJ, 345,* 819–823.

Intrator, O., Feng, Z., Mor, V., et al. (2005). The employment of nurse practitioners and physician assistants in U.S. nursing homes. *Gerontologist, 45*(4), 486–485.

Jones, M. L. (2005). Role development and effective practice in specialist and advanced practice roles in acute hospital settings: Systematic review and meta-synthesis. *Journal of Advanced Nursing, 49,*(2), 191–209.

Kitzman, H., Olds, D. L., Sidora, K., et al. (2000). Enduring effects of nurse home visitation on maternal life course. *JAMA, 283*(15), 1983–1989.

Lanksbear, A., Sheldon, T., Maynard, A. (2005). Nurse staffing and healthcare outcomes. *Advances in Nursing Science, 28*(2), 163–174.

Mackey, T. A., & McNiel, N. O. (2002). Quality indicators for academic nursing primary care centers. *Nursing Economics, 20*(2), 62–65.

Morris, & Strong, L. (2004). The impact of homelessness on the health of families. *Journal of School Nursing, 20*(4), 221–227.

National Center for Health Workforce Analysis, Bureau of Health Professions (2005). Health Resources and Services Administration (#HRSSA 230-00-0099). Retrieved on September 29, 2006, from http://www.bhpr.hrsa.gov/healthworkforce/reports

National Citizens' Coalition for Nursing Home Reform (2006). *A consumer guide to choosing a nursing home:* Consumer information sheet. Retrieved on October 8, 2006, from http://www.nursinghomeaction.org

National Respite Network. (2006). Adult day care: One form of respite for older adults. Retrieved on October 6, 2006, from http://www.archrespite.org/index.htm

Newman, D. M. (2005). A community nursing center for the health promotion of senior citizens based on the Neuman systems model. *Nursing Education Perspectives, 26*(4), 221–223.

Olds, D. L., Henderson, C. R., Jr., & Kitzman, H. (1994). Does prenatal and infancy home visitation have enduring effects on qualities of parental care giving and health at 25 to 50 months of life? *Pediatrics, 93,* 89–98.

Olds, D. L., Henderson, C. R., Jr., Tatelbaum, R., & Chamberlin, R. (1986). Improving the delivery of prenatal care and outcomes of pregnancy: A randomized trial of home visitations. *Pediatrics, 77,* 16–28.

Olds, D. L., Henderson, C. R., Jr., Tatelbaum, R., & Chamberlin, R. (1988). Improving the life course development of socially disadvantaged mothers: A randomized trial of home visitations. *American Journal of Public Health, 78*(11), 1436–1445.

Rhoads, J., Ferguson, L.A., Langford, C. (2006). Measuring nurse practitioner productivity. *Dermatology Nursing,18*(1), 32–38.

Scully, J., & Hackbarth, D. (2005). School of nursing sponsorship of a school-based health center: Challenges and barriers. *Nursing Clinics of North America, 40*(4), 607–617.

Schoenman, D. (2002). Surveillance as a nursing intervention: Use in community nursing centers. *Journal of Community Health Nursing, 19*(1), 33–47.

Solari-Twadell, P. (1999). The emerging practice of parish nursing. In P. Solari-Twadell, & M. A. McDermott (Eds.), *Parish nursing: Promoting whole person health within faith communities* (pp. 3–24). Thousand Oaks: Sage Publishing.

Strasser, P. B., Maher, H. K., Knuth, G., & Fabrey, L. J. (2006). Occupational health nursing 2004 practice analysis report. *American Association of Occupational Health Nurses, 54*(1), 14–23.

Tagliareni, M. & King, E. (2006). Documenting health promotion services in community-based nursing center. *Holistic Nursing Practice, 20*(1), 20–27.

U.S. Census Bureau. (2006). The elderly population. Retrieved on October 6, 2006, from http://www.census.gov/population/www/socdemo/age.html#older

U.S. Conference of Mayors (2006). A Status Report on Hunger and Homelessness in America. Retrieved on October 8, 2006, from http://www.usmayors.org/

U.S. Department of Health and Human Services. (2000). Healthy people 2010. National health promotion and disease prevention objectives (DHHS Publication No. 91–50212). Washington, DC: U.S. Government Printing Office.

U.S. Department of Labor. Bureau of Labor Statistics, Census of Fatal Occupation Injuries. (2006). Retrieved on October 30, 2007, from http://www.bls.gov/iif/oshwc/cfoi/cfch0005.pdf

Weis, D., Schank, M. J., & Matheus, R. (2006). The process of empowerment: A parish nurse perspective. *Journal of Holistic Nursing, 24*(1), 17–24.

Weis, D. M., Schank, M. J., Coenen, A., & Matheus, R. (2002). Parish nurse practice with client aggregates. *Journal of Community Health Nursing, 19*(2), 105–113.

Whitehead, D. (2006). The health-promoting school: What role for nursing? *Journal of Clinical Nursing, 15*(3), 264–271.

Yousey, Y., & Carr, M. (2005). A health care program for homeless children using Healthy People 2010 objectives. *Nursing Clinics of North America, 40*(4), 791–801.

L E A R N I N G ▼ A C T I V I T I E S

◆ JOURNALING ACTIVITY 11-1

Contact a nurse in a specialty area that is of interest to you. Set up an appointment to interview him or her and spend some time observing the nurse perform in the clinical role.

- Develop questions prior to the interview (at least four to eight questions about aspects of the role that interest you). Take notes during the interview or with permission from the nurse, audiotape the interview and transcribe it into written form. Complete a summary of the interview.
- As soon as you are home from the observation of the nurse, answer the following questions in your clinical journal.
  - What did you see, hear, and feel today?
  - How does it compare to what you expected?
  - What roles would you enjoy doing?
  - Which role responsibilities would you hate?
  - Is this the type of practice that you would enjoy? Why or why not?

If you are interested in this role, what is the next step that you will take to further explore this area of nursing.

◆ JOURNALING ACTIVITY 11-2

1. In your clinical journal, identify a practice setting that you would like to know more about. Identify three ways you can learn more about this setting and the roles that nurses have in it. Implement this plan.
2. Discuss the strategies you used to explore this setting and the roles of the nurse.
3. What did you learn from this experience?
4. How will you use this information?

◆ PRACTICAL APPLICATION ACTIVITY 11-3

Interview a nurse in one of the settings described in this chapter. Use the following questions as a part of the interview.

1. How do you assist your clients to improve their selfcare? Can you tell me a story about when you assisted or did not assist one of your clients to improve his or her self-care?
2. How do you alter care according to the context of the client's family, culture, and community? Can you tell me about a situation when you or someone else you work with did or did not alter care according to the context of the client's family, culture, or community?
3. How do you incorporate the concept of disease prevention and health promotion in the care you provide to your clients? Can you give me some examples?
4. How do you enhance continuity for your clients? Can you tell me about a time when you were or you weren't successful creating continuity?

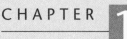

CHAPTER 12

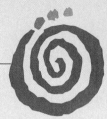

Home Health
Care Nursing

ROBERTA HUNT

LEARNING OBJECTIVES

1. Identify the purpose and goals of home care nursing.
2. Discuss types of home care agencies.
3. Outline the advantages and disadvantages of home care.
4. Discuss barriers to successful home care nursing.
5. Define the nursing skills and competencies needed in home care.
6. Describe the home visit and its main components.
7. Summarize methods the community-based nurse can use in meeting needs of the lay caregiver.

KEY TERMS

financial assessment
home care agencies
home care equipment vendors
hospital-based home care agencies

lay caregiving
official home care agencies
respite care

CHAPTER TOPICS

◆ Historical Perspective
◆ Significance of Home Health Care
◆ Agencies That Provide Home Care
◆ Acute Care Nursing Versus Home Care Nursing
◆ Challenges to Successful Home Care
◆ Nursing Skills and Competencies in Home Health Care
◆ Support of the Lay Caregiver
◆ The Future of Home Care
◆ Conclusions

┌─────────────── THE NURSE SPEAKS ───────────────┐

"Please go out and see him. He's refusing hospitalizations and hospice, so there's not much more I can do." This was a fairly common request from AIDS-specialized physicians in the early to mid-1990s, so I was not surprised to find a very cachetic, disoriented patient when I arrived. Tom was lying in soiled sheets in an upstairs bedroom. He was too weak to be walked to the bathroom by his partner, and he had fallen twice in the past 3 days. He could answer some questions but frequently drifted off to sleep midsentence. Physical inspection revealed a severely wasted male in his middle years with a stage IV decubitus ulcer on his coccyx and 4+ pitting edema bilaterally to midthigh. When he was able to talk, he conveyed a strong will to live and gratitude for a supportive partner who was willing to assist in all of his care. Tom had tried the AIDS medications, but he had stopped them because he felt too weak to keep up with the regimen.

I immediately realized Tom still had a curative versus comfort focus. I also recognized it would take the effort of many people working together if we were to pull him back from the edge of death. Complex cases require thoughtful and effective case management, and Tom's case was no exception. I pulled in as many home health aide hours as his insurance would cover. I called and got orders for a dietitian consult, which led to NG tube feedings. From there, I involved a wound care specialist, who prescribed the best products to heal the decubitus ulcer. Tom was moved to the first floor of his home, providing more space for a hospital bed, commode, and wheelchair. This also allowed his partner to get more sleep so the family did not face the frequent problem of burnout. When the insurance company balked at the cost of all these services, I reminded them of the expense that would be incurred if Tom were staying in a hospital or long-term care facility for weeks on end.

Slowly, Tom's level of strength began to return and with it his ability to take his antiretroviral medications. Three months later, I was called to the front office by our receptionist. There stood Tom with a big smile on his face and a bouquet of flowers in his hand. He gave me a warm hug and asked me to wish him luck as he returned for his first day back at his job. The combined efforts of home care professionals guided by nursing case management had indeed helped Tom follow his desire to continue to focus on living.

—Teddie M. Potter, RN, MS, Home Care Nurse,
Instructor, Minneapolis Community and Technical College

└───┘

Home health care is the provision of health services to individuals and families in their places of residence for the purpose of promoting, maintaining, and restoring health. It is one of the most rapidly growing service industries in the United States. Home care nurses must be competent communicators, teachers, managers, and physical care givers. This chapter begins with a brief introduction to the history of home health care. **Home care agencies**, the goals, advantages and disadvantages of home care, as well as the barriers to successful home care are discussed. A large section of the chapter deals with nursing skills and competencies, together with a summary of the first visit. Safety issues and lay caretaker involvement conclude the chapter.

HISTORICAL PERSPECTIVE

Home care nursing as it is practiced today is a relatively new phenomenon. However, providing health care in the home is a very old concept. Florence Nightingale is credited with developing the concept of nursing care provided in the home in the 1860s. In the United States, Lillian Wald and Mary Brewster established nursing home visiting in the late 1800s that later evolved into the New York City Visiting Nurse Association. Almost 100 years later changes in federal reimbursement for health care brought about vast growth in home health care. Figure 12-1 is a charming reminder of the long and rich history of the home care nursing profession.

Modern home care evolved from the Visiting Nurse Association (VNA), which originated at the beginning of the 20th century in New York City. The mission of home care has changed from that of the VNA in the early part of this century, when nurses were caring for mostly women who were pregnant and postpartum and their infants. In addition the VNA cared for indigent tuberculosis clients in the tenements. Physicians were involved in home care before World War II. The war produced a shortage of physicians, however, so the use of nurses for home care services expanded. In the 1940s, **hospital-based home care agencies** were established.

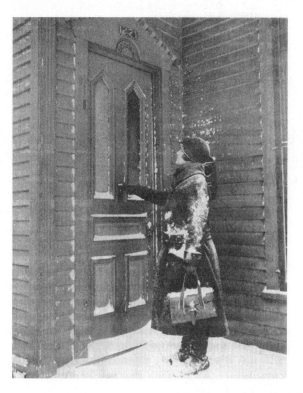

FIGURE 12-1. ▶ A Minnesota home health nurse paying a visit to a client at the beginning of the 20th century. Copyright the Minnesota Historical Society. Used with permission.

TABLE 12-1	Number of Medicare-Certified Home Care Agencies				
	Freestanding Agencies			**Facility Based**	
Year	VNA	PUB	PROP	HOSP	Total
1967	549	939	0	133	1,753
1975	525	1,228	0	273	2,242
1985	514	1,205	832	1,277	5,983
1995	575	1,182	3,951	2,470	9,120
2000	436	909	2,863	2,151	7,152
2003	439	888	3,402	1,776	7,265

Adapted from: National Association for Home Care (2006). *Basic statistics about home care*. Washington, DC: Author. Retrieved October 24, 2006, from http://www.nahc.org/04Hc-stats.pdf

A pivotal change in home care came from the 1965 Medicare and Medicaid legislation that allowed payment for home care services for qualified recipients. With this legislation, home care became more narrowly defined as a medical model alternative to extend hospital care to the home. The impact of this legislation was the first factor to contribute to the growth in the home care industry. In 1963, there were 1,100 home health agencies; today, there are more than 8,000 (Table 12-1).

The second factor that contributed to the growth in the home care industry was the implementation of diagnosis-related groups (DRGs) for Medicare during the late 1970s and early 1980s. This legislation was intended as a cost containment measure. As most hospitals and health maintenance organizations (HMOs) were required to follow Medicare's DRG reimbursement guidelines, home care began to be viewed as a vital aspect of the health care system. Again, home care became a more central aspect of health care as a cost-containment strategy. Gradually, throughout the United States, insurance companies and HMOs adopted home care as part of their standard health insurance package because of the cost efficiency of care at home versus institutional care. With the trend toward shorter hospital stays, continuing care needs, and available reimbursement for home health care, the home care boom was born. Further, the increasing number of noninstitutionalized individuals over age 65, living longer and with multiple chronic conditions, has intensified the need for more home health care services. The acceleration in development of sophisticated technology that allows people to be kept alive and relatively comfortable in their own homes has also added to the need for nursing care in the home, as has consumer demand for improved end-of-life care at home.

SIGNIFICANCE OF HOME HEALTH CARE

The goal of home health care nursing is to provide services to individuals and families and to promote, maintain, and restore health. In most cases, this is achieved through short-term, intermittent, direct nursing care made in home visits. Home care nurses provide direct services or supervise those services to assist with activities of daily living (ADL); teach clients, families, and caregivers how to provide self-care; and use communication skills to enhance continuity of care.

Governmental, private, and hospital-based programs employ home health care nurses. Home health care nurses come from all levels of educational preparation, with 40% BSN, 24% Diploma, 23% Associate, and 5% with a Master's degree. Only

6% of all home care nurses are under 30 years of age (Anthony & Milone-Nuzzo, 2005). Home health care includes not only skilled nursing care but also the services of physical, occupational, and speech therapists; social workers; and home health aides.

The National Association for Home Care and Hospice (NAHC) is the largest home care trade organization in the country. Its mission is to improve the quality of home care services. NAHC represents the interests of clients who need home care and caregivers who provide such services. Through a variety of activities and publications, NAHC attempts to be a unified voice for the home care and hospice community.

More than 69% of clients served in home care are older than 65 years and 17% are over 85 years of age. Hospitalized clients make up a large proportion of home care clients within 30 days of discharge. Diseases of the circulatory system account for almost 31% of those receiving home care services with Medicare reimbursement (NAHC, 2006). There are also an increasing number of clients requiring high-technology medical interventions (e.g., intravenous therapy, mechanical ventilation, parenteral nutrition).

AGENCIES THAT PROVIDE HOME CARE

Home health care has evolved into a major industry, with three key components: home care agencies, **home care equipment vendors**, and home infusion therapy companies. Home infusion therapy is discussed in Chapter 13. A change in the types of agencies that provide home care resulted from the federal legislation enacted in 1965 and 1983. Agency types today include official, hospital-based, and proprietary.

Official home care agencies are often housed in city and county departments and only provide service certified by federal government mandates. Hospital-based agencies have no mandate and can offer services of their own choosing, or Medicare and Medicaid service if they are certified by the federal government. They receive no tax support and operate as a unit or department of a hospital. Proprietary agencies are freestanding and for-profit home care agencies that provide services based on third-party reimbursement or self-pay.

All three types of agencies may choose to be certified by the federal government to provide services for clients with Medicare and Medicaid insurance. The services have to be skilled and provide home visits (30 minutes to 2 hours). Services include nursing; physical, occupational, and speech therapy; medical social work; and home health aide work. Most insurance companies now pay for home health care services, but few will pay for 24-hour nursing care. Few, if any, insurance carriers will pay for paraprofessional care without skilled care services. The growing managed care movement is following the Medicare guidelines for the development of home health care services, although the number of allowed visits may be fewer and may vary among insurance companies or managed care organizations.

Private duty agencies that primarily provide shift relief at health care institutions and for private clients are generally described as home care agencies. Private sources or private insurance pays for most of the care; time is scheduled in hourly blocks, and services are largely provided by paraprofessionals (aides and homemakers) and nurses. Home care is also a generic term used for the entire industry and can include all types of agencies. In this text, the term home care is used to include all at-home nursing services.

TABLE 12-2 Sources of Payment for Home Care	
Source of Payment	**Percent**
Medicare	31.9
Medicaid	13.3
State and local government	15.7
Private insurance	18.0
Out-of-pocket	18.0
Other	2.9

From National Assocation for Home Care (2006). *Basic statistics about home care*. Washington, DC: Author. Retrieved on October 24, 2006, from http://www.nahc.org/04Hc_stats.pdf

Today, most hospitals own or contract with home care agencies to create a continuum of care or an alternative to hospitalization. HMOs frequently choose home care services over hospitalization for clients because of the cost-effectiveness of home care. Medicare is the largest single payer of home care services (Table 12-2). Clients who are homebound and under the care of a physician are eligible for home care services under Medicare (Box 12-1). Three states have lifted the homebound restriction so it is important for the nurse to know the requirements where he or she is practicing. Many insurance companies follow the same criteria. For the most part, home care has become medical care in the home; clients are given care and treatment under the specific orders of a physician. Thus, in home care the nursing focus has changed from a broad public health model that characterized the role of the VNA focuses on specific needs of the individual that have to be addressed in a limited amount of time.

ACUTE CARE NURSING VERSUS HOME CARE NURSING

Because the primary setting for care has shifted to the home, the number of nurses employed outside the acute care setting has increased. This trend is expected to continue with the growing number of older persons who have functional disabilities, consumer preference for care in the home, and technological advances that bring increasingly complex treatments into the home.

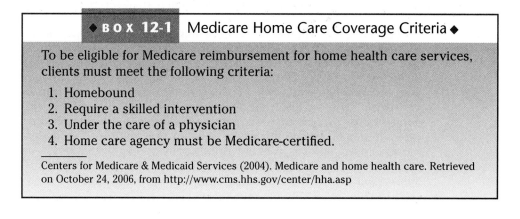

◆ **BOX 12-1** Medicare Home Care Coverage Criteria ◆

To be eligible for Medicare reimbursement for home health care services, clients must meet the following criteria:

1. Homebound
2. Require a skilled intervention
3. Under the care of a physician
4. Home care agency must be Medicare-certified.

Centers for Medicare & Medicaid Services (2004). Medicare and home health care. Retrieved on October 24, 2006, from http://www.cms.hhs.gov/center/hha.asp

There are major differences between practicing in the hospital and in the home. One obvious difference between the two settings is the environment. In the home setting, the nurse is a guest in the client's home, unlike the hospital or clinic setting, where the nurse is in control of the environment. The need to be flexible and adaptable is essential in the home setting as the nurse visits many different clients living in a variety of home situations. While hospitals recruit new graduates, home care agencies normally hire only experienced nurses because of the need for self-reliance and autonomous decision-making. When emergencies arise, unlike in the hospital where there is a large cadre of professionals to consult, there is no back-up for the nurse to consult in the home. When teaching clients in their home the nurse must be competent in developing the client and family's efficacy regarding self-care. Even charting is different in home care where reimbursement often drives all documentation (Thobaben & Sullivan, 2005).

The type and amount of family involvement is not the same in the hospital when compared to care in the home. In the acute care setting, the staff makes decisions regarding the client's care; in the home, the client and family are encouraged to participate in the decision-making process regarding care. Goals aim for long-term rather than short-term outcomes. Making decisions and setting priorities are shared activities.

Even the nurse–client relationship is not the same because in home care the client and family may be cared for over a long period of time. This allows for the development of a therapeutic relationship built on trust and caring that is much closer than in other settings.

CLIENT SITUATIONS IN PRACTICE

◆ Significance of Home Care

Rafael is a home care nurse who visits 91-year-old Norma Wilkinson three times a week. Ms. Wilkinson has several medical problems, the major ones being high blood pressure, a heart condition, and arthritis. Rafael takes Ms. Wilkinson's blood pressure, weighs her, and sometimes draws blood. He checks on Ms. Wilkinson's general well-being. Ms. Wilkinson never married and has no relatives nearby, but Ruth, a woman from her church, looks in on her now and then and takes her shopping. Ruth has a key to the apartment. Ms. Wilkinson does not always take her medications as prescribed because some of her friends tell her she is taking too many pills.

As usual, Rafael telephones before his Friday morning visit. There is no answer, but he decides to make the visit anyway. When he knocks on the door, there is no response and the door is locked. Should he leave? He knows Ms. Wilkinson has had some dizzy spells lately and has fallen several times in the apartment. Rafael decides to call Ruth to bring the key and check the apartment with him. They search the apartment, but Ms. Wilkinson is not there, and she has not slept in her bed. They realize Ms. Wilkinson did not take her pills for the previous 2 days. They begin a search of the building and discover Ms. Wilkinson in a remote part of the basement where no one ever goes. She had fallen and is confused. If the home health nurse had not made his regular visit, Ms. Wilkinson might have been in the basement for several more days before anyone discovered she was missing.

TABLE 12-3 Cost of Inpatient Care Compared With Home Care, Selected Conditions			
Condition	Hospital Costs per Patient, per Month	Home Care Costs per Patient, per Month	Savings per Patient, per Month
Low birth weight	$26,190	$330	$25,860
Ventilator-dependent adults	$21,570	$7,050	$14,520
Oxygen-dependent children	$12,090	$5,250	$6,840
Chemotherapy for children with cancer	$68,870	$55,950	$13,920
Congestive heart failure among the elderly	$1,758	$1,605	$153
Intravenous antibiotic therapy for cellulitis, osteomyelitis, others	$12,510	$4,650	$7,860

National Association for Home Care (2006). *Basic statistics about home care*. Washington, DC: Author. Retrieved on October 24, 2006, from http://www.nahc.org/04Hc_stats.pdf

Advantages of Home Health Care

There are a number of advantages to providing care in the home as opposed to the acute care setting. The primary advantage is the lower cost. Table 12-3 shows the cost of inpatient care compared with home care for selected conditions. For clients, one advantage is the less-threatening, familiar comfort of home, which enhances care and the quality of life. Home care allows for easier access to loved ones and their support, and clients are taught self-care and encouraged to be independent, which maximizes their quality of life. Being at home also removes the family burden of traveling to and from the hospital. Additionally, it contributes to the restoration of family control for the care being provided. These advantages are supported by the philosophy of community-based care, which focuses on enhancing self-care in the context of the family and the community.

Working in home care creates benefits for nurses, seen in higher job satisfaction. This is attributed to the independent nature of this type of practice as well as the opportunity to provide one-on-one care in a flexible work environment. Home care nurses also take pleasure in the health teaching aspect of this specialty. (Anthony & Milone-Nuzzo, 2005; Hartung, 2005).

Disadvantages of Home Health Care

Home care also has disadvantages. The presence of the nurse or other professional is an intrusion on the family's privacy. This may affect family decision making and interaction among members. For several decades, research has demonstrated that stress caused by multiple unfamiliar professionals coming into the home can also affect members of the family. In some instances, conflict may result if the nurse is not sensitive to the family's wishes and boundaries. Out-of-pocket expenses may accumulate as the result of home care not reimbursed by the third-party payer. These expenses may cause stress for the family. Financial pressure is often a precursor to the family assuming total responsibility for their loved one's care. In a classic study of 18 technology-dependent children, 72% of the parents indicated that financial problems were the most serious issues confronting them once the child was at home (Leonard, Brust, & Nelson, 1993). Almost 2 decades later this concern remains paramount. Further, caring for a loved one at home may also have a negative impact on siblings and may result in aggressive behavior.

Nurses cite that the amount of paperwork or documentation required in home care is excessive. Further, dealing with inclement weather and wear and tear on one's automobile is also mentioned as negative aspects of working as a home care nurse (Anthony & Milone-Nuzzo, 2005).

The advantages of home care far outweigh the disadvantages. Disadvantages of nursing care in the home are more of an issue if the family member is ill for a long period of time. In home care, although the client and family experience a loss of privacy and interruption of the normal family decision-making process, they still can enjoy a life together that is not possible if the client is hospitalized. Overall home care nurses report higher job satisfaction as compared to hospital nurses.

CHALLENGES TO SUCCESSFUL HOME CARE

Some of the disadvantages to home health care produce challenges to successful home care. For instance, family members express concerns about privacy, interruption of the family routine, loss of control, personality conflicts with the home care staff, and concerns about the competency of the nurses. Families express their difficulties with statements such as, "It changed our lives totally" as loss of privacy interrupts the family structure, function, and communication patterns.

Families may understand the importance of regularity in the client's routine. Nurses can respect this concern by arriving on time for appointments and performing procedures consistent with the family's desire as long as they are within the parameters of safe care. Families tend to resent nurses who are too pushy or who try to control everything. They want the nurse to listen to them and respect the knowledge they have accumulated from being involved in care on a 24-hour-a-day, 7-day-a-week basis.

NURSING SKILLS AND COMPETENCIES IN HOME HEALTH CARE

The basic concepts of professionalism apply to nursing care in the home as they do in every setting. Promptness is imperative to good work habits. Nursing competency is critical. Families want procedures done carefully and in a manner similar to what was performed or taught in the hospital. Common needs of the home care client and family are psychosocial and learning needs: information about community resources, physical care, and management. Thus, as in other settings, communication, teaching, managing, and hands-on caregiving are important competencies and skills. Figure 12-2 shows "Don'ts for Young Nurses," an excerpt taken from a historic 1919 text for home care nurses. It is interesting that the tips provided are just as true today as they were so many years ago.

Communication

A comfortable relationship between the nurse and the client is essential to successful home care. First and foremost, the successful nurse communicates effectively with the client and family. If the nurse can build a trusting relationship, all aspects of the care will be more effective.

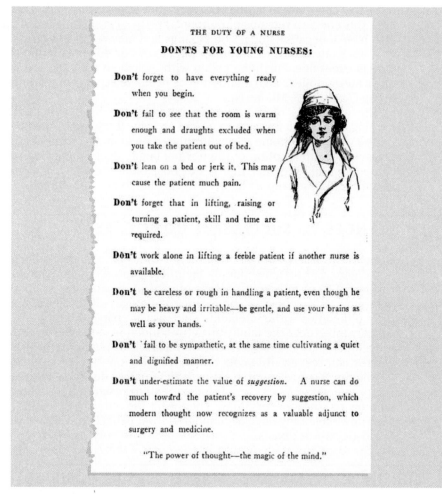

THE DUTY OF A NURSE

DON'TS FOR YOUNG NURSES:

Don't forget to have everything ready when you begin.

Don't fail to see that the room is warm enough and draughts excluded when you take the patient out of bed.

Don't lean on a bed or jerk it. This may cause the patient much pain.

Don't forget that in lifting, raising or turning a patient, skill and time are required.

Don't work alone in lifting a feeble patient if another nurse is available.

Don't be careless or rough in handling a patient, even though he may be heavy and irritable—be gentle, and use your brains as well as your hands.

Don't fail to be sympathetic, at the same time cultivating a quiet and dignified manner.

Don't under-estimate the value of *suggestion*.   A nurse can do much toward the patient's recovery by suggestion, which modern thought now recognizes as a valuable adjunct to surgery and medicine.

"The power of thought—the magic of the mind."

FIGURE 12-2. ▶ Suggestions for visiting nurses from historic visiting nurse's text. Source: South, L. H. (1919). *Nurses in the home,* 11th ed. Buffalo, NY.

The nurse must be able to deal with a myriad of psychosocial issues characteristic of the home care client. The nurse wears many hats when providing care in the home, including but not limited to: social worker, friend, spiritual comforter, psychologist, financial counselor, and translator of medical information. One home care nurse says this:

> I was not prepared for the numerous psychosocial demands of the job. I thought I was pretty good at dealing holistically with the clients I cared for in the hospital, but it was nothing like caring for someone in the home with the family present.

The psychosocial needs of the home care client primarily revolve around the client's adjustment to the illness, the anxiety it produces, and the possible social isolation that results. Nursing interventions that address the psychosocial needs of the client are primarily focused on building a trusting, therapeutic relationship. It is also helpful to elicit the client and family's thoughts and feelings about this situation, which has taken control away from them.

Health Teaching

Health teaching is a major role for the home care nurse (Fig. 12-3). Chapter 6 addresses teaching in detail. Teaching includes explaining and demonstrating care and treatment at a comprehensible level. The nurse remains open minded by listening and showing respect for the client and family's knowledge. Clients and families soon become experts and are generally accurate in their observations.

The nurse can follow the teaching principles outlined in Chapter 6 when assessing the client's learning needs, remembering that the learner may be the client, family member, or other caregiver. The learner's readiness to learn, need to learn, and past experiences are assessed. Learning needs are then placed in the affective, psychomotor, or cognitive domain. Finally, the learning need is validated, and the teaching plan is mutually developed with the learner. After instruction, the teaching and learning are evaluated for their effectiveness. Several common areas of learning needs are the disease process, treatments, and medication.

Disease Management

Most clients and families need assistance understanding the client's diagnosis and any related disease processes. Teaching about the disease process, medications, or treatments varies depending on the client's specific condition and the complexity of the diagnosis.

The client who requires only two or three home visits after routine surgery would require less information about managing his or her condition as compared to the client with multiple chronic diseases. Disease management is a relatively new reimbursable aspect of skilled nursing home care provided in the home and is discussed in more depth in Chapter 13.

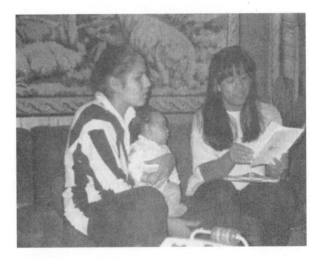

FIGURE 12-3. ▶ Teaching plays a major role in home care. Here a young woman is taught infant care by the community-based nurse involved in home care.

Treatments

Frequently, home care nurses are required to do treatments for clients and then assist the client or family to learn to be responsible for the treatment at some future date. Treatment complexity varies. In some instances, the nurse may teach a dressing change by demonstration. In other cases, the family may have to learn to administer treatments with high-tech equipment. For example, a client may have brittle diabetes with a complicating large leg ulcer. The nurse changes the dressing, monitors the diabetes, and determines the learning and teaching needs of the client and family. If the client and family are capable, the nurse teaches them to change the dressing and monitor the diabetes. It is not unusual for a client with complex technical equipment to be home with either full-time or intermittent (visits of 30 to 90 minutes) nursing care. After instruction from the home care nurse, family members often provide daily intravenous line changes and irrigation, as well as infusions of intravenous fluids, medications, or hyperalimentation through peripheral or central venous lines. They may also insert a Foley catheter or nasogastric tube or carry out tracheotomy care, including suctioning. Each year, more complex treatments and related equipment are available through home care. This trend requires home care nurses to provide teaching for increasingly complex treatments and rely on the client and family to perform procedures with a high degree of competence, identifying complicating issues and notifying the home care agency or physician appropriately.

Medication

Most of what is known about medication errors is the additional health are costs associated with preventable incidents. Medication errors in the hospital result in an annual cost of $ 3.5 billion a year, while the cost from errors in ambulatory care is estimated at $887 million a year (Aspden, et al., 2007). A thorough assessment of the client or family's ability to set up medications is the essential first step to this important intervention. The assessment is initiated with a complete review of the medications the client is taking, compared with the most recent orders from the physician(s).

The need for assistance with medications will vary from client to client according to diagnosis, age, and competency in self-care. For example, clients recently diagnosed with diabetes may have complex learning needs for medication administration. Clients may need to learn about using a sliding scale for their insulin dosage based on taking a daily blood sugar level, drawing up the medication correctly, and injecting themselves. Some clients have a large number of medications with complicated doses that they must take several times a day. The more medications prescribed, the more likely the client is to not follow the prescribed regimen. Comprehensive teaching enhances compliance with the home care client.

Case Management

As a manager of home care services, the nurse must apply leadership knowledge by performing the functions of planning, organizing, coordinating, delegating, and evaluating care for a group of clients. The nurse must coordinate, through case management, an interdisciplinary team of practitioners, the client, family, physician, and various community providers (such as Meals On Wheels and equipment vendors). The nurse's role as case manager depends on the scope of services provided by the agency and the specific providers outside the agency who are involved in the care of the client. Continuity of care is accomplished by effective communication among all members of the interdisciplinary team. To ensure comprehensive quality care, management also includes delegation and evaluation of care provided by paraprofessional caregivers, such as home health aides or homemakers and the family, as well as other professionals.

Physical Caregiving

Although one of the primary functions of the home care nurse is physical caregiving, the nurse is required to be flexible in this role. This means allowing the family to participate in caregiving whenever possible. Before doing a procedure, the nurse must explain to the client and the family what is being done and why, adjusting the instruction to their particular developmental stage and cognitive abilities (Fig. 12-4). It is essential for the nurse to know his or her own strengths and weaknesses and to master new skills before attempting them. Confidence is not instilled in the client if the nurse is inept and unable to provide skilled care proficiently.

The nurse should keep the work area neat and clean by carefully disposing of laundry, trash, and equipment. Medical researchers have known for several decades that hand washing decreases transmission of pathogens between clients. People who receive nursing care in the home are at risk of acquiring infections, just as they are in the acute care setting. Thorough hand washing on entering the home, after procedures, and before leaving the home is an essential aspect of good care.

The Centers for Disease Control and Prevention (CDC) Healthcare Infection Control Guidelines recommend either antimicrobial or non-antimicrobial soap and water must be used when hands are visibly soiled or contaminated with blood or other body fluids. An alcohol-based hand rub may be used routinely for decontaminating hands that are not visibly soiled in the following clinical situations:

◆ Before and after direct contact with clients
◆ Before and after contact with a client's nonintact skin and wound dressings
◆ Before and after using gloves

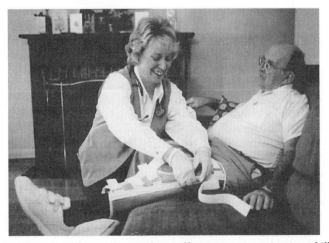

FIGURE 12-4. ▶ Home health nurses combine effective communication skills with their knowledge base of physical caregiving as they provide care for their clients.

◆ Before inserting an indwelling urinary catheter, peripheral vascular catheters, or other nonsurgical invasive devices (CDC, 2002) The Centers for Disease Control and Prevention (CDC) Healthcare Infection Control Guidelines

The Home Visit

The skill and competency central to home health care is the home visit. However, all nurses working in the community should be equipped to make home visits. Even school nurses or those in occupational health care are sometimes required to make home visits. Visiting a client in his or her home will often disclose information not obtained in other ways.

The main components of the home visit follow the nursing process. Observation of patterns of subjective and objective data helps the nurse make assessments. Skilled home nursing care reimbursed by Medicare requires following the Outcome Assessment Information Set (OASIS) format, which is explained in the next section. Nursing diagnoses (or problem statements) allow the nurse to work with the family to formulate joint plans and establish goals. Following through with these plans helps cement a therapeutic relationship.

Preparation

In preparation for the initial visit, the referral information is reviewed for basic information about the new client. Referrals come from a variety of sources, including hospitals, clinics, health care providers, physicians, nurses, individuals, and families. Home care referrals most often request intermittent or episodic care.

The client is contacted by telephone to inform him or her of the referral and to make an appointment for the first visit. The nurse identifies himself or herself, gives the name of the agency, and describes the purpose of the visit. A basic overview about the cost of services, eligibility, and alternative sources of financial support should also be discussed at this time. When applicable, the nurse must alert the client that he or she will need an insurance card or other evidence of coverage from a third-party payer, Medicare, or Medicaid on the first visit.

Unlike the acute care setting where a quick trip to the supply cart or utility room satisfies most equipment needs, the nurse must carry supplies in home health care. Before the first visit, the nurse should ask about supplies and determine what is needed. All home health care nurses use a bag to carry essential supplies to every home visit. This may consist of supplies and equipment the nurse uses daily for all clients, along with additional supplies. Each day, the nurse should review the needs of the clients to be visited that day and add specific items. Box 12-2 lists essential supplies and equipment often suggested for a home visit.

Beginning the Visit

After introductions, the visit usually begins with a short period of casual, social conversation to put the client and family at ease. The length of this introductory phase will vary depending on the cultural background of the family. In some cultures the family will place a great deal of weight on getting to know the nurse before they will allow the admission assessment to commence. One nurse who specializes in transcultural home visiting states "I know that the family is ready to begin the admission interview when they offer me tea and food." A friendly, warm manner helps as the nurse begins to ask the client questions about specific health care needs. It is important to begin building a trusting relationship from the first greeting.

> ◆ **BOX 12-2** Essential Supplies and Equipment for a Home Visit ◆
>
> - Handwashing equipment: disinfectant foam for hands, soap in container, paper towels, old newspapers (to set bag on in the home)
> - Assessment equipment: thermometer, sphygmomanometer, stethoscope, tape measure, penlight, urine and blood testing equipment
> - Treatment supplies: dressings, sterile and clean gloves, tape, alcohol swabs, scissors, lubricant jelly, forceps, syringes
> - Occupational health and safety supplies: eye shields, mask, apron, gloves, plastic bag to double bag, sharps containers, disinfectant spray and clean-up supplies for spills, disposable scrubs, airway/mask
> - Printed materials: map, agency forms, business cards
> - Laboratory supplies: specimen containers, tubes, and equipment for venipuncture, culture, or urine specimen

During the initial interview, the nurse outlines a contract stating the purpose of the visit. The nurse uses a variety of communication tools to assist the client and family to understand the need for nursing care in the home.

Assessment

Assessment on a home visit differs from that of the acute care setting (Fig. 12-5). The nurse incorporates the general elements of community-based care into the process and follows specific guidelines for documenting the status of each client receiving service. First and foremost, the nurse considers the issue of self-care by determining what the client's perceptions of his or her condition is, and what the client identifies as personal problems and strengths. The client's ability to perform self-care and the family's acceptance of responsibility for care are explored. All assessments are made in the context of the family and community resources and support. Culture must also be considered. Continuity of care among various

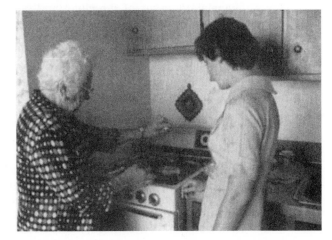

FIGURE 12-5. ▶ Home visits enable the nurse to assess whether the client can safely manage important self-care tasks such as cooking.

physicians and other professionals caring for the client is evaluated. A preventive focus, keeping in mind the principles of continuity of care, is used. The nurse assesses the client and family's knowledge of the client's condition, care, and treatment. Learning needs are assessed.

All individuals receiving Medicare-certified home care must be assessed following the OASIS guidelines. OASIS is an assessment tool developed to measure outcomes of persons receiving home health care. The OASIS data provide a consistent format and standardized time points for documenting client care status. When OASIS information between two or more visits is compared, client outcomes can be identified (Richard, Crisler, & Stearns, 2000). All certified home health care agencies use OASIS as the assessment tool for home visits.

PHYSICAL ASSESSMENT

Specifics of the physical assessment vary according to the client's needs. In most cases, the initial physical assessment will determine if the client is appropriate for home care services, what type of services are indicated, how long these services are likely to be needed, and who will pay for the care.

On the initial visit, and regularly throughout care, the nurse takes vital signs and conducts a full physical assessment of the client, including a review of all systems and a focused assessment of the client's presenting condition. During this assessment, the nurse collects information about the client's physical condition, functional status, ability to leave the home unassisted, ability to do self-care, and ability to perform ADL independently, using the OASIS format as required. Blood or urine specimens are sometimes collected and sent to the laboratory.

FAMILY ASSESSMENT

Because community-based care is provided in the context of the client's family and community, assessment of the family is an essential ingredient to the success of home care. Family structure, stage of illness, developmental stage, and family functions may be assessed. The nurse must also determine if the client is isolated physically or socially from other members of the family or if the family is a close-knit, nurturing, and supportive family or kinship network.

FINANCIAL ASSESSMENT

Information about the costs of home care services, insurance payment, and other financial concerns of the client and family should be discussed on the first visit. **Financial assessment** and options to reduce the cost of care while continuing the provision of safe, quality care should be explored. Some clients are insured 100% for home care services as long as the services are provided within the parameters of coverage. Others may have little or no insurance coverage. Clients and families may have little knowledge about their home care coverage and may be unaware that the number of visits may be limited or that they have a lifetime maximum as stipulated in the particular health insurance policy. All of these issues must be explored.

Determination of Needs and Planning Care

After assessment, the nurse, client, and family discuss the nursing care needs and develop a plan of care. They also determine who will be responsible for particular aspects of the care until the next nursing visit. The family support person may be responsible, or other professional health care or home care providers may be needed. Expected outcomes are developed and plans are made for a follow-up visit. Now and in the future, home health agencies have to demonstrate the client's progress toward achievement of desired outcomes. Medicare and insurance will not reimburse for a home visit if quality improvement and outcomes are not achieved.

Implementation

Physical care, including delegated medical functions, teaching, counseling, and referrals are completed according to the plan of care. Because home care often replaces hospitalization in meeting acute medical needs, home care focuses on physical care of the client. Short visits of 30 minutes to 2 hours focus on hands-on care of the client, incorporating a large variety of nursing skills. These include giving injections, performing venipunctures for laboratory work, doing dressing changes, giving medications, teaching the client and family how to do the care on an ongoing basis, and being the eyes and ears for the physician in observing the client's progress toward recovery. While the nurse is performing skilled nursing care, he or she is also teaching, assessing, counseling, and acting as a consultant for client and family.

Termination of the Visit

The nurse reviews the purpose of the visit, outlines what was learned in the assessment phase, and reviews the mutually agreed on plan of care. The time and purpose of the next visit are discussed and agreed on by all involved. The nurse may end the visit with a small amount of casual conversation. Especially if the client lives alone, conversation will be anticipated and appreciated.

Follow-up Visits and Evaluation

A thorough initial assessment allows for comprehensive planning for productive follow-up visits. Each visit should have specific goals with plans implemented to meet those goals. Subsequent visits allow the nurse to build a trusting relationship with the client, which may lead to identification of additional nursing needs. In community-based nursing, the overall goal of every home visit is to maximize health functioning and self-care.

The nurse, client, and family or caregivers evaluate the visit and the care plan. Physical care, teaching, counseling, and referrals are discussed, and suggestions are made for ways to improve the care provided. The client may be asked to complete an evaluation survey (Assessment Tool 12-1).

Documentation

Generally, documentation for home visits follows specific regulations. To ensure that the agency will qualify for payment for the visit, the client's needs and the nursing care given are documented. This includes the client's homebound status and the need for skilled professional nursing care with Medicare, Medicaid, and most other third-party payers. If documentation is not done correctly, the agency may not be reimbursed for the visit.

At the beginning of this chapter, the Medicare coverage criteria that must be met for home care services to be reimbursed were discussed (Box 12-1). Until just recently all states followed this requirement, but now three states do not call for homebound status for clients to receive skilled nursing care through Medicare. However, assume that generally it is absolutely imperative that all of the homebound criteria are met and documented. The nurse is responsible for documenting that the client is homebound. The primary dimensions of homebound status

ASSESSMENT TOOLS 12-1

Client Satisfaction Survey

To evaluate our services and continue our excellent standards of care, we need to hear from you. Please take a few minutes to complete this form and return it to us in the enclosed stamped envelope. Thank you!

1. Home health care services were provided in a timely manner when I needed them:

    _____ Very good   _____ Satisfactory   _____ Unsatisfactory

2. Home was the best setting for the care given to me for my comfort and recovery:

    _____ Very good   _____ Satisfactory   _____ Unsatisfactory

3. The number and frequency of visits provided were adequate to meet my needs:

    _____ Very good   _____ Satisfactory   _____ Unsatisfactory

4. The care I needed to improve my condition was received from home health care:

    _____ Very good   _____ Satisfactory   _____ Unsatisfactory

5. I am now able to care for myself with the procedures and instructions provided by the staff:

    _____ Very good   _____ Satisfactory   _____ Unsatisfactory

6. The home health care staff was courteous and respectful:

    _____ Very good   _____ Satisfactory   _____ Unsatisfactory

7. The names of community service agencies were given to me as needed and their services explained:

    _____ Very good   _____ Satisfactory   _____ Unsatisfactory

8. I felt my wishes about care were supported by the staff of the home health care agency:

    _____ Very good   _____ Satisfactory   _____ Unsatisfactory

9. I would use home health care services again:

    _____ Yes   _____ No

10. Home health care provided me with the following services:

    _____ Home health care   _____ Hospice   _____ Private duty

11. Comments (Please write on a separate sheet if more space is needed):

    _____

    _____

    _____

    _____

    _____

are that absences from the home are infrequent and, for the purpose of receiving medical treatment, that leaving home requires considerable and taxing effort. Homebound status must be documented in objective and measurable terms and include the following information about a client leaving home:

◆ How often
◆ For how long
◆ For what reason
◆ The effort and assistive devices required

Clients who leave the home to receive medical care not available in the home may still be considered for homebound status for the following reasons:

◆ Physician office visits
◆ Outpatient kidney dialysis services
◆ Attendance at adult day centers to receive medical care
◆ Outpatient chemotherapy or radiation (Zuber, 2002)

Documentation should always be focused on the client's illness and safety, centering on the: statement of the problem(s); skilled care provided to deal with the problem(s); and outcomes expected and achieved from the care provided

As discussed, OASIS is the documentation system used by Medicare. Often the perception is that following OASIS will always protect from liability. However, in some instances OASIS requires an ambiguous response, while in other instances allows staff to cover an issue without having to state precisely what should be done. To protect from liability it is necessary that documentation should clearly state what is and what is not expected. Using OASIS competently not only requires precise and consistent language and care plans but also following the documented plan of care (Newfield, 2006). A complete documentation of the care plan is important not only for reimbursement and legal issues, but it is also critical to the evaluation of competent nursing practice used in quality assurance.

Confidentiality

Confidentiality is essential to quality care in community-based settings. Sometimes nurses may work in their own community and may care for someone they know or a friend or relative of someone they know outside of their professional role. Just as in the hospital setting, nurses must never discuss individual situations or the health status of clients and families with anyone except other professional staff within professional discussions.

Safety Issues for the Nurse

The nurse should know the destination for the visit and have a route mapped out to get there. Depending on the neighborhood, asking directions can prove dangerous. When entering the client's neighborhood, the nurse begins an environmental assessment by doing a brief windshield survey (see Chapter 5). The purpose of the survey is to collect information about the community where the client lives and to determine if the neighborhood is safe. Occasionally, the nurse may not feel safe entering a client's home. In some areas, the nurse may need to be accompanied by a policeman or security officer. No nurse should ever disregard personal safety in an effort to visit a client. See Community-Based Nursing Care Guidelines 12-1 for a checklist of safety points to be followed by home care nurses.

COMMUNITY-BASED NURSING CARE GUIDELINES ▶ 12-1

Personal Safety Checklist for the Home Care Nurse

- Get to know the community, especially the differences between neighborhoods.
- Dress in sensible shoes and simple clothing, avoid long necklaces, expensive jewelry, or pins of political or religious nature.
- Get to know your client and family and determine if there is a history of violence.
- Know your agency policies and procedures and follow them.
- Keep your supervisor informed of any potential violent situations with your caseload.
- Have safety accessories in your car: a working cell phone, flashlight; and have a well-maintained car.
- Lock up equipment and your purse or valuables in the trunk of the car.
- Attend a course on safety, self-defense, or self-protection.

SUPPORT OF THE LAY CAREGIVER

Because so many clients are discharged from acute care settings earlier than in the past, with conditions more serious or less stable, the home care environment has become the site of major caretaking activities. The use of families, relatives, and support systems such as caregivers is on the rise. In fact, **lay caregiving** is one of the world's fastest-growing unpaid professions. It is estimated that almost 80% of home care services are provided by family members or other unpaid assistance. More than 40% of caregivers are men. Family caregivers care for their loved ones an average of 8 years with many being caregivers for over 10 years (National Family Caregivers Association [NFCA], 2005a; NFCA, 2005b).

Lay caregivers may have responsibilities for people at both ends of the age spectrum: children and older people with chronic health problems. "Parent caring" is the term used in the literature for sons and daughters caring for older parents. These caregivers are predominantly women. The "typical caregiver" is a middle-aged, married woman who is employed full time and is also spending about 18 hours a week caring for her mother who lives nearby (NFCA, 2005a).

Sometimes the caregiver for an older person is an older person with his or her own functional disabilities. Recent research suggests that more men are becoming active in providing care in the home for a spouse.

Caregiving includes providing emotional support, direct health services, and financial support; mediating with health and social service organizations; and sharing a household. It may include tasks such as bathing, toileting, shopping, preparing food, feeding, maintaining a household budget, and housekeeping. Family dynamics can be different from household to household. The nurse must be sensitive to this variety of family dynamics and work with the family and caregivers without being judgmental regarding their decisions.

Stress on the Caregiver

Caring for a client who has acute needs that are treated with complicated technologic devices can be difficult. Such care may weigh heavily on the family. For several decades, studies have documented the strain of caregiving on the caregiver's physical and psychologic health. For example, a wife's hospitalization increased her husband's chances of dying within a month by 35%. A husband's hospitalization boosts his wife's mortality risk by 44% (Christakis & Allison, 2006). Further, family caregivers experiencing extreme stress have been shown to age prematurely. This level of stress can take as much as 10 years off a family caregiver's life (NFCA, 2005a). As family responsibility grows, parental distress increases. The nurse may need to provide not only client care and treatment but also a great deal of support for the family. The nurse is in an ideal position to intervene.

The transition from visiting a family member in the hospital, where other people are responsible for care, to being a "paraprofessional" caregiver sometimes happens almost overnight. Suddenly the lay caregiver has 24-hour responsibility for tasks for which he or she has little or no knowledge and experience. The lay caregiver may have full- or part-time employment and other family members to care for. The strain on caregivers can be great, and risks for depression and illness are high. Other psychosocial problems raise the risk. The family may already have mounting bills with a mortgage and utilities. Safety in the community may be an issue. Transportation may be a problem, especially if the person requiring care was the family's means of transportation. Drug abuse on the part of a family member may add to the burdens. The lay caregiver may have no support person or outlets on which to rely.

The 24-hour responsibility for the client's care means more than supplying physical care for the client. It means that the lay caregiver always has the client and his or her care in mind. The role is unrelenting. The day is organized around the care activities and needs of the client, and sometimes the client must be under constant observation. Many times the client's personality, which may have changed with illness, places heavy demands on the caregiver's time and energy. The difficulty of the role has been associated with low levels of life satisfaction, high levels of depression, and symptoms of stress. If the care is to be provided temporarily, the stress may not be as great. If the length of time for care, however, is indefinite, as in chronic care, additional stress may be felt by the lay caregiver. Because the stress on these lay caregivers is tremendous, community-based nurses need to consider this fact as they plan care. Although their clients are their main concern, a holistic nursing style means that nurses also provide care for family and other support persons.

Assessment

The first home visit is an important time to discuss and clarify the relationship between the client and the caregiver. The OASIS provides items to assess caregiver presence, availability, and type of assistance needed. It is also essential to assess the caregiver's knowledge and physical and psychological status. Caregiver needs must also be assessed because of the caregiver's increased risk for health problems.

Interventions for Lay Caregivers

Nursing interventions may enhance quality of life for both the client and caregiver by ensuring that everyone has adequate preparation for ongoing care needs. Health care professionals need to be sensitive to caregivers, who handle many roles such as working outside the home or caring for other dependents in addition to being a caregiver. These individuals are often stressed, burdened, and depressed, as compared to those who have a single caregiver role.

The nurse who initially establishes rapport with both the client and caregivers and builds on that trust is the most likely to successfully intervene. Three critical components that contribute to successful family caregiving include: communication, decision-making, and reciprocity (Sebern, 2006). Successful communication and decision making is characterized by frequent interactions as problems arise with the family, attempting to solve these issues as a team. Areas where communication is essential involve signs and symptoms, feelings, and information. Decision-making include seeking information and involvement in decisions. The community-based nurse in any setting should be aware of the lay caregiver's circumstances and help the caregiver find solutions to problems.

Promoting communication and decision-making takes various forms. The nurse helps caregivers cope by sharing realistic prognostic information, discussing alternative levels of care, and providing information regarding respite care. A community day care program may be available for the client to relieve the lay caregiver of constant responsibility. Some communities help with housekeeping provisions or meal programs. Churches may have volunteers who can provide respite care. Additional resources for caregivers are found at the end of the chapter in What's on the Web.

Reciprocity encompasses the interaction between the family caregiver and individual receiving care. Mutual satisfaction is seen as both parties receive support from and provide assistance to one another. Successful reciprocity incorporates empathy, listening, and partnership. In some cases working with the client to perform more self-care activities will relieve the caregiver of some responsibilities. Providing more teaching for the caregiver may help relieve the caregiver's feeling that the responsibilities are overwhelming.

Other interventions to encourage communication, decision-making, and reciprocity skills include educational and support programs, burden-reducing programs, psychotherapeutic interventions, and self-help groups. Even a busy caregiver can find time in the schedule to attend a support group if it is deemed worthwhile. In these groups, people share their experiences and report on strategies that have or have not worked for them. Just knowing that other people are in the same situation or have the same feelings is helpful. Box 12-3 provides suggestions for identifying and intervening with caregiver stress.

Respite care provides a temporary break for the caregiver. The care may include someone coming into the house for an hour or two so the caregiver can shop, do errands, or keep his or her own doctor's appointments. Respite care is an important aspect of hospice care. Another form of respite care is the client's temporary visit to a nursing home or other facility. While the client is cared for in other surroundings, the caregiver and family are free to vacation, perform household maintenance duties, or simply relax.

┌───┐

◆ BOX 12-3 Family Caregivers: Caring for Older Adults, Working With Their Families ◆

It is not always obvious who the primary caregiver is for a client. Sometimes the person who is at the bedside is not the family member who will be responsible to for the actual care once the client goes home. Approaches for accurately identifying, sufficiently communicating with, and supporting the individual family member who will be in charge of the care at home varies by setting. For instance, for the nurse working in the hospital it may be helpful to wait until the primary caregiver arrives before providing discharge instructions to the client. If someone other than the primary caregiver is transporting the client home from the hospital the nurse may consider getting the name of the primary caregiver and calling them with discharge instructions. In the nursing home the nurse expressing appreciation for the caregiver's efforts to visit and do "little extras" for the family member may promote and support family caregiving. In ambulatory care, once permission is granted, it supports the family caregiver if that person is invited from the waiting room to the exam room to participate in the review of the client's health status and hear about new instructions for new treatments. Home care nurses may find that it is helpful to determine the client and caregiver's preferences for time, day, and method (in person, by phone, or email) of communicating. Further, the nurse may want to suggest periodic family meetings to keep all members updated on progress and changes.

Long-distance caregiving creates other trials for the caregiver, client, and nurse. Long-distance caregiving is defined as care provided by those living 1 hour or more away from the care recipient. Long-distance caregivers may only be present intermittently but may play an important role in the problem solving, decision making, and advocacy aspects of caregiving. Strategies to enhance the success of long-distance caregiving may be initiated by conducting a family assessment with the client to identify long-distance caregivers and determine their availability. Developing a plan for communicating with the long-distance caregiver is important as is providing them with contact information for the agencies and team members involved in the client's care.

Source: Schumacher, K., Beck C. A., Marren, J. M. (2006). Family caregivers: Caring for older adults, working with their families. *American Journal of Nursing, 106*(8), 40–49.

└───┘

CLIENT SITUATIONS IN PRACTICE

◆ Planning and Implementing a Home Care Visit

The discharge planning nurse calls your home care agency with the following information on a referral. Mrs. Gothie is an 85-year-old woman with severe congestive heart failure (CHF). She cared for her husband, who had dementia, for 7 years. He died 4 years ago. Mrs. Gothie has lived in the same third-floor apartment for 50 years. Although she has no children, she is close to her younger sister and brother, and numerous nieces and nephews, who all live out of state. Her family is devoted to her, visiting her frequently, but most of her lifelong friends are no longer living. She has one friend who is able to help her on a limited basis, but most of her friends are aging.

When she came to the clinic 2 weeks ago, before being admitted to the hospital, her vital signs and laboratory values were as follows:

Temperature: 98.6°F
Blood pressure: 128/88 mm Hg
Respirations: 26 breaths/min
Lung sounds: rales in all lung fields
Lab values: prothrombin 4 times normal
Digoxin level: 0.1 ng/mL

Mrs. Gothie stated the following at the clinic visit:

I have had a terrible time getting my breath, especially at night. My ankles are three times as big as they used to be. I quit taking my water pill because it made me have to go to the bathroom all the time, and I couldn't sleep at night. I don't have any appetite, but I do eat fruit. Most days, I don't even bother to get dressed or take a shower because I'm so tired. What's the use—I never go anywhere—I'm always too tired. I have had a lot of bruises on my arms and legs.

She was admitted to the hospital for acute CHF. After 3 days in the hospital, she was discharged to Happy Helpful Nurse HomeCare. After 1 week of physical therapy, she is scheduled to be discharged home. You are assigned to be the case manager for Mrs. Gothie's care. After reviewing the referral form plan your first visit with Mrs. Gothie.

- *List the points you will cover when you telephone Mrs. Gothie to set up an appointment for the first visit.*

You would call Mrs. Gothie to introduce yourself, give the name of the agency, and the purpose of the visits. If the visits are partially reimbursed by insurance, you may want to tell her that you will need to see her insurance card at the visit. You may also want to know if anyone will be home with her after she is discharged and if that person will be present at the visit. You may want to inquire if she has any concerns that she would like you to address during the visit so you can bring the appropriate supplies and educational materials.

- *Determine the primary purpose of the first visit and the focus of your physical assessment.*

The primary purpose of the first visit will be determined by the policies and procedures of the agency you are working for and the insurance coverage or Medicare requirements. In the latter case, the OASIS initial assessment would be initiated. The same goes for the focus of the physical assessment. You would be particularly concerned with the assessment of her cardiovascular status and any other assessment related to the symptoms of CHF. In her case, you would make sure that you assess her appetite as she said at her last clinic visit that she doesn't have an appetite. She states that she is too tired to go anywhere, so you assess fatigue and what helps with that. Is she depressed? What about the bruises on her legs and arms? Was there a follow-up blood test done when she was in the hospital to explore this issue? Another concern will be what kind of support she needs to be safe at home. Then, you will assess the support she has and fill in the void with referrals. Obviously, you will be very concerned about the home environment and potential safety issues.

- *Identify your key areas of concern when you do your psychosocial and family assessment.*

You will do an assessment of the family structure, developmental stage, and functions. Another question you may have is whether Mrs. Gothie is physically or socially isolated from family or whether the family or her support network is close, nurturing, and supportive. Some of her statements at her last clinic visit indicated as much.

- *List the people who can provide support for Mrs. Gothie.*

According to the referral form, her sister accompanied her home when she was discharged. She also has one friend, but many of her friends are now deceased. You may want to determine the role that her sister may take as a long-distance caregiver. You will want to assess the breadth and depth of any other support network. Does she need or want a home health aide for personal care and meal preparation?

- *Identify learning needs you will assess in the first visit.*

You note that she has had CHF for 20 years, with increased symptoms the last year. You learn that her sister will be with her for a month. You will assess the learning need of both Mrs. Gothie and her sister. The first need that you will assess will be their understanding of the disease processes of CHF, her medications, and the use of oxygen. According to the notes from Mrs. Gothie's last clinic visit, it sounds like she is not taking the furosemide (Lasix) because she says that it makes her have to go to the bathroom too frequently to get adequate sleep at night. You assess when she takes the Lasix and recommend that she do so in the morning. You will also determine what her knowledge base is regarding the high-protein diet.

- *What referrals would you make?*

Your priority concerns are as follows:

1. Can she manage at home safely and make a reasonable recovery given her support system, her abilities, and other factors related to her living situation? What will she do when her sister goes back to her home in another state?
2. Does she need assistance managing her medications? Does she need someone either in her family or in the community to do this for her?
3. Does she understand the high-protein diet? Does she need to see a nutritionist?
4. How does she do grocery shopping? Are there services in the community to help her with this?
5. Is she open to home-delivered meals, such as Meals on Wheels?
6. Is congregate dining available in her community and transportation provided to the site?

- *What social opportunities would she consider?*

She states that she has no energy to go anywhere. Once she has more energy, what referrals could you make to address her social isolation (e.g., church, community senior programs, other senior programs)?

THE FUTURE OF HOME CARE

There are several trends in home care. First, there is more focus on practice, including client care, pharmacology, best practices, and cost-saving clinical approaches to client care. Agencies are improving standards of practice through the educational strategies of practice rounds, journal clubs, increased library holdings, expansion of orientation, and teleconferences. Changes that emphasis of care to accentuate empowerment with families and clients and individualize the care plan is another trend. With this shift the home visits follow what the client and family needs rather than what is typically expected for the diagnosis is gaining more legitimacy.

With the demographic changes in the United States, it is anticipated that home care will assume an increasingly important role in community-based care in the future. The client advocate role will continue to be a central element of both as complexity of health care delivery and concern for cost containment continue. Flexibility and accountability will remain fundamental as the pressure to meet professional practice standards intersects with the pressure to contain costs. Challenges facing home care nurses will require that the nurse keep up with ever-changing regulations regarding coverage, as well as the documentation requirements that will follow. In addition, nurses will be called on to counsel, teach, and act as a consultant for clients and families as they have increasing responsibility for acutely ill family members at home. Of course as in all nursing specialties, it will be vital for home care nurses to welcome the increased use of technology.

CONCLUSIONS

The setting for the provision of health care and nursing care has shifted several times from the late 1800s to the present. Care of the ill in the home was at one point primarily physician care. Then the setting for medical care moved from the home to the hospital or acute care setting in the mid-1900s. In the last 20 years it has now relocated back to the home and community. The major roles of home care are to educate, reinforce learning, and encourage clients and families to provide ongoing self-care. In home care, the family and client experience a loss of privacy and an interruption in normal decision making, but the advantages for the client and family outweigh the disadvantages when compared with inpatient care. Regardless of the client's diagnosis, the nurse in home care encourages self-care with a preventive focus, which is provided in the context of the client's family and community and follows the principles of continuity of care.

What's on the Web

Administration on Aging (AOA)
Internet address: http://www.aoa.dhhs.gov
This Web site presents information on AOA and its programs. Resources for practitioners, statistics, and consumer information on obtaining services and age-related issues are included.

Canadian Home Care Association
Internet address: http://www.cdnhome-care.ca/
The Canadian Home Care Association is dedicated to the accessibility, quality, and development of home care and community support services that permit people to stay in their homes and communities with safety and dignity. The Web site contains information on publications, related sites, employment opportunities, and education programs, as well as information related to the organization.

Centers for Disease Control and Prevention Hand Hygiene in Healthcare Settings
Internet address:
http://www.cdc.gov/handhygiene
This site provides access to the guidelines and materials to promote hand hygiene in health care facilities.

Family Caregiver Alliance
Telephone: (800) 445-8106
Internet address: http://www.caregiver.org/
caregiver/jsp/home.jsp
This site focuses on information and services to families and professionals caring for adults with cognitive disorders, as well as fact sheets and tools kits on topics applicable to a variety of caregivers.

National Association for Home Care and Hospice
Internet address: http://www.nahc.org
The National Association for Home Care & Hospice (NAHC) is a professional organization that represents a variety of agencies providing home care services, including home health agencies, hospice programs, and homemaker or home health aide agencies. The Web site contains news and information about home care and hospice, including publications, statistics about home care and hospice, a job search vehicle, and a locator for hospice and home

care agencies and their affiliates. It also has information about NAHC membership, meetings and conferences, grassroots activities, and state associations.

National Family Caregivers Association
Internet address: http://www.nfcacares.org/
Free membership is available to any family caregiver. Both the newsletter and Web site provide good resources for "caring for the caregiver" information.

Visiting Nurse Associations of America
Internet address: http://www.vnaa.org
The Visiting Nurse Associations of America is the official national association for nonprofit visiting nurse associations. It supports community-based VNAs in their mission to provide home and hospice care through skilled nursing, therapy services (physical therapy, occupational therapy), and home health aide care to elderly, children, homebound, disabled, and other types of clients.

References and Bibliography

Anthony, A., & Milone-Nuzzo, P. (2005). Factors attracting and keeping nurses in home care. *Home Healthcare Nurse, 23*(6), 372–377.

Aspden, P., Wolcott, J., Bootman, J. L., & Cronenwett, L. R. (2007). Preventing medication errors; quality chasm series. National Academy of Sciences. Retrieved on October 24, 2006, from http://books.nap/catalog/11623.html

Centers for Disease Control and Prevention. (2002). *Guideline for hand hygiene in health-care settings. MMWR, 51*(RR16), 1-44. Retrieved June 4, 2003, from http://www.cdc.gov/mmwr/preview/mmwrhtml/rr5116a1.htm

Centers for Medicare & Medicaid Services. (2004). Medicare and home health care. Retrieved on October 24, 2006, from http://www.cms.hhs.gov/center/hha.asp

Christakis, N. A., & Allison, P. D. (2006). Mortality after the hospitalization of a spouse. *New England Journal of Medicine, 354*(7), 719–730.

Hartung, S. Q. (2005). Choosing home health as a specialty and successfully transitioning into home health nursing practice. *Home Health Care Management & Practice, 17*(5), 370–387.

Leonard, B. J., Brust, J. D., & Nelson, R. P. (1993). Parental distress: Caring for medically fragile children at home. *Journal of Pediatric Nursing: Nursing Care of Children & Families, 8*(1), 22–30.

National Association for Home Care & Hospice. (2006). *Basic statistics about home care.* Washington, DC: Author. Retrieved on October 24, 2006, from http://www.nahc.org/04HC_Stats.pdf

National Family Caregivers Association. (2005a). *What is family caregiving?* Retrieved on October 25, 2006, from http://www.thefamilycaregiver.org/what/what.cfm

National Family Caregivers Association. (2005b). Who are family caregiver; Statistics. Retrieved on October 25, 2006, from http://www.thefamilycaregiver.org/who/stats.cfm

Newfield, J. S., (2006). Documentation: Focusing on better rather than more. *Home Health Care Management & Practice, 18*(3), 247–249.

Richard, A. A., Crisler, K. S., & Stearns, P. M. (2000). Using OASIS for outcome-based quality improvement. *Home Healthcare Nurse, 18*(4), 232–237.

Sebern, M. (2006). Shared care, elder and family member skills used to manage burden. *Journal of Advanced Nursing, 52*(2), 170–179.

Schumacher, K., Beck, C. A., Marren, J. M. (2006). Family caregivers: Caring for older adults, working with their families. *American Journal of Nursing, 106*(8), 40–49.

Thobaben, M., & Sullivan, A. (2005). Transitioning from hospital-based nursing practice to home health care practice. *Home Health Care Management & Practice, 17*(5), 413–415.

Zuber, R. (2002). Assessing Medicare eligibility: Suggestions for improving processes. *Home Healthcare Nurse, 20*(7), 425–430.

LEARNING ▼ ACTIVITIES

◆ JOURNALING ACTIVITY 12-1

The Home Visit

1. In your clinical journal, reflect on a home visit you have made. Identify the nursing skills and competencies you used as you provided care.
2. What did you expect the visit to be like and how did the actual visit compare?
3. How was caring for the client in the home different from an acute care setting? How was it similar? What did you do differently in the home setting?
4. What did you learn from this experience?
5. How will you use this information in your future practice?

Lay Caregiver

1. In your clinical journal, reflect on an experience you have observed or a client you have cared for in clinical who has been cared for by a lay caregiver for an extended period of time. Outline the situation into a case study.
2. Discuss what you observed with this situation and how it applies to the theory in the text.
3. How did or would you support the caregiver based on what you learned reading the text or other reading you have done?
4. How will you use what you learned from this experience in your future practice?

◆ CRITICAL THINKING ACTIVITY 12-2

Consider the psychosocial needs of home care clients in the following situations. Comment about the likelihood of their condition to produce anxiety or social isolation. Give a reason for your answer.

1. A 50-year-old retired government employee who is caring for his 50-year-old wife who has severe dementia.
2. A 20-year-old woman caring for her 5-month-old baby, who has frequent episodes of apnea. The apnea has required frequent immediate action and, on one occasion, necessitated cardiopulmonary resuscitation to revive the baby.
3. A 70-year-old woman caring for her husband, who has terminal lung cancer.

4. An 80-year-old woman with severe chronic obstructive pulmonary disease who lives alone and is homebound.
5. A 60-year-old man with congestive heart failure who has frequent episodes of shortness of breath at night.

◆ CLIENT CARE ACTIVITY 12-3

Jose Martinez is an 85-year-old man who lives in a rural area of Texas. He was discharged 2 days ago from a hospital in Austin after breaking his hip herding his sheep into the corral behind his house. His wife died last year, and he has lived alone since then. He has eight children; all of them live in and around the small rural town where Jose has lived since he immigrated from Mexico 20 years ago.

Since fracturing his hip, Mr. Martinez has not been able to care for himself and is upset about his inability to tend to his sheep and be independent. His family has gathered to meet with the home health care nurse about plans for Mr. Martinez.

1. Discuss assessment questions related to culture that the nurse should ask when establishing a relationship with this family.
2. Identify some important questions the home health care nurse should ask during the client conference.
3. Determine what options exist for Mr. Martinez.
4. State ways the nurse can address Mr. Martinez's desire to be independent.
5. Determine Mr. Martinez's primary health care needs.
6. Given all the options, summarize the ideal place for Mr. Martinez to live.

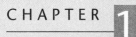

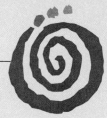

Specialized Home Health Care Nursing

ROBERTA HUNT

LEARNING OBJECTIVES

1. Identify five specialized roles for home health care nurses.
2. Outline the role responsibilities for each specialized role discussed in the chapter.
3. Utilize a pain assessment tool.
4. Identify trends for specialized roles for home health care nursing.

KEY TERMS

disease management
home infusion therapy
hospice care
hyperemesis

pregnancy-induced hypertension (PIH)
telehealth care
telehomecare
wound care

CHAPTER TOPICS

◆ **Disease Management in the Home**
◆ **Telehomecare—Telehealth in Home Care**
◆ **Infusion Therapy**
◆ **Wound Care**
◆ **Maternal–Child Home Care**
◆ **Pain Management**
◆ **Hospice Care**
◆ **Conclusions**

One day when I came in to pick up my assignments, I was asked to visit Mrs. Black, who I had just seen for the first time the day before. She had called in to triage that morning to request another visit because of increased pain from pancreatic cancer. I was relatively new to **hospice care**, so I reviewed the procedure to increase the dose of morphine on the CADD pump. As I drove to her home, I was thinking about the home visit I had made to Mrs. Black the day before for pain management and anxiety issues. I remembered that at that time, she did not want the dosage of morphine or lorazepam increased. During that visit, I noticed the sadness in her eyes and had taken time to sit down next to her and hold her hand to ask her to tell me about her life. She reached under her bed and pulled out her wedding album and talked about the joy she felt on that particular day. I could tell there was sadness and worry behind the words she spoke that she was not willing to share.

When I arrived at her home, I expected that this second visit in as many days would be very short and would be focused on increasing the morphine on the CADD pump. After a pain assessment, I decided to increase the morphine to 2 mg/hour more than she had been receiving. As we sat side by side on the sofa, I concentrated fully on the unfamiliar procedure and tuned out the words she was speaking. In fact, I remember wishing that she would be quiet so I could finish the task at hand. But there was something in the sound of her voice that jolted me into hearing her words. I realized that she was sharing deep regrets about choices she had made in her life that could not be easily rectified in the time she had left. A sudden overwhelming feeling washed over me. What could I do about this information? I stopped fumbling with the pump and listened for a long time, acknowledging her pain and her suffering but offering no solutions or answers. She seemed to gain in personal strength as she shared. This experience reminded me to never lose sight of the compassionate and caring role of the nurse in the alleviation of suffering.

—KATHLEEN DUDLEY, MSN, RN, Hospice Nurse,
Assistant Professor, College of St. Catherine

In the last 20 years, home health care has become more specialized and complex as nursing care is increasingly provided in community-based settings. As in basic home health care, nurses must be competent in communication, teaching, management, and physical and emotional caregiving. In addition, they must develop expertise in a specialized area. Specialized home health care nursing, which will be discussed in this chapter, includes home telemedicine, disease management, infusion therapy, **wound care**, maternal–child home care, pain management, and hospice care.

DISEASE MANAGEMENT IN THE HOME

Interest in disease management has increased dramatically since the mid 1990s (Huffman, 2005). **Disease management** is "an approach to delivering healthcare to persons with chronic illnesses that aims to improve patient outcomes while containing health care costs." (U.S. Department of Health and Human Services, 2003). Disease management programs encompass providers across the health care continuum, including home care. Disease management is based on the premise that coordinated, evidence-based interventions can be applied to clients with conditions that are high-cost, high-volume. The goal is to improve clinical outcomes and lower overall costs. Outcome data are the central element to the success to this approach to client care.

The Role of the Nurse in Disease Management

There are six components that are required for a full service disease management program (Disease Management Association of America, 2006). Disease management focuses on chronic conditions that are difficult to manage and costly to treat. These conditions include but are not restricted to: congestive heart failure, asthma, coronary disease, diabetes, osteoporosis, stroke, and chronic wounds. The nurse has an important role in identifying through case findings individuals who could benefit from disease management. Once the client is identified, all interventions are based on evidence–based practice guidelines for the condition(s).

As in all community-based care collaboration among physicians, care providers, client and family, and support-service, providers is key. The nurse's role in promoting the client and families' self-care skills through consultation, counseling, and health education is vital to disease management. As with any intervention, disease management necessitates evaluation of outcomes as well as application of the findings to a revised plan of care. Throughout the process of disease management, using routine reporting and feedback loops between and among all involved parties protects the integrity of the process.

Trends in Disease Management

One trend in disease management entails using technology to develop new connections with clients, particularly those who are elderly. Where home care in the past has been delivered by "high touch" through home visits, disease management uses "high tech" **telehealth** by telephone, internet, and various monitors. This trend will be more fully discussed in the next section on telehomecare.

Being a relatively new concept in home care, one of the primary trends at this time is to expand utilization of disease management with rigorous evaluation research to establish the efficacy of new programs and models. Through this process, evidence-based practice in the area of disease management will be established.

TELEHOMECARE—TELEHEALTH IN HOME CARE

Telehomecare is an interactive, two-way video process that allows home care nurses to have conversations with homebound clients to monitor clinical progress. This is accomplished by using telephones, televisions, computers, and video-conferencing to monitor vital signs, heart and lung sounds, blood glucose, and oxygen saturation. Telehomecare also allows the nurse to complete functions related to case management, chronic disease management, hospice, postsurgical care, and rehabilitation.

The main advantage of telehomecare is that of cost savings. While nurses average 4 to 8 traditional in-home visits per day it is possible to complete 20 or more telehomecare visits per day (Thobaben, 2005). Agencies receiving reimbursement under Medicare's Prospective Payment System as well as a number of health insurance plans cover telehomecare visits according to the American Telemedicine Association (2001). However, agencies may not substitute telehealth serviced for physician-ordered Medicare-covered services (Thobaben, 2005).

It is more difficult to practice relationship-based care via telecommunication. Without cautious use of thoughtfully developed guidelines, telehealth has the potential to mechanize the delivery of nursing care. Further, telehomecare creates some distinct ethical challenges, the most obvious being confidentiality and informed consent. The American Nurses Association (ANA) has developed core principles on telehealth. The first principle states that the "basic standards of professional conduct governing each health care profession are not altered by the use of telehealth technologies" (American Nurse Association, 1999).

Role of the Nurse

The role of the nurse in telehealth varies depending on the application. However, the main applications fall into three categories; monitoring, managing, and motivating (Coughlin, Pope, & Leedle, 2006). The delegated medication function of monitoring health and activities can be accomplished by the nurse 24/7, reducing emergency department visits and allowing for rapid intervention at the first sign of health changes or decline in health status. The nurse is able to act as a case manager and identify and prioritize clients requiring remote or home-based interventions with information technology. Software that contains embedded risk models can triage, review, and assess client progress. Case management allows more efficient use of both human and financial home care resources through referral and follow-up and consultation. The final role for the nurse in telehomecare involves motivating the client and family by engaging, educating, and empowering them in self-care. Motivation encompasses the nursing interventions of counseling and health teaching. As a result the client and family are able better manage the existing condition and engage in activities related to tertiary prevention (Research in Community-Based Nursing Care 13-1).

Trends in Telehealth/Telehomecare

Due to future demographic trends and economics, the value of strategies to contain cost are obvious. As the population ages and new technologies are developed, telehealth is one strategy that will be more commonly used in the next decade with wide application. However, the most common use will be as a strategy for disease management. Rapidly advancing technologies will become more widely available, and more affordable. For example, there is a small, passive sensor that can seamlessly detect and report vitals; care management systems that can improve adherence to diet and medication guidance; communication systems to improve collaborative decision making between clients, families, and caregivers. These are promising technologies that will soon become more widely available.

RESEARCH IN COMMUNITY-BASED NURSING CARE ▶ 13-1

Receptiveness, Use, and Acceptance of Telehealth by Caregivers of Stroke Patients in the Home

Stroke occurs in over 700,000 people a year and is a leading cause of mortality for elderly Americans (Heart Disease and Stroke Statistics, 2004). Often family caregivers have difficulties meeting the rehabilitation need of stroke survivors, putting them at risk for requiring long-term care. Telehealth is one cost effective approach to enhancing self-management of chronic conditions. This research identified factors that impacted the receptiveness, use, and acceptance of videophones in the home setting by 21 family caregivers of stroke patients. Videophones are advantageous for providing services to caregivers who are isolated due to physical distances or by disabilities of the client or caregiver. This research identified obstacles to receptiveness of the client or caregiver including: concerns of the caregiver about home security, very low or high degree of burden in caregiving, limited need for support from health care providers, and disinterest or awkwardness in using technology. This study found that it is important to identify possible barriers to using technology in the home prior to developing and evaluating programs using telephones for monitoring progress of rehabilitation.

Source: Buckley, K. M., Tran, B. Q., & Prandoni, C. M. (2004). Receptiveness, use and acceptance of telehealth by caregivers of stroke patients in the home. *Online Journal of Issues in Nursing, 9*(3). Retrieved on September 30, 2006, from http://nursing world.org/ojin/topic16/tpc16_6.htm

Some of these technologies allow for more comprehensive data collection, which can in turn be used to evaluate and analyze the efficacy of these interventions. All of these strategies will contribute to further developing evidence-based nursing practice in home care. This is important because the primary application of telehealth will be disease management where outcome data are the central element to client care. The challenge for the nurse will be to maintain relationship-centered care while preserving the trusting relationship that is essential to nursing care in all settings.

INFUSION THERAPY

Home infusion therapy is a broad area, incorporating chemotherapy, pain management, fluid replacement therapy, immunosuppressive drug therapy, thalassemia treatment with deferoxamine mesylate, inotropic therapy, and blood and platelet transfusion. These medications are infused by a variety of methods. The actual administration of the therapy is performed by home infusion nurses or self-administered by clients or their caregivers. Because infusion therapy has become widely utilized as a cost-containment strategy, reimbursement criteria are strict.

Preauthorization is essential before any home infusion therapy is initiated, or the result could be nonpayment for the services provided. Increasingly, family members are expected to administer medications and fluid via central line (Craven & Hirnle, 2007).

Role of the Nurse

It is imperative that nurses who seek employment in infusion therapy have sharp problem-solving and interpersonal skills, detailed knowledge of the therapies and their effects, and technical skill in working with equipment. Although all nursing roles are important in this specialized area, the primary one is that of direct caregiving or delegated medical function (Figure 13-1). Before the visit, the nurse must be sure that the visit has been preauthorized and that the medication dosage, rate, route, and site-change frequency are all indicated in the physician order. In addition, all necessary equipment and supplies must be in the home or brought to the home by the nurse. Box 13-1 details the numerous safety requirements of this type of therapy.

Another important nursing function involves completing a full assessment, including intake and output, weight, and any signs of a reaction to therapy. This assessment should also include the infusion site, operation of the infusion pump, care for the access site, signs of infection, allergic response, fluid overload, and dehydration or other signs of complications. Response to the therapy must always be assessed and documented.

Reimbursement for home care infusion therapy is often limited because it is expected that all clients and their families will assume some or all aspects of the

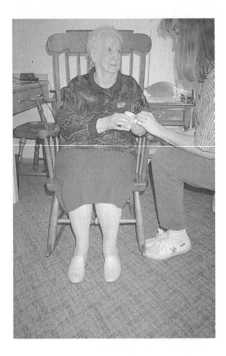

FIGURE 13-1. ▶ It is imperative never to lose sight of the importance of compassion and caring in the alleviation of suffering in our role as nurses.

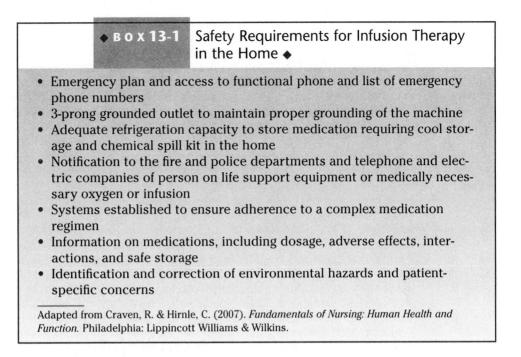

◆ **B O X 13-1** Safety Requirements for Infusion Therapy in the Home ◆

- Emergency plan and access to functional phone and list of emergency phone numbers
- 3-prong grounded outlet to maintain proper grounding of the machine
- Adequate refrigeration capacity to store medication requiring cool storage and chemical spill kit in the home
- Notification to the fire and police departments and telephone and electric companies of person on life support equipment or medically necessary oxygen or infusion
- Systems established to ensure adherence to a complex medication regimen
- Information on medications, including dosage, adverse effects, interactions, and safe storage
- Identification and correction of environmental hazards and patient-specific concerns

Adapted from Craven, R. & Hirnle, C. (2007). *Fundamentals of Nursing: Human Health and Function.* Philadelphia: Lippincott Williams & Wilkins.

care. It is more common for the infusion therapy nurse rather than the nurse in charge of discharge planning to teach the family caregiver or client how to do the infusion. It is important that the nurse teach the client and family regarding the safe infusion of the medication. In the rare case when teaching is done before discharge from the hospital, the client and family members are often so overwhelmed and anxious that they may have difficulty learning the procedure. Often the client or family is unable to complete the skill independently once they are home. The content of this teaching incorporates using proper technique for infusions and solving common problems related to intravenous (IV) therapy, site care, and use of the infusion pump, as well as the purpose, route, and dosage of the medications. The family must also know how to document the rate and time of all infusions, symptoms of IV infiltration and infection, and times to call or contact the nurse or physician (Craven & Hirnle, 2007).

Trends in Infusion Therapy

Patient safety is a major issue in infusion therapy. As previously mentioned, nurses who seek employment in this specialized area must possess a sophisticated skill set. Although not required at this time, there is some interest in requiring certification for employment as an infusion therapy nurse. Currently, the Joint Commission on Accreditation of Healthcare Organizations states that nurses must be appropriately qualified and competent in the infusion field to be employed as an infusion nurse. Orientation, training, and validation of the competency of nurses working in infusion therapy are essential for safe patient care. Competencies should include venipuncture and the assessment skills of the nurses related to the therapy and vascular access devices. This educational training is the responsibility of the agency. Some research indicates that certified nurses experience fewer adverse events and errors in care than their noncertified counterparts (Masoorli, 2005). There is a trend to require agencies to hire nurses who are certified through the Infusion Nurses Certification Corporation and maintain this certification to be reimbursed for services. The benefit is that Certified Infusion Nurses make fewer errors in administration. The downside to requiring home infusion therapy nurses to become certified is that it may create a shortage of certified nurses and consequently limit access to home infusion care.

WOUND CARE

Wounds are responsible for significant suffering and morbidity in home and hospice care (Hindelang, 2006). Wound care is a common specialized home care function. Wounds are categorized broadly as acute or chronic, with all wounds being considered acute at the onset of the injury. If the process of healing is prolonged beyond the expected trajectory the wound is classified as chronic (Whitney, 2005).

A variety of problems can occur in wound healing, stemming from a combination of factors and situations. These include the client's general health, nutritional status, skin texture and turgor, body weight, and mobility, all of which impact healing (Whitney, 2005). Wound care is not simply a technique of dressing application; there is a discipline of specialized practice for wound care that includes advanced training, education, and certification. There is a lack of wound care specialists, caused by area-specific shortages and the expense of contracting for such services.

Role of the Nurse

In wound care, the role involves an ongoing evaluation of the wound and any particular risk factors for healing. Before the first visit, the nurse must be familiar with the type of wound, wound care orders, cleaning method, and frequency of dressing change, as well as any pressure-relieving or support devices, dietary restrictions and caloric allowance, medications, and activity orders and restrictions. The nurse's main interventions fall within delegated medical functions, consultation, counseling, collaboration, and health education. Mobility enhancement and pain assessment should be initiated at the first visit and done periodically as needed. Scrupulous documentation following the Outcome and Assessment Information Set (OASIS) assessment or the agency policy is an essential aspect of wound care. For additional information on the OASIS documentation, see Chapter 12. Box 13-2 outlines other safety considerations.

It is important that the nurse is comfortable educating the client and caregivers in wound care skills. Lay caregivers must become competent in several aspects of wound care, as they often are the main care providers. They need to be able to describe and demonstrate wound care and signs and symptoms of infection. Knowledge of the importance of medicating 30 minutes before a painful dressing change is essential. Nutritional practices profoundly impact wound healing, and one way to monitor this is through a dietary log. The client should be encouraged to participate in an activity as appropriate for the condition. For those with limited mobility, caregivers must understand range-of-motion exercises and initiate them at least three times a day. Techniques for turning and positioning the client every 2 hours to alleviate pressure are also essential caregiver skills.

◆ **B O X 13-2**   Safety Considerations for Wound Care ◆

- Universal precautions for infection control and disposal of sharps and used dressings
- List available to the client and all caregivers of signs and symptoms to report to the nurse or physician
- Documentation of medications and allergies
- Identification and correction of environmental hazards and patient-specific concerns

Source: Sinkinson, G., Cammon, S., Curry, J., & Foley, M. (2001). *Pocket guide to home care standards*. Springhouse, PA: Springhouse Corporation.

Trends in Wound Care

Interdisciplinary teams and networks of wound care centers are becoming vital to the coordination of wound care. Care conferencing is where all team members meet to discuss specific cases and need for revisions to the plan of care. Most agencies have identified criteria for cases that must be examined by a care conference. It is important that these criteria explore the causes or factors contributing to the wound, and how the plan of care addresses these. The past and current status of the wound and the current orders for the dressing and treatment must also be clearly documented and must be compatible. The client or caregiver's role in the wound plan of care must be examined, as should the frequency of physical therapy visits. The barriers to wound healing should be identified and addressed. Discharge goals and timeframe should be realistic.

Through technology, new tools are being developed, along with different, targeted approaches to provide more effective care to those with wounds that require advanced care and supervision. The first trend is the use of telehealth for wound care. Home-based telewoundcare can involve teleconsulting, conferencing, reporting, and transmitting. For example, telewound care, using an ordinary digital camera to document the status of a wound for tracking and planning, is becoming commonplace. An ongoing photographic history of the wound provides excellent continuity between the home, clinic, and hospital. Cost savings of 50% have been documented as a benefit of using telewoundcare (Kinsella, 2002).

Another example of telewoundcare is specialty wound services delivered directly to the home via a computer screen. The photographs of the wound are transmitted to a specialty wound care service that provides consultation for management of difficult wounds. These virtual specialists work together with the home care nurse to assess and plan care. Both of these trends are offering hope for healing difficult wounds in a more cost-effective manner.

It is anticipated that the need for home care nurses with skills in wound care will continue to grow as the demographics shift, with an increasing percentage of the population becoming older and more obese, and developing diabetes (Sweitzer, et al., 2006).

MATERNAL–CHILD HOME CARE

Recipients of maternal-child home care fall into three main categories: high-risk pregnant women, high-risk infants, and children. The main advantage of home care for high-risk pregnancy is that it reduces costs by preventing hospitalization as well as decreases the percentage of low-birth-weight infants. With more than 9% of hospital charges attributable to pregnancy, delivery, and neonatal care, there is considerable opportunity for savings (Cross, 2006). Women who are identified as having high-risk pregnancies may require home care for several pregnancy complications, including preterm labor, **pregnancy-induced hypertension (PIH)**, and **hyperemesis** gravidarum. Increasingly, woman experiencing these complications from pregnancy require high-technology care, such as infusion therapy or telemedicine in the form of home monitoring.

High-risk infants may receive specialized home care. These include infants receiving palliative care, infants who are technology-dependent, and stable premature infants requiring intensive home support. Children with acute or chronic conditions or children requiring palliative or hospice care also may be home care recipients.

Role of the Nurse

Nursing roles depend on the client's condition. In the case of high-risk maternal visits, hyperemesis, or protracted vomiting with weight loss and fluid and electrolyte imbalance, sometimes requires IV replacement therapy at home to maintain hydration. In women at risk for preterm labor, home care prevents premature birth. Nursing roles include assessment of the mother's weight, fetal heart tones, fundal height, nutrition, psychosocial status, compliance with the plan of care, and knowledge of signs and symptoms of preterm labor.

PIH is the second leading cause of maternal mortality in the United States. Eight percent of all pregnancies are complicated by PIH (Basso, et al., 2006). PIH is a hypertensive disorder of pregnancy that includes preeclampsia, eclampsia, and transient hypertension. Home monitoring of those individuals experiencing PIH has been shown to reduce mortality and health care costs. Skilled nursing care includes assessment of the mother's weight, presence of edema and hyperreflexia, signs and symptoms of a worsening condition, fetal heart tones, compliance with the plan of care, nutrition, psychosocial status, and knowledge of symptoms.

Home Care of High-Risk Infants

As discussed in Chapter 8, the number and percentage of low-birth-weight and premature infants has increased in the United States. Low-birth-weight infants who are discharged from neonatal intensive care units may require home care services. Some low-birth-weight infants are stable at discharge but progress more successfully with intensive home support (Hummel & Cronin, 2004). Infants who are technology-dependent when they are discharged from the neonatal intensive care unit (NICU) may have need of home visiting. Infants with congenital conditions for which there is no treatment may be discharged home with palliative or hospice care. Some of the primary roles and considerations for the role of the nurse in this case are discussed in the section in this chapter on hospice care (Hummel & Cronin, 2004).

Postpartum/Well-Baby Home Care

Maternal and infant home visiting programs first began in the 19th century. Postpartum well baby care was a component of these. For several decades there has been an impressive body of research that documents the long-term value of nurse home visiting for perinatal care (Research in Community-Based Nursing 13-2). Recent international studies conclude the same benefit (Quinlivan, Box, & Evans, 2003; Fullerton, Killian, & Gass, 2005).

In the last decade, postpartum home care has become a growing area of perinatal services. It is common for insurers to reimburse at least one visit for families after early discharge in the presence of high-risk factors. These may include conditions with the infant such as hyperbilirubinemia, low birth weight, and failure to feed well or gain weight appropriately. Any woman who manifests signs of postpartum depression merits a referral for follow-up with a home care nurse after discharge. Again, the role of the nurse involves assessing and monitoring postpartum status and referring for follow-up as appropriate. A description of recent research documenting the benefits of this type of program is seen in Research in Community-Based Nursing 13-3.

Pediatric Home Care

The need for home care services for the pediatric client has grown substantially in recent years. Most of these services are for postsurgical clients released from the hospital so early that they need skilled nursing care at home through the rehabilitation phase of care. A second common group—children with chronic conditions such as bronchial pulmonary dysphasia, cystic fibrosis, and cancer—are now being

---

RESEARCH IN COMMUNITY-BASED NURSING CARE ▶ 13-2

Enduring Effects of Nurse Home Visitation on Maternal Life Course

For decades there has been evidence that nurse home visiting creates benefits for the families who receive the service. This research was designed to determine the effectiveness of prenatal or infancy home visits on the maternal life course of women in an urban setting over a 3-year period of time. Pregnant women were randomly assigned to either the control group with no visits or to weekly visits by a nurse. The 743 participants received an average of 7 visits during their pregnancy and 26 visits from birth to their child's 2nd birthday. The women who received home visits had fewer subsequent pregnancies, longer intervals between the birth of the first and second child, and fewer months of using AFDC (welfare) and food stamps. This study concluded that there are enduring effects of home visiting program on the lives of the women who participate in these programs.

Kitzman, H., Olds., D., Sidora, K., Henderson, C., Hanks, C., et al. (2000). Enduring effects of nurse home visitation on maternal life course: A 3-year follow-up of a randomized trial. *Journal of the American Medical Association*, *283*(15),1983–1989.

> **RESEARCH IN COMMUNITY-BASED NURSING CARE ▶ 13-3**
>
> ### A Home Visitation Program Welcomes Home First-time Moms and Their Infants
>
> The Welcome Home Baby! is a maternal-infant home visiting program for all-first time mothers and infants in the Northern part of San Diego County, California. The goal of this program is to ensure the health and well-being of first time mothers and infants during the critical first year of life. Unlike many maternal infant home visiting programs, this service is open to all first-time mothers who agree to participate. Numerous circumstances with infants may result in unnecessary emergency department visits or hospitalization. These episodes are expensive compared to disease prevention and health promotion activities provided through health education. Regardless of race/ethnicity or economic class all women benefit from this service. This program uses a case management, interdisciplinary model to implement the program objectives to increase parent infant safety knowledge, link infants with a health care provider, and increase longevity of breastfeeding. Evaluation of program objectives found that program objectives were met in a cost-effective way after 1 year. Based on the data from the first year, in the second year of the program a clinical pathway was used that was shown to result in a 39% reduction in program costs in the second year.
>
> Source: Hedges, S., Simmes, D., Martinez, A., Linder, C., & Brown, S. (2005). A home visitation program welcomes home first-time moms and their infants. *Home Healthcare Nurse*, 23(5), 286–289.

cared for at home rather than in the hospital setting. Children may need some of the same nursing care that has already been discussed: infusion therapy, wound care, or other high-technology care. All of the general principles and guidelines discussed in Chapter 12 that apply to the home care of adults also apply to children. It is particularly important when caring for children that all nursing functions are formulated, implemented, and evaluated in collaboration with the parents or caregiver.

Trends in Maternal–Child Home Care

Some of the trends in home care of high-risk pregnancy include use of telemedicine for the management of preterm labor (Tadir, 2004). Home monitoring devices have become increasingly sophisticated and simple to use. One example is a device that allows pregnant women to keep track of fetal heart rate (FHR) at home. This device allows the pregnant client to check the fetal heart rate whenever she has doubts about the welfare of her infant and contact the physician if she has concerns. The FHR can be transmitted to a digital display. Another new devise is a smart monitor that can be used in any setting as a wireless system. This offers nondirective supportive therapy (NST) from the client's home and may be integrated with other home telehealth services to monitor high-risk clients who otherwise would have to be admitted to the hospital.

There has been evidence in the literature for over a decade that demonstrates the cost savings of home uterine activity monitoring. In one study, the mean cost for the telemedicine group was $7,225, whereas the mean cost for the group who did not receive daily home uterine monitoring was $21,684, with an average savings of $14,459 per pregnancy using telemedicine services (Morrison, et al., 2001). A more recent example of a program that improves pregnancy and neonatal outcomes and reduces costs is a case manager model of care that saves 2 to 5 dollars for every dollar spent on home care. This is a "high touch" and "low tech" program that prevents preterm deliveries and C-section births (Cross, 2006).

Although pediatric home health care represents a small portion of all the home health care services, increasing technologic advances and the continued movement of health care from the acute care to the community setting is expected to lead to higher use.

PAIN MANAGEMENT

For many conditions, pain management is central to effective nursing care. It is common for clients and their caregivers to fear uncontrolled pain. They may need frequent reassurance that pain control can be achieved. At the same time, unfortunately, all too often, pain is underestimated and inadequately treated.

Home care nurses need ongoing pain management education as they are often the client's only advocate and source of information (Figure 13-2). The home as a setting for practice presents unique challenges (Vallerand, Hasenau, & Templin, 2004). Barriers to pain management by home care nurses are seen in Table 13-1.

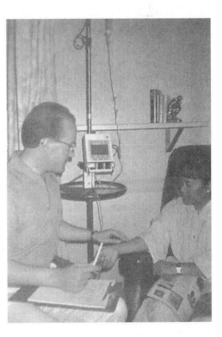

FIGURE 13-2. ▶ Intravenous therapy and other technologic treatments contribute to pain management in the home.

TABLE 13-1	Barriers to Pain Management by Home Care Nurses
Barrier	**Description**
Lack of knowledge	Persists among all nurses regardless of the area of clinical practice
Inadequate assessment skills	Believing what the client says about the level of his or her pain is less likely to be considered by the nurse compared to other data
Addiction	Concern that use of opioids will result in addiction
Respiratory depression	Concern for opioid-induced respiratory depression
Communication	Inadequate or incomplete communication with physicians and the nurse-physician relationship

Source: Vallerand, A. H., Hasenau, S. M., & Templin, T. (2004). Barriers to pain management by home care nurses. *Home Healthcare Nurse, 22*(12), 831–838.

Role of the Nurse

Many factors contribute to successful assessment and management of pain, but the relationship and trust between the nurse and client is central to this process. Caring and compassion are essential to this relationship. Effective pain management is based on a comprehensive pain assessment. In the home environment, where the nurse may see the client for very limited periods of time, it is imperative that the nurse develops skills in assessment and management of pain. Because pain is a subjective and an individual experience, the client's report of pain must be considered accurate and valid. Generally, acute pain is defined as pain that lasts less than 6 months, whereas chronic pain lasts more than 6 months. As in all community-based nursing care, prevention and early intervention is always the first consideration in the assessment and management of pain. Assessment Tools 13-1 contains a method for assessing pain.

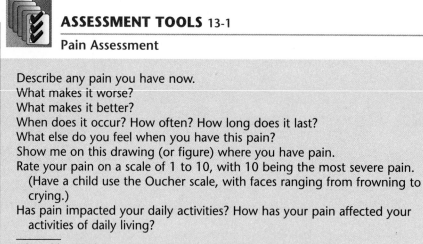

ASSESSMENT TOOLS 13-1

Pain Assessment

Describe any pain you have now.
What makes it worse?
What makes it better?
When does it occur? How often? How long does it last?
What else do you feel when you have this pain?
Show me on this drawing (or figure) where you have pain.
Rate your pain on a scale of 1 to 10, with 10 being the most severe pain.
   (Have a child use the Oucher scale, with faces ranging from frowning to crying.)
Has pain impacted your daily activities? How has your pain affected your activities of daily living?

Adapted from Weber, J., & Kelly, J. (2007). *Health Assessment in Nursing.* (3rd ed.). Philadelphia: Lippincott Williams & Wilkins.

The pharmacologic interventions for the management of pain are too numerous to address in this chapter. Most medical–surgical textbooks comprehensively discuss the common interventions for pain management, including delegated medication functions, health education, consultation, and counseling. Sometimes physical pain-relief techniques can be used with success; positioning and good hygiene often relieve pain for those individuals who spend long hours in bed. Cutaneous stimulation, such as massage, vibration, heat, and cold are often effective for temporary relief from pain. Anticipatory guidance, distraction, guided imagery, and hypnosis also contributes to pain management. There are also behavioral pain relief techniques including relaxation and meditation.

Trends in Pain Management

One trend in pain management is the increasing use of complementary therapies. A great deal of research documents the benefits of relaxation and meditation for conditions such as pain management. National Center for Complementary and Alternative Medicine (2007) authorities recommend that practitioners use relaxation and meditation for pain management, given their low cost and demonstrated health benefits, and judge them as among the best complementary therapies for widespread use.

There is considerable research at the National Institute of Health (NIH) assessing the efficacy of various pain management strategies. One area of current research focuses on chronic pain that has lasted at least 6 months. Other studies are comparing different health care approaches to the management of acute low back pain (standard care versus chiropractic, acupuncture, or massage therapy). These studies are measuring symptom relief, restoration of function, and patient satisfaction. Other research is comparing standard surgical treatments to the most commonly used standard nonsurgical treatments to measure changes in health-related quality of life among patients suffering from spinal stenosis (NIH, 2006).

As in other areas of medical research, there is a great deal of work focusing on the role of medication in pain management. Notable among these are researchers working to develop a morphine-like drug that will have the same pain-deadening qualities without the drug's negative side effects. Another group is working to develop pain medications that take advantage of the body's natural ability to block or interrupt pain signals (National Institute of Neurological Disorders and Stroke, 2006).

HOSPICE CARE

Hospice care provides an essential alternative for the terminally ill client. Dr. Cecily Saunders founded the hospice movement in London in the late 1960s. Dr. Sylvia Lack established the first hospice in the United States based on the model developed in Great Britain. Since 1982, when the Medicare hospice program was established, the number of hospices has grown dramatically. According to the Hospice Association of America (HAA, 2006) there were 31 Medicare-certified hospices in 1984. In 1985, there were 151. In 1991, there were 1,011, and by 2006, the number had increased to 2,884. In addition to all the other benefits to clients and family provided by hospice care, the daily cost is substantially less than the cost of stays in the hospital and in skilled nursing facilities.

Agencies that provide hospice care are committed to maintaining supportive social, emotional, and spiritual services to the terminally ill, as well as support for the client's family. Caring for the terminally ill includes caring for the family and caregivers (Research in Community-Based Nursing 13-4). Care varies according to the client and family's needs; however, the focus is always on the client and family as the unit of care. Hospice care is often interdisciplinary care that reaffirms the right of every individual and family to participate fully in the final stage of life.

When a client is diagnosed with a terminal illness and has 6 months or less to live, the client qualifies for hospice care through Medicare. Payment for hospice services under Medicare is based on four levels of care:

1. Routine home care
2. Continuous home care (24 hours in a crisis situation)
3. Inpatient respite care not to exceed 5 days at a time
4. General inpatient care (Hospice Association of America [HAA, 2007]).

Hospice care is offered in a variety of settings. These include the freestanding hospice house, where inpatient hospice services are provided at the end of life; hospital- and home-based services provided by freestanding hospice agencies; and home care-affiliated hospice agencies. Most of the programs in the United States are provided through autonomous, community-based, in-home hospice programs. Nurses develop and supervise many hospice agencies.

Intermittent hospice care is provided in the home by nurses; medical social workers; physical, occupational, and speech therapists; home health aides; and homemakers. Hospice programs provide short periods of continuous care in which a client is provided with shift nursing and aides for an acute episode and respite care for the family by placing the client in a nursing home for a few days. Hospice-trained volunteers provide emotional and physical support for clients and families by assisting with transportation, household care, child care, errands,

RESEARCH IN COMMUNITY-BASED NURSING CARE ▶ 13-4

The Positive Impact of Hospice Care on the Surviving Spouse

According to a recent study, hospice care not only provides benefit to the client but also to the surviving spouse. Surviving spouses of individuals who had hospice care at the end of life have lower mortality as compared to surviving spouses of those who do not have hospice care. Even receiving hospice care for 3 or 4 weeks positively affects the mortality rate of surviving spouses. This study has implications not only for the advantage of hospice care, but also for how health care affects society in broader terms. The findings of this research suggest that the type of health care received by a client impacts not only the client but also his or her family members. This study did not identify the specific hospice intervention that provided the benefit and suggests a need for further research in this area.

Christakis, N. A., & Iwashyna, T. J. (2003). The health impact of health care on families: A matched cohort study of hospice use by decedents and mortality outcomes in surviving widowed spouses. *Social Science & Medicine, 57,* 465–475.

and companionship. Volunteers also provide a vital link between the client and health care providers.

The Role of the Nurse

Death with dignity is the motto of hospice. In hospice, the focus of care shifts to palliative care and strengthening the client and family's quality of life as the client faces death. The goal of hospice in the home is to make the dying process as dignified as possible while providing physical, emotional, and spiritual comfort. Nursing care strives to assist the client and family to define their needs at the end stages of life and to have the resources necessary to carry out their wishes. Home hospice care means individuals can remain in the comfort of their own home, surrounded by family and loved ones, and die peacefully without fear of major medical intervention and resuscitative measures.

The specific role of the nurse varies according to the client's diagnosis and the wishes of the client and family. It is clear that the client is vulnerable at this time, and family members are vulnerable as their loved one is dying. It is very important in this specialization that the nurse is skilled in therapeutic communication and responding to psychological responses. It is common for the client to experience anxiety, depression, and delirium at the end of life. Each of these conditions can occur as a result of the primary disease, concurrent physical conditions, inadequate pain management, medication side effects, or a combination of all of these.

End-of-life care requires sharp assessment skills to determine necessary delegated medical functions and comfort measures. It is imperative that all hospice nurses are knowledgeable about various types of pain management techniques. Anticipating medication needs is one important role for the hospice nurse.

As in any situation providing direct physical and psychological care, the nurse must carefully assess the particular needs of the client, family members, and caregivers. This assessment should be holistic as well as follow the main premises of this book. In other words, the nurse should consider the needs of the client within the context of his or her family, culture, and community. Transcultural nursing principles related to hospice care are found in Research in Community-Based Nursing 13-5.

Even at the end of life, the focus should be on maximizing the potential of the individual and family through health promotion and disease prevention. For example, the simple intervention of good hand washing can prevent an infection that could cause pain and suffering during the client's last days. Encouraging activity that the client finds pleasurable promotes health, even when death is near. For instance, if the client enjoys animals, pet therapy may provide benefit (Fig. 13-3). Planning for medication needs even if they occur after regular pharmacy hours is another role in comfort care with end-of-life care. These situations should be anticipated before such a need arises by careful advance planning and assessment. Hospice nurses should have excellent pain management skills. Adequate pain relief is assured by the following measures:

◆ Obtaining and maintaining a standing order for analgesia that incorporates consideration of increasing pain levels
◆ Assessing for all causes of pain, including anxiety, positioning, and environment
◆ Documenting every medication dose and any changes in dose, response to medication, and nonpharmacologic interventions that are effective for pain relief for this individual

RESEARCH IN COMMUNITY-BASED NURSING CARE ▶ 13-5

Applying Principles of Transcultural Nursing to End-of-Life Issues

End-of-life care that is meaningful to each family and respects the unique perspective of each individual requires nurses to develop cultural competence. Just as health beliefs vary from one culture to another, many cultural variations exist in the dying process. Consequently, the definition of what constitutes a good death is culturally defined. The Western constructs of informed consent and individual autonomy are not consistent or valued by all cultural perspectives. Three ethical constructs important to hospice care are: 1) sharing bad news, 2) locus of decision-making, and 3) advance directives. Some cultural perspectives consider sharing news of serious illness and death as disrespectful and cruel. Locus of control or decision-making varies from one culture to another. Role responsibilities and definition of family vary related to decision-making. Some cultures are patriarchal, with a male member of the family being considered the primary decision maker. Usage of advance directives is only about 20% of the U.S. population. Usage is significantly lower in some cultural groups including Asian, Hispanic, and African American.

Source: Jenko, M., & Moffitt, S. (2006). Transcultural nursing principles: An application to hospice care. *Journal of Hospice and Palliative Nursing, 8*(3),172–180.

Following the death of the client, bereavement counseling and support for the family continue for a year. Spiritual counseling is a common aspect of care. Spirituality expressed through the religious beliefs of the client and family can be a useful tool in the care of people who are dying.

Trends in Hospice Care

Public and political consciousness, research allocation related to end-of-life issues, emphasis on personal choice, and increased public awareness of the limits of medical technology have all increased interest in hospice care. Recognition of the importance of pain management, along with the joining of forces between palliative care and hospice, has also contributed to increased availability and quality of pain management in hospice care. It is anticipated that hospice care will assume an increasingly important role in community-based care in the future (HAA, 2006).

CLIENT SITUATIONS IN PRACTICE

◆ Maria's Story of Transcultural Nursing in Hospice Care

I work for a home care agency that provides various specialized services. Most of my work is in infusion therapy and hospice care. Several years ago I cared for a woman who was Chinese American. Up to that point I had never worked with an individual with this

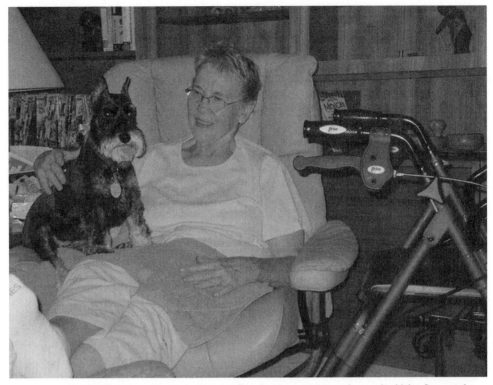

FIGURE 13-3. ▶ Pet therapy provides comfort and support at the end of life. Copyright Roberta Hunt, 2007.

cultural background. The experience was so interesting while at the same time challenging and frustrating that I decided I wanted to develop my skills in transcultural nursing.

I met May Lin on December 21st. I remember the date because she did not have a Christmas tree in her home and I concluded that May Lin was probably not Christian. I learned from the referral that May Lin was 76 years old and a widow. She had been diagnosed with breast cancer the prior January. She had a mastectomy, three rounds of chemotherapy, and radiation. In the last 3 months she had visited the clinic multiple times because she was losing weight, unable to eat, and was also very run down from the chemotherapy treatment. The referral I received was for total parenteral nutrition (TPN) infusion twice a day via central line. The treatment plan was to teach a family member to do the infusions on the first visit. I would continue to monitor May Lin a few times a week.

She appeared to understand what I saying to her but she spoke limited English. She was, however, able to communicate most of her needs and answer the questions on the admission form. In the intake interview I learned that May Lin moved to the United States in 1960. For 30 years she and her husband owned and ran a restaurant in the Chinese community where they lived in a large metropolitan city. She told me that she was the mother of two adult children. Her son, Alex, was a business lawyer with a busy practice and lived several states away from May Lin. Her daughter, Karen, lived in an apartment about 10 minutes from May Lin. Karen, a physician and neuroscientist had two teenage children, one of whom has severe asthma. Karen had a very demanding job with many responsibilities as the head of an academic department in a large university. Karen's husband had a stroke 1 year prior to her mother becoming ill. He was no longer working and had significant physical limitations.

Karen was unable to be present at the first home visit. Her son had suffered a severe exacerbation of asthma triggered from the respiratory flu and she had to take him to the emergency room. Subsequent to this visit he was hospitalized for several days. The treatment plan to teach Karen to do the infusions would not be possible for at least another week. The first visit went well, with one exception. May Lin was experiencing pain in her back. She was very stoic about the pain and I only learned about it when I noticed that when she sat down or changed positions she grimaced. When I asked if she was having pain, she denied it at first. When she continued to show nonverbal evidence of pain, and I asked again if she was uncomfortable she admitted that she had been having severe pain for several months. I suggested she try a heating pad to relieve the discomfort and make an appointment to see her oncologist later in the week.

The next week Karen became ill with the flu. Due to May Lin's compromised immune system, Karen and I decided that I would do the treatment for the next week. We scheduled a teaching session with the expectation that Karen would begin to do the infusions before and after work. During the visits in the second week May Lin continued to move very carefully, as if she was experiencing considerable discomfort with any movement. When she tried to sit during the infusion she would frequently adjust positions as if it were impossible to be comfortable. I asked if she had seen her oncologist or made an appointment about her back pain. She indicated that she had not. When I asked if she was having any difficulties sleeping she indicated that she was. I asked her if she would like my assistance to call her physician's office and she indicated that she did. I dialed the number and assisted her in making the appointment for the beginning of the next week.

The next week Karen called and said that she was not able to come to the teaching visit to learn about the central line. Her husband had fallen and broken his foot. I told her about her mother's back pain and that we had set up an appointment for her to see her physician. Karen indicated that she would accompany her mother to the visit.

A week later I received a referral from the oncologist's office that May Lin's plan of care had changed. The pain in her back was bone cancer. A magnetic resonance image (MRI) scan revealed extensive disease, with a large questionable area in her liver. Liver function tests had been done but the results were not yet available. I was to continue the infusion therapy. The family had been given information about hospice care. I was to follow-up to determine if the family had any questions about hospice.

I went to May Lin's home that day to teach Karen about the infusions. When I asked May Lin about how the clinic visit went she said it went fine and that the pain in her back was from arthritis. Puzzled that May Lin had reached a conclusion very different from the one that I had about her conditions, I looked at Karen. She did not make eye contact. I was perplexed and decided I would follow up with a phone call.

The next day I called Karen and asked what the physician had told them about the results of the tests and what her understanding was about the source of her mother's back pain. She indicated that the physician had told her that May Lin had widespread bone cancer and her liver function tests were abnormal. The physician stated that her disease was very advanced and there was no chemotherapy available for her condition. I told her that her mother told me that the source of the pain was from arthritis. I asked her if she thought that her mother understood what the physician had told them and she said, "My brother and I did not tell mother that she has a terminal disease." I was shocked and concerned by this news but I knew that I would abide by Karen's desire not to inform her mother for the time being.

I continued to care for May Lin as her primary nurse. Increasingly I was bothered by the fact that May Lin did not know that she was terminally ill. Why would this family choose not to inform their mother about her condition? Was this situation where a client is not informed about her condition ethical? Was I enabling the family to hide information from their mother, thus also practicing without following ethical practice guidelines? I decided to call Karen and meet with her. I could not continue to support the family's desires without considering my client's rights and interests. It appeared to me that she needed an advocate.

When Karen and I met I asked her, "Tell me about how you made the decision not to tell your mother about her diagnosis." She replied, "In my family's culture sharing a terminal diagnosis is unnecessarily cruel. My mother holds traditional Chinese values, and telling her that she has a terminal illness would be impolite and disrespectful." I was shocked by her response. While I had concluded that this family was secretive or denying their mother's condition and not advocating for their mother, rather their reaction stemmed from a norm in their culture that was inconsistent from what is considered "best practice" in my own culture. At that moment I realized how dominant cultural norms are to one's worldview. I had scrutinized this family's reaction through my own definition of the "right way" and made assumptions without clarifying on what basis this family had made this judgment.

I continued in my role as May Lin's primary nurse and cared for her until her death. There were several decisions related to May Lin's care that were debated in the next 3 months. Asian families are often patriarchal, which was true for May Lin's family. This meant that despite the fact that Karen was the primary family caregiver and a physician, Alex was the family decision-maker related to May Lin's end-of-life decisions. Although this meant a somewhat cumbersome communication process and patience on the part of the hospice nurses, it worked for the family. When it came to decisions related to do-not-resuscitate (DNR), Karen provided Alex with many resources to educate him about the advantages and disadvantages. At first Alex was opposed to suspending any treatments but in the end decided that May Lin should have a DNR order, to suspend any life-prolonging treatments, and shift to palliative care. May Lin died a peaceful death at home with her son and daughter at her side. Karen said, "Mother's death was dignified and the type of death she wanted."

CONCLUSIONS

Both specialized home care and hospice care will be important settings for practice in the future. The client advocate role will continue to be a central element of community care as complexity of health care delivery and concern for cost containment continue. Flexibility and accountability will remain fundamental as the pressure to meet professional practice standards intersects with pressure to contain costs. Challenges facing home care will require that the nurse keep up with ever-changing regulations regarding coverage, the documentation requirements that will follow, and the evolving certification requirements for nurses in these specialties. In addition, nurses will be called on to teach and support clients and families because of increasing responsibility for caring for acutely ill family members at home. As in all nursing specialties, it will be vital for specialized home care and hospice nurses to welcome the increased use of technology. Balancing "high tech" and "high touch" will continue to be the practice imperative in specialized home care.

What's on the Web

American Society for Pain Management Nursing (ASPMN)
Internet address: http://www.aspmn.org/
This organization of nurses is dedicated to promoting and providing optimal care for individuals with pain, including the management of its sequelae. All of this is accomplished through education, standards, advocacy, and research.

Home Care Guide: Pediatric *Home Care Guide*
Internet address:
http://www.hmc.psu.edu/hematology/homeguide/
This wonderful site outlines practical suggestions for typical issues that arise with pediatric home care for children with cancer. It takes the nurse step-by-step through nursing interventions for common symptoms that arise with cancer care.

Infusion Nurses Society
Internet address: http:/www.ins1.org/
The Infusion Nurses Society (INS) promotes excellence in infusion nursing through standards, education, advocacy, and outcome research. They are committed to supporting access to the highest quality, cost-effective infusion care for all individuals. INS achieves this mission by providing opportunities for advanced knowledge and expertise through professional development and resource networking.

Nursing: Specialties: Wound Care
Internet address: http://www.nursewebsearch.com/Specialties/Wound_Care/
This Web site lists numerous links related to the nursing specialty of wound care.

Pediatric Home Care Association of America (PedHCAA)
Internet address:
http://www.nahc.org/PedHCAA/home.html
This site provides valuable information about this affiliate of the National Association for Home Care and Hospice (NAHC). One of the goals of this organization is to strengthen communication between pediatric hospices and home care providers. It also represents the interests of pediatric hospice and home care providers to the U.S. Congress and regulatory bodies. Another goal is to develop pediatric resources and educational opportunities at national, regional, and local organization meetings.

End-of-Life Educational Consortium (ELNEC)
Internet address:
http://www.aacn.nche.edu/ELNEC/about.htm
This site provides nursing educators with training in end-of-life care. Content includes a module devoted to cultural consideration.

References and Bibliography

American Nurses Association. (1999). *ANA's core principles on telehealth.* Retrieved on October 4, 2006, from http://www.acnpweb.org/i4a/pages/Index.cfm?pageID=3471

American Telemedicine Association. (2001). *Memorandum on telehomecare under the Medicare prospective payment system.* Retrieved on October 6, 2006, from http://www.americantelemed.org/news/homecarememo012201.htm

Basso, O., Rasmussen, S., Weinberg, C. R., Wilcox, A. J., Irgens, L. M., & Skjaerven, R. (2006). Trends in fetal and infant survival following preeclampsia. *JAMA, 296*(6), 1357–1362.

Buckley, K. M, Tran, B. Q., & Prandoni, C. M. (2004). Receptiveness, use and acceptance of telehealth by caregivers of stroke patients in the home. *Online Journal of Issues in Nursing, 9*(3), 51–65.

Christakis, N. A., & Iwashyna, T. J. (2003). The health impact of health care on families: A matched cohort study of hospice use by decedents and mortality outcomes in surviving widowed spouses. *Social Science & Medicine, 57,* 465–475.

Coughlin, J. F., Pope, J. E., & Leedle, B. R., Jr. (2006). Old age, new technology, and future innovations in disease management and home health care. *Home Health Care Management & Practice, 18*(3), 196–207.

Craven, R., & Hirnle, C. (2007). *Fundamentals of nursing: Human health and function.*

Philadelphia: Lippincott Williams & Wilkins.

Cross, M. (2006). Pregnancy + birth = $$$. *Managed Care.* February. Retrieved on October 14, 2006, from http://www.managedcaremag.com/archives/0602/0602.birthcosts.html

Disease Management Association of America [DMAA]. (2006). DMAA definitions of disease management. Retrieved on October 31, 2007, from http://www.dmaa.org/dm_definition.asp

Fullerton, J., Killian, R., & Gass, P. (2005). Outcomes of a community- and home-based intervention for safe motherhood and newborn care. *Health Care for Women International, 266*(7), 561–576.

Heart Disease and Stroke Statistics—2004 Update. (Retrieved on October 6, 2006, from American Heart Association Web site at http://americanheart.org/presenter.jhtml

Hedges, S., Simmes, D., Martinez, A., Linder, C., & Brown, S. (2005). A home visitation program welcomes home first-time moms and their infants. *Home Healthcare Nurse, 23*(5), 286–289.

Hindelang, M. (2006). Caring for wounds: More than just cuts and scrapes. *Home Healthcare Nurse, 24*(2), 112–114.

Huffman, M. H. (2005). Disease management: A new and exciting opportunity in home healthcare. *Home Healthcare Nurse, 23*(5), 290–296.

Hospice Association of America (2007). Hospice facts an statistics. Retrieved on October 31, 2007, from http://www.nahc.org/haa/2007HospiceFactsStatistics.pdf

Hummel, P., & Cronin, J. (2004). Home care of the high-risk infant. *Advances in Neonatal Care, 4*, 354–364.

Jenko, M., & Moffitt, S. (2006). Transcultural nursing principles: An application to hospice care. *Journal of Hospice and Palliative Nursing, 8*(3), 172–180.

Kinsella, A. (2002). Advanced telecare for wound care delivery. *Home Healthcare Nurse, 20*(7), 457–461.

Kitzman, H., Olds, D., Sidora, K., et al. (2000). Enduring effects of nurse home visitation on maternal life course: A 3-year follow-up of a randomized trial. *Journal of the American Medical Association, 283*(15), 1983–1989.

National Alliance of Wound Care. Internet address: http://www.nahc.org/haa/2007HospiceFactsStatistics.pdf

National Center for Complementary and Alternative Medicine. (2007). Mind-body medicine: an overview. Retrieved on October 31, 2007, from http://nccam.nih.gov/health/backgrounds/mindbody.htm

National Institute of Neurological Disorders and Stroke. (2006). Pain: Hope through research. Retrieved on October 14, 2006, from http://www.ninds.nih.gov/disorders/chronic _pain/detail_chronic_pain.htm?css=print

National Institutes of Health. Fact sheet: Pain management. Retrieved on October 31, 2007, from http://www.nih.gov/about/researchresultsforthepublic/Pain.pdf

Masoorli, S., (2005). Legal issues related to vascular access devices and infusion therapy. *Journal of Infusion Nursing, 28*(3 Supplement), S18–21.

Morrison, J., Bergauer, N., Jacques, D., Coleman, S., & Stanziano, G. (2001). Telemedicine: Cost-effective management of high-risk pregnancy. *Managed Care.* Retrieved February 7, 2003, from http://www.managedcaremag.com/archives/0111/0111.peer_highrisk.html

Quinlivan, J. A., Box, H., & Evans, S. F. (2003). Postnatal home visits in teenage mothers: A randomised control trial. *The Lancet, 361*, 893–900. Retrieved on October 5, 2006, from http://www.thelancet.com

Sinkinson, G., Cammon, S., Curry, J., & Foley, M. (2001). *Pocket guide to home care standards.* Springhouse, PA: Springhouse.

Sweitzer, S. M., Fann, S. A., Borg, T. K., Baynes, J. W., & Yost, M. J. (2006). What is the future of diabetic wound care? *The Diabetes Educator, 32*(2), 197–210.

Tadir, Y., (2004). What's in the technology pipeline? *Contemporary OB/GYN,* 20–28. Retrieved on October 5, 2006, from Info-Trac. http://www.medicalagencies.com/files/GTTADIR.final.pdf

Thobaben, M. (2005). Telehomecare. *Home Health Care Management & Practice, 17*(6), 487–488.

Vallerand, A. H., Hasenau, S. M., & Templin, T. (2004). Barriers to pain management by home care nurses. *Home Healthcare Nurse, 22*(12), 831–838.

Weber, J., & Kelley, J. (2007). *Health assessment in nursing* (3rd ed.). Philadelphia: Lippincott Williams & Wilkins.

Whitney, J. D. (2005). Overview: Acute and chronic wounds. *Nursing Clinics of North America, 40*(2),191–196.

L E A R N I N G ▼ A C T I V I T I E S

◆ JOURNALING ACTIVITY 13-1

In your clinical journal, respond to the following questions.

- Discuss your own attitudes and beliefs regarding pain control. How do you think your own assumptions and beliefs could impact the way that you provide pain control for your clients? What do you think that you can do to prevent your own attitudes about pain from interfering with the needs of your clients?
- How would you handle pain control for someone who is a self-reported drug addict?
- Discuss what you thought was important content in Chapter 13 and how it fits into what you have learned so far about the role of the nurse in the community.
- How has your view of the nursing role in the community changed after reading this chapter (and observing the role of the nurse in the community)?

◆ CLIENT CARE ACTIVITY 13-2

Maureen is a 57-year-old widow who was referred to hospice home care. She was diagnosed with liver cancer 3 months ago. After extensive surgery and chemotherapy she is not improving. Her referral states that she has almost constant pain. Her daughter lives in another state and has three preschool children. Her son is living temporarily in Africa for 6 months. You are the home care nurse doing the admission intake by following the agency forms. However, you will have some particular concerns that are not addressed in the intake form given what you read on Maureen's referral form:

1. On what do you concentrate assessment beyond the admission form?
2. What questions do you use to assess these issues?
3. What combination of interventions do you use to help keep Maureen comfortable (both pharmacologic and other methods)?
4. What safety considerations do you have and how do you assess them?

◆ PRACTICAL APPLICATION ACTIVITY 13-3

Contact an agency that employs nurses to work in one of the roles described in this chapter. Arrange to observe a nurse working in the setting. After the observation, arrange for a short interview with the nurse. Develop several questions before the observation and interview. You may decide to use some of the following questions as a part of the interview.

1. What do you enjoy about this type of work?
2. What is difficult about the work?
3. How has the role changed over the last 5 years? Ten years?
4. How do you use the concept of self-care in your practice?
5. What place does health promotion and disease prevention have in your daily work?
6. What do you need to know about families, culture, and community to do this type of work?

7. What type of special training is now required or would you recommend in preparation to perform this specialized role?
8. Do you have any recommendations for a new graduate who may be interested in entering this type of work in the future?
   - Send a thank you note to the nurse and agency after the visit. (Not only is this a great strategy for getting a job in the future you are also building goodwill with some people you may work with in the future in the community. It is also just plain good manners.)
   - Summarize your observation and interview in a 2- to 3-page paper.

◆ PRACTICAL APPLICATION ACTIVITY 13-4

Find an article or book on the Internet on CINAHL or MEDLINE about one of the specialized settings and roles from the chapter that interests you. Get the article or book (pick a chapter) and respond to the following.

1. What was the main point of the article or chapter from the book?
2. What did you think was the most important aspect of the article or chapter for your learning?
3. How do you think that you can use this new information in the future?

◆ CRITICAL THINKING ACTIVITY 13-5

Identify a topic related to one of the specialized home care settings or roles discussed in this chapter. If you have discovered a specialized home care role not included in the chapter, it can also be used as the topic for this activity. Some examples could be the following:

- Should certification be required to practice in the specialty home care roles (e.g., pain management, infusion nursing, pediatric home care, high-risk obstetrics home care, hospice home care)?
- What are the current issues in one of the settings or roles? (For example, in high-risk home care, one issue is whether home uterine monitoring prevents preterm birth. In pediatric home care, one issue is how to work with the parents to plan and implement care.)
- How has the nursing shortage impacted these specialized roles?
- What issues related to funding impact the availability of specialized care?

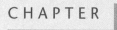

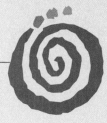

Mental Health Nursing in Community-Based Settings

MARVA THURSTON

LEARNING OBJECTIVES

1. Describe the historical evolution of mental health care.
2. Identify the behaviors of the major mental illnesses.
3. Discuss the significance of mental illness.
4. Describe the risk factors affecting those with mental illness.
5. Outline the elements of a therapeutic relationship.
6. Identify agencies that serve the mentally ill.

KEY TERMS

culture of poverty
deinstitutionalization of
   the mentally ill
professional relatedness
psychotropic medication

seriously mentally ill (SMI)
seriously and persistently
   mentally ill (SPMI)
staff splitting
stigma of mental illness

CHAPTER TOPICS

◆ Historical Perspective
◆ Significance of Community Mental Health
◆ Nursing Skills and Competencies
◆ Mental Health Assessment
◆ Community Mental Health Agencies and Related Services
◆ Challenges to Successful Implementation
◆ Conclusions

┌───┐
│   **A NURSING STUDENT SPEAKS**   │
└───┘

I recently gained fast ground with a client who was initially quite suspicious. When asked what he liked to do in his spare time, he said, "work on old cars." I took this cue to engage him in a lively discussion of 1950s and 1960s model cars (the cars that my brothers used to have and work on). I became an immediate hit when he learned that I knew what a '55 Chevy and a '69 T-Bird are. This information has never before been given in any nurse–client relationships and may never be used again, but it has won the trust of this client. And through this common ground, we have developed a connection and a springboard for dealing with his mental health issues. His doctors are delighted that since I have been working with him, he has, for the first time, been medication compliant for longer than 3 months.

—JANE ELWOOD, **University of Delaware**

HISTORICAL PERSPECTIVE

The earliest ancient civilizations attributed mental illness to possession by evil spirits or having divine or inspirational power. Later (BC) views of mental illness explained the condition as magical, caused by guilt, or created by excessive heat, cold, or moisture. Hippocratic physicians were the first to label symptoms of depression as melancholia caused by the accumulation of black bile.

Further views of mental illness in the Middle Ages included the idea of madness and demonic possession. Witches and midwives were seen as evil members of a dangerous class of sinful women. The overriding view of treatment was that of moral judgment, persecution, and degradation, with the mentally ill seen as social outcasts, living on the fringes of society in jails or poor houses. During the mid-1500s, St. Mary's of Bethlehem (Bedlam) was opened to house the insane. People were chained in rat-infested cells, where the public paid 1 penny to see the "loonies." Individuals suffering from mental illness were seen as incompetent and dangerous. They possessed no rights in society.

By the end of the 18th century, there was greater understanding of mental illness, and those who suffered from mental illness were being treated more humanely. Asylums were constructed where actual treatment protocols, however primitive, were in place. Far from anything like today, there remained great stigma, coercion, and degradation of people with mental illness. The first half of the 20th century saw the evolution of modern psychiatry, but with continued inhumane institutionalized care.

Two women in nursing known for their progressive awareness of mental illness are Linda Richards and Jane Taylor. Richards, who graduated in 1873, is designated as American's first trained nurse and is also honored as the first psychiatric nurse in the United States. Taylor was the first professor of psychiatric nursing at the Yale School of Nursing in 1926.

Not until the mid-1950s did the first **deinstitutionalization of the mentally ill** occur and a move to community-based mental health services. Unfortunately, many of the clients released from institutions were unprepared to live outside their institutions and were ill-served in the community. The deinstitutionalization caused increased stigma for mentally ill persons, but it also forced society to look at the needs of the mentally ill, who were no longer locked away, out of sight.

The 1950s and 1960s brought about other significant changes related to treatment of mental illness. Hildegard Peplau, RN, promoted the "therapeutic use of self" for nurses and brought forth the concept of "Milieu Therapy."

Medication development dramatically changed psychiatric care for the **seriously mentally ill** (SMI); in 1952, chlorpromazine (Thorazine), the first antipsychotic medication, was introduced. In 1960, haloperidol (Haldol) brought calm and order to the noisy and chaotic psychiatric wards. In 1962, the revolution of treatment of bipolar disorder occurred with the use of lithium. Currently, we are in the midst of yet another era of evolution of psychopharmacologic treatment. The neurotransmission theory has brought about major changes in the medication management of persons with depression and schizophrenia.

The 1970s brought third-party reimbursement for RNs who could bill for counseling services. Following this came prescriptive authority for mental health clinical nurse specialists.

Today, we continue to struggle with placement of our mentally ill, as well as with the **stigma of mental illness**. We still have hard questions to answer, such as these:

◆ Why are 90% percent of adults with SMI unemployed?
◆ What are the barriers that keep adults with mental illness from productive work and children with serious emotional disturbances from success in school?

Although there have been ad campaigns promoting the awareness of depression and schizophrenia, there remains much to do in terms of progress. The 1999 Surgeon General's report addresses these issues, and Healthy People 2010 further emphasizes mental illness as a major health focus (U.S. Department of Health and Human Services [DHHS], 1999). As nurses in the community at the beginning of the 21st century, we have the unique opportunity to address the mental health needs of our clients through promotion, advocacy, and education.

SIGNIFICANCE OF COMMUNITY MENTAL HEALTH

Historically in Western medicine, the mind and body have been treated as separate entities. It is over time that the mind–body connection has been made and mental and physical functioning are seen as parts of a whole. The U.S. Congress declared the 1990s the "Decade of the Brain," and DHHS published Healthy People 2010, declaring mental health among the top 10 leading indicators of health (DHHS, 2000). According to Healthy People 2010, in established market economies such as the United States, mental illness is equal to heart disease and cancer as a cause for disability. The National Institute of Mental Health (NIMH, 2007) and the Surgeon General (2001) report that mental disorders are common in the United States and internationally. The current estimate is that about 20 percent of the U.S. population is affected by mental disorders during a given year.

About 20% of children, as well, experience mental disorders. More severe functional limitations, known as "serious emotional disturbance" (SED), occur in 5–9% of children ages 9–17. The multitude of risk factors that contribute to mental illness, shown in Box 14-1, speak to the tremendous challenges in treatment and prevention that must be addressed.

◆ **B O X 14-1** Risk Factors That Contribute to
Mental Illness ◆

Emotional Factors

Self-Esteem—Many Factors Can Affect One's Self-Esteem and Impact Mental Health
- Developmental factors such as the changes that are experienced in adolescence, and middle and old age
- Relationships that are neglectful and/or abusive
- Body image, how one sees one's physical self (e.g., as in anorexia and bulimia)

General Mood
- Fluctuations in mood such as mania and depression—these are not willful, but are phenomena of mental illness
- Psychological stress
- Multiple unresolved losses

Attachment/Bonding Issues
- Research proves that lack of maternal or paternal attachment in infancy and childhood predisposes children to issues of abandonment.
- Child abuse and neglect

Biologic Factors

Neurobiologic and Genetic Factors
- Family history of mental illness
- Birth defects
- Low birth weight
- Language disabilities
- Below average intelligence

Physical Health Problems With Associated Mental Illness
- Diabetes/depression
- Heart disease/depression
- Chronic physical illness of any kind/depression

General Physical Conditions That Predispose to Mental Illness
- Traumatic injuries
- Prenatal damage due to diet, chemical abuse, or smoking
- Alcohol and drug abuse

Relationship/Role Model Factors
- Abuse/neglect
- Assault
- Manipulation
- Abandonment
- Severe family discord
- Overcrowding or large family size
- Paternal criminality
- Maternal mental illness
- Admission to foster care

(continued)

> ◆ **BOX 14-1**   Risk Factors That Contribute to
> Mental Illness (*Continued*) ◆

Support System Factors

- **Negative**—support systems that are a detriment to functioning
- **Lack of**—inability to develop relationships that are supportive in nature
- **Burn out**—due to the chronic nature of mental illness, families and friends may become exhausted in their ability to provide support. Lack of understanding of why the client can't just "get over it" leads to major frustration and ineffective treatment.

Environmental Factors

- **Climate and seasonal changes**—Seasonal Affective Disorder (SAD) is an example of a mental disorder that exists as a phenomenon of seasonal change.
- **Crime**—often mentally ill clients who are chemically dependent will resort to criminal activity such as stealing and prostitution as a means of gaining resources for survival. By virtue of their vulnerability, the mentally ill can also be easy victims of crime.
- **Stigma**—is an unjustifiable mark of shame as a result of misunderstandings and myths about mental illness. Stigma also arises from lack of knowledge about how mental illness occurs and how it can be treated.

Economic/Financial Factors

Economic stress

Poverty

Homelessness—The vast majority of people who are homeless are mentally ill, chemically dependent, or both. For some, the downhill slide into homelessness can in itself lead to symptoms of mental illness. There are numerous clients with bipolar illness and schizophrenia who find themselves homeless because of their mental illness as well as their drug/alcohol addiction used to self-medicate.

Social Factors

Racial and ethnic minorities are over-represented among the most vulnerable to be homeless, incarcerated, and have higher rates of mental disorders. Clinicians' inability to speak the language of the minority client and a lack of awareness of cultural issues of mental health in minority populations contribute to the social stigma of mental illness and fear and mistrust of treatment.

The cost of inpatient mental health treatment has also come to the forefront with a move away from high-cost, hospital-based treatment to, once again, community health management and treatment for mental illness. Health insurance and the economic challenges of payment for mental health services, while still lagging behind medical care coverage, is moving toward greater reimbursement of community mental health services. Today, in order to be hospitalized for mental health reasons, one has to be considered dangerous to one's self or others. All other mental health issues are now dealt with in the community.

The need for community mental health nurses continues to grow. A broad knowledge base and understanding of mental illness becomes the springboard for effective community-based mental health nursing.

NURSING SKILLS AND COMPETENCIES

Because of the pervasiveness of mental health issues, nurses working in all settings are called on to have skills and knowledge to work with individuals who have mental health issues. Clients with mental illness are seen in clinics, on every unit in hospitals, often in crisis at hospital emergency rooms, and everywhere in the community.

Knowledge of the major mental illnesses is important in understanding behavior and planning for intervention. A guideline for diagnosis and treatment of mental illness, published by the American Psychiatric Association, is the *Diagnostic and Statistical Manual of Mental Disorders (DSM-IV-TR)*. The manual classifies mental illnesses and provides diagnostic criteria for approximately 300 mental disorders. The diagnostic criteria for several of the major mental illness are listed along with general information relevant to quality nursing care.

As a community mental health nurse you will be called on to assess individuals in varied environments. There is the need to accurately assess and identify factors in the psychological, social, and physical environment that may contribute to mental health or illness. You will assess and make recommendations for continued care, for emergency care, and teach caretakers or family information about relevant mental illness issues as well as methods of dealing with psychiatric emergencies. In the nurse's holistic approach, other issues of need will be assessed. Such issues could be medical, social, or housing. Due to limited social support and family limitations or burn out, clients may need placement in the community.

In addition to the client and their caretakers, you may be called on to supervise, counsel, and teach paraprofessionals or other professional staff development information about mental health/illness.

A summary of several of the major diagnostic criteria with integration of nursing process information follows.

Mood Disorders

The mood disorders range from major depressive disorder to acute mania. The definitions used in relation to the mood disorders are as follows:

◆ Major depressive disorder: A major mood disorder with one or more episodes of major depression, with or without full recovery
◆ Dysthymic disorder: Depressed mood with loss of interest or pleasure in activities of daily life

Major Depression→ Dysthymia → Cyclothymia → Hypomania → Bipolar I → Bipolar II → Mania

FIGURE 14-1. ▶ The continuum of mood disorders.

◆ Cyclothymic disorder: A mood disorder of at least 2 years with numerous periods of mild depressive symptoms mixed with periods of hypomania
◆ Hypomania: Behaviors that are less than manic; a lesser degree of mania
◆ Bipolar I disorder: A major mood disorder characterized by episodes of major depression and mania (requires one or more episodes of mania or hypomania)
◆ Bipolar II disorder: A major mood disorder with the occurrence of one or more major depressive episodes with at least one episode of hypomania
◆ The continuum of mood disorders (see Fig. 14-1) further defines the dynamic nature of depression and mania.

Depression

Depression affects approximately 15 million Americans each year. The direct costs for mental health care for those suffering from depression are in the billions of dollars. Other factors to consider are the loss of productivity and the value of lost workdays. As nurses working with clients in a variety of settings, we need to look more closely for signs of depression in clients who present with physical symptoms, particularly chronic symptoms of all kinds, and those who have recently suffered major loss. We need to look at those clients who are chemically dependent and anyone with whom we come in contact who is feeling the effects of oppression or abuse. It is essential that the risk factors for depression (Box 14-2) are considered with each individual cared for, considering the pervasiveness of depression.

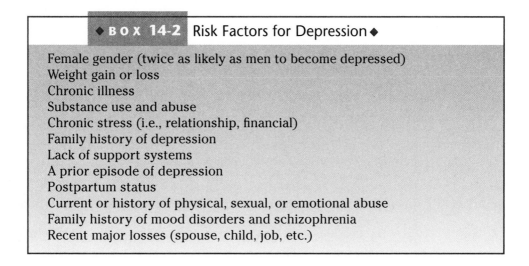

◆ B O X 14-2 Risk Factors for Depression ◆

Female gender (twice as likely as men to become depressed)
Weight gain or loss
Chronic illness
Substance use and abuse
Chronic stress (i.e., relationship, financial)
Family history of depression
Lack of support systems
A prior episode of depression
Postpartum status
Current or history of physical, sexual, or emotional abuse
Family history of mood disorders and schizophrenia
Recent major losses (spouse, child, job, etc.)

The word *depression* has a variety of definitions that can range from feelings of sadness and loss to the symptoms of major depression. The clinical definition of depression goes beyond sadness and seriously affects an individual's functioning and feelings about life and self. In addition, depression has a high rate of co-occurrence with other psychiatric disorders (anxiety disorder, substance-related disorders, eating disorders, and obsessive-compulsive disorder [OCD]), as well as with other general medical conditions such as stroke, diabetes, coronary artery disease, chronic fatigue syndrome, and a history of traumatic brain syndrome.

The major indicators of depression are summarized here and are also outlined in Assessment Tools 14-1. Behaviors include withdrawal, negativism, and unhappiness with self-deprecating; guilty or self-blaming comments; and expressions of hopelessness. The sense of hopelessness that one presents is a defining factor in clinical depression. There is decreased attentiveness to oneself, with decreased energy, an inability to concentrate, and excessive indecisiveness. Additional physical signs are changes in weight or eating patterns, changes in sleep patterns, and changes in sexual interest and activity.

Nursing interventions in depression include an ongoing assessment of behavioral symptoms related to self-care, medication compliance, general well-being, and suicidal thoughts or actions. The current outpatient treatments available for depression are antidepressant medications including the selective serotonin reuptake inhibitors (SSRIs), and electroconvulsive therapy (ECT), in conjunction with group or individual therapy. A new treatment modality approved by the U.S. Food and Drug Administration in July 2005 is vagus nerve stimulation (VNS). Originally used in the treatment of epilepsy, it is now considered for use in depression when medication trials are ineffective. The nurse should take into consideration a client's limited concentration and reaction time by waiting patiently for answers to questions. The nurse wants to provide positive feedback about a client's seeking help for depression or any improvements in the client's behavior. Try not to be overzealous, but rather calm and supportive. It may be appropriate to offer hope, particularly if you have an ongoing care-giving relationship with the individual, and to acknowledge that you understand the tremendous energy it takes when depressed to just get up in the morning or to get dressed.

Ongoing assessment of suicide is an important aspect of working with the depressed client. To be comfortable with suicide assessment, the nurse must

ASSESSMENT TOOLS 14-1

Assessing Behaviors in Major Depression

Individuals with depression may exhibit any or all of the following behaviors:
- A sense of hopelessness
- Depressed mood most of the time
- Loss of interest or pleasure in usual activities
- Changes in weight, either loss or gain
- Inability to concentrate, difficulty focusing or processing information
- Changes in sleep habits, either an increase or decrease in sleep
- Frequent thoughts of death and suicide, with or without a plan or attempt

address any misconceptions or fears he or she has about it. Suicidal thoughts or actions can occur at anytime in the course of depression. One important time in the course of treatment that is risky for suicidal clients is when they start on medications and begin to feel some energy. This energy can make them more vulnerable to the risk of acting on a suicidal plan. Awareness of the risk of suicide allows you to set up a safety net for the client during his or her most vulnerable time. The next section addresses further aspects of suicide.

Suicide

Suicide is a major public health issue. The NIMH identified suicide (in 2004) as the 11th leading cause of death in the United States. It is important to consider this information in terms of the risk factors for suicide. In addition, those who are at risk for suicide can suffer from any number of conditions. Persons who suffer from depression, schizophrenia, panic disorder, substance abuse, and chronic medical conditions may be at risk for suicide.

Signs to look for when assessing for suicide risk are recurrent thoughts of or preoccupation with death; ongoing suicidal ideation with or without a plan; a bleak, hopeless attitude toward life; or a sudden change from being depressed to being upbeat or "at peace," which may include preparations for "putting one's house in order." Other major factors are possession of means to commit suicide and a history of or recent suicide attempt.

Suicide is a very difficult and devastating type of death faced by family, friends, health care professionals, and society as a whole. For family and friends, there is overwhelming guilt for not having prevented it. For health care professionals, there can be sadness, guilt, and frustration for not seeing the signs.

As a nurse, the first aspect of suicide assessment that must be understood is that by asking someone if they are suicidal it does not give them the idea, and it does not make one any more likely to act on suicidal thoughts. In fact, the opposite is true. By asking, "Have you had or are you having thoughts of hurting yourself?" you are giving the client the opportunity to talk about it and ask for help if needed. You may also provide a great sense of relief in that someone is willing to talk about the guilt and sadness surrounding thoughts of suicide. If the client states that he or she has suicidal thoughts, the next question to ask is does he or she have a plan. If the client says he or she has a plan, you should ask about the plan, availability of the method, and lethality of the method. For example, a client who plans to shoot himself and owns a gun is at a high immediate risk compared to the client who tells you she wants to overdose but doesn't have the pills to do it. If the client presents with a lethal method and a means, immediate hospitalization may be necessary.

Less lethal means may require a contract for safety in which the client signs a document stating that he will not hurt himself, and if he feels like he will, he will have an alternative plan, such as someone to call or a place to go for help. Assessment Tools 14-2 lists guidelines for suicide assessment and includes questions to ask. Don't ever feel like you are alone in deciding what steps to take for suicidal behavior. The team approach in community mental health nursing means that you have other professionals whom you can call for consultation and support.

Mania

The primary symptoms you will observe in manic behavior are any degree of the following: a decreased need for sleep with increased motor activity or agitation, pressured speech, decreased appetite, grandiosity, and impulsivity and focus on

ASSESSMENT TOOLS 14-2

Suicide Assessment

General Questions

- Are you feeling like you want to hurt yourself?
- Are you feeling like ending it all?
- Do you have thoughts of wanting to end it all?
- Do you ever feel like it would be easier to not go on?
- Does this feel so overwhelming that you do not feel like living?

Specific Questions

If there is an answer of yes to any of the above, you want to assess frequency of thoughts and methods:

- How often do you feel this way?
- Have you had any thoughts about how you would end your life?
- What thoughts have you had about ending it all?
- When you feel this way, what do you feel like doing?

Assess Lethality

Assess how lethal the methods are and the availability of those methods. Lethality has to do with how easy it is to rescue someone as well as what access he or she has to the means.

Highly Lethal Methods	*Less Lethal Methods*
Gunshot	Driving into a tree
Jumping from a bridge	Taking pills
Hanging	Walking out into traffic

pleasurable activities, such as spending large amounts of money or promiscuous sexual behavior. The individual will exhibit a flight of ideas by jumping from one topic to another and will be easily irritated. The client may exhibit an inflated opinion of himself and a loss of normal inhibition. Because of the flight of ideas and impulsiveness, there is a lack of follow-through on meaningful activities. Psychoses may also develop in the form of delusions or hallucinations.

Nursing interventions include providing for safety from self-harm and balanced psychologic and physiologic functioning. The first-line treatment for mania is the use of **psychotropic medication**, including mood stabilizers or anticonvulsants and lithium.

Providing a safe environment with minimal stimulation is also critical. Persons with major manic behavior often need to be hospitalized because of exhaustion and the need to reinstate a treatment plan including medication compliance. Clients in the community who become manic can become extremely resistant to help because of their grandiose and expansive thinking. In addition, clients may be sexually inappropriate; they may speak so loudly and rapidly that it is impossible to get a word in, or they may be bordering on the brink of exhaustion. At any of these times, it will take a team approach that involves mental health professionals as well as other community persons who can collaborate to prevent both self-harm and harm to others. If the person is thought to be a danger to self or others, you may need to call in the police to assist with transport when hospitalization is needed.

Developing and maintaining a working relationship with professionals in the community becomes essential for a good and positive outcome. Recovery for persons with bipolar disorder requires acceptance of the illness and understanding that medication must not be stopped when a manic cycle begins and the client feels "on top of the world." This can be a lifelong learning process for individuals. Prevention of relapse is a primary goal as symptoms become worse and recovery more difficult with each successive relapse.

Anxiety Disorders

Anxiety is a normal, healthy aspect of living, alerting a person to take action in the face of danger. Someone who is experiencing mild to moderate levels of anxiety may use voluntary coping skills (getting information, avoiding situations, or seeking resources) that will decrease the anxiety (see Table 14-1). If, however, anxiety levels become unmanageable or the person lacks the coping skills to manage the anxiety, he or she may be at risk to develop any of the anxiety disorders.

Some of the more common anxiety disorders are generalized anxiety disorder, panic disorder (with or without agoraphobia), post-traumatic stress disorder (PTSD), and OCD.

Generalized Anxiety Disorder

Generalized anxiety disorder (GAD) affects about 3% to 4% of the U.S. population, and it primarily affects women. The person experiencing GAD is often on edge and easily fatigued. Chronic worry that causes one to experience irritability, muscle tension, and sleep disturbance is common. Persons with GAD are likely to present with physical symptoms and other disorders, such as major depression, panic disorder, and substance addictions. Clients do not always seek treatment, may not initially admit to feeling anxious, and may suffer for years until their physical symptoms cause them to seek medical attention. Clients with GAD may self-medicate with alcohol, other substances, or prescription medications.

Nursing interventions involve awareness of the behaviors that may indicate an underlying anxiety disorder. This means going beyond the physical symptoms, exploring a client's history, and focusing on the client's anxieties, fears, and

TABLE 14-1 Four Levels of Anxiety	
Level	**Client's Focus**
Mild—Increase in pulse, blood pressure, and heart rate	Alert, able to problem solve
Moderate—Muscle tension, sweating, increased pulse, blood pressure and breathing rate, peripheral vasoconstriction	Attention focused
Severe—"Fight or flight" responses, dry mouth	Detailed focus very narrow; no learning can occur
Panic—Continued increase in symptoms	Focus entirely on internal symptoms

concerns. Another aspect of effective nursing intervention in anxiety is awareness of the nurse's own reactions to the anxious client. Anxiety is contagious, and we can easily become excited and anxious, particularly when others are experiencing high levels of anxiety and panic. Awareness involves taking a deep breath and centering awareness on remaining calm. A nurse's ability to be calm and focused can, in itself, be the most effective nursing intervention offered.

Panic Disorder

The prevalence of panic disorder is about 1% to 2% of the U.S. population, with women being twice as likely to be diagnosed. Diagnosis of panic disorder may be difficult because of symptoms that mimic a variety of medical problems. These clients may present in a hospital emergency room with what they think is a heart attack, when in reality, it is a panic attack.

A panic attack usually lasts for only a short time (minutes) and begins suddenly with intense feelings of fear and impending doom. Symptoms can include shortness of breath, dizziness, palpitations, trembling, light-headedness, abdominal distress, numbness, chest tightness and pain, and a fear of going crazy. The individual can actually be fearful of dying. Panic attacks are time limited, usually reaching a peak within 10 minutes.

After recurrent attacks, there is a pervasive worry of having another and avoidance of the situations in which previous panic attacks occurred. In addition, a person may develop agoraphobia, which is the fear of being in places from which it might be difficult or embarrassing to escape. Common fears involve being in crowd; waiting in a line; or traveling in a car, bus, or plane. If untreated, panic disorder greatly reduces one's quality of life and ability to perform activities of daily living.

Nursing interventions with panic include first determining that it is indeed panic and not a heart attack as the client may believe it is. This will require assessing vital signs and calmly giving guidance and direction. The person in panic has no decision-making skills, as all energy is wrapped up in the fear and the symptoms. Calmly talking your client through the panic, knowing that it is time limited, and reassuring and validating what the client is experiencing are all effective interventions.

Those clients who experience panic and agoraphobia may require referral to mental health professionals to manage their symptoms.

Post-Traumatic Stress Disorder

The incidence of PTSD in the general population is about 7%, with 50% of high-risk populations experiencing PTSD. It occurs at all ages and may include symptoms of depression, chemical dependency, and anxiety.

A real and devastating event or events in one's life cause PTSD. Events that are beyond the individual's control, such as natural disasters; sexual abuse; the horrors of war; or being the witness of trauma, mutilation, or death, may cause PTSD. A primary feature of this disorder is that the person continues to re-experience the event by having recurrent, persistent, and frightening thoughts and memories of the experience.

The manner in which people relive their experiences is through nightmares, obsessive thoughts, or flashbacks that occur at random times. Fear and persistent arousal lead to sleep disturbances and hypervigilance, with exaggerated startle response that leads to difficulty concentrating and completing tasks. Symptoms of depression, feelings of emotional detachment and emotional numbness, anxiety, anger, sadness, and rage may also occur.

PTSD is treated with anti-anxiety and antidepressant medications. Psychotherapy and group therapy are needed for the individual to work through the experience and regain a sense of security. Recovery is variable, with some people recovering within 6 months. For others, it may take longer and for some, PTSD can become a chronic disorder.

Nursing interventions with PTSD require assessment to determine the magnitude of symptoms. Often referral to mental health professionals allows the client options such as medication and individual and/or group therapy.

Phobias

A phobia is a severe, persistent, and irrational fear of a specific object or situation. The person is generally aware that the fear is unreasonable, but he or she is unable to control it and will do everything he or she can do to avoid the situation or object that triggers the fear. The objects or situations that cause phobias include almost anything: animals, lightening, public speaking, and crowds, to name a few. Phobias generally start in childhood and early adulthood and affect approximately 13% of the population, making them the most common type of anxiety disorder.

Treatment includes the use of anti-anxiety medications and most often behavioral therapy in which the person is exposed to the feared object or experience and is taught to alter his or her responses.

Nursing intervention involves assessment of the disability caused by the phobia and appropriate referral for treatment along with management of day to day living.

Obsessive–Compulsive Disorder

Persons of all ages and both sexes (approximately 2% of the U.S. population) are affected by OCD. It is most often diagnosed during the teen years or young adulthood, with frequent co-occurrence of depression and panic attacks. In childhood, it may occur with other neurologic disorders.

OCD is characterized by preoccupation with recurrent, ritualistic thoughts or actions that the individual has difficulty controlling. Obsessions are persistent thoughts, impulses, or images that are intrusive and cause anxiety. Compulsions are the uncontrollable repetitive acts used to relieve the anxiety of the obsession. An example is having the obsession that your hands are always contaminated. The high level of anxiety about that contamination causes the compulsive act of hand washing. The person knows that the thoughts of contamination are irrational, and at the same time, he or she is afraid that they are true. Personal attempts to avoid the thought or the action as well as interruptions in the ritual lead to great anxiety.

CLIENT SITUATIONS IN PRACTICE

Hoarding, a form of OCD, may be something you experience in the community. Effie was a sweet, frail lady about age 80 who came to the community center for lunch nearly every day. She came to my attention by the staff due to the fact that every day she was observed not eating her food but rather asking for a container to put it in. During this process she would almost always ask for more food. For a time the staff was supplying her with about three containers of food, but when this continued almost daily, they became concerned. As the community mental health nurse, I was notified. In talking with Effie, she was pleasant and very noncommittal about what she did with her food. She would vaguely tell me that she was not hungry and was taking it back to her apartment. Getting nowhere with Effie, I approached the staff. It turns out that Effie has a friend she cares for in her apartment building who is unable to go outside. It also turns out that the staff has made visits to her apartment and, although she would not let them in, they were able to see that her home was packed high with paper and different articles so that there was only a narrow path through the rooms. My plan the next week was to make a home visit to Effie. Before I could make that visit, I was notified by the center staff that Effie had been hospitalized over the weekend with a broken hip. It was now my job to make sure that Effie gained a case manager to manage her situation. I made 3 visits to the hospital to see Effie, who, by the way, had every intention to go back to her apartment! I met with the hospital social worker and Effie's doctor. I learned that Effie's closest relatives are two nieces who live in another town. The hospital social worker learned that one of the nieces, just 2 years earlier, was called by Effie's landlord to clean out her apartment to prevent her eviction. To date, Effie is recovering from her hip surgery in an extended care center where she is finding the help and stimulation enjoyable. I met her niece at her apartment and it turned out that Effie had been saving much of the food she had received from the community center for some time. She had stacks of papers to the ceiling in most of her living room. Her kitchen table top and counters were covered with 2- to 3-foot stacks of rotting food. She did have a path from her bed to the bathroom. Interestingly, her bathtub was full of toiletries such has toothpaste, shampoo, lotions, some of them samples, many of them purchased, none of them opened or used.

The Plan: Effie's niece has made arrangements to get the apartment emptied and cleaned. Effie will not be able to move back there, as the money she has will go toward her living at the care center. I have talked with the social worker from the center and she reports that Effie has now begun to engage in activities at the center; she particularly loves bingo and the sing alongs! They have to watch her at the meal table; she often takes food from the table and from time to time takes it from others.

Because Effie does not appear affected by the removal of her food from her room by the staff and the fact that she is directable at the table, no medication for OCD is given.

Effie suffers from OCD in the type of Hoarding. She compulsively needed to collect certain things and was unable to throw anything away. This situation precipitated a real public health concern. In this case, exterminators were called in to deal with the insect and rodent issues that existed in Effie's apartment.

The antidepressant medications clomipramine and fluoxetine have been most effective in the treatment of OCD. Behavioral and family therapy tend to be the most effective modes of nonpharmacologic treatment.

One aspect of nursing care to remember when working with persons with OCD is to never interrupt their compulsions. Telling them to stop or in any way interfere with the compulsive behavior causes greater anxiety and distress. Let them complete what they are doing and then interact. In cases in which daily living is significantly affected, appropriate referral for behavioral or medication treatment is essential.

Schizophrenia

Schizophrenia is a thought disorder that is characterized by a disturbance in how one thinks, feels, and relates to others and the environment. This disorder affects 2 million people in the United States and remains one of the least understood and least accepted of the mental illnesses. It is now known that schizophrenia is a neurobiological disorder of the brain. This knowledge has led to major advances in the treatment of schizophrenia. Newer antipsychotic medications offer individuals treatment with fewer side effects, which contributes to better compliance and treatment outcomes. The DSM–IV–TR diagnostic guidelines for schizophrenia identify nine categories of illness: schizophrenia, schizophreniform disorder, schizoaffective disorder, delusional disorder, brief psychotic disorder, shared psychotic disorder, psychotic disorder due to a general medical condition, substance-induced psychotic disorder, and psychotic disorder not otherwise specified.

The positive symptoms of this illness are any variety of the following: delusions, hallucinations, disorganized speech, and disorganized or catatonic behavior. The negative symptoms of this illness are flat affect, lack of drive to perform, and lack of interest or ability for follow-through. Social and occupational dysfunctions are caused by positive or negative symptoms. Depending on the degree of functioning of the client, community management of the client can involve many facets.

Medication management is a priority, as are housing and economic management. Health issues and safety concerns may need to be addressed in relation to issues of paranoid or delusional thinking, hallucinations, lack of self-care, and vulnerability. Community-Based Nursing Care Guidelines 14-1 outlines nursing interventions specific to schizophrenia.

COMMUNITY-BASED NURSING CARE GUIDELINES ▶ 14-1

Nursing Interventions Specific to Schizophrenia

Clients with schizophrenia may exhibit unusual or bizarre behaviors; they may have very limited communication; and they may demonstrate altered thinking. These behaviors may make developing a therapeutic relationship particularly challenging.

Interventions for Developing a Relationship

Approach in a calm, genuine, and accepting manner

- Spend short periods of time with the client, even if they interact very little.
- Demonstrate interest and concern for how the client perceives their illness.
- Speak clearly and distinctly with short sentences and with one thought per sentence.
- Encourage the client to identify and discuss feelings and concerns.

Ongoing Assessment Factors to Observe

- Disturbance in the client's thought processes including the presence of hallucinations or delusional thinking
- Response and adherence with medication regimen as well as assessment of side effects from medications
- Behavioral changes in hygiene, isolation or withdrawal, and lack of motivation
- Suicide assessment

CLIENT SITUATIONS IN PRACTICE

◆ Assessing the Mentally Ill Patient

Mary Smith is a 29-year-old woman who has never been married. The history she provides is somewhat vague; however, she says that she comes from the West and that her family is very dysfunctional. She makes several references to rape and her crazy family, but there are no further details offered.

She says that she was diagnosed as bipolar when she was a teenager. Mary was taking lithium for several years, but how long she took it and how much are unclear. She dropped out of school when she was a junior because she says that the voices she was hearing in her head made it too hard to concentrate on her studies. She was diagnosed with schizophrenia and was prescribed Haldol. She took the Haldol for awhile, but because she didn't like the side effects, she was off medications for most of her 20s.

She has seen a doctor in the last month and is currently taking 200 mg of quetiapine fumarate (Seroquel). She recently became homeless for a time, but then she was able to find an apartment. I first met Mary in a group for the homeless at our clinic.

What Further Information Would You Pursue?

The issue of being raped would be an important one to consider in terms of when and what degree of assault. The diagnosis of schizophrenia and bipolar disorder would lead to questions about hallucinations or delusions and mood swings, as well as her level of functioning.

What Symptoms Is She Having and to What Degree Are They Affecting Her?

It would also be important to assess her use of her medication Seroquel. Is she taking it as prescribed? Is she having any side effects? Does she feel it is helping?

On my first community visit to Mary, I found her living in a relatively safe part of the city, in a secure building. Her room was on the top floor, which meant a four-flight walk. Her apartment was a room, about 8 × 10 feet, with a small closet with no door. She had a sink, stove, and refrigerator and two large windows that faced another building about 5 feet away. Mary had many drawings hung on the walls, and she had also painted her windows. She was pleasant and friendly. Mary was dressed in a tee shirt that did not cover her protruding stomach and blue plaid pants. She proceeded to talk about all the things she was planning to tell me and in doing so became disorganized, moving from topic to topic: "I feel great. I'm having a good day. Do you suppose we could get some milk? Could you pray for me? I am joining that rape support group, you know. My refrigerator is working good, and I have bread."

I asked Mary, "Is there any man trying to hurt you now? Are you afraid?" Mary replied, "No, oh, no, I am not dating. There is a nice man down the hall; he helped take out my garbage the other day. How do you like my apartment, isn't it nice? I really want to stay here . . . ."

What Are the Major Safety Issues for Mary?

Mary is proud of having her own apartment, meager as it is. She displays disorganized thinking. The biggest concern is for Mary's vulnerability because she is pleasant and friendly and talks to anyone. Although she appears to have been the victim of sexual assault in the past, her state of mental health does not protect her from sexual assault in the future.

What Behavior Would You Reinforce?

We decided to take a walk to a nearby grocery store. On our walk back to her apartment, I encouraged Mary to be sure to take her medicine as prescribed and to see me again in 3 days.

What Steps Would You Take?

Because my visit was on a Friday, I left the crisis line phone number with Mary in case she needed someone over the weekend. On Monday morning, I phoned a service called Early Intervention to get Mary a mental health case manager. I will also make referrals for Mary for day treatment and social programs where she can interact with others safely. After letting her psychiatrist know of my concerns, we arranged for an appointment with Mary and her psychiatrist to reevaluate her medication. My biggest concern for Mary is her vulnerability and her safety.

Personality Disorders

There are several types of personality disorder: borderline personality disorder, dependent personality disorder, narcissistic personality disorder, and sociopathic personality disorder. One of the most prevalent types of personality disorder seen in the community and talked about here is borderline personality disorder.

Borderline personality disorder is manifested by highly manipulative actions that an individual uses to get his or her needs met. Frequent eruptions of anger are common when expectations are not realized. The client has strong underlying fears of abandonment and exhibits concrete thinking, with all things categorized as being right or wrong, good or bad.

Borderline personality disorder, as with all personality disorders, often becomes evident by the emotions evoked by the client's behaviors. If you are experiencing a strong emotional reaction to a client, feeling angry, frustrated, or agitated, you are possibly dealing with someone with borderline characteristics. Assessment Tools 14-3 outlines the behaviors.

ASSESSMENT TOOLS 14-3

Assessment Criteria for Borderline Personality Disorder

- Highly manipulative actions used to get needs met, with frequent eruptions of anger when expectations are not realized
- Repeated feelings of boredom and emptiness that lead to the seeking out of repeated intense and chaotic interpersonal relationships
- Extremes in emotional reactivity; major mood swings that change from minute to minute, hour to hour, or day to day
- Impulsive behavior that is often self-damaging including cutting, burning, excessive sexual encounters, or binge drinking
- Chronic suicidal behavior such as threats with or without actions and self-mutilating behaviors such as cutting and burning areas of the body

There is a term called "**staff splitting**" that involves the manipulative behaviors of clients with borderline personality disorder. It occurs when a client with borderline personality disorder pits staff members against each other. An example of this is when a client tells you what a horrible thing another staff member did to him or her, or that you are the only person in the whole world who understands him or her because you are the best nurse to ever live. Secretive feelings about a client, feelings like you are the only one who understands him or her, or staff conflict over how to treat a client are examples of the effects of manipulation by a client with borderline personality disorder. When these issues arise, it is necessary to take a team approach to problem solving. The team's responsibility is that of processing the issues and then planning a cohesive approach to care that involves clear boundaries: which nurse does what, when, and how.

A major safety issue may be the establishment of the behavioral contract. This is a verbal or written agreement between you the caregiver and the individual experiencing self-harming behavior. The contract is most often a written document that can be put in the chart to verify that both you and the client agree on a plan for safety. See Community-Based Nursing Care Guidelines 14-2 for a summary of nursing interventions and Box 14-3 for guidelines in writing a behavioral contract.

Eating Disorders

Anorexia nervosa and bulimia nervosa have been primarily associated with White women in the middle to upper socioeconomic groups in industrialized countries, with typical onset between the ages of 12 and 22. Young men with eating disorders, while less common, do exist.

The development of eating disorders is believed to have its psychologic base in issues of coping, self-esteem, and perfectionism. The major problem is not with

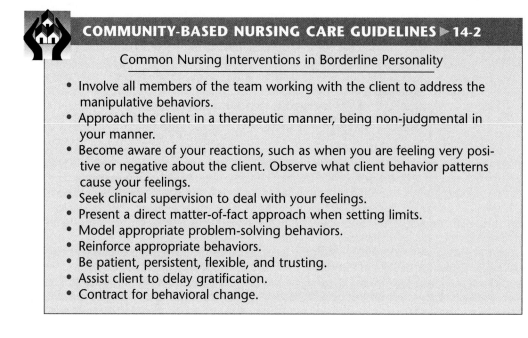

COMMUNITY-BASED NURSING CARE GUIDELINES ▶ 14-2

Common Nursing Interventions in Borderline Personality

- Involve all members of the team working with the client to address the manipulative behaviors.
- Approach the client in a therapeutic manner, being non-judgmental in your manner.
- Become aware of your reactions, such as when you are feeling very positive or negative about the client. Observe what client behavior patterns cause your feelings.
- Seek clinical supervision to deal with your feelings.
- Present a direct matter-of-fact approach when setting limits.
- Model appropriate problem-solving behaviors.
- Reinforce appropriate behaviors.
- Be patient, persistent, flexible, and trusting.
- Assist client to delay gratification.
- Contract for behavioral change.

◆ **BOX 14-3** The Client Contract ◆

The client contract is usually a written contract. It is a way of helping the client be accountable for his or her behaviors, particularly in the area of safety.

Contract for Safety

1. When I (the client) feel disturbed, I will go to a friend or family's house where I can air my (intense) feelings.
2. I will call the Crisis Center if I can't stop thinking about harming myself.
3. While I'm receiving care, I will refrain from using verbal or physical threats.
4. When I feel like lashing out, I will try to identify other ways to cope, such as
   a. Removing myself from a conflicting situation by going to another room or taking a walk away from the area.
   b. Stepping back and counting to 5 very slowly.

Signed _____
                Client

Signed _____
                Nurse

---

food but rather with issues of self-esteem, control, management of intimate relationships, and developmental expectations. The degree of regulation and use of food are expressions of the individual's difficulty in managing these issues. By focusing on food, the person's time is consumed, so that making decisions and facing the challenges and issues of life can be avoided.

Anorexia Nervosa

The anorexic client presents with poor self-image, eagerness to please, concrete all-or-none thinking, and extreme perfectionism. As the anorexic loses weight, her fear of fatness increases and she loses her ability to read her body's signals.

The primary goal of treatment for anorexia nervosa is to restore the anorexic to their normal weight. Nutritional rehabilitation, psychosocial intervention, and medication management with use of the SSRIs, a class of antidepressants, are most often employed with eating disorders in both inpatient and outpatient settings. The family dynamic is an important consideration due to the fact that alcohol or substance abuse, rape, incest, verbal abuse, and neglect are common issues of people with eating disorders.

Nursing interventions revolve around developing a therapeutic relationship that allows for disclosure of the eating disorder and support for ongoing treatment. There are both inpatient and outpatient eating disorder programs. Another intervention strategy is that of obtaining information and referral resources for the client and family and supporting their efforts toward recovery.

Bulimia Nervosa

People with bulimia tend to be of normal weight and engage in the binge–purge cycle. Bulimic clients are often tense and anxious before bingeing. During bingeing, bulimics feel a temporary sense of relief. Shortly after bingeing, the anxiety begins to mount, and the urge to purge occurs. Purging behavior most often involves vomiting, with a release of tension and a pervasive sense of relief.

The primary goal of treatment for bulimia is to reduce or eliminate binge eating and purging behaviors. As with anorexia nervosa, nutritional rehabilitation and psychosocial interventions are effective.

Substance Abuse

The economic costs to society of substance abuse costs billions per year. This number includes alcohol and drug-related loss of productivity as well as alcohol and drug-related crime. The cost to the individual who is addicted and family members, friends, and society as a whole is both devastating and immeasurable. When a person becomes addicted, emotional and maturational growth becomes limited. All actions of the addicted individual are focused on the drug of choice: how to get it, when to use it, how to get more of it. Substance abusers may lose all moral and legal judgment, engaging in behaviors of stealing, prostitution, and selling of drugs.

Three major unconscious psychologic defenses are used by persons who are addicted: denial, rationalization, and projection. Denial is the addicted person's insistence that he or she does not have a problem despite concrete evidence to the contrary. Contrary evidence such as driving under the influence (DUI) arrests, missed days of work or school, and obvious concerns of others are ignored and denied. Rationalization is a means of justifying one's addictive behavior. An example is the statement that "I am not an alcoholic or cocaine addict because I only use on weekends." Projection is the blaming of external forces, such as a nagging spouse, stressful job, or impossible boss, as a reason to use and abuse substances. These defenses affect the addicted individual, those who are part of the individual's family and social system, as well as society as a whole. As health care professionals, we must not be afraid to recognize and confront the use of these defenses and educate the individual struggling with substance abuse, as well as the family members about their importance in the dynamics of substance abuse.

Nurses need to be aware of the signs and symptoms of drug and alcohol use and abuse. Addicted persons present in every setting in health care and may present with intoxication or withdrawal at any time. Drug and alcohol withdrawal may lead to a medical emergency in some cases. See Box 14-4 for signs and symptoms of drug and alcohol intoxication and withdrawal.

The symptoms of substance disorders include the consistent use of alcohol or other mood-altering drugs until the client is high or intoxicated, or he or she has passed out. There is the inability to stop or cut down use, despite wishes to do so or negative consequences from use. There is denial that substance use is a problem despite feedback from significant others stating that the abuse is negatively affecting them. The abuse continues despite recurrent and persistent issues with physical, legal, vocational, social, or relationship problems directly related to the chemical use. Addicted individuals also consume a substance in greater amounts and for longer periods than intended.

◆ B O X 14-4 Symptoms of Drug and Alcohol Intoxication and Withdrawal ◆

All conditions of drug and alcohol intoxication and withdrawal present a medical emergency and may require hospitalization.

- Alcohol Intoxication: impaired judgment, slurred speech, double vision, dizziness, volatile emotional changes, stupor, and unconsciousness
  Alcohol Withdrawal: anxiety, insomnia, tremors, and delirium tremors (DTs), which include confusion and convulsions (a hospital emergency)
- Sedative-Hypnotic and Anxiolytic Intoxication: slurred speech; slow, shallow respirations; cold, clammy skin; weak, rapid pulse; drowsiness and disorientation
  Sedative-Hypnotic and Anxiolytic Withdrawal: anxiety, insomnia, tremors and convulsions that may occur up to 2 weeks after stopping use
- Opioid Intoxication: sedation, hypertension, respiratory depression, impaired function, constipation, and constricted pupils with watery eyes and hypertension
  Opioid Withdrawal: restlessness, irritability, panic, chills, sweating, cramps, watery eyes with dilated pupils, nausea, and vomiting
- Cocaine Intoxication: irritability, anxiety, hyperactivity, hypervigilance, slow and weak pulse, shallow breathing, sweating, and dilated pupils
  Cocaine Withdrawal: agitation, depression, and suicidal ideation; usually requires hospitalization
- Amphetamine Intoxication: agitation, hyperactivity, and paranoia, dilated pupils, headache, and chills
  Amphetamine Withdrawal: prolonged periods of sleep, disorientation, and major depression
- Hallucinogen Intoxication: bizarre behavior with mood swings and paranoia, nausea and vomiting, tremors, and panic with aggression; and possibly flushing, fever, and sweating
  Hallucinogen Withdrawal: depression, irritability, and restlessness

---

Treatment

Recovery and abstinence from drug or alcohol addiction is a lifelong process that requires changes in one's life. Old routines that activate drug use and alcoholic behaviors have to be replaced with new and productive patterns of coping. Without the use of the substance, individuals must confront long-standing anger, resentments, and unresolved grief. Changing friends, where one lives, and with whom one socializes are all aspects of the challenges of recovery. Resources for recovery tend to be highly structured, with an emphasis on self-awareness, limit setting, group therapy, skill development, and family treatment. They may include behavioral and family therapy and various group therapy options, such as involvement in a social skills group; loss and grief group; developing-structured-support

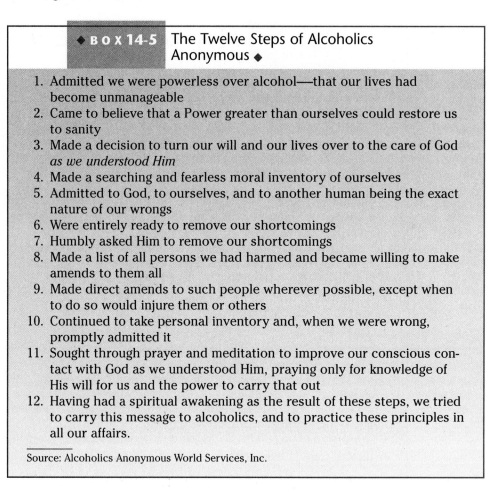

◆ B O X 14-5   The Twelve Steps of Alcoholics Anonymous ◆

1. Admitted we were powerless over alcohol—that our lives had become unmanageable
2. Came to believe that a Power greater than ourselves could restore us to sanity
3. Made a decision to turn our will and our lives over to the care of God *as we understood Him*
4. Made a searching and fearless moral inventory of ourselves
5. Admitted to God, to ourselves, and to another human being the exact nature of our wrongs
6. Were entirely ready to remove our shortcomings
7. Humbly asked Him to remove our shortcomings
8. Made a list of all persons we had harmed and became willing to make amends to them all
9. Made direct amends to such people wherever possible, except when to do so would injure them or others
10. Continued to take personal inventory and, when we were wrong, promptly admitted it
11. Sought through prayer and meditation to improve our conscious contact with God as we understood Him, praying only for knowledge of His will for us and the power to carry that out
12. Having had a spiritual awakening as the result of these steps, we tried to carry this message to alcoholics, and to practice these principles in all our affairs.

Source: Alcoholics Anonymous World Services, Inc.

group; mental illness/chemical dependency (MI/CD) group, for those with a dual diagnosis; and self-help groups. Self-help groups such as Alcoholics Anonymous (AA), Cocaine Anonymous, and Narcotics Anonymous use a 12-step program to help the addict develop a different lifestyle and lend support to those in recovery. Box 14-5 lists the 12 steps of AA, providing a road map for recovery and a life of abstinence.

MENTAL HEALTH ASSESSMENT

Establishing a framework for mental health assessment is a vital component of working with clients who are at risk. It can be particularly challenging to gather information from a client whose thought processes and communication skills are impaired. You will be called on to be creative and sensitive in your approach. Utilizing a framework such as the one outlined in Assessment Tools 14-4 can help you stay focused and aware of the basic information that is important to assess.

ASSESSMENT TOOLS 14-4

Framework for Mental Health Assessment

Client Description and Current Life Situation

Name, age, sex, race, marital status, current employment/means of financial support, current living situation

Sources of Information

Client, family, friends, health care worker, other associates

Presenting Problem

The major issue/s affecting the client at this time

Current Functioning

Mental status including appearance and self-care, attention, concentration, orientation, relating through eye contact and facial expression, thought content, delusions, hallucinations, preoccupations
Ability to have insight and judgment
Stressors, coping ability, and supports

History Including Mental Health History

Developmental, familial, and social history
Issues of trauma, losses, and abuse

Physical Health

Current health and significant health history

Current Medications

Psychotropic and other medications; known drug allergies; use of alternative substances

Chemical Health

Current use, history of use, history of chemical dependency treatment, family history

Establishing the Therapeutic Relationship

As a community health nurse, your major goal is the establishment and maintenance of the therapeutic relationship. In hospital and clinic nursing, we may see clients for one or more 8-hour shifts over a week's time, or for a 15-minute clinic visit. As a community health nurse, you may see the client for 1-hour visits, but you may see this client over time for 6 months, a year, or even longer. By being in the community, we have the unique pleasure of meeting the client on his or her turf, which can offer us a much more holistic view of our clients. Two concepts that are vital to this process are partnership and connection.

Partnership means collaborating, mutual relating, and relationship building with the client to effect the best outcome for him or her. To do so, the nurse needs to connect with his or her clients in a trusting, nonjudgmental, and nonconfrontational manner. **Professional relatedness** involves understanding, mutual relating, self-awareness, reliability, and respect for privacy.

The process of understanding involves avoiding imposing one's own will on a client and being open to the client's experience, such as what makes him or her happy, sad, scared, or anxious. Nurses should consider how life is for their clients, what impact their environments have on them, and what relationships they have. What do they care about, and what is their source of joy, fun, and peace? This process of understanding involves the professional responsibility of educating oneself to the culture of those with whom you relate. Culture as we first consider it may involve one's ethnic origin. Chapter 3 provides information on the topic of culture. It also may be important to learn about the **culture of poverty** as many of our clients may be in poverty. See Box 14-6 for additional information on the culture of poverty.

Self-awareness involves being aware of what one does not know, as well as being aware of oneself. Part of making assumptions is the process of not knowing or being aware. By making assumptions, we block reality and awareness, thinking that we know what our clients need and want without asking them. In terms of oneself, we need to be aware of our personal language and expression. Professional self-awareness is the act of self-reflection, as well as the humble act of being open to learning, to the environment, and to the impact that we as professionals have on our clients.

Mutual relating means being flexible and open in our approach, being honest, relating on the client's level, having a sense of humor, and using self-disclosure appropriately. This does not mean disclosing private and personal information, but rather, it involves sharing common ground such as hobbies or interests.

CLIENT SITUATIONS IN PRACTICE

◆ Developing a Trusting Nurse–Client Relationship

I was working with Dottie, who was very quiet and was considered "treatment resistant" by our team. Dottie had been a resident of the local homeless shelter for more than a year, but until recently, no one really knew anything about her. Dottie would come and go and did not engage in any outreach efforts. Being the new kid on the block, I was appointed to try to see what I could do to connect with her. After a couple of meetings with Dottie, I learned that she liked to knit, but she had always wanted to crochet and had never learned. I asked her if she would mind if I brought a crochet hook and some yarn to our next meeting, and she said that would be fine. I taught her how to crochet, and in the period of several weeks, we talked and she opened up to tell me about the tragic loss of three of her family members to a man who robbed their home when she was 15, the physical and sexual abuse that she endured in her first marriage, and the loss of her grandmother, who was her main support and friend.

◆ **B O X 14-6** Culture of Poverty ◆

It is essential to understand ethnic origins as well as class origins. Because so many of our mentally ill clients live in poverty, it becomes essential to understand the culture of poverty. Many nurses who serve mentally ill clients come from middle-class backgrounds and may have difficulty understanding why their clients act the way they do. There are norms within the three economic classes: wealthy, middle class, and poor. We need to understand our origins and expectations as a basis for understanding the different classes.

Social Values of the Wealthy

Political connections
Investment of money
Prestige

Social Values of the Middle Class

Work/getting ahead
Order/cleanliness
Responsibility

Social Values of the Poor

Survival/making it day to day
Relationships

Characteristics of Poverty

Jobs are about getting enough money to survive, not about climbing a career ladder
Academic achievement is not prized
Belief that fate and destiny exist over the consideration of choice
Polarized, concrete thinking where options are not considered and everything is right or wrong, black or white
Time orientation is on the present, with the focus on now
Little or no consideration of future consequences

Implications for Nurses

It becomes our ethical responsibility to not judge others based on our social values. We must educate ourselves and learn the values of the people with whom we serve. The following example illustrates this point:

When your client spends all her money the day she receives it with no consideration for the month's rent due in 2 weeks (present time orientation), has a messy disorganized home that is noisy (part of the chaos of crisis living), continually makes excuses for her children's misbehavior (because maintaining a relationship with her son is most important, and

(continued)

> ◆ **BOX 14-6** Culture of Poverty *(Continued)* ◆
>
> who knows better than she about her son's behavior), you will under-
> stand that she is operating out of the values of her class. And you will
> become aware of your middle-class values that are in direct conflict,
> because it is out of the question to not save your money to pay rent
> (responsibility with future orientation), your apartment is most often
> clean, organized, and quiet (order and cleanliness values), and you always
> hold your children accountable for their misbehavior (Who's responsible?
> Holding son accountable).
>
> ───────
>
> Adapted from Payne, R. K., DeVol, P., & Smith, T. D. (2001). *Bridges out of poverty: Strategies
> for professionals and communities.* Highlands, TX: aha! Process, Inc.

COMMUNITY MENTAL HEALTH AGENCIES AND RELATED SERVICES

Community support services are public and privately funded resources to assist
persons who are **seriously and persistently mentally ill (SPMI)** and SMI. The
resources promote mental health, prevent mental illness, and serve the needs of
the mentally ill. Some of the services provided include crisis intervention, mental
health treatment, case management, advocacy, and supportive services for living
and working. Three areas of support, including community mental health agencies, housing, and human needs support, are discussed here.

Community mental health agencies are funded primarily through public dollars
and offer a variety of services. As a community mental health nurse, you may be
employed by one of these agencies and refer any variety of services to your
clients. If you are not connected to an agency through employment, it is important
that you learn what community mental health agencies exist, what services they
offer, and how they can best serve your clients. Some of the following services are
offered through community mental health agencies:

- ◆ Individual psychotherapy
- ◆ Group therapy
- ◆ Mental health assessment, diagnosis, and treatment
- ◆ Chemical health assessment, diagnosis, and treatment
- ◆ Medication management
- ◆ Vulnerable adult protection

Housing

Housing options can be battered women's shelters, homeless shelters, halfway
houses, transitional housing, and supportive housing. Shelters for battered
women offer safety to women and their children who are in abusive living situations. These shelters offer services to both mothers and their children, including
school transportation and case management for women seeking safe housing.
Homeless shelters are of two kinds: overnight shelters with check-in from 5:00 to

8:00 PM and checkout by 7:00 AM, to 24-hour shelters where people can stay in during the day. Halfway houses and transitional housing are both temporary housing but are generally longer-term living situations than shelters for persons who are not ready to live independently. Supportive housing is long-term housing that offers intensive case management to clients who are unable to live independently. This type of housing is ideal for persons with chronic mental illness who are unable to live independently or with family support. The greatest difficulty with housing services is the acute shortage of supportive housing options available for people with mental illness.

Human Needs Support

Human support services for the mentally ill include self-help groups, community drop-in centers, clothes closets, food shelves, services to immigrants and victims of abuse and crime, legal assistance, job training and placement, education programs, advocacy programs, and programs for ex-offenders. It is your responsibility when working with mentally ill clients in the community to become knowledgeable of the resources offered in your community. Once you know the resources, you are able to refer clients when appropriate as well as knowing when you need to go outside of your community to get what is needed. More than likely, you will experience frustration with lack of services; this can be your opportunity to work to effect political awareness and change.

CHALLENGES TO SUCCESSFUL IMPLEMENTATION

The decade of the 1990s brought with it both federal and state resources that focused on the study of the brain in terms of the development and implementation of magnetic resonance imaging (MRI), positron-emission tomography (PET), and computed tomography (CT). These technologies have contributed to the understanding and validation of mental illness, but there is more to be done.

As is outlined in the Healthy People 2010, which lists objectives for mental health, the over-riding goal is to improve mental health and ensure access to appropriate, quality mental health services (DHHS, 2000). The 14 objectives developed to accomplish this goal by 2010 are found in Healthy People 2010 14-1.

The Healthy People 2010 objectives for mental health clearly speak to the major mental health issues facing life in the United States at this time. We as professional nurses need to advocate for mental health legislation that promotes the well-being of our clients. Affordable housing as well as structured housing options for our clients is a must. Insurance coverage for mental health services and manageable co-pays for medications are all-important issues.

Another issue is that the independent nature of community mental health nursing is not for every nurse. The fears of being out in the community, outside the constraints of a hospital or clinic, can be frightening. The individuals with whom we work can live in areas of poverty where it is not always safe. Those with mental illness and/or chemical dependency issues can pose major challenges to compassion and understanding.

Another major challenge to community mental health nursing can be the lack of facilities for referrals, decreases in funding with cuts in services, and heavy caseloads. There is also a need for teamwork and trust among team members that, if missing, makes this work very, very difficult.

▶ **HEALTHY PEOPLE 2010 ▶ 14-1**

Objectives for Mental Health

MENTAL HEALTH STATUS IMPROVEMENT
1. Reduce the suicide rate.
2. Reduce the rate of suicide attempts by adolescents.
3. Reduce the proportion of homeless adults who have serious mental illness.
4. Increase the proportion of persons with serious mental illnesses who are employed.
5. Reduce the relapse rates for persons with eating disorders, including anorexia nervosa and bulimia nervosa.
6. Increase the number of persons seen in primary health care who receive mental health screening and assessment.
7. Increase the proportion of children with mental health problems who receive treatment.
8. Increase the proportion of juvenile justice facilities that screen new admissions for mental health problems.
9. Increase the proportion of adults with mental disorders who receive treatment.
10. Increase the proportion of persons with co-occurring substance abuse and mental disorders who receive treatment for both disorders.
11. Increase the proportion of local governments with community-based jail diversion programs for adults with serious mental illnesses.

STATE ACTIVITIES
12. Increase the number of states and the District of Columbia that track consumer satisfaction with the mental health services they receive.
13. Increase the number of states, territories, and the District of Columbia with an operational mental health plan that addresses cultural competence.
14. Increase the number of states, territories, and the District of Columbia with an operational mental health plan that addresses mental health crisis interventions, ongoing screening, and treatment services for elderly persons.

Source: Healthy People 2010: Mental Health and Mental Disorders. Partners in Information Access for the Public Workforce, 2006. From: http://phpartners.orghp/mentalhealthand mentaldisorders.html.

Despite the multitude of obstacles facing community mental health nursing today, there is no more exciting area in which to work. The federal government is setting mental health as one of its priorities, and the 21st century has once again brought deinstitutionalization to the forefront, moving the mentally ill back into the community.

A new and exciting concept that community mental health nurses are experiencing is telehealth, also referred to as e-health, telemedicine, telecare, and telehomecare (Tschirch, 2006). This is defined as an integrated system that involves health care activities being carried out at a distance, where communication in person is not feasible. This concept involves interactive video teleconferencing with use of monitors and a dedicated telephone line to transmit images and sound between client and nurse. This technology lends itself nicely to mental health applications that emphasize communication and observation. Such innovations make possible outreach to clients who otherwise may not be served.

CLIENT SITUATIONS IN PRACTICE

John, who lives out of the city, 2 hours away, has limited resources and is unable to get into our clinic regularly. He does get to his local drop-in center three times each week. It is there that he is able to sign on to the computer and have an interactive talk with his nurse in the city. She is able to assess and observe how he is doing as well as monitor medications and conduct a therapy session if necessary. This interactive process brings mental health services out to more remote areas and in this case, John is able to access more comprehensive services.

This is both an exciting and challenging time for community mental health nursing as more people are served in the community. We as nurses are better able to know these clients holistically and within the context of their lives and their stories.

CONCLUSIONS

The evolution of mental health care has exploded in the last 2 decades. Understanding the origins of mental illness has contributed to major breakthroughs in medication management and treatment. These advances have also helped to eliminate some of the myths about mental illness. Essential to good care are strong communication skills that allow for flexibility and acceptance of a variety of behaviors. The magnitude of mental illness lends itself to assessment in every setting where a nurse is employed. As nurses, we must be able to look beyond the physical issues and consider our clients' stories and how they are coping. The gift of relationship is what community mental health nursing is all about. Being in a relationship with our clients, their families, and other mental health professionals, we are able to collaborate and achieve the best possible outcome for our client's mental health.

What's on the Web

The American Psychological Association (APA)
Internet address: http://apa.org
This professional and scientific organization for the practice of psychology has several brochures and fact sheets for consumers and health professionals. Write or call APA Public Affairs, 750 First Street, NE, Washington, DC 20002–4242; (800) 374-2721.

The National Alliance for the Mentally Ill (NAMI)
Internet address: http://www.nami.org
This site has a medical information series that provides clients and families with information on several mental illnesses and their treatments. NAMI state affiliates provide emotional support and can help find local services. Find your local NAMI on the Web site under State and local NAMIs.

The National Institute of Mental Health (NIMH)
Internet address: http://www.nimh.nih.gov
This site offers information and publications on all the mental health disorders. Contact the Information and Resources and Inquiries Branch, NIMH, Room 7C–02, MSC 8030, Bethesda, MD 20892-8030.

The National Mental Health Association (NMHA)
Internet address: http://www.nmha.org
The NMHA publishes information on a variety of mental health issues. NMHA also provides referrals and support. Write or call the NMHA Information Center, 1021 Prince Street, Alexandria, VA 22314–2971; (800) 969-6642.

References and Bibliography

Alcoholics Anonymous World Services, Inc. Twelve steps froms: http://www.alcoholicsanonymous.org/en_services_for_members.cfm?PageID=17&SubPage=68. *This resource was accessed by going to Alcoholics Anonymous, Twelve steps.*

American Psychiatric Association. (2000). Diagnostic and statistical manual of mental disorders (4th ed., text rev.). Washington, DC: Author.

Healthy People 2010: Mental Health and Mental Disorders. Partners in Information Access for the Public Workforce. (2006). From: http://phpartners.orghp/mentalthealthandmentaldisorders.html

Howland, R. H. (2006). What is vagus nerve stimulation? *Journal of Psychosocial Nursing and Mental Health Services, 44*(8), 11–14.

Howland, R. H. (2006). Vagus nerve stimulation for depression and other neuropsychiatric disorders. *Journal of Psychosocial Nursing and Mental Health Services, 44*(9), 11–14.

Lafferty, S., & Davidson, R. (2006, March). Putting the person first. *Mental Health Today,* pp. 31–33.

McAllister, M., Matarasso, B., Dixon, B., & Shepperd, C. (2004). Conversation starters: Re-examining and reconstructing first encounters within the therapeutic relationship. *Journal of Psychiatric and Mental Health Nursing, 11*(5), 575–582.

National Institute of Mental Health: The Numbers Count: Mental Disorders in America. (2007). Department of Health and Human Services Information and Resources and Inquiries Branch, NIMH, Room 7C-02, MSC 8030, Bethesda, MD 20892-8030. From: http://www.nimh.nih.gov/health/publications/the-numbers-count-mental-disorders-in-america.shtml#intro

National Institute of Mental Health: Suicide in the U.S. Statistics and Prevention. (2004). Department of Heath and Human Services Information and Resources and Inquiries Branch, NIMH, Room 7C-02, MSC 8030, Bethesda, MD 20892-8030. From: http://www.nimh.nih.gov/health/publications/suicide-in-the-us-statistics-and-prevention.sh

Osborne, U. L., & McComish, J. F. (2006). Borderline personality disorder: Nursing interventions using dialectical behavioral therapy. *Journal of Psychosocial Nursing and Mental Health Services, 44*(6), 40–47.

Payne, R. K., DeVol, P., & Smith, T. D. (2001). *Bridges out of poverty: Strategies for professionals and communities.* Highlands, TX: aha! Process, Inc.

Rydon, S. E. (2005). The attitude, knowledge and skills needed in mental health nurses: The perspective of users of mental health services. *International Journal of Mental Health Nursing, 14*(2), 78–87.

Tschirch, P., Walker, G., & Calvacca, L. T. (2006). Nursing in tele-mental health. *Journal of Psychosocial Nursing and Mental Health Services, 44*(5) 20–27.

U.S. Department of Health and Human Services and National Institutes of Health. (1999). *Mental health: A report of the surgeon general.* Rockville, MD: Author. Retrieved on December 8, 2006, from http://www.surgeongeneral.gov/substanceabuse.

U.S. Department of Health and Human Services. (2000). *Healthy people 2010: Understanding and improving health* (Chapter 18). Washington, DC: U.S. Government Printing Office. Retrieved on December 8, 2006, from http://www.healthypeople.gov/Document/HTML/Volume2/18Mental.htm

U.S. Department of Health and Human Services. (2001). *Mental health: Culture, race and ethnicity—A supplement to mental health: A report of the surgeon general.* Rockville, MD: U.S. Department of Health and Human Services, Substance Abuse and Mental Health Services Administration, Center for Mental Health Services. Retrieved from http://www.surgeon-general.gov/substanceabuse.

U.S. Department of Health and Human Services. (2001). *Mental Health: A Report of the Surgeon General: Epidemiology of Mental Illness.* Rockville, MD: U.S. Department of Health and Human Services. Retrieved from: http://www.surgeongeneral.gov/

library/mentalheath/chapter2/sec2_1.html. *Accessed this by starting with U.S. Surgeon General, then to Mental Health: A **Report** of the **Surgeon General**, then choose Chapter 2, The Fundamentals of Mental Health and Mental Illness and finally to Epidemiology of Mental Illness.*

Valente, S. M., & Saunders, J. (2005). Screening for depression and suicide. *Journal of Psychosocial Nursing and Mental Health Services, 43*(11), 22–31.

Varcarolis, E. M., Carson, V. B., & Shoemaker, N. C. (2005). *Foundations of Psychiatric Mental Health Nursing* (5th edition). Philadelphia: W.B. Saunders.

LEARNING ▼ ACTIVITIES

◆ JOURNALING ACTIVITY 14-1

Before your first clinical in mental health, respond to the following questions in your journal:

- What do you think it will be like on the mental health unit?
- What do you think the client you care for will be like?
- Describe what you think it will be like to care for an individual with mental illness.
- What previous experiences have you had with mental illness?
- What do you feel when you think about your first encounter as a nurse caring for someone who has a mental illness?

In your clinical journal, discuss a situation you have encountered in one of your clinical experiences with a client who is having difficulties with a mental illness.

- Describe your feelings and reactions to what you see and hear.
- Reflect on your preconceptions and compare them to what you see when working with individuals with mental illness.
- What was the most important thing you learned about mental illness?

◆ JOURNALING ACTIVITY 14-2

Contact a community mental health center in your community and find out about the volunteer opportunities available for nursing students. When you have found something that appeals to you, volunteer for a month, several months, or longer. Keep a journal about your experiences as a volunteer.

◆ PRACTICAL APPLICATION ACTIVITY 14-3

Visit a homeless shelter and meet the staff to discuss the issues and services available for the homeless. Before the visit, find information about homelessness in your community. The scope of the issue, trends, programs, and policy that has been developed to address the need.

◆ **PRACTICAL APPLICATION ACTIVITY 14-4**

With a group of students, assist with the serving of a meal in a homeless shelter. Before you go, identify an article in a nursing journal about homelessness, poverty, or mental illness and homelessness. While at the shelter, have at least one interaction with one of the people you are serving (e.g., ask someone if you can sit down and have a cup of coffee and visit with him or her). After the interaction, discuss the following:

- What are your feelings and reactions to what you said and heard?
- What did you expect that this experience would be like, and what did you actually experience?
- What did you learn from speaking to the person with whom you interacted?
- What evidence of mental illness, if any, did you see in any of the residents at the shelter?
- Discuss the article you read and how it relates to what you saw.
- Identify the most important thing you learned during this experience.

◆ **PRACTICAL APPLICATION ACTIVITY 14-5**

Contact a mental health nurse working in a community setting. Interview him or her and ask the following questions:

- What are your primary responsibilities as a nurse in this setting?
- What are the challenges and benefits of this type of work?
- What are the goals and missions of your agency?
- Would you recommend this type of work to a new graduate?
- What kind of additional education would be beneficial in preparation for doing this type of work?

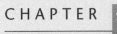
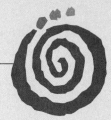

Global Health and Community-Based Care

ROBERTA HUNT

LEARNING OBJECTIVES

1. Discuss the relationship between community-based nursing and global health.
2. Identify roles that the community-based nurse has in global health.
3. Discuss the relationship between global health and environmental health.
4. Develop a global perspective on disparity.
5. Consider the global nature and global consequences of natural disasters, epidemics, and terrorism.
6. Consider the needs of immigrants, refugees, and victims of societal violence.
7. Understand the impact of the global shortage of RNs on global health.
8. Appreciate the need for nursing advocacy in global health.

KEY TERMS

advocacy
disasters
emergency preparedness
environmental health
environmental quality
globalization
global health disparity

immigrants
natural disaster
pandemic
physical environment
refugees
social environment
undocumented workers

CHAPTER TOPICS

- ◆ Developing a Global View of Nursing
- ◆ Environmental Health
- ◆ Global Health Disparity
- ◆ Emergency Preparedness
- ◆ Immigrants and Refugees
- ◆ Nursing Advocacy in Global Health
- ◆ Global Nursing Shortage
- ◆ Conclusions

Katrina Response—One Nurse's Story

Be ready for anything. Drop your job description and egos at the door. Plan to bring closure to the Operation Minnesota Lifeline service to the Gulf Coast area following the "cosmic slap" delivered by the Katrina and Rita hurricanes. Such were the instructions given us during orientation as 28 of us—health care providers, clerical and logistical workers—prepared to bus down to Louisiana to do whatever was necessary for the 16 days we were scheduled for service with evacuees of the hurricanes.

I have been a nurse for 40 years. I worked in the hospital for 5 years, 15 years in community/public health practice, and nurse educator for 20 years. This experience was an odyssey where collaboration and team-work came to life for me as never before.

The environment in which we served was every bit as tumultuous as the media portrayed. Homes, churches, and schools were totally destroyed. At the same time—6 weeks post-hurricanes—I was amazed at the resilience of people as they worked to put lives back together in the midst of turmoil. To alleviate total school disruption, districts worked together. Schools which remained intact would have classes for their respective students in the morning; schools that were destroyed would bus their students in for afternoon classes in the same intact building. The plan was to have school year round.

Amidst this backdrop our team set out each day to provide health services to the region. Working out of vans, we set up wherever there were people—trailer parks, motels, road crossings, at the local market, domes, emergency medical technician (EMT) headquarters, and campgrounds.

As one might predict, many of our "stops" included immunization "clinic." I was touched by the gratitude of all of the people who received services. After immunizing one mom and her family of four, I was hugged and mom expressed her appreciation in these words—"Honey, I loves you, I loves you like a pig loves corn!" Ah—the colloquial expressions of the Louisiana people!

As I reflect back, two areas of nursing practice stand out—that of assessment and presence. Assessment of all ages was carried out—for respiratory, skin, eye, and mental health concerns among many. We can only hope our team of primary providers made a dent in the health needs and that referrals made were indeed available and followed.

A particularly poignant experience was illustrative of the human-to-human presence that characterized much of our work among the crowds.

During one of the campground stops 7-year-old "Jimmy" came bounding up to us, followed by his dog. He grabbed our hands and asked if he could get "a shot." As we skipped along with him to find his mother, we talked about his family "camping out." He was so eager to stay with us as he told us it was kind of fun, but nobody could find his grandma. Then without missing a beat he held our hands tighter, pulled up his sleeve ready for his shot, and said "can you stay with us all day?" That encounter was one of many transforming experiences of healing presence for all of us.

—ROMANA KLAUBAUF, MSN, RN, Public Health Nurse,
Assistant Professor, College of St. Catherine

◆ B O X 1 5 - 1   Health Risks Posed by Globalization ◆

- Emerging infectious diseases, such as influenza and severe acute respiratory syndrome (SARS)
- Easier spread of disease throughout the world due to the movement of people and tainted goods as a part of the world economy
- Need to better manage international health disasters, such as tsunamis, earthquakes, and hurricanes
- Awareness of biological and chemical terror threats
- Effects of global warming
- Acquired immunodeficiency syndrome (AIDS)

Source: WHO. (2007). Nations focus on health risks posed by globalization. Retrieved on April 14, 2007, from http://www.who.int/trade/en/

Globalization is defined as the development of an increasingly integrated global economy marked especially by free trade, free flow of capital, and the tapping of cheaper foreign labor markets (Merriam Webster, 2007).

Globalization has become a major challenge for the nursing profession. An illness is no longer contained by geographic boundaries nor is anyone protected from events occurring in distance places. For example, an epidemic in New York may quickly spread to Thailand. One person with influenza who travels by plane to an international conference may be responsible for exposing numerous individuals attending the conference to the virus. If several conference attendees become ill and return home, each may serve as a vector and spread the illness to colleagues and family in their respective countries. With increasing air travel, epidemics are easily transmitted throughout the world. Another example is seen in the ways that nursing knowledge is becoming global. There has been an increase in participation in international nursing conferences as well as publications of studies conducted by nurses worldwide over the last 2 decades. As a result, nurses in Sioux Falls, South Dakota, may be using a model of practice developed in Sweden. Nurses in Budapest, Hungary may use a model of community-based care conceived by a nurse in St. Paul, Minnesota. The main health risks posed by globalization are found in Box 15-1. In this chapter, community-based nursing will be considered from the perspective of global health. Increasingly, nurses must be competent to consider health as a comprehensive concept that requires an understanding of environmental health, global health disparity, and emergency preparedness. Once health is understood as a global concept, our professional responsibility to consider and address issues of global health follows. Our scope of advocacy broadens as we develop a sense of social responsibility for the health of new Americans and citizens of other countries.

DEVELOPING A GLOBAL VIEW OF NURSING

In order to develop a global view of nursing it is helpful to look to professional standards as a guide. The *Nursing Code of Ethics* delineates professional responsibility to global health and the international community. Nursing commitment to health promotion, welfare, and safety extends to all persons. This requires consideration of not only individual clients but also to broader health concerns for community, national, and international issues. These issues may include world hunger, environmental pollution, lack of access to health care, and inequitable distribution of nursing and health care resources. To address these professional responsibilities nurses may participate in interdisciplinary planning and collaborative partnerships among health professionals and others at the community, national, and international level (American Nurses Association [ANA] Code of Ethics, 2001).

There are numerous avenues for developing a global view of nursing. First, it is important to become informed about local, national, and international health issues. Once acquainted with the issues, speaking out and informing others is the next step. Attending international conferences develops a global view of nursing, with a modest commitment of time and resources. International conferences provide ample opportunities to meet other attendees and, in some cases, begin a connection that evolves into a collaborative relationship. Volunteering internationally is a powerful way to learn both about oneself and health care from another cultural perspective. For additional resources there are some Web sites of volunteer opportunities listed at the end of the chapter. Working abroad in developing countries provides opportunities to share clinical expertise while learning new approaches to health and illness. There are numerous student exchange programs that offer study abroad. Immersion experience exposes one to the language, religion, art, customs, and traditions along with health care systems. Most universities and colleges offer study abroad programs.

ENVIRONMENTAL HEALTH

Environmental health is defined by the World Health Organization (WHO) as the study of "the effects of various chemical, physical, and biological agents, as well as the effects on the health of the broad physical and social environment, which includes housing, urban development, land-use and transportation, industry, and agriculture" (U.S. Department of Health and Human Services [DHHS], 2000 p. 83). The **environmental quality** of both the physical and social environments plays major roles in the health of individuals and communities. The **physical environment** includes the air, water, and soil through which exposure to chemical, biological, and physical agents may occur. The **social environment** consists of housing, transportation, urban development, land use, industry, and agriculture along with issues related to work-related stress, injury, and violence (DHHS, 2002).

It is not possible for individual nations to completely regulate and ensure environmental quality because some of the elements such as air and water pollution are not contained by geographical borders. Acid rain is a good example, in that the states or nations that have the highest concentration of acid rain are often those areas downwind of states or nations that are the source of the pollution. Thus, environmental quality and environment health is a global issue that depends on interstate and international cooperation and agreements. It is important to remember that the quality of both the immediate and broader environment impacts the health status of individuals, families, and communities. This chapter will discuss the concept of environmental health as it relates to the health of populations in the United States as well as globally.

Environmental Health in the United States

The goals of Healthy People 2010 discussed in Chapter 2 are to reduce health disparity and increase the quality and years of healthy life. These goals are determined and monitored through health indicators. You may remember that one of the health indicators is environmental quality. There is a relationship between the environmental quality and health.

Assessing the contribution that quality of the immediate physical environment has on health is an important role for the nurse in community settings. An example is seen when a nurse does a home assessment for the presence of lead in a home where there are infants or children living. If the nurse discovers that there is evidence of lead, an abatement process commences to improve the environmental quality of the home. Asthma is an example of a chronic condition common among children and adults in the United States that is impacted by environmental quality. Nurses play an important role in the assessment and intervention of factors that contribute to asthma in individuals, families, and populations (Research in Community-Based Nursing Care 15-1).

A commonly discussed issue related to environmental health of communities and populations is the relationship between air pollution and health. Air pollution is an environmental quality that characterizes the broader physical environment. In the United States, air pollution is associated with approximately 50,000 premature deaths and an estimated $40 billion to $50 billion in health-related costs annually (DHHS, 2000). Infants exposed to higher levels of air pollution are more likely to die of respiratory related illnesses and sudden infant death syndrome (SIDS) compared to infants living in areas with low air pollution (Ritz, Wilhelm, & Zhao, 2006). As with other health indicators, there is disparity in the ways that environmental quality impacts health. Black Americans are 79% more likely than Whites to live in neighborhoods where industrial pollution is suspected of posing the greatest health danger (Pace, 2006).

RESEARCH IN COMMUNITY-BASED NURSING CARE ▶ 15-1

Inner-City Asthma Study

Families with children ages 5 to 11 with moderate-to-severe asthma received individualized in-home evaluations and education by nurses to reduce allergens in their homes. A control group of families with children who did not receive the home visit were compared to the families who did receive the visits. Over 2 years the intervention group made significantly fewer unscheduled clinic visits and used fewer inhalers compare to the control group. Benefits may have continued beyond the 2-year study but were not measured. Nor were the indirect costs associated with asthma such as parents losing time from work and children from school calculated.

Kattan, M., Crain, E. F., Steinbach, S., et al. (2006). A randomized clinical trial of clinician feedback to improve quality of care for inner-city children with asthma. *Pediatrics*, *117*(6):e1095–1103.

Environmental Health as a Global Issue

An estimated 25% of preventable illnesses worldwide can be attributed to poor environmental quality. Air pollution has been associated with hospital admissions for respiratory disease in cities all over the world (Medina-Ramón, Zanobetti, & Schwartz, 2006). As mentioned earlier, the fact that air and water pollution are not contained by national boundaries contributes to the global nature of environmental issues. Further, as increasing numbers of people and products cross national borders, health risks such as infectious diseases and chemical hazards often follow. An example is seen in pesticides that are not registered or are restricted for use in the United States but that may be imported in the fruits, vegetables, and seafood produced abroad.

Nurses are increasingly the primary contact for clients, families, and communities concerned about health problems related to the environment both locally and globally. Nursing is well positioned to assess, prevent, and mitigate the impact of environmental hazards on the health of populations.

GLOBAL HEALTH DISPARITY

There are increasing **global health disparities** between the developed and developing world. Although there is no standard designation of "developed" and "developing" countries, in common practice, Japan, Canada, the United States, Australia, New Zealand, and Europe are considered "developed" countries. In international trade statistics, the Southern African Customs Union is also treated as a developed region and Israel as a developed country; countries emerging from the former Yugoslavia are treated as developing countries; and countries of Eastern Europe and the former USSR countries in Europe are not included under either developed or developing regions (Organisation for Economic Co-operation and Development [OECD], 2007). These disparities include differences in health and access to health care services by gender, age, race or ethnicity, education or income, disability, geographic location, or sexual orientation. An example is seen in life expectancy. Over the past 50 years, average life expectancy at birth has increased globally by almost 20 years. Although life expectancy is improving worldwide, closer examination of these statistics reveals this increase is primarily in the developed world, while in the poorest counties life expectancy is decreasing (Benatar, Daar, & Singer, 2005). Most deaths worldwide are from noncommunicable diseases, with over half from cardiovascular disease.

Although mortality from cardiovascular disease has declined steadily to 250 per 100,000 in the European Union (EU) since 1970, the rate in the former Soviet Union is almost three times this level; over 750 per 100,000. The use of cigarettes and other tobacco products are responsible for 5 million deaths in the EU each year, mostly in poor countries and poor populations. In the next 20 years, without effective intervention, this toll is expected to double. Across the world poorer children are at higher risk of dying. Child mortality rates in countries in the developed world are improving at a faster rate, while many of the poorer countries are losing ground (WHO, The World Health Report, 2003). Child mortality rates in developing countries are attributed to lack of care during pregnancy and childbirth, lack of immunizations and treatment during illness, and malnutrition (East-West Center, 2003).

Just as nurses have a role in the issue of health disparity in their own community and country, there are contributions to be made towards addressing the issue

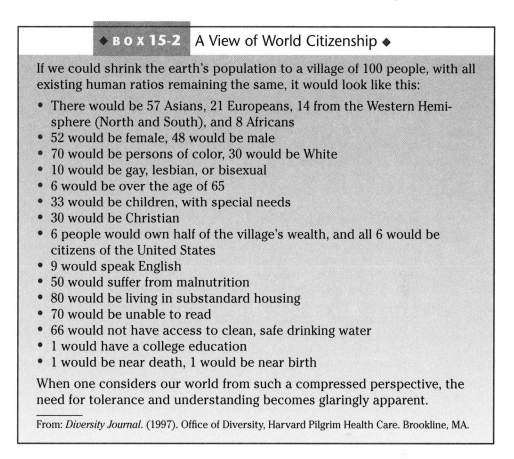

◆ **B O X 15-2**   A View of World Citizenship ◆

If we could shrink the earth's population to a village of 100 people, with all existing human ratios remaining the same, it would look like this:

- There would be 57 Asians, 21 Europeans, 14 from the Western Hemisphere (North and South), and 8 Africans
- 52 would be female, 48 would be male
- 70 would be persons of color, 30 would be White
- 10 would be gay, lesbian, or bisexual
- 6 would be over the age of 65
- 33 would be children, with special needs
- 30 would be Christian
- 6 people would own half of the village's wealth, and all 6 would be citizens of the United States
- 9 would speak English
- 50 would suffer from malnutrition
- 80 would be living in substandard housing
- 70 would be unable to read
- 66 would not have access to clean, safe drinking water
- 1 would have a college education
- 1 would be near death, 1 would be near birth

When one considers our world from such a compressed perspective, the need for tolerance and understanding becomes glaringly apparent.

From: *Diversity Journal.* (1997). Office of Diversity, Harvard Pilgrim Health Care. Brookline, MA.

of global disparity. Most obvious is to become informed about the issues, speak out, and inform others. Box 15-2 provides an interesting illustration of the magnitude of the issue of worldwide disparity.

EMERGENCY PREPAREDNESS

What does an outbreak of West Nile virus, a public water supply contaminated with potentially deadly levels of *Cryptosporidium* protozoa, a war in Iraq, an outbreak of a highly contagious spinal meningitis in a school and a bioterrorist attack have in common? All require a major population-based response. The difference in these issues is the level from which the response occurs. West Nile virus is likely to be addressed through individual city or state efforts, while public water may be within the auspice of municipalities or cities. The chaos, violence, and death created by any war may require an international response through organizations like the United Nations (UN), Red Cross, United Nations Educational, Scientific and Cultural Organization (UNESCO), or Doctors Without Borders. A school district or state or county health department would be the intervening body for an outbreak of spinal meningitis. Bioterrorism has become the focus of national governments as well as multinational efforts such as the North Atlantic Treaty Organization (NATO) and the UN.

The equivalent of prevention as it relates to natural disasters, epidemics, and terrorism is emergency preparedness. At this time, **emergency preparedness** as a defining concept across disciplines is still emerging. It may be defined as "comprehensive knowledge, skills, abilities, and actions needed to prepare for and respond to threatened, actual, or suspected chemical, biological, radiological, nuclear or explosive incidents, man-made incidents, natural disasters, or other related events" (Slepski, 2005). In the following section epidemics, natural disasters, and terrorism will be discussed. Further, the role of the nurse in addressing the related health concerns as well as the role of emergency preparedness will be outlined.

Disasters

Disasters are unpredictable but occur with regularity. **Natural disasters** include such events as earthquakes, fires, hurricanes, tornados, tsunamis, and wildfires. They take tens of thousands of lives and cause billions of dollars in damage. Man-made disasters such as airline crashes, wars, chemical explosions, and other mishaps with other hazardous material also take thousands of lives each year. Both natural and man-made disasters impact the health of individuals, families, and communities by devastating the environment and significantly disrupting daily life. To mitigate these consequences the need for preparedness is imperative.

Recent disasters have illustrated that the U.S. federal government's disaster response is not always as quick as needed, leaving much of the rescue work to local health care and emergency workers, and ordinary citizens. A good example of this would be hurricane Katrina. Therefore, communities must prepare long before disaster strikes. Nurses should be at the forefront of these initiatives. As nurses and advocates for the vulnerable it is our professional and social responsibility to educate and guide policymakers to develop emergency preparedness to minimize harm to people and property (Chaffee, 2006).

Epidemics and Pandemics

One of the great epidemics of modern times occurred during the last 6 months of World War I in 1918. In pockets across the globe, a new enemy erupted–influenza–that at first seemed as benign as the common cold but eventually became the major pandemic of modern history. A **pandemic** is an epidemic or outbreak of an infectious disease that occurs over a wide geographic area and affecting an exceptionally high proportion of the population (Merriam Webster, 2007). In the 2 years that followed, the virus infected a fifth of the world's population. Unlike the typical pattern for influenza, which is most deadly for young children and the elderly, this strain was most fatal to people ages 20 to 40. It infected 28% of all Americans. An estimated 675,000 Americans died of influenza during the pandemic, ten times as many as in the World War. Of the U.S. soldiers who died in Europe, half of the deaths were from influenza virus (Billings, 2005).

There is a great deal of concern about the increasing possibility of a major epidemic similar to the one in 1918. Influenza pandemic has the potential to cause more death and illness compared to any other major disaster. The potential for rapid transmission has increased exponentially. In our highly mobile global community, if a businessperson with a subclinical case of influenza boards an airplane in London, develops a fever and begins to cough on a flight to Beijing, a new strain of influenza has also been transported to Beijing along with the passengers and luggage. If an influenza virus with a similar virulence to that of the 1918 strain emerged today, it is estimated that, without planning and intervention, 1.9 million Americans could die and almost 10 million could be hospitalized over the course of the pandemic. Minimizing social and economic disruption will require a coordinated response between national and state governments, communities, and other public and private sector stakeholders (DHHS, 2005).

There are contributions that nurses can make to minimize the mortality, morbidity, and other losses in the event of a pandemic. An immunized health care staff is one defense strategy to minimize the spread of infectious agents. Health care workers are known to be a reservoir and vector of the influenza virus and the Centers for Disease Control and Prevention (CDC) recommends a yearly influenza vaccine (Harper, 2005). A yearly vaccine not only helps protect the nurse, but also his or her family, patients, and the community from getting the flu. Further, a yearly vaccine reduces absenteeism and allows the nurse to continue to provide patient care in the event of an epidemic or pandemic. Maintaining a low nurse/patient ratio is known to reduce mortality and improve patient outcomes (DHHS, 2005).

Once again, assessment skills are essential in early identification and intervention with emerging epidemics. Nurses are in a position to notice patterns and trends in the conditions clients present with in clinics and hospitals. An upsurge in the number of clients with respiratory illness or symptoms that follows a pattern not seen in past years always requires additional exploration. Keen clinical skills along with an open, curious attitude toward clinical care can lead nurses to question what they observe. This may lead to the early identification of a new virus as well as early vigilance with an emerging epidemic. One nurse contacting the local or state department of health with a question or concern may be enough to identify an early case of a communicable disease. Further, the nurse may intervene by investigating the disease, gathering and analyzing the information regarding the threat to the health of populations, ascertain the source of the threat, and determine control measures. These actions may serve to protect a community from a pandemic.

Another way that nurses can take part is by participating in local emergency preparedness task forces for pandemics. In addition, nurses are often the professionals who develop educational materials and participate in training. All of these actions contribute to containing an influenza epidemic. Nurses may also participate in training in behavioral techniques to cope with grief, exhaustion, stress, and fear. This expertise allows nurses to assist patients, other employees, families, and communities with the psychological aspects of care during an emergency (DHHS, 2006).

Terrorism

The events of September 11, 2001, as well as other acts of terrorism worldwide have heightened awareness of the need for bioterrorism preparedness. The most important role played by nurses is that of first responders (Baldwin, LaManitia, & Prozialeck, 2005). In terms of being a real threat to the health and welfare of large numbers of individuals bioterrorism has, up to this point, caused limited mortality as compared to natural disasters and epidemics. However, preparedness for any emergency protects the citizenry. The elements of bioterrorism preparedness and management are essentially the same as those already mentioned.

Clinical Situation: Hurricane Katrina—Failure to Rescue
Prevention is a central component to community-based care. The inadequacy of the current system seen in the lack of emergency preparedness that would have

minimized or avoided damage to New Orleans from Hurricane Katrina was not taken. Despite warnings from the Army Corps of Engineer, federal funding to shore up the sinking levee that protected New Orleans from Lake Pontchartrain was slashed. Despite enormous allocation of resources into biopreparedness, public officials were days too slow in responding. The inadequate command of the situation by the local, state, and federal officials was obvious. Likewise, the emergency response was poorly coordinated. Multiple inadequate systems and leadership compounded the devastation. The most heart-wrenching aspect of the entire disaster was seen in the photos and films of the aftermath of the event. These exemplified the disparity of services in the United States and illustrated the racial and class divide. Katrina profoundly brought to light that disparity is real in the United States. Nurses were some of the heroes of this disaster. Nurses were working around the clock in the hospitals without electricity hand-ventilating patients and in the community providing primary care and triage for the injured (Mason, (2005).

IMMIGRANTS AND REFUGEES

The plight of refugees and immigrants has been a phenomena throughout human history. Famines, floods, and other natural disasters, as well as human-created disasters of war and domination are documented in the holy books of the Old Testament and Torah. All of these events have, and do, force human relocation at great loss of life and severe disruption of quality of life.

In the United States, there are three categories of newcomers: legal immigrants, refugees, and undocumented workers. Although there are some similarities between these categories, there are important distinctions. Most newcomers to the United States are legal **immigrants** who come here by choice, while **refugees** are typically fleeing from their country of origin. In most cases, despite the harsh circumstances surrounding the immigrant or refugees' life in their country of origin, their experience is colored by loss and uncertainly following relocation (Rosenberg, Gonzalez, & Rosenberg, 2005).

There an unspecified number of **undocumented workers** in the United States who enter the country illegally mainly for employment opportunities. Most of these individuals leave their country of origin to escape abject poverty. Despite their contribution to the U.S. economy through taxes, they are barred from many rights that most citizens take for granted: the legal right to work, hold a driver's license, and collect Social Security payments. Understandably, reluctant to have any contact with government or state officials, they often avoid health or legal services.

The varied needs of this diverse population present a challenge to health care providers. One is access to systems of care. They often encounter numerous barriers to care, stemming from their own cultural norms towards certain types of care from their country of origin. This reluctance to seek care is often seen in mental health services or prenatal care. Along with many other Americans, newcomers often lack adequate health insurance. Unfortunately health care services are not always designed with a multicultural awareness, resulting in their not being appealing or appearing relevant to the newcomer. Cultural norms both of the newcomer and of the nurse create powerful barriers to care. The language barriers are often obvious but create ongoing barriers to care. Specific suggestions to deal with these obstacles are discussed in Chapters 3 and 6 (p. 179).

Nurses can learn a great deal about international health by seeking out experiences with new Americans in their own communities. One way to do this is by requesting to care for these clients when they come to the unit, clinic, or agency where the nurse works. Developing expertise in caring for new Americans in one's own community is another approach to understanding global health. Listening to the life stories of new Americans is another, as our clients are often our most important teachers.

NURSING ADVOCACY IN GLOBAL HEALTH

Advocacy is to "plead someone's cause or act on someone's behalf, with a focus on developing the individual, family's, or community capacity to plead their own cause or act on their own behalf" (Public Health Nursing Interventions, 2001, p. 262). The principles of advocacy in global health are the same whether in one's own neighborhood or in a distant land. Obviously, because issues related to global health often occur some distance away, some of the strategies for advocacy are different, as compared to those in our community. To act as an advocate for someone suffering from a famine in Africa, we may think the only way to impact their condition is to go to central Africa or to donate to a charity. Too far, we may say, to make a difference. However, awareness campaigns and membership in groups supporting international efforts are ways to participate in international advocacy. As mentioned, one way to broaden practice skills and knowledge is to become familiar with, and eventually act as advocate for, new Americans in our own community. Another strategy is to become involved in international health organizations.

There is wide variation in the size, organization, and funding of international health organizations. Sometimes getting involved in an organization creates opportunities to learn about the organizations' goals and missions. It is prudent to use care before giving time or money to any cause. The agenda of some of these organizations may be self-serving in their agenda and work against improving the health status of a population the organization seeks to serve. An example would be an organization offering free samples or selling formula to women who are breast-feeding. Unless contraindicated because of certain infectious diseases, it is generally in the infant and mother's best interest to continue breast-feeding. Another example would be if in a country where most citizens are Muslim, a Christian organization requires that recipients of humanitarian aid participate in Christian religious services.

The trend in international health organizations is to focus more on preventative services and sustainability. Agencies are concentrating on the development of rapid response teams that use short-term assignments to target specific health issues (Veenema, 2001). Once you have clarified that the agency you are interested in becoming active in represents an approach consistent with your own values, you may decide to become more involved. Some international health organizations are listed in What's on the Web at the end of the chapter.

GLOBAL NURSING SHORTAGE

The nursing shortage is a global problem. It is occurring in health systems around the world, creating a serious crisis in terms of adverse impact on heath and well-being of populations. One recent report states there is a shortfall of more than 600,000 nurses compared to need in sub-Saharan Africa. Although there have been a shortage of nurses in the past, currently the health systems are suffering from pressure exerted on both the supply and demand. Further, the future need for

◆ **B O X 15-3**   The Global Nursing Shortage: Priority Areas for Interventions ◆

- Macroeconomic and health sector funding policies
- Workforce policy and planning, including regulation
- Positive practice environments and organizational performance
- Recruitment and retention; addressing in-country misdistribution, and out-migration
- Nursing leadership

Source: International Council of Nurses. (2006). Global nursing shortage: Priority areas for intervention, a report from ICN/FNIF. Retrieved on July 27, 2006, from http://www.hrhresourcecenter.org/node/420

nurses will continue to escalate as the worldwide population ages, the health care provider workforce ages, and the growth for alternative careers for woman continues (International Council of Nurses [ICN], 2006).

Multiple critical issues contribute to the current shortage, including poor deployment practices, migration, high attrition, human immunodeficiency virus/acquired immunodeficiency syndrome (HIV/AIDS), and underinvestment in human resources.

Nurses make up the largest group of health care providers in every country in the world (ICN, 2006). Because nursing services are essential to the provision of safe and effective care, addressing these issues is imperative to thwart a major crisis in health care. The International Council of Nurses has identified five priority areas for addressing the critical issue of nursing shortage (Box 15-3). In a world where global issues become local issues, a global nursing shortage has implications for citizens in every country.

The nursing shortage brings up interesting questions related to advocacy at the global level. This plays out in a variety of ways with numerous implications. Rather than further marginalize fledgling health systems, wealthy nations could act as advocates by not actively recruiting nurses from developing countries. Perhaps nurses in developed countries have a professional responsibility to advocate, not to actively recruit nurses from developing countries into developed countries. The intent would be to avoid exacerbating disparity between developed and developing countries and prevent further marginalizing of these fledgling health systems.

CONCLUSIONS

Globalization requires that the profession of nursing expand the scope and emphasis of community-based care to include the global community. It is imperative that nurses be informed and competent in the areas of environmental health, global health disparity, and emergency preparedness. The need for international advocacy intensifies as the nursing shortage worldwide simultaneously transpires while the health needs of the world intensify. These challenges call for all nurses regardless of their nationality or ethnicity, to reflect on the world as the client.

What's on the Web

World Health Organization
Internet address: http://www.who.int/en/
The World Health Organization is the United Nations agency for health. It was established to focus on the attainment by all peoples of the highest possible level of health. Health is defined in WHO's Constitution as a state of complete physical, mental, and social well-being and not merely the absence of disease or infirmity.

International Health Volunteers
Internet address:
http://www.globalvolunteers.org/
As a non-governmental organization (NGO) in special consultative status with the United Nations, Global Volunteers mobilizes some 150 service-learning teams year-round to work in 20 countries on six continents, and is the internationally recognized leader in this field of work. Global Volunteers continues to work to help lay a foundation for world peace through mutual understanding.

Cross-Cultural Solutions
Internet address:
http://www.crossculturalsolutions.org/
Cross-Cultural Solutions offers international volunteers an opportunity to make a meaningful contribution working side-by-side with local people and sharing in the goals of a community. This experience allows one to gain new perspective and insight into the culture and themselves.

Peace Corps
Internet address: http://www.peacecorp.gov
The Peace Corps traces its roots and mission to 1960, when then-Senator John F. Kennedy challenged college students to serve their country in the cause of peace by living and working in developing countries. From that inspiration grew an

agency of the federal government devoted to world peace and friendship. Since that time, more than 182,000 Peace Corps Volunteers have been invited by 138 host countries to work on issues ranging from AIDS education, information technology, and environmental preservation.

Center for Disease Control and Prevention/ Emergency Preparedness & Response
Internet address: http://www.bt.cdc.gov/
This site provides information and links for bioterrorism, mass causalities, chemical emergencies, natural disasters, radiation emergencies, and recent outbreaks and incidents (epidemics). There are numerous other topics found on this site along with the most recent research and resources such as videos and slides.

New York Consortium for Emergency Preparedness Continuing Education (NYCEPCE)
Internet address:
http://www.nycepce.org/default.htm
The mission of the NYCEPCE is to strengthen the competency of health professionals to respond effectively to emergency events of all kinds through competency-based continuing education. There are numerous resources on the Web site that can be used for training purposes including an emergency preparedness course for hospital clinicians.

International Council of Nurses Disaster Preparedness Resource List
Internet address:
www.icn.ch/disas_relatedpubs.htm
This resource list includes over 40 links to resources for disaster preparedness geared for nurses. These include courses, conferences, discussion rooms, printed and video resources lists.

References and Bibliography

_____. (1993). The future of environmental health. *Journal of Environmental Health, 55*(4), 28–32.

American Nurses Association. The Center for Ethics and Human Rights. *Nursing Code of Ethics.* Retrieved on October 30, 2007, from http://www.med.howard.edu/ethics/handouts/american_nurses_association_code.htm

Baldwin, K., LaMantia, J., & Prozialeck, L. (2005). Emergency preparedness and bioterrorism response: Development of an educational program for public health personnel. *Public Health Nursing, 22*(3), 248–253.

Benatar, S. R., Daar., A. S., & Singer, P. A. (2005). Global health challenges: The need for an expanded discourse on bioethics. *PLoS Med, 2*(7): e143. Retrieved on July 27, 2006, from http://www.plosmedicine.org

Billings, M. (2005). *The 1918 Influenza Pandemic.* Retrieved on July 25, 2006, from http://www.virus.stanford.edu.uda/

Chaffee, M. (2006). Reality check. How prepared are we for disasters? *American Journal of Nursing, 106*(3), 13.

Diversity Journal. (1997). Office of Diversity, Harvard Pilgrim Health Care. Brookline, MA

East-West Center. (2003). Asia-Pacific population and policy. *Child survival and health care in developing countries of Asia.* Retrieved on April 14, 2007, from http://www.eastwestcenter.org

Grady, P. A., Harden, J. T., Moritz, P., & Amende, L. M. (1997). Incorporating environmental science and nursing research: An NINR initiative. *Nursing Outlook, 45*(2), 73–75.

Harper, S. A., Fukuda, K., Uyeki, T. M., et al. (2005). Prevention and control of influenza. Recommendations of the Advisory Committee on Immunization Practices (ACIP). *MMWR Recommendations Report, 54*(RR-8), 1–40.

International Council of Nurses. (2006). *Global nursing shortage: Priority areas for intervention, a report from ICN/FNIF.* Retrieved on October 31, 2007, from www.icn.ch/global/report2006.pdf

Kattan, M., Crain, E. F., Steinbach, S., et al. (2006). A randomized clinical trial of clinician feedback to improve quality of care for inner-city children with asthma. *Pediatrics, 117*(6), e1095–1103.

Mason, D. J. (2005). Failure to rescue. After hurricane Katrina, assessing the heroism and the breakdowns. *American Journal of Nursing, 105*(10), 11.

Medina-Ramón, M., Zanobetti, A., & Schwartz, J. (2006). The effect of ozone and PM10 on hospital admissions for pneumonia and chronic obstructive pulmonary disease: A national multicity study. *American Journal of Epidemiology, 163*(6), 579–588. Epub 2006 Jan 27.

Merriam/Webster. (2007). Retrieved on October 31, 2007, from www.merriam-webster.com/dictionary/globalization.

Minnesota Department of Health. Division of Community Health Services. Public Health Nursing Section. (20001). Public health nursing Interventions: Application for public health nursing practice. Minneapolis, Minnesota: Author.

Organisation for Economic Co-operation and Development (OECD). *Glossary of Statistical Terms.* Retrieved on April 14, 2007, from http://stats.oecd.org/glossary/search.asp

Pace, D. (2006). AP: More blacks live with pollution. Retrieved on July 26, 2006, from http://whttp://abcnews.go.com/Health/wireStory?id=1402266ww.comcast.net/includes/Public Health Nursing Interventions. (2001).

Ritz, B., Wilhelm, M.; & Zhao, Y. (2006). Air pollution and infant deaths in southern California, 1989-2000. *Pediatrics, 118,* 493–502.

Rosenberg, J., Gonzalez, M., & Rosenberg, S. (2005). Clinical practice with immigrants and refugees: An ethnographic multicultural approach. In: Congress, E., & Gonzalez, M. (editors) *Multicultural perspectives in working with families. 2nd ed.* New York: Springer Publishing.

Slepski, L.A. (2005). Emergency preparedness: Concept development for nursing practice. *Nursing Clinics of North America, 40*(3), 419–430.

U.S. Department of Health and Human Services. (2000). *Environmental health.* In Healthypeople 2010: I (8th ed.). Washington, DC: Author.

U.S. Department of Health and Human Services. (2005). *HHS pandemic influenza plan.* Retrieved on July 25, 2006, from http://www.hhs.gov/pandemicflu/plan/pdf/HHSPandemicInfluenzaPlan.pdf

Veenema, T. G. (2001). An evidence-based curriculum to prepare students for global nursing practice. *Nursing and Health Care Perspectives, 22*(6), 292–298.

World Health Organization. (2003). *The World Health report 2003– shaping the future.* Retrieved on July 27, 2006, from http://www.who.int/whr/2003/en/

L E A R N I N G ▼ A C T I V I T I E S

◆ JOURNALING ACTIVITY 15-1

In your clinical journal, respond to the following:

- What has surprised you about the information presented in this chapter?
- Discuss your own attitudes and beliefs regarding global health.
- Describe what you learned from reading this chapter.
- Discuss what you thought was important and how it fits into what you have learned so far about the role of the nurse in the community.
- How has your view of the nursing role in the community changed after reading this chapter (and observing the role of the nurse in the community)?

◆ CLIENT CARE ACTIVITY 15-2

Marie is a Central American woman in her mid–30s. She comes to your clinic with a wound on the top of her hand that is red, draining copious green and yellow pus.

As you remove the dirty bandage that is covering the wound you ask her what happened to her hand. She looks down and does not answer your question. You ask her again. When she does not reply, what do you do?

You wonder if she hears you or if she does not speak English.

You ask her in Spanish if she speaks or understands English. She indicates that she does not speak English but understands. You contact an interpreter.

The interpreter arrives 1 hour later. In the meantime you have cleaned and débrided the wound and applied ointment. How do you proceed with the interpreter? (HINT: see Community-Based Nursing Care Guidelines 6-1 Working with Interpreters.)

◆ PRACTICAL APPLICATION ACTIVITY 15-3

Find the WHO web site (http://www.who.int/en). Click on the Countries site. Choose two or three countries and compare the statistics, health expenditures, and provisions/coverage.

- What did you learn? What surprised you?
- What issues did you identify?
- How does this information help you in your practice?
- What do you think that nurses should or can do about the issues you have identified.

◆ PRACTICAL APPLICATION ACTIVITY 15-4

Find an article or book on the Internet on CINAHL or MEDLINE about one of the issues you identified in the previous Practical Application Activity. Respond to the following:

1. What was the main point of the article or chapter from the book?
2. What did you think was the most important aspect of the article or chapter for your learning?
3. How do you think that you can use this new information in the future?

◆ CRITICAL THINKING ACTIVITY 15-5

Find the Global Burden of Disease documents on the WHO Web site at http://www.who.int/en/. Respond to the following questions.

1. What is the intent of this initiative?
2. Explore this site to learn more about health problems based on geographic location and age-gender.
3. Why is this initiative important for global health?
4. Why is it important for the health of citizens in the United States?

◆ SIMULATION ACTIVITY 15-6: OUTBREAK AT WATERSEDGE

http://www.mclph.umn.edu/watersedge/

Follow the link and complete this interactive game. It provides an opportunity to learn about how a disease outbreak is handled by a public health agency. It is an entertaining way to learn what nurses and other public health professionals do in the event of a disease outbreak. Learn how nurses play an important role in determining the source of disease outbreaks in most communities.

Source: Centers for Public Health Education and Outreach (CPHEO) at the University of Minnesota School of Public Health.

◆ SIMULATION ACTIVITY 15-7: DISASTER IN FRANKLIN COUNTY

http://cpheo.sph.umn.edu/umncphp/franklincounty.html

Complete this simulation, where you will assume the perspective of various public health professionals responding to a natural disaster. You will make decisions as would a county public health director, a public health nurse, an environmental health specialist, and other public health professionals. By approaching the emerging public health issues from these perspectives, you will gain a deeper understanding of the issues at hand, the decisions that colleagues in other disciplines face, and how those decisions impact nursing.

Source: Centers for Public Health Education and Outreach (CPHEO) at the University of Minnesota School of Public Health.

◆ LEARNING MODULE ACTIVITY 15-8: WHAT IS PUBLIC HEALTH?

http://cpheo.sph.umn.edu/mclph/course/wiph.html

Complete this module and acquire an in-depth background of the core functions of public health and their impact on primary, secondary, and tertiary prevention of disease and injury. One of the sections discusses the role of public health in emergency preparedness and response. Another provides information about working with diverse populations that will help you build your skills in working with refugee and immigrant populations.

Source: Centers for Public Health Education and Outreach (CPHEO) at the University of Minnesota School of Public Health.

◆ LEARNING MODULE ACTIVITY 15-9: ENVIRONMENTAL HEALTH ONLINE

http://cpheo.sph.umn.edu/mclph/courses/ehn.html

Complete the first section, *Introduction to Environmental Health and Nursing.* This will assist you to develop a framework for integrating environmental health concepts into nursing practice.

Source: Centers for Public Health Education and Outreach (CPHEO) at the University of Minnesota School of Public Health.

IMPLICATIONS FOR FUTURE PRACTICE

N ursing is a profession that is constantly evolving. Any nurse, whether he or she has practiced for years or is just entering the profession, needs to think ahead. What will the trends and patterns in society hold for the future of community-based nursing care? How can you best prepare yourself to give quality care in your future practice?

Chapter 16 reviews anticipated future trends in health care and implications for community-based nursing care. The role of the nurse, including educational preparation, is discussed at length. Cost containment will remain a prominent deciding factor in health care delivery, but it must also be weighed in relation to maintaining quality care. The implications of technologic development and the information age, and their profound impact on everyday nursing care, are discussed. All of these issues are considered in light of the shift in demographics in the United States.

CHAPTER 16 ◆ **Trends in Community-Based Nursing**

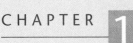
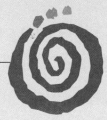

Trends in Community-Based Nursing

ROBERTA HUNT

LEARNING OBJECTIVES

1. Discuss how current trends in community-based nursing will affect the role of the nurse in the future.
2. Determine how market-driven economic policy affects the delivery of nursing care.
3. Discuss the implications of technologic development on health care in general and on the nursing profession specifically.
4. Identify trends in knowledge explosion related to alternative and complementary therapies.
5. Outline how the shift in demographics affects the role of the nurse.
6. Discuss the importance of the nursing competency of civic responsibility.
7. Develop a plan for your personal goals as a nurse in community-based settings.

KEY TERMS

alternative therapies
civic responsibility
complementary therapies
health care organization
integrated health care system
knowledge explosion
market-driven economy

pharmacogenomics
seamless care
service learning
underserved population
underinsured
uninsured

CHAPTER TOPICS

◆ Trends in Health Care
◆ The Future of Nursing Care
◆ Cost Containment
◆ Technology and Information
◆ Alternative and Complementary Therapies
◆ Shifting Demographics
◆ Civic Responsibility
◆ The Future of Community-Based Nursing Care
◆ Conclusions

THE NURSING STUDENT SPEAKS

Completing a rotation in the community has definitely made me realize that I am no longer going to be Elizabeth Wright. I am going to be Elizabeth Wright, RN, and along with that title comes that piece of responsibility. I am no longer just a name; I am a person with a title. In other words, when you think of Dr. Smith, you automatically think that there is an air of power with that title, and I fully intend to use my new power. This is something that became more apparent to me this last semester when I was doing my community rotation. Yes, people look up to someone with a title. I am a role model for people. And I have to be very careful and deliberate in my actions. But it is also very exciting. I always wanted to be a nurse, and I have always wanted to do good and make a positive difference. I have always known that that was possible through nursing. But I think being at a shelter and working as a student in the community has made it much more real for me.

—ELIZABETH WRIGHT, **Nursing Student, College of St. Catherine**

TRENDS IN HEALTH CARE

Forces affecting health care in the future will also affect the role of the nurse. One can only speculate about what that future will be. Some broad changes can almost certainly be predicted. These include: emphasis on cost containment resulting from market-driven economic policy; advancements in technology; knowledge explosion; expanded use of alternative and complementary therapies; and demographic shifts.

Anticipating these trends is imperative to maintaining quality and appropriate nursing service. Curricula in schools of nursing and staff education in the service arena are faced with preparing nurses to meet these changing requirements. Content related to cost containment will be essential. It will be a given that nurses are technologically competent. This means not only being computer competent, but also being able to keep up with new ways of accessing and using information. The knowledge explosion requires that nurses develop skills in evaluating the legitimacy, efficacy, and importance of information and new treatments. All of these changes will occur within the context of shifting demographics as nurses care for a population that is older, more diverse, and living with more chronic conditions. A shortage of nurses and nurse educators creates additional challenges. In this chapter all of these are addressed within the context of community-based care.

THE FUTURE OF NURSING CARE

Several broad competencies will be demanded of nurses in practice in the 21st century. These include critical thinking and clinical judgment skills, effective organizational and teamwork skills, service orientation and cost awareness, accountability for clinical outcomes and quality of care, continuous improvement of health care, population-based approaches to care, an ethic of social responsibility, and commitment to continual learning and development (Bellack & O'Neil, 2000).

Nurses must be prepared to use critical thinking skills to solve problems and make independent clinical judgments regarding care based on the most recent evidence. They must be knowledgeable about making age-appropriate referrals to other disciplines and community agencies. Because more acute care will be provided in the home and clinics, nurses must be more technically advanced in their skills, able to practice autonomously, and adept at detailed documentation to ensure payment for services. As a larger number and percentage of the population are living with chronic conditions and managing symptoms at home, there will be a need for competent, skilled nursing practitioners who are comfortable practicing independently in the area of disease management.

Flexibility will be important because cost-containment measures require decreased specialization. Administrators are introducing multi-skilled health care providers who are cross-trained to practice in a "seamless care" environment, in which practitioners provide care in different facilities or settings. With the trend away from specialization of health care personnel, nurses will be called on to perform more tasks and to cross discipline lines. In home care nursing, this is evidenced by nurses doing venipunctures (a laboratory technician's role) and teaching and monitoring administration of oxygen (a respiratory therapist's role). To prepare for the home care role, nurses must be competent case managers and health educators.

Nurses have a responsibility for advocating for our clients as well as taking the lead in shaping health care in the future. Nurses are fortunate to belong to a profession that commands a high level of credibility and respect seen in the fact that they have consistently been the highest rated profession in Gallup's "honesty and ethics" survey since 1999 (Artz, 2006). This high degree of public support begs the question: "How can nurses use this asset to advocate on behalf on our profession and our clients?" Every day elected officials make decisions that impact our profession and the clients we care for. Registered nurses have the largest number of professionals of all health care professions. There is power in numbers. If nurses were to become involved in the political, legislative, and regulatory processes of government, they could have a significant impact on policy. Nurses should not only know who their elected Congresspeople and Senators are, but also educate these officials about health and the status of health care. Nurses observe on a daily basis clients and families without insurance and the impact that poor health has on individual and family life. Nurses may be forced, because of policy or lack of insurance, to discharge clients home with inadequate resources. Nurses often hear antidotes from clients and families of hospitalizations because of the lack of sufficient health teaching, case management, or continuity. Both anecdotal accounts of what is seen in practice as well as research findings can be shared with officials to affect future legislation on health care reform (Fig. 16-1).

In the last decade, our profession has made major progress in several areas of public policy. The issue of delegating duties to nonlicensed personnel has been addressed and continues to need clarification. Today, advanced practice nurses (APNs) can bill directly through Medicare and in most states can prescribe medication. In some states hospitals are mandated to maintain a safe level of staffing registered nurses based on the research on staffing ratio and hospital mortality. Increasingly, concern about the number and the percentage of Americans without health insurance has lead more states to devise plans to provide primary care to the underinsured or uninsured. All of these policies were shaped by the lobbying efforts of various nursing organizations and numerous individuals.

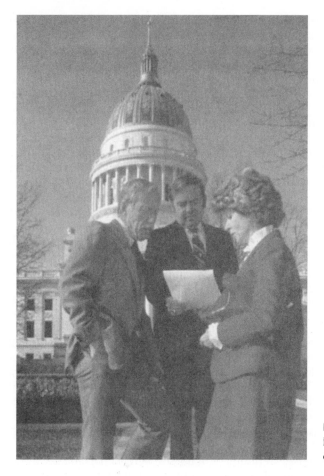

FIGURE 16-1. ▶ Nurses are invaluable sources of health care information for legislators.

There are several ways that nurses can be involved in the political process. The first is to be informed about issues that impact health care and the nursing profession. Visit http://nursingworld.org/MainMenuCategories/ANAPoliticalPower/ ANAPAC.aspx or http://nursingworld.org/MainMenuCategories/ANAPoliticalPower .aspx. Obviously, once informed, everyone must remember to vote. "If only a fraction of our nation's 2.9 million RNs became invoked, our collective voice would be an unstoppable force for change for our profession, our patients, and our nation's crumbling health care system" (Artz, 2006, p 91).

Educational Preparation and Advanced Practice Nursing

If current trends continue, future nurses will perform a wider range of responsibilities. This will require both increased knowledge and skill because community-based care demands a more proficient and autonomous practitioner. The current number of nurses educated at each level of preparation does not support this growing demand. Forty-two percent of all new nurses graduate from an associate degree program; 31% receive baccalaureate degrees and 4% from hospital-based programs (U.S. Department of Health and Human Services [DHHS], 2006b). The need for nurses with a baccalaureate degree will exceed the supply in the first 2 decades of the 21st century. There is a need for more nurses with baccalaureate degrees. The fastest growing nursing programs for undergraduate preparation are those offering a BA/BS in nursing for registered nurses with an ADN degree, and those offering a major in nursing for individuals who have already completed a BS or BA in another discipline.

Currently, there is a great deal of support for APNs or RNs with specialty training at the master's degree level to provide primary care. As early as the 1980s, studies have shown that when comparing the same type of clients, nurse practitioners have as good or better outcomes as physicians. These studies are discussed in Chapter 11. During the early 1990s, state laws broadened the authority of nurse practitioners by allowing prescriptive authority and third-party billing. As a result, nurse practitioners can establish independent practices paralleling those of primary care physicians. This trend is expected to continue.

Specialty areas of nurse practitioners have expanded to numerous subspecialties in the last 3 decades. These include adult, gerontologic, neonatal, occupational, pediatric, psychiatric, school or college student, and women's health. Nurse practitioners work in both rural and urban areas, from rural North Dakota to New York City. They practice in diverse settings such as community health centers, hospitals, college student health clinics, physician offices, nurse practitioner offices, nursing homes and hospices, home health care agencies, and nursing schools.

The most severe shortage of graduate prepared nurses is in nursing education. With a large percentage of nurse educators anticipated to retire in the next decade, this trend is expected to continue and accelerate. Further there is an established need for practitioners with an interest in research and advanced practice at the master's and doctoral levels. Nursing administrators must be educated and trained in management, finance, and the economic and social implications of our changing population as it affects the health care system.

Trends call for all nurses to be well prepared for the current and future practice roles. Nurses must view education as a lifelong process, not limited to a job entry degree. Continuing education is essential as the care delivery system demands more education, including baccalaureate, graduate, and postgraduate degrees. In most areas of the country, the curriculum at each level lays the groundwork for the next level of education, facilitating ongoing nursing education.

COST CONTAINMENT

The U.S. health care system is the most expensive in the world, using over 15% of the gross national product (GNP), yet ranks behind most other industrialized countries in virtually every measure of health (Johnson, 2006). Further, only half of U.S. adults receive preventive and screening tests. Every industrialized nation except the United States has a national health plan in place that covers all citizens. However, in the United States, health care is not a right but a commodity available to those who can purchase it, sold as a part of a **market-driven economy**. In a market-driven economy, consumer demand drives production regarding what services will be created and consumed and in what quantity. Keeping costs down and profits up is always a key aspect of a market-driven economy. Managed care has increasingly become an important provider of care because its central element is cost containment. Thus, cost containment as an important element of health care is here to stay. Consequently, nurses must continue to be aware of the financial aspects of the work they do, whatever the setting or position, now and in the future.

TECHNOLOGY AND INFORMATION

Technologic Development

The health care system of the future will be driven by technology and information. Technology is the tool to extend human abilities. Technology will be used to manage information and make decisions about care. Such technology may include medications, procedures, devices, and electronically-based systems that support care delivery. Already clients are wearing programmable medication administration pumps. Nurses will need to program and troubleshoot such machines. These models will evolve constantly. The most promising advances are those related to high-speed telecommunications and portable computers. At present, it is possible to link a desktop computer to a modem and standard telephone line to transmit radiographs, computed tomography images, electrocardiograms, electroencephalograms, and health histories instantly. The potential for improving continuity is important.

Several trends are shaping technology in health care. One trend is that of globalization. This started at the beginning of the 20th century with the invention of the telephone and was expanded at the end of the 20th century with expansion of personal computers and the creation of the Internet. Gradually, the world's borders have dissolved as the world has become one. Thanks to telephones, telecommunications, and telemedicine, nurses are now able to practice across geographic and national borders. Physicians and health care organizations are using globalization to export expertise, a practice that has accelerated because of concerns for cost and profit. Through the construction of systems, health care providers, intermediaries, and consumers are able to collaborate and share information. Further, through technology, we now have the capability to maintain comprehensive health care databases for creating disease-management programs and clinical protocols. In addition, through telemedicine and remote-monitoring technologies, health care providers are able to access health information 24 hours a day, 7 days a week.

Personal health records are one important application of multiple technologies. The value of personal health records was evident after Hurricane Katrina in 2005 when hundreds of thousands of health records were destroyed. There are three major approaches to electronic personal health records. One is a provider-owned and -maintained digital summary of clinically relevant health information available to clients and providers. A second is a client-owned software program designed for individuals to enter, organize, and retrieve health information and capture client concerns, problems, symptoms, and emergency contact information. A third type of personal health record is a portable, interoperable digital file that allows clinically relevant health data to be managed, secured, and transferred. This portable personal health record may be operated on smart cards, personal digital assistants, and cellular phones (Endsley, et al., 2006).

For the last 4 decades, the focus of health care has been the aggressive treatment of acute episodes of illness. We have enhanced this capacity through technology. Although "recovery" from an acute situation may result in a long-term chronic condition, technologic assistance is continuing to be developed to enhance care for the rest of a client's life. What occurred in the intensive care unit yesterday may occur at home tomorrow. With the increase in available technology, care can be provided at an ever higher level of sophistication in the home. If respirators, intravenous therapy, and home dialysis are now common, what will technology allow in the future? It is anticipated that advancements in technology will improve the quality and efficiency of client care, raise the general health care status of the nation's population, and reduce the overall cost of health care.

Knowledge Explosion

The **knowledge explosion** has produced what is often referred to as the information age. Genetics is one area in which the information explosion is particularly evident. Because of the completion in 2000 of part of the Human Genome Project, which has mapped the human genetic code, treatments will be possible that were not even considered within the realm of possibility 10 years ago. For example, **pharmacogenomics** is the technology of developing and producing medications tailored to specific genetic profiles. The physician or nurse practitioner would give a genetic blood test that would indicate which medication was right for each person. This has led to an increased integration of diagnostics and pharmaceuticals. With this emergence of co-developed products between the areas of diagnostics and drugs there will be a need for new regulatory models. For example, biotech companies are developing blood tests that reveal disease–gene mutations that forecast an individual's chances of developing a certain condition or disease. The rapid development of technology in health care creates numerous ethical questions. Often the technology is ready for use before these ethical issues are fully explored (Phillips, 2006). Further, the exponential availability of medical technology drives consumer expectations and demands.

Major scientific developments have been occurring so quickly that knowledge overload is common. In the past, clients and families have consulted their nurses, nurse practitioners, or physicians for information regarding health and illness. The health care provider has carried that information in his or her head, or has known where to go to explore the question. Now, an almost infinite amount of information is available to anyone who is computer-literate. This causes difficulty for the consumer as well as the health care provider. Not only is the amount of information overwhelming, but also it is difficult to discern what is outdated, incorrect, or unproven information, and what is not. Therefore, it is important for the health care provider and the consumer to realize that being information-literate is an ongoing process.

Nursing Implications

Computer technology has freed the nurse from some paperwork, allowing more time for client care and teaching about self-care. The expanding implementation of computer-based client records allows the preservation of a client's history from birth to death.

Automation in home care is viewed as a way to improve efficiency. Recent developments in information technology offer a variety of alternatives for documentation. For instance, the use of handheld computers for field staff is a growing trend. Here, the practitioner inputs clinical, financial, and administrative data, and the system produces appropriate reports and forms. These systems are capable of redefining the data content, structure, and preconceptions about clinical information, client assessment, care planning, and care delivery. Nurses chart information directly on a terminal or laptop computer with no need for writing copious notes, charting from memory, or carrying around stacks of papers. Data entry is done through the keyboard, mouse, touch screen, voice activation, bar code, or pen touch. The system can alert nurses about inconsistencies in the data or the need to collect more information, generate a time-based report, or create a task list for each client. A growing number of manufacturers produce this developing technology that integrates data with a central system, facilitates the tracking of specific costs, and allows the client to interact with the system and retrieve information regarding care.

Imagine working as a home health care nurse, transmitting pertinent diagnostic data directly to the attending physician and having a three-way interaction with the client, physician, and nurse instantly. It has become common for nurses to electronically connect with client databases to obtain information from the client's complete nursing, medical, diagnostic, medication, and treatment history. Nurses are also able to order online prescriptions or home care equipment.

As a result of the explosion in information, people have access to near-infinite amounts of information. Many diagnostic kits will become available in the consumer market. The nurse may be called on to interpret or explain the results. Misinformation and misunderstanding by the consumer may be possible, which will require another service of the nurse. As self-care becomes a social norm, many individuals are finding information related to health promotion, disease prevention and management on the Web. There are numerous benefits to this type of resource for health education. At the same time, there are issues including quality and validity of the information on the various Web sites. Box 16-1 provides a guide for evaluating health resources on the Web.

There are some important questions to ponder regarding use of technology. Are educational programs for nurses preparing adequately for using technology? Are nurses comfortable moving into a present and future dominated by information systems? Educational institutions must have exit criteria that at a minimum ensure computer skills including ability to use the Internet for accessing health information. Faculty members benefit from continually updating their skills in

---

◆ **B O X 16-1** Things to Know about Evaluating Health Resources on the Web ◆

- Who runs the site?
- Who pays for the site?
- What is the purpose of the site?
- Where does the information come from?
- How is the information selected?
- How current is the information?
- How does the site choose links to other sites?
- What information about you does the site collect, and why?
- How does the site manage interactions with visitors?

Source: National Center for Complementary and Alternative Medicine. (2006). *Get the facts: 10 things to know about evaluating medical resources on the web.* Retrieved on November 1, 2007, from http://nccam.nih.gov/health/webresources/

computers and other technology. The profession of nursing has to have an impact on the future of home care.

ALTERNATIVE AND COMPLEMENTARY THERAPIES

Twenty years ago, **alternative** and **complementary therapies** were considered fringe treatments by most Western health care practitioners. However, consumers wanted more choices for treatment and more control over their care. As a result of unpleasant side effects from conventional therapies and a growing skepticism about Western medicine, consumers have turned in larger numbers to other treatment modalities. Large numbers of individuals have used alternative therapies for at least the last 2 decades, as seen in the classic studies done in 1993 and 1998 by Eisenberg and colleagues (Eisenberg, et al., 1993, 1998). These studies reported that one third of persons contacted in a national survey had used unconventional therapy in the past year. Total out-of-pocket expenditure for alternative therapies was estimated at $10.3 billion in 1990, compared with $12.8 billion for all hospital care in the United States that year. In 1998, Eisenberg found that the out-of-pocket expenditure for alternative therapies was $21.2 billion. Alternative therapies are increasingly being valued and used by nurses and other health care providers.

Alternative therapies are generally defined treatment that is an alternative to Western modalities, while complementary therapies complement other treatments. However, in this discussion they will be used interchangeably. There is a basic distinction between alternative and complementary therapies and Western medicine. Western medicine bases care on the disease model and the nature of pathology, whereas alternative therapies address holistic functioning within the social and environmental context, not focusing only on the function of the organs.

Nursing Implications

To follow the holistic perspective, nurses must be knowledgeable about alternative therapies. With such knowledge, they can monitor care and treatment and provide information about benefits and potential harm for clients. The National Institutes of Health has categorized alternative modalities and therapies into major types of modalities seen in Box 16-2. Nurses benefit from education and training in multiple alternative/complementary therapies.

It is always essential that the client discuss with his or her primary caregiver any over-the-counter medication, or alternative or complementary therapies he or she may be taking concurrently with Western medicines or treatments. Many alternative or complementary therapies may either potentiate or diminish the impact of medications or other treatments. To ensure maximum efficacy of all treatment modalities, the use of alternative or complementary therapies and Western medicine should always be coordinated with the primary health care provider.

Alternative and complementary therapies have gained respect and recognition from the general public and medical professionals as more is known about efficacy. Medical and nursing educators are beginning to integrate alternative and complementary therapies into medical and nursing curricula. In the future, nurses will increasingly be called on to provide knowledge about and use of alternative therapies. Therefore, it is imperative that nurses continue to build their knowledge and skill base about alternative therapies. As the population becomes more

> ◆ **BOX 16-2** Major Types of Complementary and Alternative Therapies ◆
>
> **Alternative Systems** are systems built on theory and practice that have evolved apart from and earlier than the conventional medical approach used in the United States. Examples include homeopathic and naturopathic medicine, and traditional Chinese medicine.
>
> **Mind–Body Therapies** are techniques designed to enhance the mind's capacity to affect bodily function and symptoms. These include the commonly used patient support group and cognitive-behavioral therapy as well as meditation, prayer, mental healing, and creative arts such as art, music, or dance.
>
> **Biologically Based Therapies** are those substances found in nature, such as herbs, foods, and vitamins. Examples include dietary supplements and herbal products.
>
> **Manipulative and Body-Based Methods** are therapies that are based on manipulation and/or movement of one or more parts of the body. Examples include chiropractic or osteopathic manipulation and massage.
>
> **Energy Therapies** consist of two types. One is biofield therapies that are intended to affect energy fields that purportedly surround and penetrate the human body. Examples are qi gong, Reiki, and Therapeutic Touch. Bioelectromagnetic based therapies involve the unconventional use of electromagnetic fields, alternating current or direct current fields.
>
> Source: National Center for Complementary and Alternative Medicine. National Institute of Health. *What is complementary and alternative medicine?* Retrieved on November 21, 2006, from http://www.nccam.nih.gov/health/whatiscam/

diverse ethnically, it is anticipated that more methods of promoting health and treating illness will be necessary.

For the person who feels intimidated and dehumanized by the sterility and businesslike environment of most Western medical facilities, the warm, personal caring and concern of alternative practitioners may be therapeutic (Fig. 16-2). Because stress and anxiety are major factors in many illnesses, the soothing environment and supportive attitude of alternative practice and practitioners have contributed to their appeal.

Research provides evidence that some alternative therapies enhance health and promote recovery from illness for both the client and family caregivers (Research in Community-Based Nursing Care 16-1). While some caregivers still support only Western methods of health care and continue to ignore or repudiate the value of more traditional or alternative methods, the use of these practices has persisted and grown because people find them useful. Acknowledging the full breadth of services that individuals use, and working with them, is more productive than ignoring what the client chooses to do in the quest for wholeness and health.

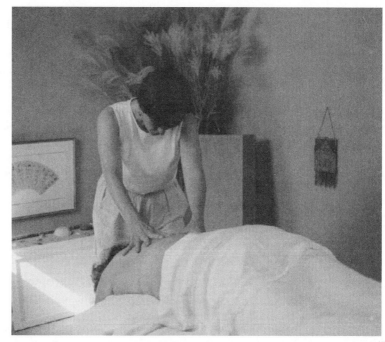

FIGURE 16-2. ▶ One complementary therapy is neuromuscular and therapeutic massage.

RESEARCH IN COMMUNITY-BASED NURSING CARE ▶ 16-1

Transcendental Meditation May Improve Blood Pressure and Insulin Resistance

In a randomized clinical trial, stable individuals with coronary heart disease (CHD) practiced transcendental meditation (TM), while the control group received health education matched for frequency and time. The TM group participated in two introductory lectures, a personal interview, personal instruction, three group meetings and follow-up meetings twice a week for 4 weeks, and then weekly meetings. Participants receiving health education attended the same number of sessions focused on stress management, diet, and exercise, facilitated by experienced health educators. Blood pressure, lipoprotein profile, and insulin resistance were compared before and after both interventions. After 16 weeks, the group practicing TM had beneficial changes in blood pressure and insulin resistance when compared to the group receiving health education.

Source: Paul-Labrador, M., Polk, D., Dwyer, J. H., et al. (2006). Effects of a randomized controlled trial of transcendental meditation on components of the metabolic syndrome in subjects with coronary heart disease. *Archives of Internal Medicine, 166,* 1218-1224.

However, because alternative and complementary therapies are an unregulated industry, care should be taken before recommending or utilizing them. One study designed to determine the chemical components of herbal medicines found that 20% of the samples purchased in the United States contained levels of lead, mercury, and arsenic high enough to cause heavy metal toxicity (Kales, et al., 2004). The authors recommended that testing of herbal medicine for toxic heavy metals should be mandatory. Empirical research of the benefit and harm of complementary and alternative medicine is in its infancy. The potential for harm should always be a part of the risk-benefit analysis, with some interventions such as massage and acupuncture presenting less risk as compared to those ingested, such as herbal medications. Nurses can begin to broaden their perspectives about different health care therapies by addressing their own bodies, minds, and spirit issues. It is possible to work successfully with clients who use alternative approaches.

CLIENT SITUATIONS IN PRACTICE

◆ When the Nurse Has Not Been Exposed to Alternative Therapies

Lisa is a 29-year-old woman who delivered a healthy, 9-lb, 10-oz baby boy 2 weeks ago. The home health care nurse makes a home visit. Lisa complains about continued perineal discomfort with no unusual discharge or odor. The nurse suggests hydrocortisone cream and suppositories. Lisa says that she wants to avoid steroid creams and asks if there is an alternative. The nurse is concerned but states that she cannot provide her with any other suggestions. The only things that work, she says, are hydrocortisone and time, and Lisa should adhere to the medications that are known to be effective. Lisa is left feeling insecure and unsatisfied, without a remedy for her discomfort.

Aromatherapy, the use of essential oils with diverse medicinal qualities, was shown over a decade ago to help in the treatment of a range of conditions, including perineal discomfort (Dale & Cornwell, 1994). If the home health care nurse had interest and training in alternative therapies, she may have been better equipped to care for her client. When the nurse is willing to acknowledge the client's philosophy and values, the client may be willing to consider what the nurse has to offer for the client's care.

SHIFTING DEMOGRAPHICS

The number and proportion of older people continues to increase. Life expectancies at ages 65 and 85 have increased over the past 50 years. People who live to age 65 can expect to live, on average, nearly 18 more years. Since 1900, the percentage of the population older than 65 years has tripled, and this growth is expected to continue. In 1994, about one in eight Americans were elderly but about one in five will be elderly by the year 2030 as the postwar baby boom generation will move into the 65-and-older age group. In addition, the elderly population will continue to be more and more diverse (Hobbs, 2006).

In North America, cultural diversity continues to increase. In 1900, about one out of eight Americans was of a race other than White. By 2000, about one out of four Americans was of a race other than White. Figure 16-3 shows the change in

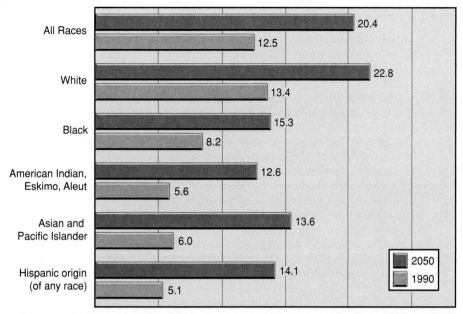

FIGURE 16-3. ▶ Percent of the elderly by race and Hispanic origin: U.S., 1990 and 2050. Source: Hobbs, F. (2006). *The elderly population.* United States Census Bureau. Retrieved on October 20, 2006, from http://www.census.gov/population/www/pop-profile/elderpop.html.

the percentage of the population by race from 1950 projected to 2050. At the same time, between 1960 and 2005, the health disparity between Whites and Blacks in the United States as seen in the mortality rates has changed very little and worsened for Black infants and Black men age 35 and over (Satcher, et al., 2005). If the Black-White health disparity gap were closed it would eliminate 83,000 excess deaths per year among African Americans.

People living longer with more chronic conditions require an increased use of health care resources. It is estimated that over half of the older population reported having a least one disability, with more than 37% reporting at least one severe disability. Because the percentages with disabilities increase sharply with age, disability takes a heavier toll on the very old. Of people older than 70 years, 80% have one or more chronic conditions. This is one of the rationales for more emphasis on health promotion and disease prevention; because without intervention, it is likely that as this group ages, the percentage of the elderly population with chronic conditions will increase exponentially (Administration on Aging, 2005). This growing segment of the population has health care needs that are different from those of other segments of the population.

The nursing shortage is the latest demographic trend that will impact community-based care in the future. One national survey of RNs indicated that 82% of nurses reported a shortage in their hospital or community. These nurses did not have positive expectations of the impact of the shortage on work conditions, believing that some tasks currently assigned to nurses will shift to other staff. They anticipate the shortage will result in nurses leaving nursing for non-nursing jobs, thus intensifying the shortage. These changes could result in lower quality of care provided (Buerhaus, et al., 2006).

Nursing Implications

Because community-based nursing practice will be central to the care of a population of aging and chronically ill people, nurses will be confronted with many challenges. Providing nursing care to diverse populations has been discussed throughout this text and will increasingly be an issue for nurses.

In the future, regardless of the nurse's own ethnic background, the nurse must be proficient at transcultural nursing to be an effective caregiver. Nurses will play a major role in promoting self-care and addressing health promotion and disease prevention issues for elderly clients. A larger proportion of the nurse's caseload will include individuals with chronic, disabling conditions. Promoting self-care and health promotion and disease prevention with this population entails skills and knowledge that are different from those needed for clients having an acute episode of a resolvable condition.

Continuity is more complex in cross-cultural nursing. Every decision hinges on the cultural context of the issue. Also, it is often more difficult to enhance continuity with older clients who may have a weak support system or multiple chronic conditions that impair mobility or sensory perception than it is for a middle-aged client with a spouse.

Collaboration is even more important when working with diverse populations. Collaboration across disciplines is always challenging, but it is particularly so if the interdisciplinary team members are from several cultural backgrounds.

CIVIC RESPONSIBILITY

The Pew Health Professions Commission's 21 competencies for the 21st century are shown in Box 1–2 in Chapter 1. It is easy to see how these competencies follow the trends discussed in this chapter. The first competency is "embrace a personal ethic of social responsibility and service." Health care is a commodity that a growing number of individuals and families have limited or no access to. This growing **underserved population** would benefit from additional access to nursing service. The competency of **civic responsibility** is intended to serve individuals who are **uninsured** or **underinsured**.

One way to cultivate this competency is through volunteerism. Nurses, students, and nursing faculty must make a sustained commitment to community well-being through direct service. By carefully exploring options, students may find that by volunteering in a community-based setting, they expand their skills and knowledge base in ways that they do not in a traditional clinical setting.

A second way to develop the competency of social responsibility is through **service learning** experiences that are structured to combine learning and volunteering. Service learning experiences can be valuable to develop empathy, social awareness, and social and cultural competence. Students can take the initiative to learn while volunteering by taking an internship or independent study in an area of community health that interests them.

Another way to becoming more socially responsible is by understanding the impact that public policy has on the individuals included or excluded from that policy. For example, a nurse volunteers in his community with homeless youth. He see first-hand the positive impact that having emergency housing in his community has on directing some of the homeless youth he works with to access community resources. He notes that youth who are referred to certain services in the community are less likely to become permanently homeless, more likely to complete high school, and more likely to adopt a more stable lifestyle. When the funding in his state for emergency housing for homeless youth is scheduled to be cut, the nurse sends a letter to his State Legislator and Governor. In this letter the nurse describes the lives that he has seen changed through participation in the programs at the emergency shelter. He includes some numerical data that supports his observations (i.e., number of teens that graduate from high school or technical training as a result of participating in the programs). The nurse relates the impact that the program cuts will have on the youth who do not receive assistance. If the funding for homeless youth in this example was affected by federal policy, the nurse may contact his Senator or Congressman with similar information.

There is a large number and percentage of the population, including individuals of all ages, in many cities, states, and the United States at large who do not receive the basic services and opportunities necessary to sustain health. Basic services include sufficient food, a livable-wage job, safe housing, adequate education, and access to health care. Volunteering provides the opportunity to consider the context in which some of the social issues facing our society develop and what our responsibility as a registered nurse is to right these wrongs. Ask yourself what system issues contribute to social issues in my community?

THE FUTURE OF COMMUNITY-BASED NURSING CARE

Cost containment will continue to be a driving force for health care services, challenging nurses to be flexible, autonomous, and creative in their thinking. The current decrease in specialization calls for flexibility in the performance of roles across disciplines and the articulation of nursing as a profession. This requires the nurse to encourage clients and families to maximize their independence and follow through with self-care in all aspects of their lives. The educational preparation of the nurse will determine tasks; however, this may involve a broad range of activities from the simple to the complex. More education will be necessary for some who are required to perform, teach, and oversee complicated care. Further, as in most professions, nurses benefit from continually updating their skills and knowledge related to emerging technology in health care.

Self-Care

In the future, the number of clients requiring assistance with self-care will grow as the percentage of the population with chronic disease increases. Self-care requires the nurse to recognize that assessment, planning, intervention, and evaluation revolve around the question, "How much care can the client and caregivers safely provide on their own?"

Self-care is especially challenging when the client is older or is from a culture different from the nurse. The nurse of the future must be equipped to enhance the self-care skills of the client who is likely to be aging, from a different culture, and coping with several chronic conditions.

Self-care in the future will require mastery of an increasingly complex technology. To manage at home with a chronic health problem, the client and family caregiver will have to use complicated monitors and life-sustaining medical equipment, while the nurse uses sophisticated telecommunications devices to access information and transmit client data to the agency, attending physician, or nurse practitioner.

Preventive Care

The future focus of health care will be on treatment efficacy rather than technologic imperative. This promotes preventive nursing care, as discussed in Chapter 2. Community-based nursing considers all three levels of prevention. Focusing on prevention will be particularly challenging as the percentage of the population ages and is living with chronic conditions. Growing trends in alternative health therapies allow more culturally sensitive options in preventive care.

Health care's focus on cost-containment challenges the nurse to use prevention strategies to reduce costs. This is as true in the hospital as in other community-based settings. Rather than being seen as expensive baggage that can be eliminated, nurses need to be seen as the key to holding down health care costs. This concept has been discussed throughout this book but will require numerous initiatives of creative application in the future.

There are different ways that nurses can operationalize the concepts of health promotion and disease prevention in community-based nursing. Nurses can position themselves as the first link between clients and the hospital, thus developing long-term relationships. This involves developing systems and models of care that require periodically contacting clients with chronic problems. For example, nurses can develop telephone triage services for the hospital by fielding calls, referring clients to more cost-effective services, and reducing the number of unnecessary visits to emergency departments. In addition, nurses can be proactive by contacting clients about immunizations and screening programs or fielding calls about medication administration, dressing changes, or proper diet. They can help correct problems before they become serious or identify already serious problems that need immediate care rather than postponed service. For example, nurses can develop and implement educational programs on drug counseling, substance abuse, birth control, diet, and prenatal and well-baby care, as well as self help groups. Or nurses can contact aging clients routinely to identify health problems at early stages and to eliminate some physician visits that are motivated by loneliness and boredom.

Care Within the Context of Community

Earlier chapters explained the value of the community in providing health care, and Chapter 3 discussed the cultural aspects of community-based nursing. Nursing care must be provided within this cultural context, taking into consideration the strengths and resources of the client, family, and community. As the population ages, this challenge will be further complicated by the demands of technology. Acceptance of alternative methods of care will allow care within the context of the client's family and community, including, in many cases, popular and folk healers. Because the racial and ethnic face of the nation is changing, nurses will be required to speak languages other than English or to be knowledgeable about using interpreters. The nurse may need to carry a card explaining to non–English-speaking clients that it is their right to have interpretation services provided at no charge. Nurses should also encourage representatives of minority groups to enter the nursing profession.

Continuity of Care and Collaborative Care

The hospital of the future may be known as a **health care organization** or an **integrated health care system**. These systems already exist in many parts of the country. More community-based care programs will come from these integrated systems. Another term used is **seamless care**, in which all levels of care are available in an integrated form. Continuity allows quality care to be preserved in a changing health care delivery system. It is an essential component of cost containment and prevents duplication of services, re-hospitalization, and inappropriate use of services. An older, more diverse population will provide challenges to the nurse as continuous care becomes the expected norm.

As a result of increased use of alternative therapies, the importance of continuity is evident. It will be essential for traditional and nontraditional providers to respect one another's contributions to the client's care and to communicate and coordinate care effectively.

CONCLUSIONS

Cost-effective and quality health care accessible to everyone remains at the forefront of health care goals for the 21st century. In addition, flexibility will be an important aspect of community-based care. Ongoing professional development will be imperative to keep pace with the professional demands of community-based nursing. The nurse of the future must be equipped to care for the client who is likely to be aging, from a different culture, and coping with several chronic conditions. It will be essential for traditional and nontraditional providers to respect one another's contributions to the client's care and to communicate effectively. Trends in alternative methods of healing allow more culturally sensitive options.

The nature and scope of nursing are broader than any one setting in which care is offered. Nursing care has remained constant in its philosophy over the decades. However, nurses must now adapt their care delivery models to include clients in acute care settings, long-term care, ambulatory settings, and the home. Nurses follow the standards of nursing care in all settings. In the future, this will require a more educated, autonomous, and competent nurse.

What's on the Web

Alternative Medicine Homepage
Internet address:
http://www.pitt.edu/~cbw/altm.html
This site, maintained by the Falk Library of the Health Sciences at the University of Pittsburgh, is a starting point for sources of information on alternative therapies.

American Botanical Council
Internet address:
http://www.herbalgram.org
This site is dedicated to providing current and accurate information on herbal medicine. There is an educational link that consumers may find helpful. On this site are a variety of accredited continuing education modules for professionals interested in learning more about the safety and efficacy of herbal products.

American Medical Informatics Association
Nursing Informatics Work Group
Internet address: http://www.amia.org/mbrcenter/wg/ni/news.asp
This organization's goal is to promote the advancement of nursing informatics within an interdisciplinary context. This goal is pursued in professional practice, education, research, and governmental and other service.

Online Journal of Issues in Nursing
Internet address:
http://www.nursingworld.org/ojin
This online publication provides a forum for discussion of current issues in nursing.

National Center for Complementary and Alternative Medicine (NCCAM)
NCCAM Clearinghouse
P.O. Box 7923
Gaithersburg, MD 20898
Telephone: (888) 644-6226
TTY/TDT: (888)464-3615
Fax: (301) 495-4957
Internet address:
http://www.nccam.nih.gov
The NCCAM at the National Institutes of Health (NIH) conducts and supports basic and applied research on complementary and alternative therapies. This site disseminates information on complementary and alternative interventions to practitioners and the public. This is an excellent site for current, reliable information based on research.

General Web Resources
Internet address: http://www.adam.com
This is a commercial site that provides health and wellness information.

Aetna InteliHealth
Internet address:
http://www.intelihealth.com
This site provides physician-reviewed, consumer-friendly articles; online communities; and a medical dictionary. The "Ask the Expert" feature is popular.

American Heart Association
Internet address:
http://www.americanheart.org
This Web page contains information related to heart health, support group links, licensed products and services, and science and research. There is an excellent client and caregiver education area, "Heart Failure," at http://www.americanheart.org/presenter.jhtml?identifier=1486

American Lung Association
Internet address: http://www.lungusa.org

This site contains information on lung disease in all forms, with special emphasis on asthma, tobacco control, and environmental health.

The Body: The Complete HIV/AIDS Resource
Internet address: http://www.thebody.com
This site is a comprehensive resource with information on the disease processes of acquired immunodeficiency syndrome (AIDS) and human immunodeficiency virus (HIV). It discusses safe sex, support group treatment, mental health, and legal and financial issues from a variety of sites and links.

National Cancer Institute
Internet address:
http://www.cancernet.nci.nih.gov
Maintained by the National Cancer Institute, this site has extensive credible information on cancer, reviewed by oncology experts and based on research.

Health on the Net Foundation
Internet address: http://www.hon.ch
This international initiative has a multilingual search engine for information on health and health care.

Health Promotion Online
Internet address: http://www.hc-sc.gc.ca/hppb/hpo/index.html
This Canadian site addresses a wide range of health promotion and disease prevention programs. It also offers content in French.

Health Resources on IHP Net
Internet address:
http://www.ihpnet.org/4listserv.htm
Designed to save time, this site provides direct routes to health information.

Healthfinder
Internet address:
http://www.healthfinder.gov
This site from the DHHS leads to publications, clearinghouses, databases, Web sites, and support and self-help groups, as well as providing reliable information.

Healthy People 2010
Internet address:
http://web.health.gov/healthypeople
This site provides access to all of the
Healthy People 2010 (DHHS, 2000a)
documents and initiatives.

Lippincott Williams & Wilkins
Internet address: http://www.lww.com
Lippincott Williams & Wilkins leads in the
world of information resources for nursing, medical, and allied health professionals and students.

March of Dimes
Internet address: http://www.modimes.org
This organization focuses on issues
related to prenatal care and prevention of
birth defects, infant mortality, and low-
birth-weight infants. The Web site includes
information on research, programs, and
public affairs.

MayoClinic.com
Internet address:
http://www.mayohealth.org
Sponsored by the Mayo Clinic, this site
features reliable information on a variety
of health issues with resources for each.

McGill Medical Informatics
Internet address: http://www.mmi.mcgill.ca
This Canada-wide database for medical
teaching and learning has a wide variety of
medical information.

Medscape
Internet address:
http://www.medscape.com
This commercial site is a professional
site built around practice-oriented
information.

National Institutes of Health (NIH)
Internet address: http://www.nih.gov
The NIH Web site is an excellent all-
around resource for nurses from all
specialties. It contains news and events,
health information, grants, scientific
resources, and links to other sites, including the National Institute of Nursing
Research and the W.G. Magnuson Clinical
Center Nursing Department.

National Institutes of Health
Warren Grant Magnuson Clinical Center
Nursing Department
Internet address:
http://www.cc.nih.gov/nursing
This site provides links to federal
resources, Internet search engines, and
other useful resources. This nursing-
specific site provides information from
universities, the Centers for Disease
Control and Prevention, and the National
Institute of Nursing Research.

National League for Nursing
Internet address: http://www.nln.org
A resource for nursing education, practice,
and research, this site has the latest
information about the organization and
nursing in general.

National Women's Health Information
Center (NWHIC)
Internet address:
http://www.womenshealth.gov
The NWHIC is a free information and
resource service on women's health issues
for consumers, health care professionals,
researchers, educators, and students. This
bilingual site (English and Spanish) contains a wealth of information on health
issues that is free of copyright restrictions
and may be copied.

OncoLink
Internet address:
http://www.oncolink.upenn.edu
This site is maintained by the University
of Pennsylvania's Abramson Cancer Center. It contains news, education on treatment options, reporting on clinical trials,
psychosocial support through an active
online community, and resources such as
associations, support groups, online
journals, and book reviews.

Planned Parenthood
Internet address:
http://www.plannedparenthood.org
In both Spanish and English, this Web site
includes legislative updates, statistics,
newsletters, and a library with information
on family planning.

PubMed
Internet address:
http://www.ncbi.nlm.nih.gov/entrez/
query.fcgi
This search service of the National Library of Medicine provides access to more than 10 million citations.

RealAge
Internet address: http://www.realage.com
This commercial site provides news, an online support community, and interactive health assessment tools.

Sudden Infant Death Syndrome and Other Infant Death (SIDS/OID) Information Web Site
Internet address: http://sids-network.org
At this site, you will find up-to-date information about SIDS.

Transcultural Nursing
Internet address:
http://www.culturediversity.org

This site's goal is to provide information about transcultural nursing to help other nurses understand behavior and its cultural basis.

U.S. Department of Health and Human Services
Internet address: http://www.dhhs.gov
This site provides links to numerous health resources from the federal government.

U.S. National Library of Medicine
Internet address: http://www.nlm.nih.gov
The U.S. National Library of Medicine is the world's largest medical library.

World Health Organization
Internet address: http://www.who.int/en
This is the Web site of the international World Health Organization, which is committed to the attainment of the highest possible level of health for everyone worldwide.

References and Bibliography

Administration on Aging. (2005). *A profile of older Americans: 2005.* Retrieved on October 20, 2006, from http://www.aoa.gov/PROF/Statistics/profile/2005/2005profile.pdf

Artz, M. (2006). Ask not what nursing can do for you... Nurses have a lot of power. *American Journal of Nursing, 106*(9), 91.

Bellack, J. P., & O'Neil, E. H. (2000). Recreating nursing practice for a new century. Recommendations and implications of the Pew Health Professions Commission's final report. *Nursing and Health Care Perspectives, 21*(1), 15–21.

Buerhaus, P. I., Donelan, K., Ulrich, B. T., Norman, L., & Dittus, R. (2006). State of the registered nurse workforce in the United States. *Nursing Economics, 24*(1), 6–12.

Dale, A., & Cornwell, S. (1994). The role of lavender oil in relieving perineal discomfort following childbirth: A blind randomized clinical trial. *Journal of Advanced Nursing, 19*(1), 89–96.

Eisenberg, D. M., Davis, R. B., Ettner, S. L., et al. (1998). Trends in alternative medicine use in the United States, 1990–1997: Results of a follow-up national survey.

Journal of the American Medical Association, 280(18), 1569–1575.

Eisenberg, D. M., Kessler, R. C., Foster, C., et al. (1993). Unconventional medicine in the United States. Prevalence, costs, and patterns of use. *New England Journal of Medicine, 328,* 246–252.

Endsley, S., Kibbbe, D. C., Linares, A., & Colorafi, K. (2006). An introduction to personal health records. *Family Practice Management, 13*(5), 57–62.

Hobbs, F. (2006). *The elderly population.* United States Census Bureau. Retrieved on October 20, 2006, from http://www.census.gov/population/www/pop-profile/elderpop.html

Johnson, T. (2006). U.S. not getting good value for its health care investment. *The Nation's Health, 36*(9), 6.

Kales, S. N., Paquin, J., Burns, M. J., et al. (2004). Heavy metal content of ayurvedic herbal medicine product. *Journal of the American Medical Association, 292*(23), 2868–2873.

National Center for Complementary and Alternative Medicine. National Institutes of Health. (2006a). *What is CAM?* Retrieved November 22, 2006, from http://www.nccam.nih.gov/health/whatiscam/

National Center for Complementary and Alternative Medicine. (2006b). Get the facts: 10 things to know about evaluating medical resources on the web. Retrieved on November 22, 2006, from http://nccam.nih.gov/health/webresources/

Paul-Labrador, M., Polk, D., Dwyer, J. H., et al. (2006). Effects of a randomized controlled trail of transcendental meditation on components of the metabolic syndrome in subjects with coronary heart disease. *Archives of Internal Medicine, 166*, 1218–1224.

Phillips, K. A. (2006). The intersection of biotechnology and pharmacogenomics: Health policy implications. *Health Affairs (Millwood), 25(5)*, 1271–1280.

Satcher, D., Fryer, G. E., Jr., et al. (2005). What if we were equal? A comparison of the black-white mortality gap in 1960 and 2000. *Health Affairs (Millwood), 24(2)*, 459–464.

U.S. Department of Health and Human Services. (2000a). *Healthy people 2010* (Conference edition I & II). Washington, DC: U.S. Government Printing Office.

U.S. Department of Health and Human Services. (2006). *Preliminary Findings: 2004 National Sample Survey of Registered Nurses.*. Retrieved on November 15, 2006, from http://www.bhpr.hrsa.gov/healthworkforce/reports/rnpopulation/preliminaryfindings.htm

LEARNING ▼ ACTIVITIES

◆ JOURNALING ACTIVITY 16-1

1. In your clinical journal, identify a future trend in health care. Find at least two articles about this trend and summarize each.
2. Follow the summary with two paragraphs in which you discuss the implications for health care, the nursing profession, and nurses' daily practice. What further education needs come from these implications?

◆ CLIENT CARE ACTIVITY 16-2

The year is 2025—the future is here. You are a case manager in a busy, urban nursing clinic. You have a caseload of clients who live in the community where your center is located. Most of the clients have multiple chronic conditions. You see your clients in the ambulatory clinic, in the client's home or you communicate with them via computer. Today, one of your clients, Alfred Martinez, who is 64 years old, is having a sigmoid bowel resection with a temporary colostomy by laparoscopic laser surgery at the day surgery center. Home care will be provided by his wife, who will be assisted by their three adult sons on a rotating basis. It is your responsibility to coordinate the disciplines involved in his health care and manage his nursing care.

1. Identify factors that must be addressed when you plan for Mr. Martinez's post-operative recovery at home.
2. List five questions you will ask Mr. Martinez when you assess his care needs. Review the questions.
   * Do these questions view the client holistically?
   * Are they indicative of a contextual approach to identifying the client's needs?

3. Organize topics you will include when you teach Mrs. Martinez and her sons about Mr. Martinez's postoperative care. Compare and contrast current care from the care that would have likely been provided in 1997.
4. State alternative treatments or nursing interventions you included in the plan of care. How would you determine if they are paid for by a third-party payer?
5. Analyze how technology will assist you in Mr. Martinez's care (e.g., in making the assessment, communicating, maintaining a therapeutic relationship, and implementing the plan of care).

◆ PRACTICAL APPLICATION ACTIVITY 16-3

Interview a nurse who has been employed for at least 10 years. The longer the nurse has been working, the more interesting the discussion will be. Use the following questions as a basis for the interview:

- When did you first start working as a registered nurse?
- What was nursing like when you first started working?
- How has health care changed in the last 10 years?
- How is nursing different now?
- How many clients did you care for when you first started working as a nurse?
- How are the clients different now than when you first started working as an RN?
- What were your responsibilities for client care when you first started working and how have those responsibilities changed?
- What concerns do you have about how nursing has changed over the last 10 years?
- What is better about how nursing care is provided now?
- Summarize the interview in a two page paper. What did you learn?

◆ PRACTICAL APPLICATION ACTIVITY 16-4

Interview an elderly client or family member who has had a chronic condition over a long period of time (at least 10 years). Ask that person the following questions:

- How have health care services changed over the last 10 years (or however long you have had your health condition)?
- What differences are of particular concern to you and why?
- Has your family taken over more of your care in the last 10 years?
- What has that been like for you to have a chronic illness?
- What has that been like for your family members?

Nutrition Questionnaires for Infants, Children, and Adolescents

NUTRITION QUESTIONNAIRE FOR INFANTS

1. How would you describe feeding time with your baby? *(Check all that apply.)*

❑ Always pleasant

❑ Usually pleasant

❑ Sometimes pleasant

❑ Never pleasant

2. How do you know when your baby is hungry or has had enough to eat?

3. What type of milk do you feed your baby? *(Check all that apply.)*

❑ Breastmilk

❑ Iron-fortified infant formula

❑ Low-iron infant formula

❑ Goat's milk

❑ Evaporated milk

❑ Whole milk

❑ Reduced-fat (2%) milk

❑ Low-fat (1%) milk

❑ Fat-free (skim)

4. What types of things can your baby do? *(Check all that apply.)*

❑ Open mouth for breast or bottle

❑ Drink liquids

❑ Follow objects and sounds with eyes

❑ Put hand in mouth

❑ Sit with support

❑ Bring objects to mouth and bite them

❑ Hold bottle without support

❑ Drink from a cup that is held

5. Does your baby eat solid foods? If so, which ones?

6. Does your baby drink juice? If so, how much?

7. Does your baby take a bottle to bed at night or carry a bottle around during the day?

8. Do you add honey to your baby's bottle or dip your baby's pacifier in honey?

9. What is the source of the water your baby drinks? Sources include public, well, commercially bottled, and home system–processed water.

10. Do you have a working stove, oven, and refrigerator where you live?

11. Were there any days last month when your family didn't have enough food to eat or enough money to buy food?

12. What concerns or questions do you have about feeding your baby?

Source for all questionnaires: *Bright Futures at Georgetown University.* (2006). Retrieved on July 10, 2006, from http://www.brightfutures.org/nutrition.

NUTRITION QUESTIONNAIRE FOR CHILDREN

1. How would you describe your child's appetite?

   ❏ Good

   ❏ Fair

   ❏ Poor

2. How many days does your family eat meals together per week?

3. How would you describe mealtimes with your child?

   ❏ Always pleasant

   ❏ Usually pleasant

   ❏ Sometimes pleasant

   ❏ Never pleasant

4. How many meals does your child eat per day? How many snacks?

5. Which of these foods did your child eat or drink last week? *(Check all that apply.)*

   Grains

   ❏ Bread   ❏ Noodles/pasta/rice

   ❏ Rolls   ❏ Tortillas

   ❏ Bagels   ❏ Crackers

   ❏ Muffins   ❏ Cereal/grits

   ❏ Other grains: _____

   _____

Vegetables

❏ Corn   ❏ Green salad

❏ Peas   ❏ Broccoli

❏ Potatoes   ❏ Green beans

❏ French fries   ❏ Carrots

❏ Tomatoes

❏ Greens (collard, spinach)

❏ Other vegetables: _____

_____

Fruits

❏ Apples/juice   ❏ Bananas

❏ Oranges/juice   ❏ Pears

❏ Grapefruit/juice   ❏ Melon

❏ Grapes/juice   ❏ Peaches

❏ Other fruits/juice: _____

_____

Milk and Other Dairy Products

❏ Whole milk   ❏ Yogurt

❏ Reduced-fat (2%) milk   ❏ Cheese

                          ❏ Ice cream

❏ Low-fat (1%) milk   ❏ Flavored milk

❏ Fat-free (skim) milk

❏ Other milk and dairy products:

_____

_____

Meat and Meat Alternatives

❑ Beef/hamburger   ❑ Sausage/bacon

❑ Pork   ❑ Peanut butter/
nuts

❑ Chicken

❑ Turkey   ❑ Eggs

❑ Fish   ❑ Dried beans

❑ Cold cuts   ❑ Tofu

❑ Other meat and meat alternatives:

_____

_____

Fats and Sweets

❑ Cake/cupcakes   ❑ Candy

❑ Pie   ❑ Fruit-flavored
drinks

❑ Cookies

❑ Chips   ❑ Soft drinks

❑ Doughnuts

❑ Other fats and sweets: _____

_____

6. If your child is 5 years old or younger, does he or she eat any of these foods? *(Check all that apply.)*

   ❑ Hot dogs   ❑ Whole grapes

   ❑ Pretzels and
   chips   ❑ Popcorn

   ❑ Marshmallows

   ❑ Raw celery or
   carrots   ❑ Round or hard
   candy

   ❑ Nuts and seeds   ❑ Peanut butter

   ❑ Raisins

7. How much juice does your child drink per day? How much sweetened beverage (for example, fruit punch, and soft drinks) does your child drink per day?

8. Does your child take a bottle to bed at night or carry a bottle around during the day?

   ❑ Yes   ❑ No

9. What is the source of the water your child drinks? Sources include public, well, commercially bottled, and home system–processed water.

10. Do you have a working stove, oven, and refrigerator where you live?

    ❑ Yes   ❑ No

11. Were there any days last month when your family didn't have enough food to eat or enough money to buy food?

    ❑ Yes   ❑ No

12. Did you participate in physical activity (for example, walking or riding a bike) in the past week? If yes, on how many days and for how long?

    ❑ Yes   ❑ No

13. Does your child spend more than 2 hours per day watching television and videotapes or playing computer games? If yes, how many hours per day?

    ❑ Yes   ❑ No

14. What concerns or questions do you have about feeding your child?

NUTRITION QUESTIONNAIRE FOR ADOLESCENTS

1. Which of these meals or snacks did you eat yesterday? (Check all that apply.)

   ❑ Breakfast   ❑ Afternoon snack

   ❑ Morning snack   ❑ Dinner/supper

   ❑ Lunch   ❑ Evening snack

2. Do you skip breakfast three or more times a week?

   ❑ Yes   ❑ No

   Do you skip lunch three or more times a week?

   ❑ Yes   ❑ No

   Do you skip dinner/supper three or more times a week?

   ❑ Yes   ❑ No

3. Do you eat dinner/supper with your family four or more times a week?

   ❑ Yes   ❑ No

4. Do you fix or buy the food for any of your family's meals?

   ❑ Yes   ❑ No

5. Do you eat or take out a meal from a fast-food restaurant two or more times a week?

   ❑ Yes   ❑ No

6. Are you on a special diet for medical reasons?

   ❑ Yes   ❑ No

7. Are you a vegetarian?

   ❑ Yes   ❑ No

8. Do you have any problems with your appetite, like not feeling hungry, or feeling hungry all the time?

   ❑ Yes   ❑ No

9. Which of the following did you drink last week? (Check all that apply.)

   ❑ Regular soft drinks   ❑ Fat-free (skim) milk

   ❑ Diet soft drinks   ❑ Coffee/tea

   ❑ Fruit-flavored drinks   ❑ Tap/bottled water

   ❑ Whole milk   ❑ Juice

   ❑ Reduced-fat (2%) milk   ❑ Sports drinks

   ❑ Low-fat (1%) milk   ❑ Beer/wine/hard liquor

   ❑ Flavored milk (for example, chocolate, strawberry)

10. Which of these foods did you eat last week? (Check all that apply.)

    Grains

    ❑ Bread   ❑ Cereal/grits

    ❑ Rolls   ❑ Popcorn

    ❑ Bagels   ❑ Noodles/pasta/rice

    ❑ Crackers   ❑ Tortillas

    ❑ Other grains: _____

    _____

    Vegetables

    ❑ Corn   ❑ Green salad

    ❑ Peas   ❑ Broccoli

    ❑ Potatoes   ❑ Green beans

    ❑ French fries   ❑ Carrots

    ❑ Tomatoes

    ❑ Greens (collard, spinach)

    ❑ Other vegetables: _____

    _____

    Fruits

    ❑ Apples/juice   ❑ Peaches

    ❑ Oranges/juice   ❑ Pears

    ❑ Grapefruit/juice   ❑ Berries

❑ Grapes/juice   ❑ Melon

❑ Bananas

❑ Other fruits/juice: _____

_____

Milk and Other Dairy Products

❑ Whole milk   ❑ Yogurt

❑ Reduced-fat (2%) milk   ❑ Cheese

❑ Ice cream

❑ Low-fat (1%) milk   ❑ Flavored milk

❑ Fat-free (skim) milk

❑ Other milk and dairy products:

_____

_____

Meat and Meat Alternatives

❑ Beef/hamburger   ❑ Sausage/bacon

❑ Pork   ❑ Peanut butter/ nuts

❑ Chicken

❑ Turkey   ❑ Eggs

❑ Fish   ❑ Dried beans

❑ Cold cuts   ❑ Tofu

❑ Other meat and meat alternatives:

_____

_____

Fats and Sweets

❑ Cake/cupcakes   ❑ Chips

❑ Pie   ❑ Doughnuts

❑ Cookies   ❑ Candy

❑ Other fats and sweets: _____

_____

11. Do you have a working stove, oven, and refrigerator where you live?

❑ Yes   ❑ No

12. Were there any days last month when your family didn't have enough food to eat or enough money to buy food?

❑ Yes   ❑ No

13. Are you concerned about your weight?

❑ Yes   ❑ No

14. Are you on a diet now to lose weight or to maintain your weight?

❑ Yes   ❑ No

15. In the past year, have you tried to lose weight or control your weight by vomiting, taking diet pills or laxatives, or not eating?

❑ Yes   ❑ No

16. Did you participate in physical activity (for example, walking or riding a bike) in the past week? If yes, on how many days and for how long?

❑ Yes   ❑ No

17. Do you spend more than 2 hours per day watching television and videotapes or playing computer games? If yes, how many hours per day?

❑ Yes   ❑ No

18. Do you take vitamin, mineral, herbal, or other dietary supplements (for example, protein powders)?

❑ Yes   ❑ No

19. Do you smoke cigarettes or chew tobacco?

❑ Yes   ❑ No

20. Do you ever use any of the following? *(Check all that apply.)*

❑ Alcohol/beer/wine

❑ Steroids (without a doctor's permission)

❑ Street drugs (marijuana/speed/ crack/heroin)

Implications for Teaching at Various Developmental Stages

Age	Physical Development	Language (Cognitive) Development (based on Piaget)	Psychosocial Development (based on Erikson)	Nurse's Approach to Teaching
Overview of birth to 1 y		*Sensorimotor stage of development*	*Developmental task: trust vs. mistrust.* Learns to trust and to anticipate satisfaction. Sends cues to mother/caretaker. Begins understanding self as separate from others (body image).	Involve caretaker in all aspects of care
1–3 y	Begins to walk and run well. Drinks from cup, feeds self. Develops fine motor control. Climbs. Begin self-toileting. Kneels without support. Steady growth in height/ weight. Adult height will be approximately double the height at age 2. Dresses self by age 3.	*Preoperational stage of development.* Has poor time sense. Increasing verbal ability. Formulates sentences of 4 to 5 words by age 3. Talks to self and others. Has misconceptions about cause and effect. Interested in pictures. *Fears:* • Loss/separation from parents— peak • Dark • Machines/ equipment • Intrusive procedures • Bedtime Speaks to dolls and animals. Increasing attention span. Knows own sex by age 3.	*Developmental task: autonomy vs. shame and doubt.* Establishes self-control, decision making, independence (autonomy). Extremely curious and prefers to do things himself. Demonstrates independence through negativism. Very egocentric; believes he or she controls the world. Attempts to please parents. Participates in parallel play; able to share some toys by age 3.	Be flexible. Begin any intervention with play period to establish rapport. Be honest. Praise for cooperation. Begin slowly; speak to child. Involve caretaker/ parent. Let child hold security object. Allow child to play with stethoscope, tongue blade, flashlight before using on child if possible.

(continued)

Age	Physical Development	Language (Cognitive) Development (based on Piaget)	Psychosocial Development (based on Erikson)	Nurse's Approach to Teaching
4–6 y	Growth slows. Locomotion skills increase and coordination improves. Tricycle/bicycle riding. Throws ball but difficulty catching. Constantly active, increasing dexterity. Eruption of permanent teeth. Skips, hops, jumps rope.	*Preoperational/thought stage of development continues.* Language skills flourish. Generates many questions e.g., How, Why, What? Simple problem solving. Uses fantasy to understand and problem solve. *Fears* • Mutilation • Castration • Dark • Unknown • Inanimate • Unfamiliar objects Causality related to proximity of events. Enjoys mimicking and imitating adults.	*Developmental tasks: initiative vs. guilt.* Attempts to establish self like his or her parents, but independent. Explores environment on own initiative. Boasts, brags, has feelings of indestructibility. Family is primary social group. Peers increasingly important. Assumes sex roles. Aggressive, very curious. Enjoys activities such as sports, cooking, shopping. Cooperative play. Likes rules. May stretch the truth and tell large stories.	Establish rapport through talking and play. Introduce self to child. Have parent present but direct conversation to child. Games such as "follow the leader" and "Simon says" can be used to elicit necessary behaviors. Explain each intervention in simple language. Ask for child's help and use flattery. Use pictures, models, or items he or she can see or touch. Reserve genital examination for last; drape accordingly.
6–11 y	Moves constantly. Physical play prevalent; sports, swimming, skating, etc. Increased smoothness of movement. Grows at rate of 2 inches/7 lb a year. Eyes/hands well coordinated.	*Concrete operations stage of development.* Organized thought; memory concepts more complicated. Reads, reasons better, Focuses on concrete understanding. *Fears* • Mutilation • Death • Immobility • Rejection • Failure	*Developmental task: industry vs. inferiority.* Learns to include values and skills of school, neighborhood, peers. Peer relationships important. Focuses more on reality, less on fantasy. Family is main base of security and identity. Sensitive to reactions of	Explain all procedures and impact on body. Encourage questioning and active participation in care. Be direct about explanation of procedures, based on what child will hear, see, smell, and feel. (In addition,

(continued)

Age	Physical Development	Language (Cognitive) Development (based on Piaget)	Psychosocial Development (based on Erikson)	Nurse's Approach to Teaching
			others. Seeks approval and recognition. Enthusiastic, noisy, imaginative, desires to explore. Likes to complete a task. Enjoys helping others.	explain body part involved, and use anatomical names and pictures to explain step by step.) Be honest. Reassure child that he or she is liked. Provide privacy. Involve parents, but give child choice as to whether parent will stay during exam. Reason and explain. Allow child some choice as to direction of assessment. May be able to proceed as if assessing adult. Praise cooperation.
12–18 y	Well developed. Rapid physical growth (early adolescence: maximum growth). Secondary sex characteristics.	*Formal operations stage of development.* Abstract reasoning, problem solving. Understanding of of multiple cause-and-effect relationships. May plan for future career. *Fears* • Mutilation • Disruption of body image • Rejection by peers	*Developmental task: identity vs role confusion.* Predominant values are those of peer group. Early adolescence: outgoing and enthusiastic. Emotions are extreme, with mood swings. Seeking self-identity; sexual identity. Wants privacy and independence. Develops interests not	Respect privacy. Accept expression of feelings. Direct discussions of care and condition to child. Ask for child's opinions and encourage questions. Allow input into decisions. Be flexible with routines. Explain all procedures/ treatments. Encourage continuance

(continued)

Age	Physical Development	Language (Cognitive) Development (based on Piaget)	Psychosocial Development (based on Erikson)	Nurse's Approach to Teaching
			shared with family. Concern with physical self. Explores adult roles.	of peer relationships. Listen actively. Identify impact of illness on body image, future, and level of functioning. Correct misconceptions. Involve parent in assessment only if child requests presence.
19–30 y		*Formal operations*	*Developmental task: intimacy vs. isolation.* Intimate relationships are ultimate.	Involve significant other in care and consider how the client's condition affects the relationship.
30–60 y		*Formal operations*	*Developmental task: generativity vs. stagnation.* Concerned with parenthood, mentoring and guiding the next generation.	Work, family, and children are priorities. Teach with this concern in mind.
60 y to death		*Formal operations*	*Developmental task: integrity vs. despair.* Reviews life to bring life events into an integrated life theme.	Use life review to help client reduce anxiety and blocks to learning.

Adapted from Weber, J. (2008). *Nurses' handbook of health assessment* (6th ed.). Philadelphia: Lippincott Williams & Wilkins.

Cognitive Stages and Approaches to Patient Education With Children

Cognitive Stage	Approach to Teaching
Ages Birth to 2 y—Sensorimotor Development	
Begins as completely undifferentiated from environment	Orient all teaching to parents.
Eventually learns to repeat actions that have effect on objects	Make infants feel as secure as possible with familiar objects in home environment.
Has rudimentary ability to make associations	Give older infants an opportunity to manipulate objects in their environments, especially if long hospitalization is expected.
Ages 2–7 y—Preoperational Developments	
Has cognitive processes that are literal and concrete	Be aware of explanations that the child may interpret literally (e.g., "The doctor is going to make your heart like new" may be interpreted as, "He is going to give me a new heart"); allow child to manipulate safe equipment, such as stethoscopes, tongue blades, reflex hammers; use simple drawings of the external anatomy because children have limited knowledge of organs' functions.
Lacks ability to generalize	Do not compare child to other children; this is not helpful, nor is it meaningful to compare one diagnostic test or procedure to another.
Has egocentrism predominating	Reassure child that no one is to blame for his pain or other problems; belief that he causes events to happen may result in guilty thoughts that he caused his own pain, hospitalization, and so forth;
Has animistic thinking (thinks that all objects possess life or human characteristics of their own)	Anthropomorphize and name equipment that is especially frightening.
Ages 7–12 y—Concrete Operational Thought Developments	
Has concrete, but more realistic and objective, cognitive processes	Use drawings and models; children at this age have vague understandings of internal body processes; use needle play with dolls to explain surgical techniques and facilitate learning.
Is able to compare objects and experiences because of increased ability to classify along many different dimensions	Relate his or her care to other children's experiences so he or she can learn from them; compare procedures to one another to diminish anxiety.

(continued)

Cognitive Stage	Approach to Teaching
Ages 7–12 y—Concrete Operational Thought Developments	
Views world more objectively and is able to understand another's position	Use films and group activities to add to repertoire of useful behaviors and establish role models.
Has knowledge of cause and effect that has progressed to deductive logical reasoning	Use child's interest in science to explain logically what has happened and what will happen; explain medications simply and straightforwardly (e.g., "This medicine [insulin] unlocks the door to your body's cells just as a key unlocks the door to your house. By unlocking the door to the cell, the insulin can deliver the food and energy in your blood to the cell.").

Sources: London, F. (1999). *No time to teach: A nurse's guide to patient and family education.* Philadelphia: Lippincott Williams & Wilkins. Adapted from Petrillo, M., & Sanger, S. (1998). *Emotional care of hospitalized children* (pp. 38–50). Philadelphia: Lippincott-Raven; and Kolb, L. C. (1977). *Modern clinical psychiatry* (9th ed., pp. 90–91). Philadelphia: Saunders.

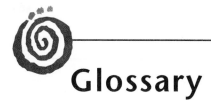

Glossary

acculturation: Individuals or groups from one culture learning the ways to exist in a new culture.

activities of daily living (ADL): Normal tasks of daily life.

acute care: Short-term medical or nursing care.

adult foster care homes: Small residential sites that provide housing and protective oversight; also known as board and care homes or family care homes.

advance directive: Written guide that allows people to state in advance what their choices for health care would be if certain circumstances should develop.

advanced practice nurse: Registered nurse who has completed graduate study in a specialty area according to specific academic requirements.

advocacy: Protection and support of another's rights.

affective interventions: Those teaching and nursing interventions that facilitate changes in attitudes, values, and feelings.

affective learning: Changes in attitudes, values, and feelings.

agoraphobia: Fear of being in places from which it might be difficult or embarrassing to escape.

alternative therapies: Interventions that focus on body, mind, and spirit integration; may be used in addition to conventional treatments. Examples include relaxation, imagery, prayer. See complementary therapies.

ambulatory care center: Any health care setting that provides a wide variety of services, including those related to medical, surgical, mental health, or substance abuse. See outpatient services.

assessment: A dynamic, ongoing process that uses observations and interactions to collect information, recognize changes, analyze needs, and plan care.

assimilation: Individuals or groups from one culture identifying more strongly with the dominant culture in values, activities, and daily living.

assisted-living facilities: Multiple dwellings that provide help with activities of daily living, such as being reminded to take medication, assistance with dressing and bathing, and meal preparation.

barriers: Factors that may adversely affect a process, (e.g., referral process).

behavioral interventions: Teaching or nursing interventions that assist clients to change their own behavior.

boarding care homes: Homes for the disabled or older person who needs meal service and housekeeping only and can manage most personal care.

care manager: Individual who manages the care of the client.

care of the caregiver: Nursing interventions intended to assist the individual providing care for the client.

case finding: A set of activities used by the nurse working in community settings that identifies clients who are not currently receiving health care, but who could benefit from such care.

case management: A systematic process used by nurses to ensure that clients' multiple health and service needs are met. These include assessing client needs, planning and coordinating services, referring to other appropriate providers, and monitoring and evaluating progress.

civic responsibility: A personal ethic of social responsibility and service.

client advocacy: Intervening or acting on behalf of the client to provide the highest quality health care obtainable.

clinical nurse specialist: A registered nurse with a graduate degree in a specialty or subspecialty area of nursing who usually practices in acute care settings, providing direct or indirect client care.

cognitive interventions: Teaching or nursing actions that enhance the client's ability to intellectually process information.

cognitive learning: The ability to intellectually process information, including remembering, perceiving, abstracting, and generalizing.

collaboration: Purposeful interaction between nurse, clients, and other professional and community members based on mutual participation and joint effort.

community: People, location, and social systems.

community assessment: The process of determining the real or perceived needs of a defined community of people.

community-based nursing: Nursing care within the context of the client's family and community with a prevention focus that enhances the client's ability for self-care; a collaborative effort to maintain continuity of care.

community health problem: The health need identified in community assessment.

community resources: A collection of health care providers or supportive care providers who share common interests or a sense of unity.

complementary therapies: Interventions that focus on body, mind, and spirit integration (e.g., relaxation, imagery, prayer); may be used in addition to conventional therapies. See alternative therapies.

constructed survey: A time-consuming and expensive method of collecting information about a community with a valid and reliable survey, using a random sample of a targeted population where the data collected are analyzed for patterns and trends.

consultation: An interactive problem-solving process between the nurse and the client continuity of care: coordination of services provided to clients before they enter a health care setting, during the time they are in the setting, and after they leave the setting.

coordinated care: The coordination of interdisciplinary sources of care and support to provide successful continuity of care.

coordination: Harmonious adjustment or working together.

cultural assessment: Considers the cultural beliefs, values, and practices of an individual, group, or community to determine needs and interventions within a specific cultural context.

cultural awareness: Self-awareness of one's own cultural background, influences, and biases.

cultural blindness: Lack of recognition of one's own beliefs and practices or of the beliefs and practices of others.

cultural care: Health care in a cultural context, acknowledging the client's cultural beliefs about disease and treatment.

cultural encounter: Direct contact with members of cultural communities.

cultural knowledge: Familiarity with a culturally or ethnically diverse group's world view, beliefs, values, practices, lifestyles, and problem-solving strategies.

cultural sensitivity: The considerate, respectful, compassionate, empathic, and sensible response to a person or situation.

cultural skill: The ability to collect relevant cultural data regarding the client's health history.

culture: A set of values, beliefs, and attitudes that characterizes a group and provides guidance in determining one's behavior.

day surgery centers: Ambulatory services that provide preoperative, operative, and postoperative care on an outpatient basis.

deinstitutionalization: Discharge from an inpatient mental health facility into the community where ongoing treatment can be provided by community-based mental health services.

demographics: Statistics related to age-specific categories, birth and death rates, marital status, ethnicity.

Denver Developmental Screening Test (DDST): The most widely used tool to assess development; used to screen children from 1 month to 6 years, covering the topics of gross motor skills, fine motor skills, language development, and personal/social development.

detoxification center: Facility that provides individuals safe detoxification of chemicals; the focus is on immediate health care needs and discharge planning.

developmental family assessment: Determination of family developmental stage and the ability to meet the developmental tasks of that stage.

developmental task: The usual and expected psychosocial, cognitive, or psychomotor skills at certain periods in life; failure to master the developmental task can lead to unhappiness and difficulty with later tasks.

diagnosis-related groups (DRGs): Classification of clients by major medical diagnosis for the purpose of standardizing health care costs.

discharge planning: Coordinating, planning, and arranging for the transition from one health care setting to another.

diversity: The condition of being different.

documentation: The process of obtaining and recording information used for communication, reference, and legal issues.

dual diagnosis: Coexistent mental health and other disorders (often an addictive disorder).

emergency preparedness: Comprehensive knowledge, skills, abilities, and actions needed to prepare for and respond to threatened, actual, or suspected chemical, biological, radiological, nuclear or explosive incidents, man-made incidents, natural disasters, or other related events.

emic care: Care determined by the local or insider's views and values.

employee assistance programs: Provision of assistance to an employee when emotional or physical illness threatens to interfere with the employee's health.

employee wellness programs: Plans that focus on keeping employees healthy and preventing illness and accidents.

environmental assessment: Evaluation of the client's home and neighborhood environment.

environmental health: The study of the effects of various chemical, physical, and biological agents on health, as well as their effects on the health of the entire physical and social environment.

environmental quality: The quality of the physical and social environments that play major roles in the health of individuals and communities.

epidemic: Disease occurrence that exceeds normal or expected frequency in a community or region.

ethnicity: Cultural differences based on heritage.

ethnocentrism: Belief that one's own cultural beliefs and values are best for all.

etic care: Care determined by the professional's or outsider's views and values.

extended care facilities: Synonymous with nursing homes; provide care for individuals who need daily care generally for the rest of their lives.

extended family: Nuclear family and other related people.

family developmental tasks: The usual and expected family psychosocial, cognitive, or psychomotor skills at certain periods in life; failure to master a developmental task can lead to unhappiness and difficulty with later tasks.

family functions: Activities or behaviors of family members that maintain the unity of the family and meet the family's needs.

family health: How well the family functions together as a unit; the family's ability to carry out usual and desired daily activities.

family roles: Expected set of behaviors associated with a particular family position.

family structure: The characteristics of individuals (age, gender, number) who make up the family unit.

family systems theory: A theory that says the family is a collection of people who are integrated, interacting, and independent, and that the actions of one member impact the actions of other members.

fee-for-service: Retrospective method of reimbursing medical care where each service requires payment.

fetal alcohol syndrome (FAS): A set of birth defects in infants/children caused by the mother's excessive ingestion of alcohol during pregnancy.

financial assessment: Evaluation of a client's ability to pay for service.

function: Subjective and objective evidence of ability to perform activities of daily living.

functional assessment: Determination of level of health defined by one's ability to carry out usual and desired daily activities.

genogram: An assessment to show family structure.

gerontology nursing: The nursing care of older adults, particularly those older than 65 years.

global health disparity: Differences in health and access to health care services between developed and developing countries.

globalization: Expanding the scope of community-based nursing care to include the global community, as illnesses are no longer contained to geographic boundaries.

health: State of physical, mental, and social well-being and not merely the absence of disease or infirmity.

health disparity: Differences in health and access to health care by gender, race, or ethnicity, education or income, disability, living in rural localities, or sexual orientation.

health indicator: Reflects the major public health concerns and illuminates factors that affect the health of individuals and communities.

health maintenance organizations (HMOs): Health care systems that provide comprehensive health service delivered by a defined network of providers to their members, who pay a fixed premium.

health promotion: Activities that enhance the well-being of an already healthy individual.

health protection: Environmental or regulatory measures that confer protection on large population groups.

health-illness continuum: Health described in a range of degrees from optimal health at one end to total disability or death at the other.

health teaching: Communicating facts, ideas, and skills that change knowledge, attitudes, values, beliefs, behaviors, and practices regarding the health of individuals, families, systems, and/or communities.

health literacy: The degree to which individuals have the capacity to obtain, process, and understand the information and services they need to make appropriate health decisions.

healthy family functioning: Optimal level of family health as defined by the family's ability to carry out usual and desired daily activities.

holism: A way of viewing the person as an integrated whole of mind, body, and spirit; reflects the interactive process that occurs in all of us.

holistic assessment: Considers not only physical and psychosocial factors, but also cultural, functional, nutritional, environmental, and spiritual aspects of the client.

home care agencies: Official, hospital-based, or proprietary organizations that provide health care in the client's residence.

home health care: Component of comprehensive health care whereby health services are provided to individuals and families in their places of residence for the purpose of promoting, maintaining, or restoring health.

home infusion therapy: A broad area of chemotherapy that incorporates intravascular chemotherapy performed by home infusion nurses or self-administered by patients or their caregivers.

home visit: Assessment, diagnosis, planning, and evaluation of nursing care in the client's home.

homeless shelter: Facility that provides food and shelter for individuals without homes.

hospice care: Holistic services provided to dying persons and their loved ones to provide a more dignified and comfortable death.

hospital-based home care agency: An operating department of a hospital that has no mandates and no tax support to determine which services to provide.

hyperemesis: Protracted vomiting with weight loss and fluid and electrolyte imbalance.

immigrant: An individual who moves to another country for permanent residence.

infant mortality rate: Rate of death per 1,000 infants defined as 1 month to 1 year of age.

informant interviews: Asking community residents who are either key informants or members of the general public about their observations and concerns regarding their community.

instrumental activities of daily living (IADL): Ability to plan and prepare meals, travel, do laundry, do housekeeping, shop, and use the telephone.

integrated health care system (also called seamless care): A health care system in which all levels of care are available in an integrated form.

lay caregiving: Care provided by families, friends, or other medical nonprofessionals in the home.

lead poisoning: Chronic ingestion or inhalation of lead; causes adverse effects on the central nervous system, kidneys, etc.

learning domains: Three areas (cognitive, affective, and psychomotor) in which teaching and learning occur.

learning need: A deficit in knowledge, skills, or attitude that interrupts functioning.

learning objectives: Expected outcome for the client, including a subject, action verb, performance criteria, target time, and special conditions.

lifeways: Beliefs about dress, diet, and other activities of daily living.

living will: Written advance directive specifying the medical care a person desires to refuse should he or she lack the capacity to consent or refuse treatment at some point.

low birth weight (LBW): Weight less than 2,500 g or 5.5 lb; the leading cause of preventable neonatal death.

market-driven economy: A system in which consumer demand drives production regarding what services will be created and consumed and in what quantity.

medication safety: Concern with taking medication the correct way and avoiding taking medication with other drugs and substances that cause harmful interactions.

minority: Race, ethnic, or cultural group that does not belong to the dominant group.

morbidity rates: Rates of illness or injury.

mortality rates: Rates of causes of death.

natural disaster: Events such as earthquakes, fires, hurricanes, tornados, tsunamis, and wildfires.

need to learn: Perception that information or skill is relevant or necessary for immediate or delayed application.

neural tube defects (NTDs): Occur when the neural tube does not form correctly during the first month of gestation.

nuclear family: Mother, father, and children living together.

nurse midwife: A nurse who provides independent care for women during normal pregnancy, labor, and delivery.

nurse practitioner: (See Advanced Practice Nurse)

nursing centers: Clinics that deliver primary health care, managed and served by nurses, practitioners, and other advanced practice nurses.

nursing functions: Those activities that enable the nurse to fulfill the roles of caregiver, manager, educator, planner, and advocate.

occupational health nurse: Registered nurse employed in a work setting who focuses on the health and well-being of people in the workplace.

official home care agency: Agency mandated to offer a particular group of services and supported by tax dollars.

outpatient services: Also called ambulatory care centers or clinics; provide a broad range of health care services for the client who does not require inpatient care.

pandemic: An epidemic (outbreak of an infectious disease) that spreads worldwide or at least across a large region.

parish nurse: Registered nurse employed by a religious organization to provide nursing care to members of the congregation.

participant observations: Examination of formal and informal social systems at work for the purpose of community assessment.

pharmacogenomics: The technology of developing and producing medications tailored to specific genetic profiles.

physical environment: An aspect of environmental health that includes the air, water, and soil through which exposure to chemical, biological, and physical agents may occur.

polypharmacy: The prescription of more than one medication.

population-based care: Care that occurs through partnerships between all constituents, just as nursing care of the individual and family is a mutually formulated process.

power system: A group of people who determine how control is distributed throughout a community or social system.

preferred provider organizations (PPOs): A network of physicians, hospitals, and other health-related services that contract with a third-party payer organization to provide comprehensive health services to subscribers on a fee-for-service basis.

pregnancy-induced hypertension (PIH): Hypertensive disorder of pregnancy that includes preeclampsia, eclampsia, and transient hypertension; the second leading cause of maternal mortality in the United States.

preventive services: Services attempting to avoid disease or injury or minimize the consequences.

primary prevention: Actions that avoid the initial occurrence of disease or injury.

professional relatedness: Professional phenomenon that involves understanding, mutual relating, self-awareness, reliability, and respect for privacy.

proprietary home care agency: A freestanding for-profit home care agency; services are provided based on third-party reimbursement schedules or by self-pay.

prospective payment: Payment for health care services in advance, based on rate derived from predictions of annual service costs.

psychomotor learning: Physical skills that can be demonstrated.

race: A distinct human type characterized by traits that are transmitted by descent.

readiness to learn: Emotional state, abilities, and potential that allow learning to occur.

referral process: A dynamic process between community resources that ensures continuity of care for the well-being of a client.

refugees: Individuals that have fled their country of origin to avoid danger or persecution.

rehabilitation centers: Either residential or outpatient facilities providing services to individuals requiring either physical or emotional rehabilitation; residence is generally limited to the achievement of goals.

reimbursement requirements: Governmental or proprietary requirements that must be met before a service is paid for.

residential centers: Supervised group facilities with various levels of independence, including, among other levels, retirement communities, assisted living facilities, board and care, skilled nursing facilities, and subacute rehabilitation centers.

respite care: Services to a family or caregivers to temporarily relieve caregiving demands.

retirement communities: Homes or apartments with supportive services provided by the retirement community, providing a community-living style for individuals who choose to live with other seniors.

school nurse: A registered nurse charged with the health care of school-age children and school personnel in an educational setting.

secondary data: Records, documents, or any previously collected information.

secondary prevention: Actions providing early identification and treatment of disease or injury with the purpose of limiting disability.

self-care: The actions of individuals, families, and communities to preserve and promote their own health, life, and sense of well-being.

service learning: Experiences that are structured to combine learning and volunteering.

skilled nursing facilities: Provision of nursing, medical, and therapy services for the individual who does not require acute care, but requires ongoing care; generally transferred to extended care or to home.

sliding fee scale: Payment schedule based on the client's ability to pay for service.

social environment: An aspect of environmental health that consists of housing, transportation, urban development, land use, industry, and agriculture along with issues related to work-related stress, injury, and violence.

social system: The various components of a community, including economic, educational, religious, political, legal, and methods of communication.

specialized care centers: Facilities that provide health care for a specific population group.

spiritual assessment: Allows the nurse to determine the presence of spiritual distress or identify other spiritual needs and incorporate them into the plan of care.

spirituality: A flowing, healing, dynamic balance that allows and creates health and well-being; sometimes involves organized religion.

staff splitting: Manipulative behaviors by which a client pits health care staff members against each other.

stereotyping: A mental picture or an assumption about a person based on a characteristic that comes from myths, or generalizations based on the perceived membership in a group.

structural family assessment: Family assessment that maps out the composition of the family, such as a genogram.

subacute rehabilitation centers: Limited-time residence; discharge usually occurs when the client has met certain goals.

sudden infant death syndrome (SIDS): Death of an apparently healthy infant, usually less than 1 year of age, for no apparent reason; usually occurs during sleep.

support services: Services that help people avoid problems or solve problems that interfere with their well-being.

technology: A tool to extend human abilities.

tertiary prevention: Actions to maximize recovery and potential after an injury or illness.

transcultural nursing: A body of knowledge and practice for caring for people from other cultures.

transferring: Moving from one tertiary care setting to another.

transitional housing: Temporary service often used between acute illness episodes or a personal housing crisis and permanent housing.

underserved populations: Individuals and families who do not have access to health care.

undocumented workers: Individuals who enter the country illegally, mainly for employment opportunities.

vital statistics: Information related to ongoing registration of births, deaths, adoptions, divorces, marriages, causes of death, and other statistics that reflect the vital signs of a community.

wellness promotion: To encourage or promote a healthy state.

windshield survey: Motorized equivalent of a simple observation where the observer drives through a chosen neighborhood and uses the power of observation to conduct a general assessment of that neighborhood.

work site health promotion: Programs that focus on the health of employees within business and industry.

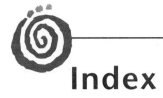

Index

A "t" following a page number indicates a table; an "f" indicates a figure; and a "b" indicates a box.